Hormones and Brain Plasticity

Oxford Series in Behavioral Neuroendocrinology

Series Editors

Gregory F. Ball, Jacques Balthazart, and Randy J. Nelson

Hormones and Brain Plasticity

LUIS MIGUEL GARCIA-SEGURA

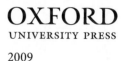

UNIVERSITY PRESS

2009

OXFORD
UNIVERSITY PRESS

Oxford University Press, Inc., publishes works that further
Oxford University's objective of excellence
in research, scholarship, and education.

Oxford New York
Auckland Cape Town Dar es Salaam Hong Kong Karachi
Kuala Lumpur Madrid Melbourne Mexico City Nairobi
New Delhi Shanghai Taipei Toronto

With offices in
Argentina Austria Brazil Chile Czech Republic France Greece
Guatemala Hungary Italy Japan Poland Portugal Singapore
South Korea Switzerland Thailand Turkey Ukraine Vietnam

Copyright © 2009 by Luis Miguel Garcia-Segura

Published by Oxford University Press, Inc.
198 Madison Avenue, New York, New York 10016
www.oup.com

Oxford is a registered trademark of Oxford University Press

Library of Congress Cataloging-in-Publication Data

Garcia-Segura, Luis Miguel.
Hormones and brain plasticity / Luis Miguel Garcia-Segura.
p. ; cm.—(Oxford series in behavioral neuroendocrinology ; 1)
Includes bibliographical references and index.
ISBN 978-0-19-532661-1 (cloth : alk. paper)
1. Neuroendocrinology.   2. Neuroplasticity.   I. Title.
II. Series. [DNLM: 1. Brain—physiology. 2. Neuronal Plasticity—physiology.
3. Aging—physiology. 4. Brain—growth & development.
5. Hormones—physiology. WL 300 G216h 2009]
QP356.4.G37 2009
612.8—dc22
2008042771

To my mentor, Alfredo Carrato Ibáñez (1911–1994)
For his gift of the light of science in times of deep darkness
In memoriam

Contents

Preface and Acknowledgments

One of the most fascinating developments in the field of neuroscience in the second half of the twentieth century was the discovery of the endogenous capacity of the brain for reorganization during adult life. Morphological and functional mechanisms underlying brain plasticity have been extensively explored and characterized. However, our understanding of the functional significance of these plastic changes is still fragmentary. I have attempted to approach this question by the examination of the cross talk between the brain and the endocrine glands. I had two main aims in writing this book. The first was to show that brain plasticity plays an essential role in the regulation of hormonal levels. The second aim was to propose that hormones orchestrate the multiple endogenous plastic events of the brain for the generation of adequate physiological and behavioral responses in adaptation to and prediction of changing life conditions.

To adequately address these aims, some conceptual clarifications are necessary. The first one is on the concept of brain plasticity. Originally, brain plasticity was thought to represent the manifestation of neuronal plasticity, either morphological, functional, or both. However, new advances in the understanding of the communication between neurons, glial cells, and blood vessels call for a reconsideration of nonneuronal cells in the plastic mechanisms of the brain. We know today that functional and morphological modifications of glial cells and endothelial cells are essential to sustain the plastic changes of neuronal and neuroglial networks during physiological and pathological conditions. In addition, another important conceptual change has been promoted by the discovery of the capacity that certain regions have in the adult brain to generate new neurons from neuronal precursors. Together with the known capacity of the adult brain to generate new glial and endothelial cells, the result is that adult nervous tissue is composed by cellular elements that are not permanent, but replaceable. Transient generation and elimination of neurons, glial cells and endothelial cells sustain transient building and demolishing of specific neuronal–glial networks and specific brain structures. Metaplasticity, the plasticity of plasticity, is another concept used and elaborated in the book. Plastic changes in the central nervous system, including cellular replacement, are not linear and are subjected to many regulations and modifications over time that may impact on future manifestations of plasticity. Therefore, the hormonal regulation of a specific form of brain plasticity in a given moment may affect the regulation of this specific form (and of other forms) of brain plasticity in the future.

To develop these arguments, I have organized the book into ten chapters. The first is an introduction in which the conceptual backgrounds of the book are presented. Chapter 2 is devoted to the analysis of the role of brain plasticity in the regulation of the activity of endocrine glands. Chapters 3 to 5 examine different hormonal influences on brain plasticity. Then, Chapters 6 to 10 cover the interactions of hormones and brain plasticity along the life cycle under physiological and pathological conditions. Because of space limitations, I have restricted my analysis to vertebrates, with particular emphasis on mammals. In addition, the influence exerted on brain plasticity by pheromones and by environmental endocrine disruptors, two topics partially related with the main theme of the book, have not been covered.

The initiative of this book corresponds to the Behavioral Neuroendocrinology Series, edited by Gregory Ball, Jacques Balthazart, and Randy Nelson. In particular, I have to acknowledge the persistent insistence of Jacques Balthazart, who convinced me to accept the challenge. This book has been also possible thanks to the fruitful discussions with my students, collaborators and colleagues. Special mention is due to Frederick Naftolin, who introduced me to the topic of hormones and brain plasticity more than 25 years ago. Without him and his endless new ideas and thoughts, I would never have been able to write this book. Parts of the manuscript were also read at some stage by Iñigo Azcoitia, Julie Ann Chowen, Muriel Darnaudery, Javier DeFelipe, Lydia L. DonCarlos, Miguel Garcìa-Diaz, Ana Guadaño-Ferraz, Tamas L. Horvath, Janice M. Juraska, Roberto C. Melcangi, Arpad Parducz, Vincent Prevot, Antonio Ruiz-Marcos, Carmen Sandi, José Luis Trejo, Marìa Paz Viveros, and Catherine Woolley. I am extremely grateful to all of them for their precious comments, corrections, and improvements. I want also to credit and acknowledge George Barreto, Gloria Patricia Cardona-Gomez, Tamas L. Horvath, María Llorens-Martín, Arpad Parducz, Vincent Prevot, Dionysia T. Theodosis, José Luis Trejo, Catherine Woolley, and Josué G. Yague, who provided original images from their work to illustrate the book. I am also extremely grateful to Catharine A. Carlin and Nicholas Liu from Oxford University Press, for their excellent editorial assistance and to Newgen Imaging Systems for careful editing of the text. Finally, the most important and heartfelt thanks are due to my wife Paz, without whose love, enthusiastic support, and permanent encouragement, this work could never have been completed.

Hormones and Brain Plasticity

Chapter 1

Hormones and the Mutable Brain

INTRODUCTION: ENDOCRINE GLANDS, BRAIN PLASTICITY, HOMEOSTASIS, ALLOSTASIS, AND HOMEODYNAMICS

One of the most fascinating problems in evolutionary biology is the origin of multicellular organisms. While it is relatively easy to imagine the generation of multicellular colonies formed by the association of individual cells with the same morphological and functional characteristics, it is much more difficult to define the steps necessary for the origin of an organism formed by multiple cell types organized in specialized tissues and organs. However, there is no doubt that among other essential evolutionary acquisitions, the generation of adequate systems of intercellular regulation is indispensable for the viability of a multicellular organism. These systems should integrate information originated from different cell types within a tissue, different tissues within an organ, and different organs within the organism to maintain a coordinated activity and the equilibrium of the internal environment.

The concepts of homeostasis and homeodynamics are essential for the arguments in this book. The term "homeostasis" (from Greek: "homoios"—similar, like—and "stasis"—fixed, immobile) was introduced by Walter Bradford Cannon (1878–1945) to define the maintenance of the constancy and stability—or steady state—of the internal environment (Cannon, 1929), which for Claude Bernard (1813–1878), the founder of experimental medicine, was an indispensable condition for life (Bernard, 1878, 1879). Several mechanisms have evolved to maintain homeostasis in multicellular organisms, including cells that move from one organ to another, such as red blood cells or immune cells; chemical intercellular signals; and nerve communication. These mechanisms involve numerous modifications in the structure and function of cells, body tissues, and organs, not only to compensate for the changing conditions in daily life to maintain body constants but also in the prediction of future changes in life conditions. Therefore, homeostasis is achieved through change. Peter Sterling and Joseph Eyer, in 1988, proposed the term "allostasis" to refer to the maintenance of stability of body function through body changes in response to and in prediction of the changing conditions of daily life (Schulkin, 2003; Sterling, 2004; Sterling and Eyer, 1988). Furthermore, stability does not mean immutability. Biological systems are dynamically stable: their stability is dynamic (Yates, 1994). The so-called physiological constants in fact show fluctuations in adaptation to changing life conditions. For instance, body temperature changes in many animals in adaptation to external temperature, and heartbeat adapts as a consequence and in prediction of physical activity. In addition, stable body conditions are different during fetal development, early postnatal life, puberty, adult reproductive life, and aging, not to mention adaptive alterations in body conditions associated with pathology. Therefore, the steady state of the internal environment is not fixed and immobile, but rather dynamic. In consequence, it has been proposed that the term "homeodynamics" (Lloyd et al., 2001; Yates, 1994) reflects the process of maintenance of satiability of body function with more precision than the term homeostasis.

Although homeostasis is an accepted term, I will preferentially use the term homeodynamics in this book. In my opinion, homeodynamics reflects with more accuracy the result of the plastic structural and functional modifications that the organism undergoes in adaptation and in prediction of new life events to maintain stable, but not immutable, internal environmental conditions. There is no doubt that most molecular, cellular, and physiological regulations are based on homeostatic mechanisms. However, considering the whole organism, the stability of the internal environment implies predictions of future changing conditions; the result is a dynamic and not static equilibrium. In this book, I will focus on two main homeostatic and homeodynamic regulators: the endocrine and the nervous systems. Many chemical signals, including growth factors and cytokines, are involved in cell-to-cell and tissue-to-tissue communication to generate homeostatic mechanisms that maintain body homeodynamics. These molecules may act by means of autocrine or paracrine actions within a given organ. In addition, long-distance communication by chemical messengers integrates the function of different organs. Some of these long-distance chemical messengers are called "hormones" and are produced by specialized organs: the endocrine glands. Another main mechanism for long-distance communication, which is adequate for rapid responses, is the transfer of information by membrane depolarization in chains of intercommunicated specialized cells that cover long distances with their cell bodies and cell processes. This is the mechanism used by the nervous system that, in addition, uses chemical messengers as well, called neurotransmitters, gliotransmitters (molecules released by glial cells that modulate synaptic function), and neuromodulators, for local cell-to-cell communication. Through evolution, the same molecules have been used for multiple functions, and sometimes it is difficult to determine whether a molecule should be classified as a hormone, a cytokine, or a neurotransmitter. For instance, the same molecule used for cell-to-cell signaling by the nervous system may be used as a long-distance messenger by the endocrine system. We will see in several chapters of this book that this is an important cause of difficulty if we want to determine whether the action of some molecules, produced both by the brain and the endocrine glands, represents an autocrine, a paracrine, or an endocrine action.

Plants and animals use chemical signals called hormones, but their spatial range of action may be different. In plants, the action of hormones may be limited in space by diffusion constraints, while in animals, hormones may reach different organs in a relatively short time via the circulatory system. Animals also have a nervous system that allows for rapid communication between different regions of the body and the generation of quick behavioral responses. In animals, hormones and the nervous system contribute to body homeodynamics with different time ranges. Neuronal activity may change in milliseconds, while the more rapid hormonal actions may take minutes, and many hormonal actions, involving gene expression, may take hours or days. However, these different time scales are integrated. Slow hormonal actions regulate plastic modifications in the nervous system that predetermine many aspects of quick neuronal activity. In turn, rapid changes in neuronal activity impact the function of endocrine glands, regulating plastic homeodynamic changes in hormonal release.

Although this book is about the interaction between hormones and the nervous system in vertebrates, this is not a text on neuroendocrinology. I will not cover neural mechanisms involved in the control of hormonal secretions. My aim is to specifically address the question of the interaction between hormones, or endocrine glands, and the plastic properties of the neural tissue.

Evolutionary selection has provided the nervous system the capacity of adaptation to modifications in external temperature, food availability, social interactions, activity of predators, and many other external factors. In addition, the nervous system is also able to adapt its functional activity to the changing inner conditions of the organism. The adaptation of the nervous system to changes in the external and internal environments is achieved by modifications in the morphological and functional organization of neuronal circuits and its associated glial cells and blood vessels. Hormones play a major role in the adaptation of the nervous system to new environmental and internal situations by regulating brain plasticity. The interaction of hormones and the nervous system is essential for the regulation of basic homeostatic and homeodynamic mechanisms, including metabolism, body temperature, and immune responses. In addition, the cross talk between hormones and the brain impacts the higher levels of homeostatic regulation, such as drivers, motivations, emotions, and feelings (see Damasio, 2003, for a discussion on emotions, feelings, and homeostasis), and affects cognition and behavior (Fig. 1.1). Using hormones as messengers, the body sends essential information to the brain, allowing an adequate neural response to challenging transformations of an inner and outer world that is in permanent mutation. Hormones influence brain function and affect motivation, emotions, feelings, affection, learning, memory, and behavior. Hormones shape our personality, our capacity to interact with the external world, and also, very importantly, regulate the interaction of our brain with the internal milieu. Recent research findings tell us that hormones exert these actions, at least in part, by regulating the

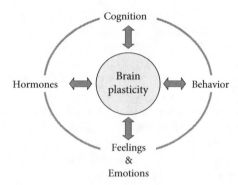

Figure 1.1. Brain plasticity is considered to be a central element in the communication of the body and the brain. Hormonal signals carry information from the body to the brain and regulate brain plasticity. Hormonally regulated brain plastic modifications may then impact feelings, emotions, cognition, and behavior. In turn, changes in emotions, cognitive function, and behavioral responses contribute to the functional plastic regulation of brain regions involved in hormonal control.

remodeling of the structure and function of the nervous system. In turn, feelings, emotions, cognitive changes, and behavioral responses modulate hormonal levels by affecting brain plasticity (Fig. 1.1).

Brain and spinal cord remodeling during and after the developmental period is always accompanied by significant hormonal changes. Hormones and the central nervous system maintain constant cross talk during the life span, and brain remodeling both regulates and is regulated by hormonal modifications (Fig. 1.1). Fetal development, early postnatal development, and puberty are periods of substantial brain remodeling and hormonal adjustments. In adulthood, brain remodeling and hormonal modifications are associated with a large variety of life events, including circadian, seasonal, and reproductive cycles; pregnancy; motherhood; lactation; feeding; social interactions; and behavioral performance. Furthermore, the interaction between brain remodeling and the activity of endocrine glands is modified during pathological conditions and with aging. In all these circumstances, brain remodeling affects hormonal secretions, and in turn, changing hormonal levels regulate brain remodeling. There is, therefore, a continuous feedback between the endocrine glands and the brain to adjust the physiological homeodynamic equilibrium to each particular life event, and in the prediction of future events (Fig. 1.2). The adjustment may originate from changes in the brain or peripheral glands, and it may have exteroceptive or interoceptive causes, but it always involves a cross talk between the endocrine glands and the brain.

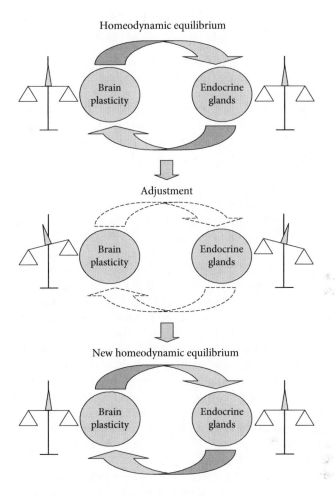

Figure 1.2. The cross talk between the brain and endocrine glands is in constant readjustment in adaptation to the changing homeodynamic demands. Homeodynamics is reached by functional plastic modifications in the brain regions that regulate endocrine secretions. In turn, hormones released by the endocrine glands exert a constant regulation of brain plasticity and metaplasticity, adapting the threshold for brain plasticity during life to the precise homeodynamic needs of each moment and function to maintain the homoedynamic equilibrium. Alterations in the external environment and/or internal physiological conditions require a readjustment of the communication between the brain and endocrine glands. Plastic reorganization of brain circuits interact with plastic modifications in the activity of endocrine glands, readjusting the brain–endocrine cross talk to sustain a new homeodynamic equilibrium.

THE NERVOUS SYSTEM IS IN A CONSTANT STATE OF REMODELING: CELLULAR PLASTICITY AND CELLULAR REPLACEMENT

The major structural components of the nervous system (neurons, glial cells, and blood vessels) are in permanent structural reorganization in adaptation to the variable functional requirements of ever-changing external and internal environments during a life span. Many of the modifications that occur in the nervous system under physiological conditions are transient, and in some structural and functional aspects, reversible. Indeed, some neuroplastic events are cyclic in nature, such as seasonal brain plasticity. However, the morphological and functional organization of the nervous tissue never goes back to previous states. The nervous system is never in the same structural and functional situation twice throughout life.

With no doubt, the formation of the nervous system itself during embryonic and early postnatal developmental stages is the period of the most prominent plastic reorganization of neural tissue. The developing brain and spinal cord are characterized by an incessant movement of cells and cellular processes that produce a continuous state of remodeling of the neural structure. These changes are initiated with the folding of the neural plate in the ectoderm to form the neural tube and neural crest. Neuroepithelial germinal cells then proliferate and differentiate to produce neurons and glial cells. These newly generated cells migrate to their final destination, to be organized into multicellular anatomical and functional assemblies within the brain and spinal cord. The final neuronal and glial cytoarchitectonics of the neural structures is the result of several waves of migrating cells, which are also accompanied by several steps of cellular replacement in transitory networks. Therefore, the developing nervous system shows an incessant traffic of cells moving in different directions.

Unlike traffic on a highway, the movement of cells in the developing nervous system is in three dimensions. Cells move according dorsoventral, lateral, and anteroposterior cues. In addition, there are cellular and regional specific temporal patterns for migration. Thus, different cell groups have different temporal and spatial migratory routes. In parallel to cell movements, axons and dendrites grow and retract while exploring the intercellular environment in search of adequate cellular partners to establish interneuronal contacts. Finally, functional synapses mature and then polarized neuronal circuits emerge. This activity is not linear, and in many cases there are transitory steps in the structural and functional organization of the nervous tissue that will be followed by phases of reorganization. For instance, cells may migrate to transient positions before reaching their final destination, and axons and dendrites may establish transient synaptic connections that will be replaced later by new ones. These events of organization and reorganization represent the steps of an astonishing transformation of a small fragment of the ectoderm into the most highly complex and sophisticated biological machinery. The nervous system will never be as mutable as in the developmental period.

Although the developmental period is when the nervous system has the highest capacity for mutability, the neural tissue maintains a remarkable capacity of reorganization during the life span of the individual. The structural modifications of neural tissue under physiological conditions in adult life may be subtle and consist of modest alterations in cell morphology, such as the reorganization of the branching of dendrites, receptive processes of neurons, or small changes in the number, size, and form of synaptic terminals (the points where information is transmitted from one neuron to another). In the long run, these small modifications in the structure and function of neural cells may result in macroscopic changes, such as modifications in the receptive fields of neurons or the reorganization of the functional specialization of the somatosensory or motor cerebral cortical regions. In addition to neurons, other cellular components are involved in the plastic reorganization of the nervous system. Blood vessels experiment modifications to adapt regional blood flow to the changing neuronal requirements of glucose and oxygen. Changes in cell morphology of glial cells (oligodendroglia, astroglia, and microglia) in the brain and spinal cord, and Schwann cells in the peripheral nervous system also contribute to the remodeling of neural tissue. In addition, blood vessels, glial cells, and neurons maintain cross talk via different chemical messengers that coordinate their plastic modifications.

The role of glial cells and neurons in the reorganization of neural tissue structure under physiological conditions in adult life is supported not only by their ability to extend and retract their cellular processes but also by their ability to migrate and proliferate. New neurons are generated during adult life in the brain of vertebrates. Adult neurogenesis is considerably active in the hippocampus, the olfactory bulb, and other brain regions in the mammalian brain, and it is even higher in the brain of some nonmammalian vertebrates, including songbirds, reptiles, and fish (Zupanc, 2001). Indeed, the brain of these vertebrate groups maintains a considerable capacity for growth and regeneration in adult life. The new neurons generated during adult life integrate into functional neuronal networks, and may die and be replaced, maintaining these circuits in a continuous structural and functional state of remodeling (Fig. 1.3).

Microglia, astroglia, oligodendroglia, and Schwann cells maintain proliferative activity during the life span and new glial cells are continuously generated from glial precursors and migrate to all regions of the nervous system. Glial cells die and are replaced by other glial cells during adult life as well. Endothelial cells also proliferate within the brain and contribute to the remodeling of blood vessels. Therefore, cells within the nervous system are able to change not only in shape during adult life but also in number and position. Thus, new neurons, glial cells, and endothelial cells may be generated during adult life and replace previous cells in neuronal networks, glial networks, and blood vessels. This represents a different form of brain plasticity that we may call "cellular replacement." I use this term to indicate that different cellular elements are replaced by other cellular elements in the nervous system.

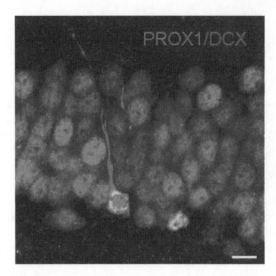

Figure 1.3. Incorporation of new neurons in the granule cell layer of the dentate gyrus of the hippocampus. The figure corresponds to a young adult (4 months old) female mouse. Newly incorporated neurons are immunolabeled in red for doublecortin (DCX), a cytoskeletal maker of immature differentiating neurons. Granule cells are immunolabeled in green for the prospero-related homeobox 1 gene (Prox 1), a granule cell–specific transcription factor. The colocalization of green and red labeling indicates that the newly incorporated neurons are granule cells. Scale bar, 10 μm. (Courtesy of María Llorens-Martín and José Luis Trejo. Based on Llorens-Martín et al., 2007.)

We may then distinguish at least two forms of brain plasticity or mutability in the nervous system (Fig. 1.4). One form of brain plasticity, cellular plasticity, is provided by modifications in cell shape, in the extension of neuronal and glial cell processes, and in the number, location, and function of intercellular contacts. Another form of brain plasticity, cellular replacement, is provided by the capacity of neuronal, glial, and endothelial cell precursors to proliferate, change its position within the nervous system, integrate into preexisting cellular assemblies, and finally, be replaced by other cells. Both forms of brain plasticity—changes in cell shape and cellular replacement—contribute to the functional plasticity of the nervous tissue, including the functional modifications of synaptic function. I will consider in this book the terms "brain plasticity," "neuroplasticity," and "mutability" as synonymous; and I will consider cellular plasticity and cellular replacement as two specific forms of morphological brain plasticity that finally result in functional plasticity of synaptic circuits. We will now briefly consider the concepts of cellular plasticity and cellular replacement within a historical perspective.

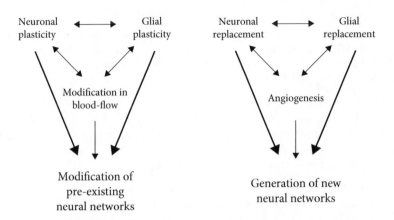

Figure 1.4. Differences between two forms of brain plasticity: cellular plasticity and cellular replacement. Cellular plasticity is the result of (i) modifications in dendritic branching, in the number of dendritic spines, in the growth of axons, and in the number and function of synapses (neuronal plasticity); (ii) changes in the shape and extension of glial processes and in functional modifications of glial cells (glial plasticity); and (iii) functional modification in local blood flow. Cellular plasticity results in the morphological and functional modification of preexisting neural networks. In contrast, according to the concept of cellular replacement, neuronal and glial networks and their associated blood vessels are not permanent unalterable structures integrated by the same cellular elements but are structures showing substitutions of their cellular components. Cellular replacement is provided by the capacity of neuronal precursors and glial cells to proliferate, to change its position within the nervous system, and to integrate into preexisting cellular assemblies to form new neural networks. Endothelial cells may also proliferate and new blood vessels may be formed (angiogenesis) according to the metabolic demands of the new neural networks. Both forms of brain plasticity, cellular plasticity and cellular replacement, are regulated by hormones.

The Classic Concept of Brain Plasticity: Cajal's Heritage

All living cells and all living tissues are in a constant molecular, morphological, and functional remodeling in adaptation to changing physiological conditions. The nervous tissue is not an exception. However, we do place emphasis on brain plasticity since, for many years, it was considered that the structure of the central nervous system was in essence unalterable after the end of the developmental period. Although this view has dramatically changed only in recent decades, a prediction of the plastic activity of the brain was formulated around the turn of the twentieth century in several papers from Santiago

Ramón y Cajal, the founder of modern neuroscience. Using his poetic and metaphoric prose, beautifully translated to English by Javier DeFelipe and Edward G. Jones (DeFelipe and Jones, 1988), Cajal exposed in the Cronian Lecture of 1894 his vision on the plastic capacity of the brain:

> ...the cerebral cortex is similar to a garden filled with trees, the pyramidal cells, which, thanks to intelligent culture, can multiply their branches, sending their roots deeper and producing more and more varied and exquisite flowers and fruits. (Ramón y Cajal, 1894)

Cajal considered that both the retraction and the growth of cellular processes were involved in intellectual activity, learning, and sleep. He postulated that mental activity results in an enrichment of neuronal connectivity and promoted the growth of neuronal processes, dendrites, and axons, in a similar way as physical exercise promotes muscle growth:

> It can be admitted as very probable that mental exercise leads to a greater development of the dendritic apparatus and of the system of axonal collaterals in the most utilized cerebral regions. In this way, associations already established among certain groups of cells would be notably reinforced by means of the multiplication of the small terminal branches of the dendritic appendages and axonal collaterals; but, in addition, completely new intercellular connections could be established thanks to the new formation of [axonal] collaterals and dendrites. (1894)

These predictions of Cajal on the plastic modification of dendritic arbors and axonal collaterals have been extensively confirmed by more recent investigations. The dendritic arbors are indeed plastic, and dendrites grow and retract during normal physiological conditions (Purves and Hadley, 1985). Plastic changes in the structure of dendritic trees are functionally important since, in addition to resulting in modifications in the space available for the formation of synaptic connections, they affect neuronal firing properties (Mainen and Sejnowski, 1996; Schaefer et al., 2003).

Further, Cajal considered that the growth and retraction of glial cell processes could have an important impact in the regulation of blood flow, neuronal activity, and neuronal interactions (DeFelipe, 2006; Garcia-Marin et al., 2007; Garcia-Segura, 2002). Therefore, Cajal also recognized the importance of glial plasticity for normal physiological brain function. Indeed, it is well demonstrated that glial cells play an important physiological role providing metabolic support for neurons and regulating the functional cross-coupling between neuronal activity, blood flow, and neuronal metabolism (Magistretti, 2006). In addition, glial cells form interconnected cellular networks and release glial transmitters that affect the activity of other glial cells, as well as the activity of neighboring neurons. Neuronal activity, on the other hand, via the release of neurotransmitters, affects the activity of glial cells. Therefore, there is a bidirectional communication between glial cells and neurons that play an active role in the regulation of neuronal activity, synaptic transmission, and synaptic plasticity (Araque et al., 1999, 2001; Jourdain et al., 2007;

Ni et al., 2007; Perea and Araque, 2007; Volterra and Meldolesi, 2005; Wigley et al., 2007).

Both oligodendroglial and astroglial cells show different forms of molecular, morphological, and functional plasticity, including reversible modifications in the extension of their cellular processes in adaptation to neuronal metabolic demands, in response to functional modifications in neuronal activity and in parallel to neuronal morphological changes. The growth and retraction of astrocytic processes may influence the intercellular environment, including the extracellular levels of potassium and neurotransmitters, which in turn will affect neuronal excitability and synaptic transmission. In addition, growth and retraction of astroglial cell processes is associated with modifications in the glial coverage of the neuronal cell bodies and neuronal processes and in the transient connection and disconnection of presynaptic terminals on postsynaptic structures (Garcia-Segura et al., 1994a, b; Theodosis et al., 2006a, 2008). Microglial cells, the macrophages of the brain, also show dramatic modification in cellular form. Resting microglial cells have a highly ramified phenotype, and after activation, cellular processes become thicker and retract, and finally the cell may acquire an amoeboid shape and a phagocytic function. These morphological modifications are accompanied by marked changes in the levels of expression of different membrane molecules and in the release of cytokines that affect the function of other cellular elements in the nervous system and contribute to the regulation of plastic remodeling of neural processes and synapses (Aldskogius et al., 1999; Bessis et al., 2007; Bruce-Keller, 1999).

A key contribution of Cajal, with important implications for synaptic plasticity, was the discovery of dendritic spines (Garcia-Lopez et al., 2007). Dendritic spines are small protrusions emerging from the neuronal dendritic processes and represent specialized postsynaptic structures. Using, after some improvements, the silver staining method invented by Camillo Golgi, the "reazione nera," Cajal discovered in 1888 the presence of these small structures in the dendrites of Purkinje cells of the cerebellum (Ramón y Cajal, 1888). He confirmed their existence in 1896, using another staining technique based on the use of methylene blue (Ramón y Cajal, 1896 a, b), and he showed that dendritic spines were present in the dendrites of many neuronal types. Cajal postulated that dendritic spines were points of contact between axons and dendrites and considered them as dynamic structures that grow and retract in association with modifications in neuronal function and neuronal activity (Ramón y Cajal, 1891, 1899).

Today we know that dendritic spines, which contain the contractile molecule actin, are highly motile structures. Spines grow, split, change their form and volume, and retract in parallel with physiological plastic changes in synaptic function (Alvarez and Sabatini, 2007; Cesa and Strata, 2005; Segal, 2005; Trachtenberg et al., 2002). In addition, the morphological modifications of dendritic spines are accompanied by a parallel reorganization of presynaptic elements (De Paola et al., 2003; Muller and Nikonenko, 2003). Plasticity of dendritic spines occurs under many physiological and pathological conditions, and these concepts will be frequently considered in this book.

One of the most important consequences of cellular plasticity is the generation of functional synaptic changes. Therefore, in addition to the morphological plasticity of dendritic spines and their associated presynaptic terminals, I will also consider different forms of functional synaptic plasticity in the next chapters. Lorente de Nó (1933) proposed that reverberating closed neuronal circuits forming cell assemblies could be the substrates for memory traces. Donald O. Hebb elaborated on this idea and postulated that changes in synaptic strength as a result of repeated coincidence in pre- and postsynaptic activity were the substrate for learning and memory (Hebb, 1949). The work of Eric Kandel and Ladislav Tauc in *Aplysia* (Kandel and Tauc, 1965) and of Terje Lømo and Tim Bliss in the hippocampus of rabbits (Bliss and Gardner-Medwin, 1973; Bliss and Lømo, 1973) provided experimental support to Hebb's ideas, showing long-term changes in synaptic efficacy associated with repeated neuronal activity. Bliss and Lømo analyzed extracellular recordings of neurons in the hippocampal dentate gyrus in vivo after stimulation of afferent axons from the entorhinal cortex. Axons were stimulated in a region of the hippocampus named the perforant path and the amplitude of the population excitatory postsynaptic potential and the amplitude and latency of the population spike were recorded in the dentate gyrus. They observed that high-frequency stimulation of the axons in the perforant path enhanced the postsynaptic response in the dentate gyrus to subsequent single-pulse stimulation of the perforant path for several hours (Bliss and Gardner-Medwin, 1973; Bliss and Lømo, 1973). This functional modification in synaptic activity, which received the name "long-term potentiation of synaptic transmission" (usually refereed to as LTP), has been confirmed by numerous studies and has been detected in different brain regions (Malenka and Bear, *2004*).

Some forms of long-term synaptic potentiation involve the intracellular traffic of highly mobile AMPA receptors, which are increased in the membrane (Malinow and Malenka, 2002; Perez-Otano and Ehlers, 2005). However, other forms are independent of AMPA receptors (Kullmann and Lamsa, 2007; Malenka and Bear, *2004*). Long-term synaptic potentiation is accompanied by an increased transmitter release and is thought to be essential for some forms of learning (Barnes et al., 1994; Brun et al., 2001; Gruart et al., 2006; Gruart and Delgado-García, 2007).

Another form of functional synaptic plasticity that will also be frequently mentioned in this book is long-term depression of synaptic function, which is also an activity-dependent form of plasticity that may be induced by the application of a low-frequency train of synaptic activity (Artola et al., 1990; Artola et al., 1996; Artola and Singer, 1993; *Malenka and Bear, 2004*). Functional and morphological synaptic plasticity are probably interrelated, and changes in the shape and number of dendritic spines are associated with modifications in functional synaptic plasticity (Engert and Bonhoeffer, 1999; Harris et al., 2003; Muller et al., 2002; Toni et al., 1999; Yuste and Bonhoeffer, 2001).

Cellular Replacement: A New Concept

The concept of brain plasticity that we have inherited from Cajal is supported by modifications in cellular form, such as changes in the shape, length, number and position of axons, dendrites, dendritic spines, and glial cell processes. Although Cajal discovered the capacity of glial cells to proliferate in the adult brain (Ramón y Cajal, 1913), he considered that, unlike glia, neurons were unable to proliferate in the adult brain. Therefore, for Cajal, the basic organization of neuronal circuits was immutable in the adult brain:

> Cerebral gymnastics are not capable of improving the organization of the brain by increasing the number of cells, because it is known that the nerve cells after the embryonic period have lost the property of proliferation. (DeFelipe and Jones, 1988; Ramón y Cajal, 1894)

Thus, for Cajal, the main limitation of brain plasticity was that new neurons are not generated during adult life, and therefore, new neurons cannot be incorporated into the existing neuronal circuits. This point of view was challenged by Joseph Altman, who in the 1960s detected evidence of neurogenesis in the brain of adult mammals (Altman, 1962). In the strict sense, Cajal was right: adult differentiated neurons do not divide, and therefore, differentiated neurons do not proliferate during adult life. However, we know today that neuronal progenitors remain in the adult tissue and that new neurons are generated in several regions of the vertebrate brain throughout the life span (Cameron and Dayer, 2008; Gould, 2007). These newly generated neurons migrate to their final destination and are incorporated into functional synaptic circuits (Abrous et al., 2005; Christie and Cameron, 2006; Gould, 2007; Nottebohm, 2002). For instance, neurons generated in the subventricular zone in rodents migrate rostrally and are incorporated in neuronal circuits in the olfactory bulb. Thus, neurons, as glial cells, may also change in number and position in the adult brain.

Several examples of adult neurogenesis will be mentioned in next chapters. Indeed, adult neurogenesis is one of the manifestations of brain plasticity that will be repeatedly appearing in this book. Adult neurogenesis is of functional significance—for instance, changes in the rate of adult neurogenesis in the brain of songbirds are correlated with the manifestation of song behavior (Nottebohm, 2002) and changes in the rate of neurogenesis in the dentate gyrus of the hippocampus in mammals are correlated with modifications in cognition and affection (Abrous et al., 2005; Dupret et al., 2007; Llorens-Martín et al., 2007; Sahay and Hen, 2007; Trejo et al., 2007). Furthermore, spatial learning and spatial relational memory in rodents require hippocampal adult neurogenesis (Dupret et al., 2007, 2008).

The role of adult neurogenesis is not simply to add new neurons to preexisting neuronal circuits but to induce a functional reorganization of these circuits by the addition and substitution of cellular elements (Lledo and Lazarini, 2007). The reorganization of the synaptic circuits is transient, since many newly generated neurons will finally die. However, these transient synaptic circuits are functionally relevant, and the selective elimination of neurons within the synaptic circuits may allow for their rapid functional modification (Lledo and Lazarini, 2007). In addition, there is good evidence indicating that both addition and removal of new hippocampal neurons is necessary for spatial learning (Dupret et al., 2007). Thus, adult neurogenesis represents a process of neuronal replacement. Consequently, cellular replacement in the adult nervous system is limited not only to glial cells, but also to neurons, at least in specific neuronal circuits.

Since glial cells form functionally organized cellular networks that respond to changes in neuronal activity and that regulate synaptic transmission and synaptic plasticity (Araque et al., 1999, 2001; Perea and Araque, 2007), glial replacement may also potentially impact the processing of information within the nervous system. In addition, oligodendroglia replacement is essential for remyelination and reorganization of neuronal connectivity mediated by myelinated axons. Proliferation of endothelial cells and angiogenesis are also necessary for the remodeling of blood vessels in adaptation to neuronal activity (Fig. 1.4). Thus, according to the concept of cellular replacement, neuronal and glial networks and their associated blood vessels are not permanent unalterable structures integrated by the same cellular elements but are structures showing substitutions of their cellular components. This form of plasticity may have important consequences for brain physiology and pathology.

ROLE OF HORMONES ON BRAIN MUTABILITY: PLASTICITY AND METAPLASTICITY

The nervous system is therefore mutable; but what are the causes of its mutability? Brain plasticity is regulated by exteroceptive and interoceptive signals (Fig. 1.5). Incoming information from the external world is one of the factors that participate in the regulation of plastic modifications in the sensory neuronal circuits and the associated glial cells and blood vessels. For instance, the configuration of cortical representation maps is under the continuous influence of peripheral inputs. Therefore, deprivation or stimulation of the information from one region of the skin results in the retraction or enlargement, respectively, of its representation area in the cerebral cortex (Kaas and Florence, 2001; Merzenich et al., 1983a, b). Another well-characterized example of plastic modifications in the adult cerebral cortex in response to sensory stimulation is provided by the representation of whiskers in the barrel cortex of mice. Stimulation of whiskers, which are sensory organs, results in plastic modifications in their representation maps in the barrel cortex (Ferezou et al., 2007; Kossut, 1998; Welker et al., 1992).

The visual cortex is also plastic during adult life, and visual cortex synaptic circuits in adult mammals are affected by perceptual learning and visual deprivation (Hofer et al., 2006; Karmarkar and Dan, 2006). Motor activity also impacts brain plasticity. Motor activity and the feedback information received from muscles and tendon sensory organs contribute to reorganize the structure and function of neuronal circuits involved in motor control and physical exercise promotes the generation of new neurons in the hippocampus (Cotman and Berchtold, 2002; Kempermann et al., 2000).

Behavioral activity and the associated feedback information from the external environment provided by sensory organs contribute to regulate brain plasticity in the cerebral cortex and other brain regions. Thus, exposure to an enriched physical and social environment increases the complexity of dendrites and neuronal connectivity in the brain (Faherty et al., 2003; Mora et al., 2007; Rosenzweig and Bennett, 1996; Volkmar and Greenough, 1972). Furthermore, there is evidence that behavioral activity engaged in by an individual feeds back to increase the probability that new formed neurons will survive in the high vocal center of the brain of songbirds (Li XC et al., 2000). Therefore, many external influences participate in the regulation of brain plasticity. Interoceptive signals from the body also affect brain plasticity (Fig. 1.5). These influences are mediated by the autonomous nervous system and by hormonal secretions. As we will see in the next chapters, many hormones reach the brain and modulate neuronal and glial plasticity.

Although exteroceptive and interoceptive information affect brain plasticity, this information does not seem to be the origin of plastic activity, since mutability seems to be an intrinsic property of the nervous system (Fig. 1.5). One of the theses of this book is that the brain and spinal cord are genetically programmed to be mutable and that their endogenous plastic activity is constantly generating modifications in neuronal circuits and associated cellular elements. According to this concept, the inner mutability of the central nervous system allows the adaptation of neuronal structure and function to provide adequate behavioral and inner regulatory responses to the changing external and internal conditions. For this purpose, the brain and spinal cord use the incoming information to organize its endogenous plastic activity. Exteroceptive and interoceptive information is therefore essential for the adaptation of endogenous brain plasticity to the changing social, biological, and physical context (Fig. 1.5), but it is not the cause of plasticity.

If the nervous system has an endogenous capacity for remodeling, the consequence is that hormones are not necessary for the induction of brain plasticity. Indeed, different forms of plasticity, including modifications in the number and size of dendritic spines, the induction of long-term synaptic potentiation, or the induction of long-term synaptic depression, may be provoked in brain slices in vitro by experimental manipulations, in absence of hormonal influences. This indicates that the brain does not need hormones to be mutable. Why is it then necessary to dedicate a book to the subject of hormones and brain plasticity? I consider this topic important because hormones play an essential role in the adjustment of the endogenous and permanent plastic capacity of the nervous system to the changing conditions in the body and in the external physical, biological, and social context. In other words, hormones do not induce brain plasticity but contribute to give "biological and contextual meaning" to brain plasticity. In fact, hormonal signals allow the brain

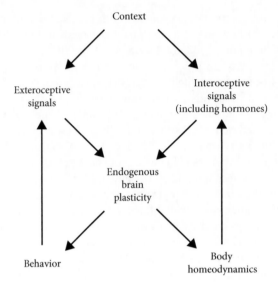

Figure 1.5. Brain plasticity is regulated by signals from the external world (exteroceptive) and from the body (interoceptive). Hormones are among the interoceptive
signals that regulate brain plasticity. Incoming exteroceptive and interoceptive information is essential for the adaptation of endogenous brain plasticity to the changing social, biological, and physical context. Exteroceptive and interoceptive signals
(including hormones) are not necessary for the induction of brain plasticity (which is
an endogenous property of brain tissue), but they give biological or contextual "meaning" to brain plasticity. The regulation of brain plasticity by exteroceptive and interoceptive signals allow the maintenance of the homeodynamic equilibrium of the inner
milieu (body homeodynamics) and the generation of adequate adaptive behavioral
responses.

to integrate external environmental information with the internal homeodynamic needs of the organism to generate adequate plastic modifications in the
nervous system. In turn, brain plasticity is essential to integrate exteroceptive
and interoceptive signals with body homeodynamics by the regulation of hormonal secretions and behavior. Therefore, the cross talk between endocrine
glands and brain plasticity maintains a homeodynamic equilibrium in adaptation of body needs to an ever-changing external and internal environment
(Figs. 1.2 and 1.5).

   Another important point to consider is that hormones do not seem to regulate specific mechanisms of plasticity. They appear to coordinate, in space (i.e.,
different brain regions) and through time, plastic modifications in adaptation to homeodynamic needs. A given hormone may facilitate the induction of
long-term depression of synaptic transmission or reduction in the branching of
dendritic arbors in a given brain structure, and at the same time may facilitate

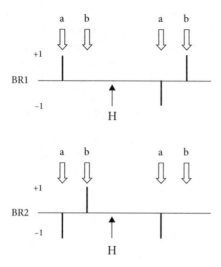

Figure 1.6. Schematic representation of an example of the regulation of brain meta-plasticity by hormones. An exteroceptive or interoceptive signal (a) facilitates the induction of a positive plastic event in brain region 1 (BR1) and a negative plastic event in brain region 2 (BR2). Another signal (b) facilitates the induction of a positive plastic event in BR2. After a hormonal action (H), the plastic event elicited by the first signal is modified in BR1 but not in BR2. In addition, the hormonal action facilitates the induction of a plastic event in BR1 by the second signal that was not observed before. In contrast, the plastic event elicited by the second signal in BR2 is inhibited. Thus, hormones do not induce specific forms of brain plasticity but regulate brain plastic events in a specific regional and temporal manner. Therefore, hormones regulate metaplasticity.

the induction of long-term synaptic potentiation or growth of dendritic arbors in another brain region (Fig. 1.6). Even within the same brain region, a given hormone may facilitate one form of synaptic plasticity and repress another mechanism of plasticity. We will examine examples of this in the next chapters. In addition, depending on the biological context, a given hormone may have different effects on brain plasticity. Therefore, hormones act as master regulators of brain plasticity, adapting endogenous mechanisms of plasticity to the immediate biological needs. Hormones, then, regulate plastic modifications of brain plasticity (Garcia, 2001, 2002; Kim and Yoon, 1998).

The term "metaplasticity," the plasticity of plasticity, was introduced to define the modification in the ability of synapses to exhibit functional synaptic plasticity in response to synaptic activity (Abraham and Bear, 1996; Deisseroth et al., 1995). Synaptic plasticity is dependent on the previous history of synaptic activity. For instance, previous N-methyl-D-aspartate receptor activation may result in an inhibition of the induction of long-term synaptic potentiation and a facilitation of long-term synaptic depression. In contrast, prior metabotropic glutamate receptor activation may facilitate the induction of long-term synaptic potentiation (Abraham and Bear, 1996; Abraham and Tate, 1997; Deisseroth et al., 1995; Perez-Otano and Ehlers, 2005). Therefore, metaplasticity is caused by a change in the threshold for the induction of synaptic plasticity, which is caused by the previous history of synaptic activity. We may extend the concept of metaplasticity to morphological synaptic plasticity and to neuronal and glial replacement and to the associated changes in angiogenesis, since the induction of these plastic events and its consequences for cognition, emotions, and behavior (Post et al., 1998) is also variable over long timescales and depends on the biological context and previous history of plasticity. We will see in this book several examples on how hormones regulate metaplasticity—adapting the threshold for brain plasticity during life to the precise homeodynamic needs of each moment.

Chapter 2

Brain Plasticity Regulates Hormonal Homeodynamics

INTRODUCTION: BRAIN PLASTICITY REGULATES THE ACTIVITY OF ENDOCRINE GLANDS

As mentioned in the previous chapter, in the context of the cross talk between the brain and endocrine glands, we should consider not only the neuroplastic actions that hormones exert in the brain but also the consequences that brain remodeling has for hormonal production and release. Exteroceptive and interoceptive signals, including hormones, regulate the plasticity of the nervous system. In turn, neuronal and glial plasticity in the brain centers involved in endocrine control is associated with the regulation of hormonal levels under physiological and pathological conditions (see Chapter 9 for the effects of pathological brain remodeling on hormonal levels). Thus, brain remodeling is a consequence and a cause of hormonal changes. Brain plasticity contributes to the adaptation of the activity of endocrine glands to homeodynamic needs and hormones participate in the interoceptive regulation of brain plasticity (Fig. 2.1).

Modifications of plasticity in cognitive areas or in brain regions involved in the modulation of emotions and feelings may regulate hormonal secretions, either by modifications of behavior or by the indirect innervation of the hypothalamic regions controlling the release of pituitary hormones. For instance, alterations in plasticity in the prefrontal cortex and hippocampus may be the result and the cause of an impaired secretion of stress hormones (see Chapter 3). However, we have very limited information on the link between plasticity in these cortical regions and the control of hormonal release. Therefore, here I will limit my analysis to plasticity associated with neuronal networks, which are known to be directly involved in the regulation of hypothalamic neurosecretory neurons.

The hypothalamic neurosecretory neurons constitute a very heterogeneous population of cells that may be classified into two main groups: magnocellular and parvocellular. In addition to obvious differences in cell volume, which justify their names, the most important difference between the two types of neurosecretory neurons is that the axons of magnocellular cells transport their neurosecretory products to the neurohypophysis to be released into the bloodstream, while the axons of parvocellular neurons reach the median eminence where the hormonal products are released into the hypophyseal portal

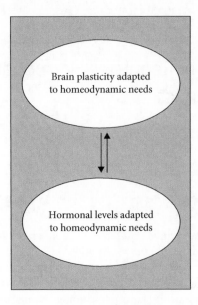

Figure 2.1. Brain plasticity regulates hormonal levels and hormones regulate brain plasticity. The brain adapts its activity to the changing environmental and physiological conditions with plastic modifications in neurons and glial cells, according to the information transmitted by a variety of exteroceptive and interoceptive signals, including hormones. In turn, the plastic reorganization of brain regions involved in hormonal control regulates the activity of endocrine glands to adapt hormonal secretion to the changing homeodynamic needs.

system, which connects the hypothalamus with the anterior lobe of the pituitary gland. Magnocellular neurons release two important hormones, vasopressin and oxytocin. Among other functions, vasopressin is involved in the control of water homeodynamics and blood pressure. Oxytocin regulates milk ejection, uterine contraction, and maternal behavior, and affects sexual behavior. In addition, both oxytocin and vasopressin have cognitive effects and are involved in social behavior and in the regulation of affection. Parvocellular neurons release a variety of hormones, such as thyrotropin-releasing hormone, corticotropin-releasing hormone (or corticotropin-releasing factor), gonadotropin-releasing hormone, growth hormone–releasing hormone, and somatostatin, among others. These parvocellular hypothalamic hormones are released in the median eminence and reach the anterior pituitary through the portal blood to regulate the secretion of anterior pituitary hormones. Structural and functional plastic remodeling of neurons and glial cells associated with modifications in hypothalamic hormonal release has been detected in the hypothalamus, the neurohypophysis, and the median eminence. In this chapter, I will first examine neuroglia and synaptic plasticity in the soma and dendrites of magnocellular neurosecretory neurons in the hypothalamus and the associated neuroglial plasticity in the neurohypophysis. Then, I will consider plastic events in parvocellular hypothalamic neurons and the associated plastic reorganization of glia and parvocellular neurosecretory endings in the median eminence.

NEUROGLIAL REMODELING ASSOCIATED WITH HORMONAL SECRETION BY HYPOTHALAMIC MAGNOCELLULAR NEURONS

Studies on oxytocin and vasopressin magnocellular neurons located in the supraoptic and paraventricular hypothalamic nuclei have provided clear examples on how neuroglial plastic remodeling may participate in the regulation of endocrine secretions (Hatton, 1990, 1997; Miyata and Hatton, 2002; Theodosis, 2002; Theodosis et al., 1995; Theodosis and Poulain, 1987, 1993). This neuroglial remodeling is also a paradigm for the involvement of glial cells in morphological and functional synaptic plasticity. Cell bodies and dendrites of magnocellular neurons in the supraoptic and paraventricular nuclei are tightly packed. Under basal conditions, thin, lamella-like astrocytic processes separate the perikaryal and dendritic plasma membranes from adjacent magnocellular neurons. In addition, the stimulation of magnocellular hormonal release produces a dramatic retraction of astrocytic processes in the supraoptic and paraventricular nuclei, allowing the direct juxtaposing of plasma membranes from adjacent neuronal somas and adjacent dendrites (Fig. 2.2). This synaptic and glial remodeling is transient and disappears when stimulation ceases. Neuroglial and synaptic remodeling associated with magnocellular neurons has been detected during different physiological conditions associated with an increased hormonal demand, such as osmotic stimulation (Chapman et al., 1986; Gregory et al., 1980; Miyata et al., 1994a; Tweedle and Hatton, 1976, 1977), parturition (Hatton et al., 1984; Montagnese et al., 1987; Theodosis and Poulain, 1984a), lactation (Hatton et al., 1984; Montagnese et al., 1987; Theodosis et al., 1986a; Theodosis and Poulain, 1984a), and chronic stress (Miyata et al., 1994b). I will present in this section a brief account of these studies.

In the early seventies, Glenn I. Hatton, from Michigan State University, analyzed the morphology and physiology of supraoptic neurons by dehydration and rehydration in rats. He was interested in parameters such as the number of nucleoli, cell volume, and cell firing rate that could be related to neurosecretory activity (Hatton and Walters, 1973; Walters and Hatton, 1974). Together with James K. Walters he found that firing rates and cell size increased in supraoptic neurons as a consequence of dehydration. Cell size changes in supraoptic neurons were measurable early in dehydration and continued as long as the deprivation conditions persisted (Hatton and Walters, 1973). By this time, Miguel Lafarga and collaborators in Barcelona, through electron microscopic studies, demonstrated interruptions in the glial wrapping of magnocellular perikarya in the supraoptic nucleus. Lafarga and collaborators proposed that

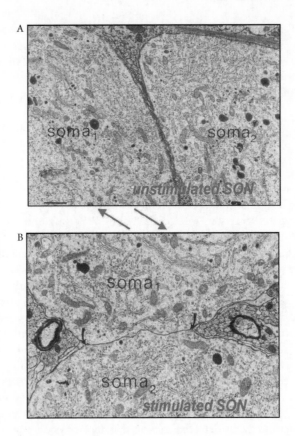

Figure 2.2. Glial and neuronal plastic remodeling in magnocellular neurons associated with the release of oxytocin in the adult supraoptic nucleus (SON). A: Under basal unstimulated conditions, neuronal somas are separated by multiple astrocytic processes. B: Under conditions of high hormonal release, glial processes retract, and the proportion of magnocellular somas in juxtaposition with other somas (black arrows) is increased. These plastic modifications are interpreted as a mechanism to facilitate synchronization of hormonal release by magnocellular neurons. When activity is back to basal conditions (red arrows), astrocytic processes again separate neuronal profiles. (Courtesy of Dr. Dionysia T. Theodosis. Based on Theodosis and Poulain, 1987.)

neuronal juxtapositions between contiguous cell bodies at sites where the glial wrapping was interrupted may be related to the synchronization of supraoptic nucleus neuronal activity for hormonal release (Lafarga et al., 1975). Then, in collaboration with Charles D. Tweedle, Hatton performed a quantitative ultrastructural analysis of the nucleus circularis (a group of magnocellular elements arranged in a ring around a capillary bed) and supraoptic nucleus. They studied rats under normal and water-deprived conditions and found that dehydration produced not only an increase in neuronal size but also a retraction of fine glial processes located between the neuronal somas in these two nuclei. This was accompanied by an increase in the percentage of neurons with direct soma-somatic juxtapositions and an increase in the amount of plasma membranes of adjacent neuronal somas showing juxtapositions. These findings suggested that remodeling of specific hypothalamic structures could be involved in the control of water homeodynamics. Tweedle and Hatton detected that the morphological plasticity associated with magnocellular hypothalamic neurons was transient, since rehydration reversed the changes (Tweedle and Hatton, 1976, 1977). Further studies from Hatton's laboratory revealed that the percentage of plasma membrane from neuronal somas in soma-somatic appositions increased in the primarily vasopressin-containing lateral portion of the rat paraventricular nucleus with 12 hours of dehydration, indicating that the neuroglial plasticity associated with water deprivation was also present in magnocellular paraventricular neurons (Gregory et al., 1980).

In 1981, Dionysia T. Theodosis, Dominique A. Poulain, and Jean-Didier Vincent, working in a unit of the INSERM (Institut National de la Santé et de la Recherche Médicale) in Bordeaux, France, reported very similar plastic changes in the supraoptic nucleus of female rats during lactation. These investigators were searching for a possible morphological basis for the synchronized electrical activation of oxytocin neurons during suckling-induced reflex milk ejections. The results of a detailed quantitative morphometric analysis of the supraoptic nucleus revealed that the proportion of magnocellular somas in juxtaposition with other somas or with dendritic profiles significantly increased in lactating rats compared to normal male and virgin females. The supraoptic nucleus of lactating rats also showed a higher incidence of presynaptic terminals contacting more than one postsynaptic element (Fig. 2.2), either soma or dendrite (Theodosis et al., 1981). The double synapses were characterized, in subsequent studies, as being mainly GABAergic, but a certain amount were identified as glutamatergic (El Majdoubi et al., 1996, 1997; Gies and Theodosis, 1994; Theodosis et al., 1986c). These plastic morphological changes were interpreted as a possible mechanism to facilitate synchronization of neuronal firing.

The findings of Theodosis and her colleagues were soon confirmed by Hatton and Tweedle by an analysis of the ultrastructure of the supraoptic nucleus in virgin female rats, female rats at the last day of pregnancy, postpartum rats, and 14-day lactating rats (Hatton, 1986; Hatton et al., 1984; Hatton and Tweedle, 1982). They detected significant increases in the percentage of magnocellular neuronal profiles in the supraoptic nucleus in soma-somatic apposition and in the amount of juxtaposed neuronal membranes by the last day of pregnancy and in lactating rats. In addition, Hatton and Tweedle reported a significant increase in the percentage of supraoptic magnocellular neurons showing presynaptic terminals making synaptic contact with two postsynaptic neurons in lactating rats, and to a minor extent in postpartum rats (Fig. 2.2). As Theodosis and her colleagues proposed, the double synapses were also interpreted as a mechanism of synchronization of oxytocin cells for hormonal release. Formation and retraction of new synapses was also detected in the supraoptic nucleus by dehydration and rehydration (Tweedle and Hatton, 1984). In addition, neuroglial plasticity was also observed in the dendritic zone of the supraoptic nucleus, located in the ventral glial laminar area, after dehydration and during pregnancy, parturition, and lactation (Perlmutter et al., 1984, 1985). High hormonal demand was associated with (i) an increase in the number of dendrites with plasma membranes in direct apposition with adjacent dendrites, (ii) an increase in the amount of dendritic membrane in direct apposition, and (iii) an increase in the percentage of dendrites contacted by double synapses. Similar findings were obtained by Theodosis and Poulain (1984a) when they analyzed neuroglial changes in the supraoptic nucleus during the transition from pregnancy to lactation. The percentage of neuronal profiles, either dendrites or somas, in direct apposition and the incidence of double synapses was low 2 weeks after the beginning of pregnancy but showed a striking increase the day prior to parturition and remained increased during lactation. The incidence of direct appositions and double synapses diminished gradually after weaning to reach, by 2 months after the end of lactation, the basal situation observed in virgin animals. These findings clearly demonstrated that neuroglial and synaptic plasticity in the supraoptic nucleus are associated with modifications of the pattern of neurosecretory activity of magnocellular neurons in response to changing physiological conditions.

There is a point of controversy on whether the plastic changes are specific for a magnocellular population, the oxytocin neurons, or whether the changes affect both oxytocin and vasopressin cells. Theodosis and Poulain, using pre-embedding immunocytochemistry and electron microscopy, detected that the proportion of oxytocin neuronal profiles in juxtaposition and the incidence of double synapses on oxytocin neurons were higher in lactating rats compared to virgin rats. Therefore, they concluded that the neuroglia remodeling in the supraoptic nucleus during lactation affects the magnocellular neurons secreting oxytocin (Theodosis and Poulain, 1984b). Further studies comparing the modifications of oxytocin and vasopressin immunoreactive neurons revealed that the plastic changes during lactation exclusively affect the oxytocinergic neurons (Theodosis et al., 1986a). Furthermore, simultaneous increases in the number and extent of direct neuronal appositions and in the number of presynaptic terminals contacting two neurosecretory cells as a result of osmotic stimulation were also observed to affect oxytocin but not vasopressin neurons (Chapman et al., 1986). In addition, prolonged intracerebroventricular infusions of oxytocin and not vasopressin were able to induce the neuroglial and synaptic changes in the supraoptic nucleus associated with an increased oxytocin release (Theodosis et al., 1986b). These findings, together with previous observations of synaptic contacts of oxytocin cells with other oxytocin cells within the supraoptic nucleus (Theodosis, 1985), suggested that oxytocin enhances its own release by promoting structural plastic reorganization in the supraoptic nucleus and that the neuroglia and synaptic changes were specific to oxytocin neurons.

Very different results were reported by Hatton's laboratory (Marzban et al., 1992). Hatton and his colleagues used postembedding immunogold immuno-cytochemistry to detect oxytocin and vasopressin immunoreactive neurons in the supraoptic nucleus at the electron microscopic level. After chronic dehy-dration, both vasopressin and oxytocin immunoreactive neuronal perikarya increased in size. Furthermore, both cell types showed an increase in soma-somatic/dendritic membrane contact, indicating that both vasopressin and oxytocin cells undergo morphological changes during chronic dehydration. Therefore, these findings, obtained with a different immunocytochemical approach, were clearly different to those reported by the group of Theodosis. The reason for this discrepancy is unclear. However, there are other evidences indicating that vasopressin and oxytocin neurons do not suffer the same mor-phological plastic changes. Indeed, the analysis of dendritic trees of oxytocin and vasopressin neurons in the supraoptic nucleus has revealed a different remodeling in these two cell types during lactation. The dendritic trees of oxy-tocin neurons show a prominent reduction in dendritic branching and total dendritic length. In contrast, the dendritic trees of vasopressin neurons show an increase in branching and total dendritic length during lactation (Stern and Armstrong, 1998). Interestingly, functional synaptic plasticity is also different on oxytocin and vasopressin neurons. Short-term plasticity, either synaptic facilitation or synaptic depression, has been detected on GABAergic inputs to magnocellular neurons. Short-term facilitation was observed preferentially in oxytocin neurons, while short-term depression was predominant in vaso-pressin neurons (Baimoukhametova et al., 2004). The different physiologi-cal conditions are probably associated with a different synaptic remodeling in vasopressin and oxytocin magnocellular neurons. Thus, the laboratory of Theodosis using a morphometric analysis on semithin sections detected that lactation, which involves an increased secretion of oxytocin, is associated with an increased innervation of supraoptic and paraventricular oxytocin magno-cellular somas by noradrenergic inputs (Michaloudi et al., 1997) and with an increase in the number of glutamatergic terminals making synaptic contact simultaneously onto two or more oxytocinergic elements (El Majdoubi et al., 1996). In contrast, using confocal microscopy, Mueller and collaborators detected a decrease in the number of dopamine β-hydroxylase synaptic bou-tons in apposition of vasopressin neurons of the supraoptic nucleus of juvenile rats upon salt loading, which involves an enhanced vasopressin release. This suggests that noradrenergic/adrenergic innervation decreased in magnocel-lular vasopressin neurons under these conditions. In contrast, the number of GABAergic and glutamatergic inputs in apposition to vasopressin neurons increased (Mueller et al., 2005).

In addition to marked morphological plastic changes observed in the para-ventricular and supraoptic nucleus, there are more subtle molecular changes in magnocellular neurons, which may underlie functional synaptic plastic-ity. These may include switches in GABA(A) receptor subunit composition around parturition (Brussaard et al., 1997) and in N-methyl-D-aspartate

(NMDA) receptor subunit composition after osmotic stress (Curras-Collazo and Dao, 1999). A variety of functional plastic changes have been detected in the supraoptic nucleus. I have already mentioned the induction of synaptic facilitation or synaptic depression on GABAergic inputs to magnocellular neurons (Baimoukhametova et al., 2004). Furthermore, chronic osmotic stimulation increases the frequency of spontaneous excitatory and inhibitory postsynaptic currents in magnocellular supraoptic neurons, an effect that is probably due to increased numbers of release sites. Moreover, chronic dehydration induces a marked enhancement of the facilitatory effect of norepinephrine on glutamate release and an inhibitory effect on GABA release (Di and Tasker, 2004). In addition, glutamate afferents to the supraoptic nucleus, in particular those originating in the organum vasculosum of the lamina terminalis, exhibit NMDA receptor-dependent long-term potentiation and long-term depression (Panatier et al., 2006b).

As has been mentioned already, the morphological and functional remodeling associated with magnocellular neuronal stimulation is accompanied by gross morphological alterations in astroglia. I have already commented on the changes in the extension of glial processes between adjacent neuronal somas and dendrites that are associated with an increased hormonal demand. In addition, during lactation, the increased physiological activation of magnocellular neurons results in a redistribution of astroglial cytoskeleton in the supraoptic nucleus, detected by a reduction in glial fibrillary acidic protein (GFAP) immunoreactivity (Salm et al., 1985). Similar changes have been detected in GFAP immunoreactivity in the supraoptic nucleus during dehydration and are reversible after rehydration (Hawrylak et al., 1998). The astrocytes of the ventral glial limitans also show marked plastic changes in the supraoptic nucleus after osmotic stimulation. The ventral glial limitans decreases in thickness, and astrocyte nuclei are detected at a closer distance from the pial surface in chronic dehydrated animals compared to controls. In addition, astrocytes were reoriented from a perpendicular to a parallel orientation to the pial surface after dehydration. These changes were reversed by rehydration (Bobak and Salm, 1996).

Morphological glial changes may have important consequences for synaptic function. The studies by Theodosis and colleagues have shown that the decreased extension of glial processes is always associated with an increased formation of new synapses on oxytocin neurons. Furthermore, modifications in the contact between glia and neurons may affect neuronal membrane properties. In addition, modifications in the extension of astrocytic processes in the supraoptic nucleus of lactating and chronically dehydrated animals may affect the uptake of neurotransmitters by glia, including glutamate, and may control the level of activation of presynaptic metabotropic glutamate receptors on glutamatergic terminals, which inhibit transmitter release (Oliet et al., 2006; Oliet and Piet, 2004). Furthermore, the morphological changes in the morphology of astrocytes may affect the tortuosity of the extracellular space and the spatial local availability of neurotransmitters released by neurons, such as glutamate and GABA, and of other factors released by neurons and glia that may regulate synaptic function. One such glial factors is D-serine, the endogenous ligand for the glycine-binding site of the NMDA receptor. Changing levels of D-serine modulate NMDA receptor activation, and astrocytes are the only source of D-serine in the supraoptic nucleus. Therefore, long-term synaptic potentiation and long-term synaptic depression in glutamatergic afferents to the supraoptic nucleus is controlled by the release of D-serine by astrocytes (Panatier et al., 2006a). Another factor released by astrocytes that may affect functional synaptic plasticity is ATP. Astrocytes release ATP in response to noradrenergic stimulation. ATP then acts on neurons, promoting the insertion of AMPA receptors in postsynaptic membranes, which in turn increases postsynaptic efficacy (Gordon and Bains, 2006; Gordon et al., 2005).

Several cell adhesion molecules could participate in the mechanisms of glial and synaptic plasticity. For instance, cell surface molecules, and in particular those belonging to the immunoglobulin superfamily, appear to be involved in neuronal–glial interactions and in the establishment of neuronal connections. The best studied model is the family of neural cell adhesion molecules (N-CAMs), which are widely expressed by both neurons and glial cells. N-CAMs exist in a variety of isoforms, differing in the length of their cytoplasmic domain and/or their carbohydrate content, with these isoforms being differentially expressed according to the developmental stage and/or the cell phenotype.

In an embryonic brain, N-CAM contains more than 30% polysialic acid (PSA). During the perinatal and early postnatal periods, this embryonic N-CAM isoform (PSA-N-CAM) is gradually replaced by isoforms containing less PSA. However, expression of PSA-N-CAM persists in the adult rat in several brain areas that maintain the capacity for neuroglial plasticity, such as the hypothalamo-neurohypophysial system, the arcuate nucleus, and the median eminence (Bonfanti et al., 1992; Theodosis et al., 1991). PSA reduces cell adhesion, allowing cellular morphological plasticity. Thus, it has been proposed that polysialylation is a permanent feature of certain brain areas that permits the cells in these areas to undergo morphological remodeling in response to the appropriate stimuli (Theodosis et al., 1994). Glial and neuronal remodeling in the supraoptic and paraventricular nuclei appears to be facilitated by the high expression of PSA-N-CAM in these structures. Theodosis and her collaborators have shown that the specific enzymatic removal of PSA from N-CAM, by intracerebral microinjection of endoneuraminidase, blocks neuroglial plasticity in magnocellular nuclei normally induced by lactation and dehydration (Theodosis et al., 1999).

NEUROGLIAL REMODELING IN THE NEUROHYPOPHYSIS

Neuroglial changes associated with water deprivation and rehydration, similar to those observed in the hypothalamic regions where magnocellular neurons are present, have been observed in the neural lobe of the rat pituitary

(Theodosis and MacVicar, 1996). The neuronal lobe of the pituitary, also known as the neurohypophysis, is a central nervous system structure where the axons of magnocellular hypothalamic neurons release their content into the systemic blood circulation. Specialized glial cells of the neurohypophysis, the pituicytes, engulf neurosecretory axons from magnocellular hypothalamic neurons and probably regulate the release of magnocellular hormones.

Tweedle and Hatton observed that the number of pituicytes that completely enclosed neurosecretory axons was dramatically decreased after 24 hours of water deprivation and returned to normal levels after 24 hours of rehydration (Tweedle and Hatton, 1980). This finding suggested that plastic remodeling of pituicytes could be involved in the physiological regulation of hormonal secretions by magnocellular hypothalamic neurons (Hatton, 1988). Moreover, the observations of Tweedle and Hatton also suggested that a synchrony of neuroglial plasticity in the hypothalamus and pituitary is essential for the coordination of magnocellular hormonal secretion. This was further supported by the observation that parturition, lactation, and all other stimuli leading to increased hormone release were also associated with a marked decrease in the number of pituicytes, with neurosecretory axons completely surrounded by their cytoplasm and by an increased occupation of the basal lamina by nerve terminals (Tweedle and Hatton, 1982, 1987).

The morphological plasticity of axons and glial processes in the hypothalamus and neurohypophysis can be reproduced in in vitro preparations. These in vitro models have been used to analyze the mechanisms involved in the regulation of the plastic changes, such as the role of neurotransmitters (Langle et al., 2003; Luckman and Bicknell, 1990; Miyata et al., 1997) and cell adhesion molecules (Monlezun et al., 2005).

NEUROGLIAL REMODELING ASSOCIATED WITH PARVOCELLULAR HYPOTHALAMIC NEURONS

The hormonal products of parvocellular hypothalamic neurons reach the anterior pituitary, or adenohypophysis, and regulate the secretion of hormones by this key endocrine organ. In addition, the parvocellular neurons innervate broad areas of the brain. In contrast to magnocellular neurosecretory cells, the parvocellular neurons are a very heterogeneous neuronal population, having only in common the fact that they release their hormonal secretions in the portal blood of the median eminence. The complete variety of hormonal products released by parvocellular neurons is still unknown. We expect that hormones secreted by parvocellular neurons may exceed in number the hormones secreted by the anterior pituitary, since it is probable that the parvocellular hormonal system secretes at least one inhibitory and one stimulatory hormone for each hormone produced by the adenohypohysis. Therefore, the parvocellular hormones already identified may represent only a fraction of the total hormonal production by parvocellular cells. Even for the parvocellular hormones already identified, we have limited information on the mechanisms regulating their secretion. In particular, synaptic plastic events on parvocellular neurosecretory neurons have not been studied with so much detail as has been the case for magnocellular neurons. A wide, unexplored field is waiting for new innovative research projects.

One of the main problems in detecting plasticity associated with the neurosecretory activity of parvocellular neurons is caused by the dispersion of parvocellular cells and by the fact that their morphology is not, in general, very different from the surrounding neurons that are not neurosecretory. This problem may be solved by using specific promoters to drive the expression of genes that would allow the identification of specific parvocellular neuronal populations. One example is the use of gonadotropin-releasing hormone (GnRH) promoter-driven transgenics in the mouse for the identification of single, living GnRH neurons in acute brain slice preparation. This procedure allows electrophysiological recordings and gene profiling of GnRH cells (Clasadonte et al., 2008; Herbison et al., 2001) and has demonstrated to be a very valuable tool for the characterization of the morphology, physiology, and synaptic connectivity of GnRH neurons.

These approaches will probably give much information in the future on the synaptic plastic changes associated with parvocellular neurosecretory activity. Today, the information available is limited to a few systems. One system that provides plastic responses in response to the neurosecretory activity is the hypothalamic pituitary adrenal axis. In the next chapter (and other chapters of this book) I will analyze how stress affects plasticity in different brain structures. These plastic changes may in turn affect the ability of the central nervous system to properly regulate hormonal secretions.

Chronic stress may produce permanent alterations in the hypothalamic control of parvocellular neuronal secretions, and this may be associated with a remodeling of the circuits involved in such control. For instance, synaptic plasticity has been detected on parvocellular neurons secreting corticotropin-releasing hormone and located in the paraventricular hypothalamic nucleus. These neurons receive an abundant GABAergic innervation. Following adrenalectomy, which increases the synthesis and secretion of corticotropin-releasing hormone, there is a marked increase in the number of GABAergic inputs to corticotropin-releasing hormone neurons (Miklos and Kovacs, 2002). This suggests that the secretion of parvocellular neurosecretory cells may be controlled by plastic changes in their synaptic inputs. However, one of the best studied populations of parvocellular neurons in this regard is the one that produces the hormones that regulate the release of gonadotropins by the anterior pituitary. For instance, seasonal breeders show seasonal modifications in responsiveness of GnRH neurons to the negative feedback influence of gonadal steroids (see following text). This seasonal variation probably reflects a plastic modification of neuronal circuits controlling GnRH neurons.

Evidence from a number of different species suggests that the brain is capable of undergoing annual synaptic remodeling in the GnRH system of seasonal breeders (see also Chapter 8). The GnRH system exhibits a remarkable degree of seasonal plasticity, especially in non-mammalian vertebrates such as birds. In songbirds, seasonal changes in brain GnRH immunoreactivity are associated to changes in song control nuclei volumes (Hurley et al., 2008). The GnRH system show also seasonal plasticity in mammals. In the ewe, the number of synaptic inputs to GnRH neurons shows seasonal changes, suggesting that neuronal plastic changes in GnRH-producing neurons may participate in seasonal changes in GnRH levels (Lehman et al., 1997). For instance, preoptic GnRH neurons in breeding season ewes receive more synaptic inputs in somas and dendrites than GnRH neurons in anestrus animals (Jansen et al., 2003; Xiong et al., 1997). In particular, neuropeptide Y inputs to GnRH neurons increase during the breeding season, and β-endorphin inputs are increased during anestrus on GnRH somas and on GnRH dendrites during the breeding season (Jansen et al., 2003). GABAergic inputs also show seasonal plastic changes—they increase during the breeding season in a subpopulation of GnRH neurons (Jansen et al., 2003). However, the proportion of GnRH neurons contacted by GABAergic inputs shows a decrease (Pompolo et al., 2003).

In addition, there are seasonal variations in the ewe brain involving the association between GnRH neurons and the cell adhesion molecule PSA-N-CAM, which, as I have already mentioned, is involved in plastic neural remodeling (Viguie et al., 2001). The neuronal remodeling of synaptic inputs on GnRH cells is also associated with marked modifications in GFAP density and in the thickness of glial fibrils. Furthermore, GnRH proximal dendrites are much more heavily associated with glia during the breeding season than during anestrus (Jansen et al., 2003). In addition to direct changes in neuropeptide Y, GABA, and β-endorphin inputs, dopaminergic cells located in the hypothalamus and estrogen receptor–containing cells in the arcuate hypothalamic nucleus, which project to the median eminence, may also regulate GnRH synaptic plasticity. Interestingly, the activity of these neuronal networks regulating GnRH also shows seasonal modifications (Lehman et al., 1996; Stefanovic et al., 2000) and neuronal plasticity has been detected in the A15 dopaminergic cell group in the retrochiasmatic area, which mediate estrogen negative feedback to GnRH cells during anestrus. A twofold increase in synapsin-positive close contacts onto A15 neurons and a significant increase in dendritic length have been detected in the anestrus period with confocal microscopy (Adams et al., 2006). This finding suggests that synaptic plastic remodeling to control GnRH secretion involves not only direct inputs to GnRH neurons but also other neuronal components of the circuits controlling the activity of GnRH neurons.

Remodeling of synaptic inputs to GnRH neurons also appears to be involved in the regulation of GnRH release in nonseasonal breeders and may participate in the regulatory effects of gonadal hormones on GnRH secretion (Garcia-Segura et al., 2008). In primates, the initiation of the pubertal increase in pulsatile GnRH release is associated with a decrease in the number of synaptic inputs to GnRH neurons (Perera and Plant, 1997). Furthermore, a marked remodeling of the dendritic tree with puberty has been detected in GnRH neurons in mice (Cottrell et al., 2006), suggesting possible modification in synaptic inputs on dendrites. Nitric oxide release by neuronal networks associated with GnRH neurons may regulate GnRH neuronal plasticity and synchronize GnRH release (Clasadonte et al., 2008; d'Anglemont de Tassigny et al., 2007). In adult primates, an ovariectomy increases the apposition of glial processes to GnRH neuronal perikarya and decreases the number of synaptic inputs to GnRH neurons, while ovarian hormone replacement has the opposite effects, decreasing the glial ensheathment and increasing the innervation of GnRH neuronal somas (Witkin et al., 1991). In rats, astrocytes that are directly apposed to GnRH neurons in the rostral preoptic area show morphological changes associated with gonadotropin release. Their surface area and the number of their cell processes decrease from the morning of proestrus, before the initiation of the GnRH-induced luteinizing hormone surge, to the afternoon of proestrus. In the afternoon of proestrus, there is a significant decrease in the surface area and the number of astrocytic processes in parallel to the increase in luteinizing hormone concentration in plasma. The following day, on estrus, both the surface area and the number of processes per astrocyte return to levels similar to those seen on proestrus morning (Cashion et al., 2003).

As in seasonal breeders, synaptic and glial remodeling associated with the regulation of GnRH release is not limited to the direct inputs on GnRH neurons. Diurnal oscillation of GFAP immunoreactivity has been detected in a hypothalamic region, dorsal to the suprachiasmatic nucleus and close to the third ventricle. The oscillation is enhanced by estradiol administration to ovariectomized rats, which also causes an increase in luteinizing hormone rhythm (Fernandez-Galaz et al., 1999b). These results suggest that the perisuprachiasmatic nucleus area could be an important locus for structural plastic remodeling, linking circadian rhythms with the estrogen-induced luteinizing hormone surge. In addition, in adult female rodents the hypotalamic arcuate nucleus, which appears to be involved in the control of GnRH neurons, exhibits a natural phasic neuroglia and synaptic remodeling during the estrus cycle that is induced by estradiol and is linked to GnRH release (Olmos et al, 1989; see Fig. 2.3 and Chapter 8). The surge of luteinizing hormone on the afternoon of proestrus is coincident with a decrease in the number of inhibitory axosomatic synapses, an increase in glial coverage of neuronal somas, and an increase in the innervation of dendritic spines (Csakvari et al., 2007; Garcia-Segura et al., 1994a, b; Parducz et al., 2002).

Similar neuroglia remodeling occurs in infundibular neurons of monkeys (Naftolin et al., 1993). The neurons affected by these plastic reorganizations may form part of the circuits controlling GnRH neuronal innervation. In addition, some of the neurons affected by the remodeling of axosomatic synapses induced by estrogen are dopaminergic neurons that project to the median eminence and, therefore, probably are parvocellular neurosecretory neurons involved in the regulation of the release of prolactin (Csakvari et al.,

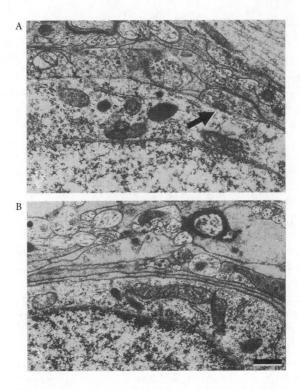

Figure 2.3. Modifications in glial processes (highlighted in yellow) and axosomatic synaptic terminals (arrow) in the rat arcuate nucleus during the estrus cycle. The electron micrographs show two arcuate neuronal somas. (A) In the morning of proestrus, before the peak of estrogen in plasma. (B) In the morning of estrus. The number of axosomatic synaptic inputs decreases from proestrus to estrus. In parallel, there is an increased warping of arcuate neuronal somas by glial processes. Scale bar, 0.5 μm. (Microphotographs from the author.)

2008; Parducz et al., 2003; see Fig. 2.4). Indeed, plasticity of GABAergic and β-endorphin neurotransmission on tuberoinfundibular dopaminergic neurons may, in part, be involved in the regulation of prolactin secretion (Racagni et al., 1984; Voogt et al., 2001).

NEUROGLIAL REMODELING IN THE MEDIAN EMINENCE

In parallel to the synaptic and glial remodeling in the GnRH neurons and in the arcuate nucleus, tanycytes in the median eminence suffer plastic morphological and biochemical changes that may be linked to the regulation of GnRH release into the portal blood vessels of the median eminence (Fig. 2.5). Tanycytes are specialized bipolar glial cells, located in the arcuate nucleus and the median eminence, that play a key role in neuroendocrine regulation.

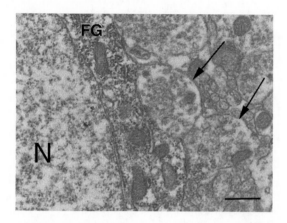

Figure 2.4. Arcuate nucleus neurons that project to the median eminence are identified by retrograde labeling with the tracer fluorogold. The tracer fluorogold is injected in the median eminence, and arcuate neurons projecting to this structure are retrogradely labeled. This electron micrograph shows an arcuate neuronal soma from an ovariectomized rat injected with fluorogold in the median eminence. Fluorogold immunoreactive precipitates (FG) are observed in the cytoplasm. Cell nucleus (N). Axosomatic synapses (arrows). With this method Parducz et al. detected estrogen regulation of synaptic connectivity in a specific subpopulation of dopaminergic arcuate neurons projecting to the median eminence. Scale bar: 1 μm. (Courtesy of Dr. Arpad Parducz; based on Csakvari et al., 2008, and Parducz et al., 2003.)

Tanycytes share some properties with astrocytes, radial glia, and Schwann cells, and are often classified as astroglia, but clearly constitute a distinct and specialized type of glia (Rodriguez et al., 2005).

Tanycytic processes are closely associated with GnRH fibers in the median eminence (Baroncini et al., 2007; King and Rubin, 1994; Kozlowski and Coates, 1985; Saldanha et al., 2001; Silverman et al., 1991) and participate in the release of GnRH to the portal blood by providing different signals to the GnRH neurons, including the excitatory neurotransmitter glutamate (Roth et al., 2006). In addition, tanycytes may contribute to the regulation of GnRH release by plastic extension and retraction of their end feet processes that are intermingled between GnRH synaptic terminals and the portal vasculature in the median eminence (King and Letourneau, 1994; King and Rubin, 1994; Kobayashi et al., 1972; Kozlowski and Coates, 1985; Prevot et al., 1999; Ugrumov et al., 1985, 1989). In rodents, tanycytic processes extend and retract following hormonal changes during the estrus cycle. Growth of tanycytic processes results in the ensheathment of GnRH terminals, preventing GnRH release. In contrast, during the preovulatory stage of the cycle, tanycytic processes retract, allowing the contact of GnRH terminals with portal capillaries (King and Letourneau, 1994; Prevot et al., 1999).

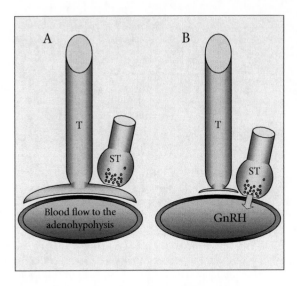

Figure 2.5. Neuroglial plasticity associated with the release of gonadotropin releasing hormone (GnRH) into the blood flow in the median eminence. The cellular processes of tanycytes (T), specialized bipolar glial cells, are closely associated with gonadotropin-releasing hormone fibers in the median eminence. Tanycytic processes extend and retract following hormonal changes during the estrus cycle in rodents. (A) Growth of tanycytic processes results in the ensheathment of gonadotropin-releasing hormone synaptic terminals (ST), preventing gonadotropin-releasing hormone release in the blood flow to the adenohypohysis. (B) Retraction of tanycytic processes during the preovulatory stage of the estrus cycle, allows the contact of gonadotropin-releasing hormone terminals with portal capillaries and the release of gonadotropin-releasing hormone to the blood flow.

Soluble factors such as epidermal growth factor–related peptides, neuregulins, transforming growth factor α, and prostaglandin E2 are also involved in the regulation of morphological plastic changes of tanycytes (Prevot, 2002; Prevot et al., 2007). For instance, estradiol increases the expression of transforming growth factor α in hypothalamic astrocytes in vitro (Galbiati et al., 2002). Furthermore, during the period encompassing the preovulatory surge of gonadotropins, there is an enhanced expression of transforming growth factor α on the hypothalamus, followed by an increase in the expression of prostaglandin E2 and transforming growth factor β (Ma et al., 1992). Transforming growth factor α released by astrocytes may act on tanycytes located in the arcuate nucleus and the median eminence. Vincent Prevot and his collaborators in the laboratory of Sergio Ojeda have shown that tanycytes in primary cultures respond to transforming growth factor α via the activation of erbB-1 receptor, by releasing prostaglandin E2. Neuregulins also induce the release of prostaglandin E2 by astrocytes, acting on erbB-4 receptors (Prevot,

2002; Prevot et al., 2007). In turn, prostaglandin E2 induces the release of transforming growth factor β1 by tanycytes. Prostaglandin E2, and transforming growth factors α and β1 regulate the morphology of tanycytes. Prevot and his collaborators have shown that prostaglandin E2 causes acute cytoplasmic retraction in cultured tanycytes. In addition, cultured tanycytes respond to transforming growth factors α and β1 with opposite morphological plastic changes. Transforming growth factor β1 induces the retraction of tanycytic processes, while short exposure to transforming growth factor α increases the outgrowth of tanycytic processes and migration of tanycytes, which showed remarkable changes in motility, extending and retracting filopodia as they migrate outwardly from their initial site of seeding. However, prolonged exposure to transforming growth factor α, for more than 12 hours, results in the retraction of tanycytic processes, an effect mediated by transforming growth factor β1 (Prevot et al., 2003). Indeed, an antibody against transforming growth factor β1 blocks the cellular retraction of tanycytes induced by a long exposure to transforming growth factor α. Thus, transforming growth factor α induces first the cellular extension of tanycytes and the release of prostaglandin E2. Then, prostaglandin E2 induces the release of transforming growth factor β1, and this factor finally induces the cellular retraction of tanycytes. Therefore, transforming growth factor α may regulate the extension and retraction of tanycytic processes, by direct actions and by actions mediated by transforming growth factor β1, respectively, imitating the reversible morphological changes that occur in these cells during the estrus cycle (Fig. 2.6).

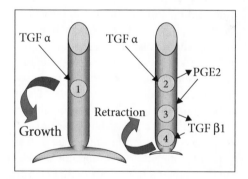

Figure 2.6. Transforming growth factor α (TGFα) regulates the extension and retraction of tanycytic processes in the median eminence in association with the release of gonadotropin-releasing hormone. TGFα first induces the cellular extension of tanycytes and the release of prostaglandin E2 (PGE2). Then, PGE2 induces the release of transforming growth factor β1 (TGFβ1); this factor finally induces the cellular retraction of tanycytes. TGFα released by astrocytes acts on tanycytes (1) and induces the growth of tanycytic processes. Tanycytes also respond to TGFα (2) by releasing PGE2. In turn, PGE2 induces the release of TGFβ1 by tanycytes (3). Then, TGFβ1 induces the retraction of tanycytic processes (4). (Based on Prevot, 2002; Prevot et al., 2003, 2007).

As for the synaptic changes in magnocellular neurons, PSA-N-CAM may also be involved in the plastic changes on tanycytes and GnRH terminals, since PSA-N-CAM immunoreactivity increases in the median eminence in the proestrus phase of the cycle compared to the diestrus phase (Kaur et al., 2002; Parkash and Kaur, 2005, 2007). In addition, Sergio Ojeda and his collaborators (Mungenast and Ojeda, 2005; Ojeda et al., 2006) have identified several additional adhesion molecules that may participate in neuroglia interactions in the median eminence. By using DNA microarrays to analyze genes expressed in the hypothalamus of the female rhesus monkey at different phases of pubertal development, Ojeda and his collaborators have identified three families of adhesion molecules, which may participate in the regulation of cell-to-cell adhesion and, at the same time, interact with intracellular signaling. These molecules, which include components of the contactin-dependent neuronal–glial adhesiveness complex, may regulate the remodeling of tanycytes and the associated GnRH terminals in the median eminence. In addition, using quantitative proteomics, Ojeda and his collaborators have identified SynCAM, an immunoglobulin-like adhesion molecule required for synapse formation, as another important molecule involved in the communication of glial cells and GnRH neurons (Ojeda et al., 2006). SynCAM expression is decreased in DNerbB4 mice, which have delayed puberty. SynCAM molecules in the membranes of glial cells may establish homophilic interactions with other SynCAM molecules expressed by adjacent neurons. In contrast, contactin expressed by GnRH neurons and axons may establish heterophilic interactions with the short form of the receptor protein for tyrosine phosphatase β located in glial membranes. This receptor activates intracellular signaling, and transmits to glial cells contact information after the interaction with contactin.

Other molecules that regulate cell-to-cell interactions may also be involved in the plastic changes in the median eminence during the estrus cycle. For instance, the activity of Zn^{2+} metalloproteinases varies in the median eminence during the estrus cycle, showing high levels of activity in proestrus, when cellular processes of tanycytes retract and GnRH terminals are in contact with portal capillaries (Estrella et al., 2004). Zn^{2+} metalloproteinases may be involved in the interactions of GnRH terminals and tanycytic processes since the blockade of metalloproteinase activity abolishes the effect of transforming growth factor β1 on tanycytes (Prevot et al., 2003). Endothelial cells may also express molecules that regulate its interactions with GnRH terminals. For example, endothelial cells may play a role in the regulation of neuroglia plasticity in the median eminence by the release of Sema3A, a chemotrophic factor that binds its cognate receptor (neuropilin-1) expressed in GnRH nerve terminals, and that may regulate GnRH axon sprouting and/or collapse during the estrus cycle (Campagne et al., 2006). Thus, it seems that endothelial cells may play a role in the regulation of neuroglia plasticity in the median eminence by the release of Sema3A and the induction of the sprouting of GnRH terminals.

Further studies by Prevot and his collaborators at INSERM in Lille (Prevot et al., 2007) have shown that endothelial cells participate in the plastic

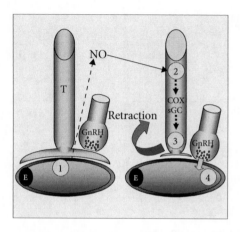

Figure 2.7. Endothelial cells (E) may also play a critical role in regulating the extension and retraction of tanycytic processes in the median eminence in association with the release of gonadotropin-releasing hormone (GnRH). Endothelial cells of the median eminence use nitric oxide (NO) to promote cytoarchitectural changes in tanycytes (T). The stimulatory effect of NO on tanycyte plasticity involves the participation of soluble guanylyl cyclase (sGC) and cyclooxigenase (COX) activities. NO released by endothelial cells (1) acts on tanycytes (2), causes retraction of tanycytic processes (3), which enables GnRH nerve terminals to directly contact the pericapillary space (4). (Courtesy of Dr. Vincent Prevot. Based on De Seranno et al., 2004; Prevot et al., 2007).

morphological modifications of tanycytes by releasing nitric oxide (Figs. 2.7 and 2.8). Using co-cultures of endothelial cells from the median eminence and tanycytes in a culture system in which both cell types are not in direct contact but share the culture medium, Prevot and his colleagues have found that endothelial cells induce rapid morphological modifications of tanycytes. This effect is mediated by the release of nitric oxide by endothelial cells. Interestingly, estradiol causes a rapid retraction of tanycytic processes in co-cultures of tanycytes and endothelial cells from the median eminence, and the inhibition of nitric oxide with L-NAME blocks the effect of estradiol (De Serrano et al., 2004). Interestingly, Prevot and his colleagues have also shown that the administration of L-NAME in the median eminence in vivo blocks estrus cyclicity. Further studies have revealed that estrogen-mediated acute cellular retraction of tanycytes in co-cultures with endothelial cells from the median eminence requires eNOS activity, and that eNOS expression is increased by estradiol. In addition, estradiol increases the sensitivity of tanycytes to nitric oxide, an effect that is probably mediated by an increased expression of Cox-1 and Cox-2 in tanycytes in response to the hormone (De Serrano et al., 2005).

The genomic and proteomic analyses carried out by Sergio Ojeda and collaborators have identified several other genes that may potentially be involved

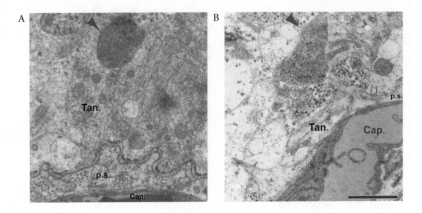

Figure 2.8. Activation of endogenous NO secretion in the media eminence induces structural changes, allowing gonadotropin-releasing hormone (GnRH) nerve terminals to form direct neurovascular junctions. Representative electron micrograph of GnRH-immunoreactive terminals (large arrowhead, green) in the external zone of the median eminence in close proximity of the fenestrated capillaries (Cap, red) of the portal vasculature in absence (A) or presence (B) of L-arginine, the precursor of NO. (A) Under basal unstimulated conditions, GnRH nerve terminals (labeled with 15 nm gold particles) are entirely embedded in tanycytic end feet (Tan, yellow), which prevent them from contacting the pericapillary space (p.s., pink) delineated by the parenchymatous basal lamina (white arrow). (B) GnRH nerve terminals forming neurovascular junctions (i.e., directly contacting the pericapillary space; white arrow) in median eminence explants after incubation for 30 minutes with L-arginine. Very few tanycytic processes (yellow) remain around GnRH nerve endings that have direct access to the pericapillary space (black arrows), suggesting that tanycytic end feet underwent retraction. Scale bar: 0.5 μm. (Courtesy of Dr. Vincent Prevot. Based on De Seranno et al., 2004)

in the initiation of the structural and functional remodeling of the median eminence and GnRH neurons at puberty and during estrus cyclicity. Some of these genes may act as master genes or upper-echelon genes, which coordinate the expression of a network of other regulatory genes and maintain the hierarchical structure of the network. Among the candidates to function as upper-echelon genes, the laboratory of Sergio Ojeda has identified Oct-2, thyroid transcription factor-1 (TTF-1), and enhanced at puberty-1 (EAP-1). Oct-2 is a transcriptional regulator of the POU-domain family of homeobox-containing genes, which may regulate transforming growth factor α and SynCAM transcription. The expression of Oct-2 increases in the hypothalamus during juvenile development, and the blockade of Oct-2 synthesis delays the age at first ovulation. In contrast, sexual precocity is associated with an increased hypothalamic expression of Oct-2 (Ojeda et al., 1999, 2006). TTF-1, the second candidate for upper-echelon gene, is, as Oct-2, a homeobox gene. TTF-1 enhances the transcriptional activity of genes required for the facilitatory control of puberty, such as GnRH, erbB2, and KiSS1, and suppresses the expression of genes inhibitory to the pubertal process, such as the preproenkephalin gene. TTF-1 is expressed by GnRH neurons and tanycytes, and its expression increases at puberty in the hypothalamus. TTF-1 disruption is associated with delayed puberty, disruption of initial estrus cyclicity, and decreased reproductive capacity (Ojeda et al., 2006). The third candidate, EAP-1, encodes a nuclear protein expressed in GnRH neurons and in neuronal subpopulations involved in the control of GnRH release, such as glutamatergic, GABAergic, proenkephalinergic, and KiSS1 neurons. Hypothalamic EAP-1 mRNA levels increase in both monkeys and rats during female puberty. As with TTF-1, EAP-1 enhances the transcriptional activity of genes that facilitate the initiation of puberty and suppresses the expression of genes that inhibit the pubertal process and its knocking down in the hypothalamus delays puberty and disrupts estrus cyclicity (Heger et al., 2007; Ojeda et al., 2006). Acting as upperechelon genes, Oct-2, TTF-1, and EAP-1 may potentially coordinate the plastic functional and structural neuroglial reorganization of the median eminence and the hypothalamus, including the reorganization of synaptic connectivity in the arcuate nucleus, associated with GnRH release.

BRAIN PLASTICITY AND THE CONTROL OF HORMONAL HOMEODYNAMICS: A RECAPITULATION

The literature reviewed in this chapter indicates that neuroglial and synaptic remodeling may participate in the regulation of hormonal release by magnocellular and parvocellular hypothalamic neurons. Glial plastic remodeling may have different consequences for the activity of neurosecretory cells by affecting the release or availability of different factors involved in synaptic function and synaptic plasticity, by modulating neuronal membrane properties and ion channels, or by regulating in an active or permissive manner the number of excitatory and inhibitory synaptic inputs. As we have seen, this regulation may occur at different levels. Synaptic and glial remodeling may involve neurons participating in the circuits controlling the afferents to neurosecretory neurons, having an indirect effect on the activity of neurosecretory neurons. Neuroglia remodeling may also be directly associated with neurosecretory neurons, controlling their activity by the regulation of the number of synaptic inputs on their somas and dendrites. Finally, an important site for the regulation of hormonal release is the axon terminal of neurosecretory neurons. There, in the median eminence for parvocellular neurons and in the neurohypophysis for magnocellular neurons, morphological reorganization of glial cells coordinated to modifications in axonal retraction and extension are coupled to the release of different factors by glia, and may play an essential role in the regulation of hormonal release.

Chapter 3

Hormonal Influences on Brain Plasticity: I. Melatonin, Thyroid Hormones, and Corticosteroids

INTRODUCTION: A LARGE VARIETY OF HORMONES REGULATE
BRAIN PLASTICITY

In the previous chapter, I have examined examples of how brain plasticity is involved in the regulation of hormonal secretions. We have seen that brain plastic changes participate in the control of body homeodynamics by safeguarding an adequate hormonal equilibrium. In turn, as has already been mentioned in the previous two chapters, hormones contribute to the regulation of brain plasticity, regulating neuronal and glial activity, and promoting the remodeling of several neural structures. This is part of the mechanisms by which hormones contribute to homeodynamic regulation, acting on different body organs, including the brain, spinal cord, and peripheral nervous system. Thus, brain plasticity regulates the activity of endocrine glands, which in turn relays feedback to the brain, at least in part via hormonal signals. This cross talk is in a continuous adjustment during a person's lifespan (see Fig. 1.2) and integrates the information originating from multiple endocrine glands and multiple brain regions. Here, and in the next two chapters, I will focus my scrutiny on the endocrine feedback to the central nervous system and will consider the hormonal signals that have been identified as modulators of neuronal and glial plasticity.

Hormones regulate the expression or activity of ion channels, neurotransmitter receptors, cytoskeletal proteins, adhesion molecules, growth factors, neuromodulators, neurotransmitters, and an additional variety of molecules participating in neural function in the central nervous system. Consequently, hormones affect neural and glial metabolic activity, glial and neuronal proliferation, cellular morphology, intercellular communication, neuronal firing, blood flow, and many other aspects of nerve cell biology in the brain and spinal cord. In many cases, as a result of these hormonal actions, neural tissue suffers a considerable morphological and functional transformation. The hormonally regulated plastic changes in the adult central nervous system may include modifications in microvascular density, glial and neuronal density, the pattern of extension and ramification of neuronal and glial processes, the pattern of neuronal connectivity, the rate of neurogenesis and gliogenesis, and functional plasticity of synapses. These modifications have many functional outcomes for neuronal activity that, in turn, determine new adjustments for the neural control of the internal milieu and the interactions of the individual with the external environment. Hormonally regulated brain remodeling, therefore, results in new patterns of hormonal release and in the initiation of new programs for the execution of specific behaviors. Hormonal effects on neural plasticity also have a considerable impact on emotions, motivations, learning, memory, and cognition.

For certain aspects, we have considerable information on how hormones modulate the endogenous functional and morphological plastic capacity of the central nervous system. Indeed, for some hormones and for some regions of the central nervous system we have a notable picture of the mechanisms of hormonal-induced plasticity, and we know that hormones may act as permissive or modulatory factors for neural mutability. However, our information is also very limited in many other aspects. To begin with, not all hormones have been examined in relation to their possible effects on neuronal plasticity. For a minor number of hormones, such as sex steroids (see Chapter 4), we have considerable information on their plastic effects in the brain and spinal cord; for some hormones, we have a relatively less number of studies showing their capacity to regulate functional and morphological plastic changes in a small selection of brain regions; and for a considerable number of hormones, our information on their possible neuroplastic activity is nonexistent. Therefore, today we cannot have a detailed picture on the impact of endocrine signals on neural remodeling. On the other hand, only a few brain regions have been examined as potential targets for hormonal plastic actions. The hippocampus is one of the brain regions that have been studied with more detail in this regard, given its implication in cognition and its relatively well-known anatomy and physiology. Other brain regions have been selected for their implications of hormonal effects on behavior, emotions, neuroendocrine regulation, reproduction, feeding, energy balance, or motor control. However, many regions of the brain and the spinal cord remain unexplored as targets for plastic actions of hormones. In spite of this fact, we know that hormonal actions converge and diverge within the brain to coordinate brain plasticity (Fig. 3.1). Thus, multiple hormones may regulate a single plastic event in a particular brain region, while a single hormone may target multiple plastic events in multiple brain regions. In the next sections of this chapter and the following chapters of this book we will see numerous examples of the integration of convergent and divergent regulatory actions of hormones on brain plasticity for the control of homeodynamics. In addition, this convergent and divergent regulation of brain plasticity by hormones over time results in a coordinated regulation of metaplasticity in different brain regions.

The neurological consequences of pathological alterations in hormonal levels are an important source of information on how endocrine secretions, acting directly or indirectly, may affect the function and plasticity of the central and peripheral nervous system. Transient pathological deficits in the levels

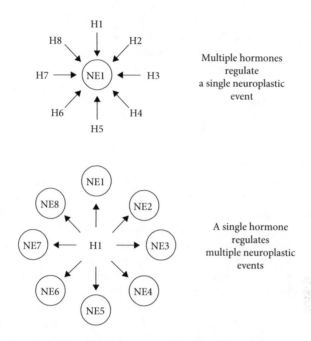

Figure 3.1. Convergent and divergent regulation of brain plasticity by endocrine signals. The action of multiple hormones (H1–H8) may converge in a particular region of the brain to regulate a single neuroplastic event (NE1). In turn, a single hormone (H1) may regulate a variety of neuroplastic events (NE1–NE8) in a single region or in multiple regions of the brain. The integration of the convergent and divergent hormonal actions over time allows for the coordination of metaplasticity between brain regions.

of some hormones are accompanied by transient modifications or impairments in brain function and neural plasticity. In extreme conditions, chronic pathological modifications in endocrine secretions may represent a risk factor for the development of neurodegenerative diseases, such as Alzheimer's and Parkinson's diseases (see Chapter 9). The neurological effects of some hormonal deficiencies are well known and have been studied for a long time. For instance, we know that the deficiency in the function of thyroid glands during development causes important neurological impairments and cognitive deficits. There is also substantial evidence of pathological neural alterations as a consequence of thyroid hormone alterations in adult life. Indeed, we know that pathological deficits in the levels of thyroid hormone in adults have an important impact on neural function and may result in cognitive deficits and depressive symptoms. We are now just starting to understand the cellular and molecular basis for the neurological consequences of these hormonal deficits. For instance, we know now that the effects of hypothyroidism in adult life include an impairment of hippocampal neurogenesis and hippocampal morphological and functional synaptic plasticity.

Another good example of how pathological alterations in hormonal secretion and signaling may affect neural function and plasticity is diabetes. Insulin deficiency or decreased responsiveness to insulin results in degenerative alterations in the peripheral and central nervous system. Neurodegenerative alterations in the retina are common in diabetes and are associated with a remodeling of dendrites. Diabetes may also impact brain cognitive regions, such as the hippocampus, causing impairments in memory, attention, and cognitive skills. Remodeling of dendrites and synapses, alterations in functional synaptic plasticity, and impairment of adult neurogenesis in the hippocampus may all be involved in the cognitive effects of diabetes. In addition, diabetes results in plastic remodeling in other central nervous system structures, including the hypothalamus and the spinal cord. Insulin therapy reverses some of the effects of diabetes in the nervous system and insulin is also able to modulate synaptic plasticity in nondiabetic animals.

Growth hormone is also an important regulator of brain plasticity by direct effects in the brain or by modulating the plasmatic and brain levels of insulin-like growth factor (IGF-I).

Deficits in growth hormone with aging are associated with cognitive decline, and growth hormone and/or IGF-I enhance cognition and modulate functional synaptic plasticity, regulate dendritic morphology, increase adult neurogenesis, and promote remodeling of brain microvasculature. IGF-I may mediate effects of physical exercise on brain remodeling and may interact with estradiol in the regulation of hypothalamic plasticity associated with the estrus cycle.

Another hormone that may induce remodeling of brain microvasculature, regulate dendritic plasticity, and promote adult neurogenesis is erythropoietin. This hormone enhances red blood cell production when oxygen levels are low, and recent studies have shown that it protects the brain and spinal cord from ischemia and other pathologies. Hormones regulating food intake and energy balance, such as leptin and ghrelin, in part exert their actions by promoting mutability and functional synaptic plasticity in the circuits controlling feeding. In addition, these hormones have an impact on cognition and promote plasticity in brain cognitive areas, such as the hippocampus.

Brain plasticity is also associated with circadian and seasonal rhythms and to specific life cycle conditions. Melatonin is an important modulator of circadian rhythms that may have an impact on circadian and seasonal neural plasticity. Other hormones, such as prolactin and sex steroids, may regulate brain plasticity in relation with different reproductive and life cycles. Glucocorticoids and gonadal hormones are potent modulators of synaptic plasticity. For these hormones, we have a much better knowledge of the behavioral correlates of their neural plastic effects than for other endocrine secretions. In addition, their cellular and molecular mechanisms of action have been also studied with more detail. Stress and glucocorticoids play an important role in the association of emotions with memory consolidation and produce severe modifications in the structure and function of adult neuronal networks in several limbic and cortical regions. Acute activation of physiological stress produces transient synaptic plastic modifications and facilitates learning and memory. In contrast, chronic stress and chronic high glucocorticoid levels cause permanent synaptic alterations, dendritic and synaptic remodeling, and decreased adult neurogenesis. These effects of chronic stress and glucocorticoids may result in impaired neural function and memory disturbances.

Sex hormones regulate synaptic plasticity in many regions of the brain and spinal cord, affecting dendritic morphology, number of dendritic spines, number of synapses, extension of glial processes, adult neurogenesis, and different forms of functional synaptic plasticity. Compared to other hormones analyzed in this chapter and in Chapter 5, we understand better the plastic effects and mechanisms of action of sex hormones because more studies have been devoted to their analysis and in a larger variety of anatomical localizations within the central nervous system. Therefore, the analysis will be in some aspects more detailed for sex hormones than for other hormones. However, this longer extension does not imply that sex hormones have necessarily a stronger impact on brain plasticity than other hormones. Certainly, sex hormones have an impressive capacity to induce the remodeling of neurons and glial cells in a large variety of central nervous system structures and during different phases of the life cycle. However, we ignore whether other hormones exert similar extensive plastic actions. My personal opinion is that we still have too many aspects to discover on the actions of a variety of hormones on brain plasticity. Indeed, Chapter 5 presents evidence indicating that hormones that have so far received relatively poor attention for their neural plastic effects, such as gonadotropin-releasing hormone, insulin, growth hormone, IGF-I, leptin and ghrelin, are in fact powerful modulators of brain remodeling.

In this chapter I will analyze the impact on brain plasticity of three non-peptide hormones: melatonin, thyroid hormones, and glucocorticoids. The next chapter will be completely devoted to sex hormones. Then, in Chapter 5, I will consider the role of several peptide hormones on brain remodeling.

HORMONES OR PARACRINE FACTORS?

Before starting our analysis on hormonal regulation of brain plasticity, there is an important aspect that we need to consider: the duality of several molecules as hormones and local factors. We will see in the following pages that several hormones affecting brain plasticity are also locally produced in the central nervous system, acting as local paracrine or autocrine factors. Examples include peptide hormones, such as oxytocin, corticotropin-releasing factor, prolactin, insulin, IGF-I, growth hormone, and erythropoietin. For some of these molecules, the balance between their hormonal and local effects varies with development and with physiological conditions. For instance, during early embryonic and postnatal development, local production of IGF-I by neurons and glial cells is probably the main source of the molecule for neural tissue. In contrast, the expression of IGF-I is dramatically reduced in the central nervous system in adults (Andersson et al., 1988; Garcia-Segura et al., 1991b ; Rotwein et al., 1988), with the exception of the hypothalamus and the median eminence where IGF-I levels increase with puberty (Dueñas et al., 1994; Garcia-Segura et al., 1996; Miller and Gore, 2001). Therefore, in adult life, IGF-I acting in the brain may predominantly be hormonal IGF-I that cross the blood–brain barrier (Carro et al., 2000, 2001; Torres-Aleman, 1999; Trejo et al., 2001).

A similar situation occurs for steroid hormones that are also locally produced by the nervous system, including estradiol and progesterone. For instance, local production of estradiol by the embryonic mouse neocortex stimulates progenitor cell division in the ventricular and subventricular zones (Martinez-Cerdeno et al., 2006), and local production of estradiol and progesterone by Purkinje cells in the cerebellum of postnatal rodents contributes to the development of its dendritic arbor, the growth of dendritic spines, and the formation of synaptic contacts (Tsutsui, 2006; Tsutsui et al., 2004). In Purkinje cells, progesterone is synthesized from pregnenolone, which in turn is synthesized from cholesterol. Therefore, we should assume that pure paracrine or autocrine actions are responsible for the developmental actions of progesterone on Purkinje cells. Testosterone, the precursor of estradiol, may also be locally produced from cholesterol metabolism in the cerebral cortex and cerebellum of rodents and other vertebrates. Thus, the action of estradiol in these systems may also represent a paracrine or autocrine effect. Local production of estradiol by the neural tissue may also affect brain plasticity in adult life. In addition, estradiol acting as a hormonal signal may regulate plasticity in different brain regions. On the other hand, there are many evidences indicating that local conversion to estradiol and dihydrotestosterone is involved in the neuroplastic actions of testosterone in several regions of the rodent brain and spinal cord. Local production of active metabolites is also essential for the neuroplastic effects of thyroid hormones. Finally, some peptide hormones may affect brain plasticity by modulating the rate of steroid synthesis in the brain. For instance, gonadotropin-releasing hormone may regulate synaptic plasticity in the hippocampus by the modulation of local estradiol synthesis (see Chapter 5). Although autocrine, paracrine, and hormonal actions are not always easy to delineate, in this and the following chapters we will mainly focus our analysis to the hormonal regulation of brain plasticity, either direct or mediated by hormone metabolites.

MELATONIN

Animal behavior and most internal physiological processes in the body are adapted to light/dark daily cycles, as well as to the seasonal modifications in the duration of the light and dark periods (see also Chapter 8). In vertebrates, a specialized endocrine organ, the pineal gland, adjusts biological rhythms

to changes in environmental lighting by the secretion of the hormone melatonin. Melatonin secretion is regulated by information provided by the master clock located in the suprachiasmatic nucleus of the hypothalamus, which
receives direct information from the retina (Chang and Reppert, 2001). The
suprachiasmatic nucleus expresses several clock genes that play a key role in
the generation of circadian rhythms. Both clock gene expression and neuronal
activity show circadian rhythms with different phases among different genes
and different neuronal subpopulations (Schaap et al., 2001, 2003). This complex multioscillator system controls the rhythmic daily secretion of hormones
by several mechanisms. Neurons in this nucleus directly project to hypothalamic neurosecretory neurons to control their activity. In addition, suprachiasmatic neurons set the phase of clock genes expressed by neurosecretory
cells (Kriegsfeld and Silver, 2006). Furthermore, the suprachiasmatic nucleus
controls body rhythms via the parasympathetic and sympathetic autonomous
nervous system. Via the sympathetic system and the superior cervical ganglia,
the suprachiasmatic nucleus controls the release of melatonin by the pineal
gland. Melatonin, in turn, may modulate synaptic plasticity in the suprachiasmatic nucleus, affecting long-term synaptic potentiation. Long-term potentiation of synaptic transmission can be induced in suprachiasmatic neurons by
high-frequency stimulation of the optic nerve. Interestingly, Kohji Fukunaga
and colleagues have found a potent inhibitory effect of melatonin on this form
of long-term potentiation. Treatment with melatonin totally prevents long-
term potentiation in the suprachiasmatic nucleus of rats without changing
basal synaptic transmission. The inhibitory effect of melatonin on synaptic
plasticity appears to be mediated by a decrease in Ca^{2+}/calmodulin-dependent
protein kinase II autophosphorylation (Fukunaga et al., 2002).

Melatonin may also be implicated in brain plastic changes associated with
annual reproductive cycles in vertebrates. The most dramatic of these changes
reported so far are those occurring in several telencephalic nuclei involved
in song learning and song production in songbirds. These nuclei show seasonal plasticity in coincidence with seasonal peaks in reproductive activity
(see Chapter 8). These reversible plastic modifications include changes in the
number and volume of cells in the song nuclei, which are associated with
modifications in the total volume of the nuclei. Seasonal increases in gonadal
hormones, in particular testosterone and its metabolites, which promote the
increase in the volume of song nuclei, are the main cause of these plastic modifications. In addition, other factors may also affect the volume changes of
song nuclei. One of these factors is melatonin, which has been shown to be
involved in this plastic remodeling of the song system and to exert an opposite
effect of testosterone in the regulation of nuclear volume. As a consequence
of the circadian fluctuations in melatonin, with high levels during the dark
phase and low levels during the light phase, the levels of the hormone also
vary in plasma during seasons. Short days of fall and winter are associated
with longer durations of high melatonin levels, while long days of spring and
summer are associated with shorter durations of high melatonin secretion.

In addition, song nuclei showing seasonal plasticity, such as the telencephalic high vocal center (HVC), the lateral magnocellular nucleus of the anterior nidopallium, the area X, and the nucleus robustus, express melatonin receptors. George E. Bentley and colleagues assessed the role of melatonin in seasonal brain plasticity of European starlings. The songbirds were castrated to remove the influence of gonadal hormones and were exposed to different photoperiods. As expected, changes in photoperiod caused volumetric changes in the HVC. Long days were associated with an increase in the volume of the HVC, and melatonin administration attenuated this effect (Bentley et al., 1999). These findings strongly suggest that melatonin is involved, by direct or indirect mechanisms, in the seasonal remodeling of the brain song system in songbirds.

Melatonin and circadian rhythms may also influence synaptic plasticity in cognitive brain regions. There is evidence that an endogenous circadian oscillator modulates functional synaptic plasticity in the hippocampus of mice (Chaudhury et al., 2005). In addition, hippocampal synaptic plasticity is affected by melatonin. Mice hippocampal pyramidal neurons exposed to melatonin change their excitability in response to repetitive stimulation (El-Sherif et al., 2003), and melatonin perfusion of rat hippocampal slices prevents the induction of tetanically induced long-term potentiation of synaptic transmission recorded in the CA1 dendritic layer (Collins and Davies, 1997). The effect of melatonin on synaptic plasticity in the hippocampus is selective for some specific circuits. Thus, in mouse hippocampus brain slices, melatonin inhibits long-term synaptic potentiation in the Schaffer collateral-CA1 pathway but has a minor effect on synaptic plasticity in the mossy fiber–CA3 synapses (Ozcan et al., 2006). The regulatory actions of melatonin on hippocampal synaptic plasticity appear to be mediated by melatonin receptors, in particular by the subtype MT(2), since mice lacking melatonin MT(2) receptors show impaired memory and altered hippocampal long-term synaptic potentiation induced by theta burst stimulation (Larson et al., 2006). A role for melatonin MT(2) receptors in the hormonal effects on hippocampal synaptic plasticity is also suggested by the studies of Wang et al. (2005), showing that the application of melatonin to mice hippocampal slices produced a concentration-dependent inhibition of the induction of long-term potentiation, measured by stimulating the Schaffer collaterals and recording the field excitatory postsynaptic potential from the CA1 dendritic layer. In this study, the inhibitory actions of melatonin were prevented by the application of the melatonin MT(2) receptor subtype antagonist 4-phenyl-2-propionamidotetraline or by forskolin, an activator of adenylyl cyclase, suggesting that melatonin may decrease synaptic plasticity in the hippocampus via a mechanism involving melatonin MT(2) receptors and the adenylyl cyclase–protein kinase A pathway. Melatonin may also affect functional synaptic plasticity in the neocortex. Intraperitoneal administration of melatonin in rats has been shown to prevent the induction of long-term potentiation in the visual cortex, determined in anesthetized rats by potentiating transcallosal evoked responses with a tetanizing train.

In parallel, intraperitoneal administration of melatonin impairs visuospatial performance (Soto-Moyano et al., 2006).

THYROID HORMONES

The central nervous system is a well-characterized target of thyroid hormones. As in other tissues, local metabolism of thyroid hormones in the brain plays an important role in their actions. Thyroxine (T_4) is metabolized in the brain to triiodothyronine (T_3) by the type II iodothyronine deiodinase enzyme, which is expressed in glial cells. T_3 modulates the activity of thyroid hormone receptors on target glial cells and neurons, affecting neuronal and glial development. In contrast, the type III iodothyronine deiodinase enzyme inactivates T_4 and T_3 by removing an iodine molecule, transforming T_4 into 3,3',5'-triiodothyronine and T_3 into 3,3'-diiodothyronine.

For many years it has been known that thyroid hormone deficiency during critical periods of brain development causes strong cognitive alterations. Thyroid hormones (thyroxine or T_4; triiodothyronine or T_3) play an important role in neuronal and glial proliferation, migration, and maturation in the developing brain (see Chapter 6). Hypothyroidism during fetal or early postnatal development may result in permanent alterations of neural function, including permanent modifications in synaptic plasticity during adult life. More recently, several laboratories have assessed the effects of adult-onset thyroid hormone deficiency for brain function and plasticity. Insufficiency of thyroid hormones in adulthood causes alterations in learning and memory, psychological changes, and mood disorders (see Chapter 9).

Hypothyroidism during adult life affects synaptic plasticity. Adult-onset hypothyroidism has been reported to alter long-term synaptic potentiation and other forms of synaptic plasticity. For instance, adult-onset hypothyroidism partially blocks early long-term synaptic potentiation in the CA1 region of the hippocampus. Furthermore, the combination of adult-onset hypothyroidism with stress eliminates early long-term synaptic potentiation in this brain region (Gerges et al., 2001). In contrast, 6 weeks of thyroxin replacement therapy fully restored long-term synaptic potentiation impaired by hypothyroidism (Alzoubi et al., 2005). Adult-onset hypothyroidism also impairs posttetanic potentiation and long-term synaptic potentiation in the superior cervical sympathetic ganglion induced by brief high-frequency stimulation of the preganglionic nerve. However, adult-onset hypothyroidism does not affect basal synaptic transmission in the superior cervical sympathetic ganglion (Alzoubi et al., 2004). Similar results have been reported in the dorsal hippocampo-medial prefrontal cortex pathway of male rats, where 4 weeks of hypothyroidism did not affect basal synaptic transmission but significantly reduced paired-pulse facilitation and long-term synaptic potentiation (Sui et al., 2006). These functional synaptic changes may be at least in part related to morphological modifications in the number of synapses, since Antonio Ruiz-Marcos, Gabriela Morreale de Escobar, and their collaborators have reported that adult-onset hypothyroidism results in a rapid decrease in the number of dendritic spines in layer V pyramidal neurons of the visual cerebral cortex. Interestingly, the morphological modification is reversible after thyroxine therapy (Ruiz-Marcos et al., 1982a,b; 1988). These findings suggest that thyroid hormones contribute to maintain the synaptic architecture of cortical neurons in adult life and indicate that changes in the plasma levels of thyroid hormones in adult life result in plastic modifications in cortical dendritic spines. Thyroid hormone levels in adulthood also regulate glial plasticity. For instance, hyperthyroidism enhances the number and length of cellular processes of oligodendrocytes, while hypothyroidism appears to delay oligodendrocyte differentiation in adult rats (Fernandez et al., 2004a).

Several laboratories have also assessed whether adult-onset hypothyroidism affects adult neurogenesis. Their findings indicate that periods of hypothyroidism in adult life may alter adult cell replacement. In the subventricular zone, thyroid hormones have been reported to affect proliferation and differentiation of neural stem cells and oligodendrocyte precursor cells in adult rats. One study reported that hypothyroidism increases and hyperthyroidism decreases cell proliferation in the subventricular zone (Fernandez et al., 2004a). In contrast, another study reported that hypothyroidism increases the number of cells that synthesize DNA in the subventricular zone but do not reenter the cell cycle, and reduces neural stem proliferation and migration (Lemkine et al., 2005). Lynette A. Desouza, Vidita A. Vaidya, and their collaborators at the Tata Institute of Fundamental Research in Mumbai, India, have reported that adult-onset hypothyroidism causes a significant decrease in the survival and neuronal differentiation of cells that incorporated the analog of thymidine 5-bromo-2-deoxyuridine (used in the detection of proliferating cells) in the subgranular zone of the dentate gyrus. The effect was abolished by euthyroid status. In contrast, they observed that adult-onset hyperthyroidism did not influence hippocampal neurogenesis. Desouza et al. interpreted the lack of effect of hyperthyroidism as an indication that the effects of thyroid hormone are optimally permissive for neurogenesis at euthyroid levels (Desouza et al., 2005). Similar results were obtained by Patrizia Ambrogini and her collaborators at the universities of Urbino and Genova, in Italy. They observed that hypothyroidism decreased the survival of newly generated neurons. In addition, neuronal differentiation of new neurons was delayed (Ambrogini et al., 2005). Furthermore, Ana Guadaño-Ferraz and her collaborators at the Instituto de Investigaciones Biomédicas in Madrid found that a short period of hypothyroidism in adult rats is able to cause a 30% reduction in the number of proliferating cells in the subgranular zone of the dentate gyrus and a decrease in the morphological maturation of new neurons. Chronic treatment of hypothyroid rats with thyroid hormones restores the number of proliferative cells and induced growth of their dendritic trees (Montero-Pedrazuela et al., 2006). These effects in neurogenesis were correlated with a reversible depressive-like disorder. All these findings suggest that thyroid hormones maintain an adequate level of neurogenesis in the adult hippocampus by pro-moting cellular proliferation, neuronal survival, and differentiation of newly generated neurons. The effect of thyroid hormones on hippocampal neuro-genesis may be related to hormonal effects on spatial learning, memory, and depressive behavior.

STRESS, CORTICOSTEROIDS, AND BRAIN PLASTICITY

Stress has two faces: acute and chronic. The response to acute stress is an essential adaptive mechanism, finely tuned by evolution, for immediate physi-ological reaction to quick adaptive changes in the external milieu. An example of an acute stress stimulus is the unexpected manifestation of a predator in the close environment. The acute stress response is initiated by the detection of the predator by the olfactory, visual, or other sensory systems. Thus, the brain plays a key role in the acute stress response, eliciting the activation of the adequate reactions, including those of the endocrine and autonomic nervous systems. The acute response to stress is associated with emotional experiences that will have an important impact in future brain responses, facilitating learning and memory consolidation. It involves a transient temporal modi-fication of the interaction between the nervous system and endocrine glands, and its finalization sets the system back to equilibrium. Chronic unpredictable stress, in contrast, represents a very different situation in which the interac-tion between the brain and endocrine glands may not reach an adaptive equi-librium. Social interactions (see Chapter 8) are a common source of chronic unpredictable stress in humans, but not the only one. Under chronic stress conditions, the brain may be unable to properly regulate and terminate stress hormone response, and the system may enter in a phase of nonadaptive, per-manent disequilibrium that may ultimately lead to cognitive and emotional impairments and other brain disturbances.

Although the concept of stress is highly popular and familiar to us today, it is a relatively modern one. It was developed by Hans Hugo Bruno Selye, who originally presented it under the name of "general adaptation syndrome" in a short but highly influential paper published in *Nature* in 1936. When he was still a second-year student at the University of Prague medical school, Selye started to develop his ideas on the existence of universal mechanisms to cope with the pressures of disease and injury. He observed similar symptoms in patients with a variety of diseases and considered that these symptoms reflected a nonspecific response of the body to the demands caused by the state of being ill. As an undergraduate student, he was not able to do much to develop his thoughts; however, he would come back to his ideas several years later, when he was doing experiments with rats at the McGill University in Montreal. In 1934, at the age of 28, he was trying to identify a new hormone by injecting ovarian extracts into rats. The rats developed a series of common symptoms after the injections, including an enlargement of the adrenal cor-tex; atrophy of the thymus, spleen, and lymph nodes; and deep bleeding ulcers in the lining of the stomach and duodenum. These symptoms could not be attributed to the known sex hormones, and he believed to be in the path of discovery of a new ovarian hormone. However, he soon realized that extracts from other organs, including the placenta, pituitary, kidney, and spleen, had the same effect. Finally, he observed the same responses when injecting an unspecific agent, formalin.

By then, it was obvious that he had failed to discover a new hormone and that the symptoms developed by the rats in response to the injections of tissue extracts were due to an apparently unspecific reaction. What was this unspecific reaction? It was at this moment when he connected his recent experimental observations with the symptoms of patients in the Prague hospital and began to reconsider his earlier ideas of a stereotyped syndrome of response to injury reflecting a nonspecific reaction of the body to damage of any kind. He published his ideas in 1936, in a paper entitled "A Syndrome Produced by Diverse Nocuous Agents" (Selye, 1936). In this paper, he introduced the concept of the general adaptation syndrome, the process by which the body copes with a variety of "noxious agents," what he later called *stress*. Selye described three stages of coping with stress. The first is characterized by a "general alarm reaction" or preparation for the response. It is the moment to quickly decide: fight or flight? The second stage is a phase of adaptation, when a resistance to the stress is built. A third stage appears when the duration of the stress is sufficiently long. Then the body eventually enters a stage of exhaustion that may contribute to the development of new diseases. During the next years, Selye was able to identify the hypothalamus–pituitary–adrenal system as being responsible for the stress response, providing a biological and scientific basis for the general adaptation syndrome.

Selye was influenced by Walter Bradford Cannon, who, as mentioned in Chapter 1, introduced the concept of homeostasis (Cannon, 1929). Cannon also coined the term "fight-or-flight response" to refer to the emergency response of an animal when strongly aroused, which has many similarities to the general alarm reaction of Selye. Another important influence was that of Claude Bernard, who introduced the concept of "internal milieu" (Bernard, 1878, 1879). Homeostasis is the process of maintaining the internal body environment or internal milieu in a steady state (see Chapter 1 for the differences between homeostasis and homeodynamics). The general alarm reaction defined by Selye is, in its acute form, a homeostatic response. The brain initiates this response and receives the feedback from the adrenal glands. During this process, the brain alters the secretion of stress hormones, and these hormones, in turn, exert severe modifications in the structure and function of neuronal networks in several limbic and cortical regions that are involved in the generation, maintenance, and termination of the stress response. In addition, these regions also play an important role in the association of emotions with memory consolidation.

Another important concept for understanding the mutual influence of brain plasticity and hormones, not only stress hormones, is the concept of allostasis (McEwen, 2002, 2008; McEwen and Wingfield, 2003). This concept was introduced by Peter Sterling and Joseph Eyer (Sterling and Eyer, 1988) to refer to the maintenance of stability through change. This means that many body systems have to change in response to and in prediction of the changing conditions of daily life to maintain stable body function (Schulkin, 2003; Sterling, 2004). These systems include the brain, the endocrine system, autonomic nervous system, and immune system. We may then consider brain plasticity as one of the allostatic responses that maintain stable body function. In this context, we may consider brain remodeling in response to acute actions of glucocorticoids as an example of allostatic response. Glucocorticoids exert a feedback action in the brain to restore physiological and behavioral homeodynamics after exposure to acute stress (de Kloet et al., 2005). However, chronic exposure to glucocorticoids may exceed the capacity of the plastic response of the brain to respond to allostatic demands. We will be then facing an example of what is called "allostatic load," which may result in the development of pathological alterations.

The action of corticosteroids in the brain is mediated by two different receptors: the type 1 or mineralocorticoid receptors, of high affinity, and the type 2 or glucocorticoid receptors, of lower affinity. Both receptor types are expressed in the limbic neuronal networks involved in the stress response. Stress and glucocorticoids generate plastic reorganization of these circuits, an effect that is linked to further modifications in neuroendocrine regulation. Acute activation of physiological stress systems produces a transient synaptic reorganization and facilitates learning and memory consolidation, and may be considered an allostatic response. In contrast, chronic exposure to stress or glucocorticoids induces permanent synaptic alterations that may be involved in the transition from normal vigilance responses to pathological anxiety and may finally result in neuronal atrophy and cell loss, impaired neural function, and memory disturbances. Furthermore, the long-term brain remodeling induced by chronic stress may trigger or exacerbate neuropsychiatric disorders, including schizophrenia, depression, and anxiety-related syndromes such as panic and posttraumatic stress disorder (see also Chapters 6 and 9). Glucocorticoid and mineralocorticoid receptors have opposite roles on the regulation of brain modifications induced by stress. While the sustained activation of glucocorticoid receptors may result in brain functional impairment, mineralocorticoid receptors appear to be neuroprotective. Mineralocorticoid receptors are important for the survival of hippocampal granule neurons in rodents, while the activation of glucocorticoid receptors in the absence of mineralocorticoid receptor activation may induce dendritic atrophy and impairments of synaptic plasticity (Sousa and Almeida, 2002; Sousa et al., 2008). Thus, mice over-expressing mineralocorticoid receptors in the forebrain show reduced neuronal death after transient cerebral global ischemia induced by bilateral common carotid artery occlusion. In addition, these animals have better spatial memory retention and reduced anxiety compared to normal mice (Lai et al., 2007).

One of the brain regions that are a target for corticosteroids is the hippocampal formation, and an important aspect of the hippocampal plasticity that is affected by these hormones is the generation of new granule neurons during adult life. Stress decreases adult hippocampal neurogenesis and the generation of new granule neurons (Darnaudery et al., 2006; Gould et al., 1992, 1997; Mirescu et al., 2004; Pham et al., 2003; Tanapat et al., 2001); glucocorticoids seem to be involved in this effect of stress. Indeed, adrenalectomy increases, while administration of corticosterone decreases, hippocampal neurogenesis (Mirescu and Gould, 2006). Once more, the effect of glucocorticoid receptors and mineralocorticoid receptors appear to be different, since the activation of mineralocorticoid receptors promotes the survival of newly generated granule neurons (Sousa and Almeida, 2002). The effect of glucocorticoids and stress on hippocampal neurogenesis has been observed in a variety of species, such as the mouse, rat, tree shrew, and marmoset; it has been detected after different modalities of stress paradigms; it is induced by both acute and chronic stress; and it occurs in both young and adult animals (Mirescu and Gould, 2006). Therefore, decreased hippocampal neurogenesis seems to be a generalized response to stress and glucocorticoids. Depending on the stress paradigm, the effect on neurogenesis may be transient or permanent. Transient changes on hippocampal neurogenesis may represent an adaptive response to stress and glucocorticoids, although we have not yet obtained a clear understanding of the significance of these changes. Permanent changes in neurogenesis may cause a reduction in the total number of granule neurons (Pham et al., 2003) and may impair hippocampal function. Furthermore, chronic glucocorticoid exposure may affect the adequate balance between addition and removal of new hippocampal neurons, which is essential for spatial learning (Dupret et al., 2007).

In addition to affecting the generation of new neurons, stress and glucocorticoids also cause plastic reorganization of synaptic circuits. Stress or glucocorticoid administration to rats causes the reorganization of dendrites in the medial prefrontal cortex, the hippocampus, and the amygdala. The amygdala is a key component in the neuronal network that coordinates stress responses: it integrates information from different brain regions involved in the hormonal, behavioral, and autonomic components of the stress response, and regulates the activity of these brain regions. The amygdala is involved in the effects of stress on emotions, affective states, and memory-related processes, and shows plastic synaptic changes associated with stress. Dendritic reorganization after repeated stress has been detected in the basolateral nucleus of the amygdala. Thus, 10 days of immobilization stress causes a permanent hypertrophy of dendritic trees in pyramidal-like and stellate neurons of this nucleus, resulting in an increase in the length and branching of dendrites (Vyas et al., 2002, 2004). Acute corticosterone treatment produces similar effects to chronic stress, inducing dendritic hypertrophy in the basolateral amygdala and heightened anxiety (Mitra and Sapolsky, 2008). The remodeling of dendrites in the amygdala may be related to the effects of chronic stress and chronic glucocorticoids on the control of fear and anxiety responses, and modifications in the volume of the basolateral amygdala in mice are associated with differences in fear conditioning and glucocorticoid responses to stress (Yang et al., 2008).

Repeated stress or repeated glucocorticoid administration also results in the remodeling of dendrites in the anterior cingulate and prelimbic cortical areas of the rat prefrontal cortex. The remodeling affects pyramidal neurons from cortical layers II/III and, in contrast to what has been observed in the amygdala, basically consists of a retraction of the apical dendritic tree (Cook and Wellman, 2004; Liston et al., 2006; Radley et al., 2004; Wellman, 2001). Apical dendritic length and spine density in apical dendrites are significantly reduced by stress in cortical neurons (Liston et al., 2006; Radley et al., 2005; Radley and Morrison, 2005). In addition, Radley and collaborators have provided evidence that repetitive stress may result in a failure of dendritic spines to mature and stabilize in the rat medial prefrontal cortex (Radley et al., 2008). The changes in dendritic structure in the prefrontal cortex are reversible after a period of absence of stress (Radley et al., 2005; Radley and Morrison, 2005). Reversible changes in synaptic plasticity in the medial prefrontal cortex may contribute to the adaptive homeodynamic response to stress. However, prolonged stress and prolonged imbalances in the corticosteroid environment may result in permanent alterations in synaptic plasticity and neuronal atrophy linked to cognitive impairments (Cerqueira et al., 2005, 2007).

Similar stress-associated dendritic remodeling has been observed in the rat hippocampus. Repeated stress or chronic administration of glucocorticoids results in remodeling of the dendritic arbor of CA3 pyramidal neurons. As in the medial prefrontal cortex, the remodeling is characterized by a decrease in the number of dendritic branches and the retraction of apical dendrites, which are the targets of mossy fiber projections (Magariños and McEwen, 1995; McKittrick et al., 2000; Sousa et al., 2000; Watanabe et al., 1992; Woolley et al., 1990b). Studies by electron microscopy have revealed that these dendritic changes after repeated stress are associated with a depletion of synaptic vesicles in mossy fiber synapses. This depletion of synaptic vesicles is accompanied by an increase in the area of the terminal occupied by mitochondrial profiles, changes that have been interpreted as reflecting an enhancement of the function of mossy fiber synapses (Magariños et al., 1997). In addition, repeated stress results in a decrease in the number of dendritic spines and axodendritic synapses on CA3 pyramidal neurons, although complex spines are unaffected (Magariños et al., 1997; Sandi et al., 2003; Sousa et al., 2000; Stewart et al., 2005). Chronic corticosterone treatment also reduces the number of CA3 synapses (Tata et al., 2006), while chronic restraint stress results in a significant increase in postsynaptic density surface area and postsynaptic density volume in axospinous synapses in CA1 stratum lacunosum-moleculare (Donohue et al., 2006).

Several mechanisms may mediate the effects of glucocorticoids on dendritic and synaptic remodeling in the cortex and hippocampus and may involve the participation of excitatory amino acids, changes in intracellular calcium levels, expression of neurotrophins, and cytoskeletal remodeling. For instance, stress is associated with an increase in glutamate neurotransmission in rodents, and a sustained exposure of neurons to glutamate may result in the sustained activation of extracellular regulated kinase (ERK) signaling. Interestingly, repeated stress induced a prominent increase in the phosphorylation of ERK1/2 in the apical dendrites of pyramidal neurons in the cortical areas showing dendritic remodeling (Kuipers et al., 2003; Trentani et al., 2002). The endocannabinoid system, which regulates glutamateric neurotransmission and short- and long-term synaptic plasticity in diverse brain regions, has been proposed to be an important mediator of the effect of stress on emotional responses (Viveros et al., 2007) and may mediate the effect of stress hormones on synaptic plasticity.

Another molecule that may play an important role in synaptic remodeling associated with stress is tissue plasminogen activator, a serine protease that appears to be involved in tissue remodeling, neuronal plasticity, and learning. Tissue plasminogen activator is present in brain structures involved in the stress response, including the hippocampus, the amygdala, and the hypothalamus. Tissue plasminogen activator is upregulated in the central and medial amygdala by acute restraint stress, and this is associated with neuronal remodeling and anxiety behavior. The inhibition of the activity of tissue plasminogen activator, or the disruption of its gene, inhibits synaptic remodeling and anxiety behavior in response to stress (Bennur et al., 2007; Matys et al., 2004; Pawlak et al., 2003). Disruptions of the tissue plasminogen activator gene, or of the plasminogen gene, also prevent the modifications in synaptic plasticity in the hippocampus induced by chronic stress (Pawlak et al., 2005).

The facilitation of synaptic remodeling by tissue plasminogen activator is probably caused, at least in part, by modifications in cell adhesion; other molecules may participate in this process. Neuronal cell adhesion molecules of the immunoglobulin superfamily regulate cell-to-cell interactions in the brain and are also important participants in the plastic brain remodeling associated with stress. Carmen Sandi's group has provided considerable and convincing evidence of the involvement of the neural cell adhesion molecule (N-CAM) in the plastic remodeling induced by stress in the brain. As mentioned in Chapter 2, N-CAM may be polysialylated. The polysialylated form of NCAM (PSA-N-CAM) may confer a reduced stability of cellular interactions, allowing synaptic remodeling and neuritic growth. High levels of PSA-N-CAM expression are observed in brain areas with a high degree of structural remodeling, such as the hippocampus, the olfactory bulb, or the hypothalamus. Brain lesions may induce the expression of PSA-N-CAM in what is considered an endogenous mechanism to facilitate repair or tissue remodeling after injury. Chronic stress also results in the induction of PSA-N-CAM expression in some brain areas, an effect that may be considered a response to compensate for the neural damage induced by the stress and that may participate in the remodeling of brain tissue after stress injury. Sandi and her colleagues have shown that PSA-N-CAM is necessary for the plastic synaptic events underlying the learning process (Venero et al., 2006), and N-CAM-knockout mice or mice deficient in polysialyltransferase-1, an enzyme which attaches PSA to N-CAM, show impaired long-term synaptic potentiation in the CA1 and CA3 hippocampal subregions (Sandi, 2004) and hippocampal-related learning and memory impairments (Markram et al., 2007). Repeated exposure to stress induces a long-lasting but transient increase in PSA-N-CAM expression in the dentate gyrus of the hippocampus (Sandi et al., 2001). Chronic stress has similar effects on PSA-N-CAM expression in the piriform cortex (Nacher et al., 2004). However, PSA-N-CAM expression is reduced in the amygdaloid complex after chronic restrain stress (Cordero et al., 2005). Thus, changes in PSA-N-CAM may be involved in the plastic dendritic remodeling regulated by stress and glucocorticoids. However, the precise role of glucocorticoids in the stress-induced changes in PSA-N-CAM is still unclear. Glucocorticoids may indeed regulate PSA-N-CAM expression in the brain; however, oral administration of corticosterone to rats for 21 days has the opposite effect of chronic restraint stress and results in a reduction in PSA-N-CAM-immunoreactive cells in the piriform cortex and dentate gyrus (Nacher et al., 2004).

An important consideration about the mechanisms of synaptic plasticity mediating the effects of stress and glucocorticoids is that the plastic changes present different characteristics depending on the brain region. As we have seen before, in the medial prefrontal cortex and the hippocampus, stress is associated with a retraction of apical dendrites in specific neuronal populations. In the amygdala, in contrast, stress increases the growth and branching of dendrites. This suggests that stress, other than affecting basic parameters of dendritic architecture and synaptic remodeling in an unspecific manner, induces a specific and selective functional modification of the different synaptic networks involved in the stress response. A similar conclusion may be reached when analyzing functional synaptic plasticity associated with stress. Indeed, the morphological remodeling of dendrites and synapses induced by stress is accompanied by functional modifications in synaptic transmission. Several studies have shown that acute and chronic stress and corticosterone impair long-term synaptic potentiation (Diamond et al., 1992; Foy et al., 1987; Kim et al., 1996; Mesches et al., 1999; Pavlides et al., 1996; Shors et al., 1989) and facilitate long-term synaptic depression (Kim et al., 1996; Pavlides et al., 1995; Xu et al., 1997, 1998). As we have seen in Chapter 1, long-term potentiation and long-term depression are functional modifications of synapses that are believed to be involved in the storage mechanisms of memory. Therefore, it has been argued that stress may affect memory consolidation by affecting these forms of functional synaptic plasticity (Kim et al., 2006).

An important aspect that needs further clarification is the precise role of stress hormones and glucocorticoid and mineralocorticoid receptors on the changes in long-term synaptic potentiation induced by stress. For instance, rats exposed to an acute stress by placing them in an elevated platform show increased plasma levels of corticosterone, an increased baseline activity in the amygdala, and an inhibition of amygdalar long-term synaptic potentiation in response to stimulation of the entorhinal cortex. An increased baseline activity was also detected in the amygdala after corticosterone administration, suggesting that acute changes in corticosterone levels mediate the effects of acute stress on amygdala activity. However, corticosterone did not induce changes in long-term synaptic potentiation in the amygdala, indicating that inhibition of amygdalar long-term potentiation by acute stress may not be exclusively explained by changes in corticosterone levels in plasma (Kavushansky et al., 2006). Glucocorticoid and mineralocorticoid receptors also have complex roles in the effects of stress on functional synaptic plasticity in the hippocampus. Thus, corticosterone administration impairs long-term synaptic potentiation in the hippocampus (Diamond et al., 1992; Pavlides et al., 1996), and serum corticosterone concentration has an inverted U-shaped correlation with primed burst potentiation, a long-lasting increase in the amplitude of the CA1 population spike, and excitatory postsynaptic potential slope in response to the stimulation of the hippocampal commissure (Alfarez et al., 2002). Primed burst potentiation showed a peak at intermediate serum levels (11–20 µg/dL) of corticosterone and was impaired at low and high corticosterone levels. Corticosterone and the glucocorticoid receptor agonist dexamethasone increase long-term synaptic depression in CA1 elicited by the activation of group 1 metabotropic glutamate receptors, by a mechanism involving local glucocorticoid receptors (Chaouloff et al., 2008). Accordingly, the glucocorticoid receptor antagonist RU38486 prevents the induction of long-term synaptic depression and the impairment of long-term synaptic potentiation in hippocampal slices from rats subjected to inescapable behavioral stress, induced by the placement of the animals on an elevated platform for 30 minutes (Xu et al., 1998). The administration of RU38486, before the exposure to acute swim stress, also facilitates synaptic long-term potentiation after hippocampal perforant path stimulation. In contrast, the injection of spironolactone, an antagonist of mineralocorticoid receptors, before the acute swim stress enables only short-term synaptic potentiation that finally reverses to long-term synaptic depression (Ahmed et al., 2006). Therefore, glucocorticoid receptors appear to impair long-term synaptic potentiation and promote long-term synaptic depression in the hippocampus, while mineralocorticoid receptors have the opposite effects. Furthermore, the blockade of both mineralocorticoid and glucocorticoid receptors results in the impairment of long-term synaptic potentiation (Avital et al., 2006). Therefore, both mineralocorticoid and glucocorticoid receptors appear to be involved in the effect of corticosteroids on functional synaptic plastic changes induced by acute stress in the hippocampus, although with opposite roles.

The relationship of stress and long-term synaptic potentiation is therefore complicated by the different effects of mineralocorticoid and glucocorticoid receptors. Another source of complexity is that different forms of stress may have a different effect on long-term synaptic potentiation in the same brain area. For instance, swim stress may decrease long-term potentiation in the basolateral amygdala (Kavushansky et al., 2006), while acute predator stress enhances long-term potentiation in this structure (Vouimba et al., 2006). In particular, chronic or repetitive stress may have very different effects on functional synaptic plasticity than acute stress. While acute swim stress may enhance long-term potentiation in the hippocampus and facilitate memory consolidation (Ahmed et al., 2006), chronic stress impairs long-term potentiation and decreases memory consolidation. For instance, long-term potentiation is markedly impaired in hippocampal explants taken from rats exposed to uncontrollable or repetitive stress (Foy et al., 1987; Shors et al., 1989). Chronic stress also produces suppression in long-term potentiation in the hippocampus in vivo (Pavlides et al., 2002).

Another factor of complexity in the relationship of stress and long-term synaptic potentiation is that the same form of stress does not affect synaptic plasticity in the same way in all brain structures involved in the stress response. For instance, rats subjected to chronic restraint stress showed a significantly lower long-term potentiation in the medial perforant input to the dentate gyrus and also in the commissural/associational input to the CA3, but not in the mossy fiber input to CA3 (Pavlides et al., 2002). Therefore, different hippocampal regions respond with a different synaptic plastic response to the same form of stress. Regional differences in the response to stress have also been detected with acute predator stress. Vouimba et al. (2006) have shown that acute predator stress blocks long-term potentiation in the CA1 region of the hippocampus and enhances long-term potentiation in the basolateral nucleus of the amygdala. Thus, the same form of acute stress has opposite effects in these two brain regions. Another example of regional differences in synaptic plasticity in response to stress was provided by Kavushansky et al. (2006), who assessed the effect of controllable and uncontrollable stress on long-term synaptic potentiation using the Morris water maze test as a source of stress. The Morris water maze test is commonly used to assess spatial memory, and the animals should locate a hidden underwater platform using spatial cues. However, the test per se supposes a stressful experience for rats and Kavushansky and collaborators assessed the effect of this form of stress. They trained one group of rats to locate a visible platform and a second group to locate an invisible platform. In both cases, the stress was controllable for the animals by escaping from the water when they found the platform. A third group of animals were introduced in the water for the same time as the average exposure of the first group, but these animals did not have a platform to escape from the water. Both controllable and uncontrollable stress in this paradigm impaired long-term potentiation in hippocampal CA1, although the effect was stronger with the uncontrollable stress. In contrast, the uncontrollable stress enhanced long-term potentiation in the dentate gyrus, and both forms of stress decreased long-term potentiation in the amygdala. Thus, in this case the dentate gyrus shows a different plastic response to stress than the amygdala and CA1.

The diverse regulation of long-term synaptic potentiation in response to the same form of stress in different brain regions indicates that stress is not affecting the basic mechanisms of synaptic plasticity in an unspecific way. On the contrary, it seems that the brain responds to stress by coordinated, and in some cases, opposite changes in functional synaptic plasticity in different brain areas involved in the stress response. This is also valid for other manifestations of synaptic plasticity. We have seen before that morphological synaptic remodeling also shows regional differences in response to stress. For instance, chronic stress induces hypertrophy of dendritic trees in the basolateral amygdala, and dendritic pruning in the prefrontal cortex and hippocampus. In addition, a corticosteroid imbalance induces neuronal loss and an atrophy of layer II of the infralimbic, prelimbic, and cingulate regions of the prefrontal cortex but does not induce morphological alterations in the retrosplenial or motor cortices (Cerqueira et al., 2005). Therefore, both functional synaptic plasticity and morphological remodeling regulated by stress and corticosteroids show regional differences, further supporting the concept that stress is causing an adaptive selective reorganization of functional interconnected synaptic circuits rather than affecting the same molecular, electrophysiological, and morphological synaptic properties in all brain regions (Fig. 3.2).

In addition, within a given brain region, stress and corticosteroids may have a different effect on different mechanisms of synaptic plasticity. Stress and corticosteroids regulate long-term synaptic plasticity by affecting the levels of serotonergic receptor activation and the expression of growth factors, such as brain-derived neurotrophic factor, or of other key proteins involved in the regulation of synaptic plasticity, such as calmodulin and calmodulin-dependent protein kinase II. Stress also affects the activation/phosphorylation levels of kinases involved in the regulation of synaptic plasticity, such as phosphatidylinositol 3-kinase, calmodulin-dependent protein kinase II, mitogen-activated protein kinase 2, and p38 mitogen-activated protein kinase; as well as the phosphorylation of cAMP response element-binding protein or the levels of expression or activation of phosphatases, such as calcineurin (Ahmed et al., 2006; Aleisa et al., 2006; Yang et al., 2004; Yang et al., 2008). Stress and corticosteroids may have different effects on these molecular mechanisms in different brain regions and within the same brain region. For instance, corticosterone has opposite effects on the regulation of long-term synaptic plasticity mediated by N-methyl-D-aspartate (NMDA) receptors than in the long-term synaptic plasticity mediated by voltage-dependent calcium channels (Krugers et al., 2005). The final plastic response to stress and corticosteroids probably integrates actions of different mechanisms of plasticity and at different brain levels. Furthermore, stress affects plasticity in the connections between different brain regions, such as the hippocampus and the prefrontal cortex (Cerqueira et al., 2007); plastic changes in one brain region may determine the nature of the plastic modifications in another brain area. For instance, the activation of the basolateral amygdala seems to be essential for

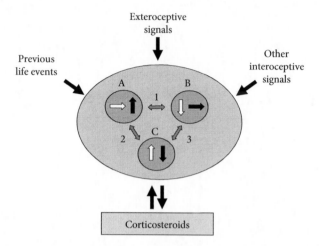

Figure 3.2. Corticosteroids and stress regulate metaplasticity in the brain. In different brain regions (A, B, C) corticosteroids may facilitate (black and white up arrows), impair (black and white down arrows), or have no effect (black and white horizontal arrows) on different forms (black vs. white arrows) of morphological and functional synaptic plasticity. Within a given brain region, corticosteroids may have different effects on different mechanisms of synaptic plasticity (black vs. white arrows). Corticosteroids may also affect plasticity in the connections between different brain regions (1, 2, 3); plastic changes regulated by corticosteroids in one brain region may determine the nature of the plastic modifications in another brain area. In addition, the effect of corticosteroids on synaptic plasticity depends on the memory of previous life events and on the updated information on the environmental and physiological context that the brain receives via exteroceptive signals and other interoceptive inputs, including other hormonal signals. Therefore, corticosteroids regulate metaplastic changes in brain plasticity in adaptation to the homeodynamic needs.

modifications in the hippocampus. Finally, it is important to consider that the effect of corticosterone on functional synaptic plasticity depends on the social and environmental conditions; is influenced by previous life events, such as previous stress or maternal care (Alfarez et al., 2008; Champagne et al., 2008; Joëls and Krugers, 2007); and is also influenced by other interoceptive signals, including other hormones and cytokines from the immune system (McEwen, 2007). Thus, the final plastic modifications in different brain regions represent an integrated brain response to stress, depending on the previous history and the present biological context. In other words: stress and corticosteroids regulate metaplasticity (Fig. 3.2; see also Chapter 1).

Chapter 4

Hormonal Influences on Brain Plasticity: II. Sex Hormones

INTRODUCTION: SEX HORMONES AND BRAIN REMODELING

The hormones produced by the ovaries and the testes exert a variety of regulatory effects in the nervous system. Gonadal hormones influence the development of numerous regions of the brain and spinal cord, affecting the survival and differentiation of specific neuronal and glial populations, as well as the establishment of synaptic connectivity. These hormonal actions result in permanent changes in the structure and function of the central nervous system, which are the foundation of sex differences in neuroendocrine regulation and behavior (see Chapter 6). Gonadal hormones also regulate the expression of morphological and functional synaptic and glial plasticity in specific regions of the brain and spinal cord during puberty (see Chapter 7) and adulthood (see Chapter 8). Effects of gonadal hormones on synaptic remodeling are well documented in neural circuits that are involved in the control of reproductive and neuroendocrine events. Indeed, there is abundant literature available on the effects of gonadal hormones on the synaptic circuits that control the innervation of muscles involved in copulation and on the brain centers that control reproductive behavior. However, gonadal hormones also influence synaptic remodeling in brain regions involved in affection and cognition, such as the amygdala, the hippocampal formation, and the cerebral neocortex. Gonadal hormones also have an important impact on brain mutability by the modulation of cell replacement, including the regulation of neuron generation in the hippocampus. I will review in this chapter these actions of gonadal hormones on synaptic plasticity and cellular replacement, and the potential mechanisms involved in the hormonal actions. I will first examine the actions of ovarian hormones, estradiol and progesterone, on neural plasticity and then analyze the effects of testicular androgens. Although this chapter is devoted to gonadal hormones, for convenience I will discuss the neuroplastic effects of the adrenal androgen dehydroepiandrosterone (DHEA), when analyzing the effects of testicular androgens.

THE FIRST EVIDENCE

The first direct evidence demonstrating that gonadal hormones regulate synaptic plasticity in the adult central nervous system was obtained by two

Japanese investigators, Akira Matsumoto and Yasumasa Arai, from the Juntendo University School of Medicine in Tokyo. Their seminal paper, published in 1979, undoubtedly showed that estrogen promotes synaptic reinnervation in a deafferented brain area. They surgically isolated in vivo the arcuate nucleus of ovariectomized rats, using a Halasz knife. This procedure eliminates the synaptic afferents and resulted in an approximately 50% decrease in the number of axodendritic synapses. The treatment with estradiol benzoate for 3 weeks from the day of surgery restored the axodendritic synaptic population (Matsumoto and Arai, 1979). This very early observation was highly revolutionary in its time and is still extremely relevant today to interpret estrogen effects in damaged brain tissue and in the aging brain. Matsumoto and Arai also discovered the existence of a sexual dimorphism in the number of synaptic contacts in the arcuate nucleus (Matsumoto and Arai, 1980) and the possibility of altering synaptic development by neonatal estrogen treatment (Arai and Matsumoto, 1978). When Matsumoto and Arai published their pioneering findings, Dominique Toran-Allerand, from Columbia University in New York, had already reported an increased neuritic growth in explant fetal hypothalamic cultures incubated with estradiol (Toran-Allerand, 1976). These early observations by Toran-Allerand, highly ahead of her time, as many other of her discoveries, suggested that the ovarian hormone was able to promote axonal growth during development in specific brain areas. Yet, the findings of Matsumoto and Arai still added another crucial step in the understanding of how sex hormones act in the brain, showing that estrogen is also able to promote axonal growth, and therefore regulate plasticity, in the adult brain.

Evidence for plasticity in the arcuate nucleus regulated by estrogen was also obtained by James R. Brawer, from the McGill University School of Medicine, and his collaborators. They reported in 1978 that the injection of high doses of estradiol valerate to young adult cyclic female rats resulted in persistent vaginal estrus, small polyfollicular ovaries, and pathological changes in the hypothalamic arcuate nucleus, which showed numerous reactive microglia, reactive astrocytes, and degenerating elements in the neuropil (Brawer et al., 1978). In 1982, two investigators from Argentina, Hugo F. Carrer and Agustín Aoki, working at the Instituto de Investigación Médica Mercedes y Martín Ferreyra and the center for electron microscopy of the Universidad Nacional de Córdoba, reported dramatic ultrastructural changes induced by estrogen in another hypothalamic region: the ventromedial hypothalamic nucleus. They injected estradiol (100 µg estradiol benzoate/kg body weight) to ovariectomized rats and studied the effect on the ventromedial hypothalamic nucleus using light and electron microscopy. Ventromedial neurons in animals treated with estradiol showed enlarged cell and nuclear volume, a marked increase in rough endoplasmic reticulum, enlarged Golgi apparatus, presence of pleomorphic mitochondria, and condensation of nucleolar material (Carrer and Aoki, 1982). All these modifications were indicative of an increased metabolic activity. These findings extended the results of a previous electron microscopic analysis from the laboratory of Donald W. Pfaff, at Rockefeller University, that had already revealed that estradiol injected into ovariectomized rats was able to induce stacking of the rough endoplasmic reticulum and increases in the number of dense-cored vesicles in ventromedial neurons (Cohen and Pfaff, 1981). However, Carrer and Aoki made a further decisive discovery—they found that the synaptic contacts per unit area were increased after estrogen treatment in the ventrolateral division of the nucleus (Carrer and Aoki, 1982). These findings suggested that physiological variations of plasma estrogen levels could induce metabolic activation linked to synaptic remodeling of specific hypothalamic neuronal populations.

Inspired by these previous studies, Frederick Naftolin, at the University of Geneva (on a sabbatical leave from Yale University), performed similar analyses by electron microscopy in the arcuate nucleus. Naftolin was fascinated by some specialized modifications of the endoplasmic reticulum that are observed in neurons in the arcuate nucleus and other brain areas such as the ventromedial hypothalamic nucleus (Cohen and Pfaff, 1981). These specializations of the endoplasmic reticulum consist of concentric sheets of cisterna and are known as *whorl bodies*. Previous studies had shown that whorl bodies in arcuate neurons were responsive to the endocrine conditions and that their number and size were affected by gonadal hormones. For instance, their number markedly increases after a gonadectomy. Naftolin observed that arcuate neuronal profiles, which contain whorl bodies, received a significantly increased number of axosomatic presynaptic terminals (Naftolin et al., 1985). Since neuronal profiles with whorl bodies were much less numerous in intact animals, the findings of Naftolin suggested that the number of axosomatic synapses was increased after castration in a subpopulation of arcuate neurons. In addition, since whorl bodies fluctuate during the estrus cycle (King et al., 1974), the observations of Naftolin predicted that synaptic changes might also occur in arcuate neurons during the estrus cycle. I had the good fortune of collaborating with Naftolin in this work, and in 1986 we finished the characterization of synaptic inputs in the arcuate nucleus of female rats treated with a high dose (20 mg/kg) of estradiol valerate (Garcia-Segura et al., 1986). We observed that the number of axosomatic and axodendritic synapses on dendritic shafts was significantly decreased in the arcuate nucleus by 8 weeks after estradiol valerate treatment. In contrast, the number of axodendritic synapses on dendritic spines was unaffected. The loss of synaptic inputs on perikarya and dendritic shafts was compatible with the degenerative images previously found by Brawer and Naftolin in the arcuate nucleus of female rats treated with estradiol valerate. Indeed, we observed a massive appearance of neuronal degenerative images by 3 weeks after estradiol valerate injection, preceding the decrease in the number of synapses. Interestingly, by 32 weeks postinjection, the number of axosomatic and axodendritic synapses had returned to control values, indicating that estradiol administration had facilitated a process of circuitry remodeling in the arcuate nucleus.

Our findings, together with those of Matsumoto and Arai (1979) obtained in the deafferented arcuate nucleus model, indicated that estrogen was able to modulate synaptic plasticity in this brain area. However, in both the cases, nonphysiological conditions were studied. Matsumoto and Arai studied rein-nervation in a denervated nucleus. In our case, we were using high doses of estradiol, which Brawer et al (1978) showed to induce constant estrus and imi-tate ovarian failure during reproductive aging. However, as mentioned before, Hugo Carrer and Agustín Aoki had already reported that estrogen increases the number of synaptic contacts in the ventromedial hypothalamic nucleus in ovariectomized rats (Carrer and Aoki, 1982). Furthermore, in 1987, Momoko Miyakawa and Yasumasa Arai reported an increase in the number of axoden-dritic synapses in the lateral septum of adult female rats after treatment for 4 weeks with estradiol (Miyakawa and Arai, 1987). These reports, one from Argentina and one from Japan, suggested that estrogen might affect synaptic inputs in the central nervous system under physiological conditions. However, the question still unanswered was whether physiological fluctuations of ovar-ian hormones were able to modulate synaptic plasticity. Therefore, together with my students Gabriel Olmos, Julio Perez, and Pedro Tranque, we decided to perform a quantitative analysis of synapses in the arcuate nucleus of female rats during the 4 days of the estrus cycle (Olmos et al., 1989). Every 4 days throughout the ovarian cycle of the rat there is a rise in circulating levels of estradiol, which peaks on the morning of proestrus. This estrogen surge sig-nals the maturation of the ovarian follicles and results in an abrupt increase in luteinizing hormone on the afternoon of proestrus. The rise in gonadotro-pins is associated with an increase in progesterone levels and a decrease in circulating estradiol levels, which then remain low throughout the following estrus day and do not rise again until the next group of follicles begins their maturation (Naftolin et al., 1972b). Our findings indicated that the number of axosomatic synapses per length of perikaryal membrane was significantly decreased in estrus, compared to other days of the estrus cycle. The reduction in the number of synapses in estrus was accompanied by a decrease in the per-centage of the average length of perikaryal membrane covered by presynaptic terminals and by an increase in the percentage of membrane in close apposi-tion of glial processes. Since the average perikaryal perimeter was not signif-icantly changed during the estrus cycle, these results indicate a net decrease in the number of arcuate nucleus axosomatic synapses between proestrus and estrus, with a reinnervation of arcuate neurons between estrus and metestrus. These results were the first demonstration of a physiological synaptic turn-over in the brain during the estrus cycle (Olmos et al., 1989). Shortly after, Elizabeth Gould, Catherine S. Woolley, Maya Frankfurt, Annabell C. Segarra, and Bruce S. McEwen at the Rockefeller University, using the Golgi method to stain neurons, reported that similar plastic changes occur in the dendritic spines of ventromedial hypothalamic neurons (Frankfurt et al., 1990; Segarra and McEwen, 1991) and of CA1 pyramidal hippocampal neurons (Gould et al., 1990; Woolley, 1998; Woolley et al., 1990a). This latter finding was the first evidence of the regulation of synaptic plasticity by ovarian hormones in brain regions involved with cognitive processing.

In the next sections of this chapter I will review the cellular and molecular mechanisms involved in the regulation of neural plasticity by estradiol and progesterone. The plastic modifications regulated by ovarian hormones in the physiological context of reproductive cycles are analyzed with more detail in Chapter 8.

REGULATION BY ESTRADIOL AND PROGESTERONE OF SYNAPTIC AND GLIAL REMODELING IN THE ARCUATE NUCLEUS

The role of estradiol and progesterone in the regulation of synaptic plasticity has been studied in the hypothalamic arcuate nucleus. Administration of a single dose of 17β-estradiol to ovariectomized rats results in a significant and reversible decrease in the number of arcuate axosomatic synapses (Perez et al., 1993a). However, the simultaneous administration of progesterone and estradiol inhibits the effect of estradiol (Perez et al., 1993a). The axosomatic synapses affected by estradiol in the arcuate nucleus include inhibitory GABAergic synapses. The administration of estradiol to ovariectomized rats results in a significant decrease in the number of GABA-immunoreactive axosomatic synapses (Parducz et al., 1993). In addition, estradiol increases the number of excitatory synapses in dendritic spines, suggesting that the hormone may increase neuronal excitability by decreasing the number of inhibitory inputs in the perikarya and increasing the number of excitatory inputs in dendritic spines. Indeed, electrophysiological recordings reveal an increased frequency of neuronal firing in a subpopulation of arcuate neurons in response to estradiol (Parducz et al., 2002).

Estradiol-induced synaptic changes in arcuate neurons of adult rats are accompanied by a prominent morphological modification of arcuate astroglia and changes in the expression and distribution of the astroglial cytoskeletal marker glial fibrillary acidic protein (GFAP) (Garcia-Segura et al., 1994a, b; Kohama et al., 1995). GFAP mRNA, the surface density of GFAP-immunoreactive cell perikarya and processes, the number of astroglial profiles in the arcuate neuropil, and the amount of neuronal perikaryal membrane covered by glial processes (Fig. 4.1) exhibit a rapid and reversible increase when ovariectomized rats are injected with 17β-estradiol. In the same experimental paradigm, a similar time frame is observed for the changes that occur in synaptic connectivity. One hour after the administration of a single dose of 17β-estradiol to ovariectomized rats, some axosomatic synapses become detached from the neuronal surface by the interposition of glial processes between the pre- and postsynaptic membranes. One day after the administration of the hormone, a multiple layer of glial processes covers a majority of the surface of arcuate neuronal perikarya (Fig. 4.1). Synaptic terminals remain in the proximity of neuronal perikarya, although glial processes are interposed between the pre- and postsynaptic membranes, preventing the formation of synaptic contacts (Fig. 4.2). At this stage, GFAP immunoreactivity reaches the highest intensity in the arcuate nucleus and median eminence. The effect of

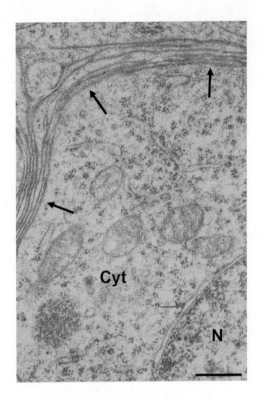

Figure 4.1. A neuron of the hypothalamic arcuate nucleus from an ovariectomized rat killed 24 hours after the administration of 17β-estradiol. The neuronal surface is covered with a multiple layer of glial processes (arrows). Cytoplasm (Cyt); cell nucleus (N). Scale bar: 0.6 μm. (Microphotograph from the author; based on Garcia-Segura et al., 1994b.)

estradiol on glia is dose dependent and, as observed for the synaptic changes, is blocked by the simultaneous administration of progesterone. Thus, there is not only a precise temporal correlation between synaptic and glial changes in the arcuate nucleus of adult animals but also a similar hormonal dependence. This suggests that coordinated glial and synaptic modifications are involved in the cellular mechanism by which estradiol modulates the activity of arcuate neurons.

Although the link between astroglial and synaptic changes in adult animals has been studied most extensively in the hypothalamus of rodents, hormonally induced astrocytic ensheathing of hypothalamic neurons is also associated with modifications in the number of synaptic inputs to the hypothalamic neurons in adult primates. Joan W. Witkin, Ann-Judith Silverman, and their collaborators at Columbia University in New York showed that an ovariectomy of the rhesus monkey results in a significant decline in the number of

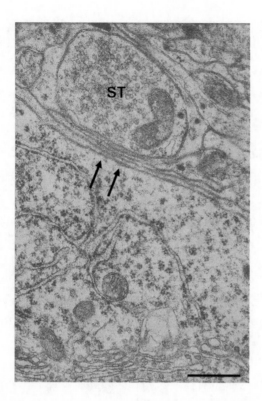

Figure 4.2. Detail of a synaptic terminal (ST) on the proximity of an arcuate neuronal soma from an ovariectomized rat killed 24 hours after the administration of 17β-estradiol. The synaptic terminal is surrounded by glial profiles and is separated from the neuronal soma by a multiple layer of glial processes (arrows). Scale bar: 0.6 μm. (Microphotograph from the author; based on Garcia-Segura et al., 1994b.)

axosomatic synaptic inputs to gonadotropin-releasing hormone (GnRH) neurons in the mediobasal hypothalamus. This decrease in the number of synaptic appositions is accompanied by increased coverage of neuronal perikarya by glial processes, and these changes can be prevented by estrogen replacement (Witkin et al., 1991). It is interesting to note that, in this case, estradiol decreases the glial coverage of neuronal perikarya and increases the number of axosomatic synaptic inputs (Fig. 4.3). Thus, the effect of estradiol on synaptic and glial plasticity associated with GnRH neurons of monkeys is the opposite of that exerted on rat arcuate neurons, where the hormone increases glial coverage and decreases axosomatic synaptic inputs. This suggests that estradiol facilitates the onset of plasticity, rather than promoting an identical plastic modification in all brain structures. The hormonal facilitation of plasticity will result in an increased or a decreased glial coverage or in synaptic

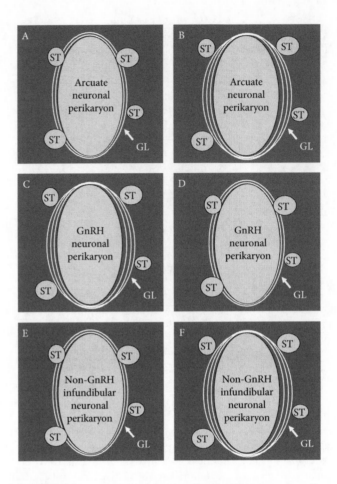

Figure 4.3. Glial and synaptic plasticity associated with neuronal perikarya in the arcuate nucleus of adults rats (A, B); in gonadotropin-releasing hormone (GnRH) neurons in adult rhesus monkeys and adult African green monkeys (C, D); and in non-GnRH neurons in the infundibular/arcuate nucleus of adult African green monkeys (E, F). (A and B) The perikaryon of arcuate neurons from ovariectomized rats treated with vehicle (A) have less wrapping by glial lamellae (GL) and an increased number of contacts with axosomatic synaptic terminals (ST) compared with the perikarya from ovariectomized rats treated with estradiol (B). In estradiol-treated rats, there is a detachment of axosomatic synaptic terminals by the interposition of glial processes between the pre- and the postsynaptic membranes (based on Garcia-Segura et al., 1994b; and Perez et al., 1993a). (C and D) In monkeys, an ovariectomy (C) increases the apposition of glial lamellae to GnRH neuronal perikarya and decreases the number of inhibitory axosomatic synaptic terminals. An ovarian hormone replacement regimen (which mimicked the menstrual cycle) had the opposite effects (D), decreasing the glial ensheathment of neuronal somas and increasing the innervation of GnRH perikarya (based on Witkin et al., 1991; and Zsarnovszky et al., 2001). (E and F) Non-GnRH neuronal perikarya in the infundibular/arcuate nucleus of ovariectomized

formation or retraction depending on the specific function of the synaptic circuit and/or the brain region involved.

This hypothesis was directly tested by the analysis of synaptic and glial changes in the infundibular nucleus of African green monkeys, a hypothalamic region with a similar function to the rat arcuate nucleus. However, unlike rats, where GnRH neuronal perikarya are not located in the arcuate nucleus, in monkeys some GnRH perikarya are present in the infundibular/arcuate nucleus. Therefore, in the infundibular/arcuate nucleus of monkeys, it is possible to analyze synaptic and glial changes on GnRH and non-GnRH neurons in parallel. The morphometric analysis revealed that the effects of estradiol on the apposition of synapses and glial processes on neuronal perikarya in most infundibular/arcuate nucleus of monkeys were similar to those observed in the arcuate neurons of rats. Most infundibular/arcuate neurons of ovariectomized monkeys showed a significant increase in the length of neuronal soma membrane in contact with glial processes and a significant decrease in the number of axosomatic synapses after estradiol treatment (Naftolin et al., 1993). Since GnRH neurons in the infundibular/arcuate nucleus of monkeys are a minor population, the observed changes likely reflect the effect of estradiol on non-GnRH neurons. Indeed, the analysis of the synaptic connectivity in GnRH and non-GnRH neurons revealed that the changes in response to estradiol in the number of axosynaptic inputs were different in the two neuronal populations (Fig. 4.3E, F). One day after estrogen treatment, the number of inhibitory axosomatic synapses increased in GnRH neurons, while axosomatic inhibitory synapses on non-GnRH neurons decreased compared to control conditions (Zsarnovszky et al., 2001). Thus, plastic changes in most infundibular/arcuate neurons in monkeys parallel those observed in the arcuate neurons of rats, while the synaptic changes in the specific population of GnRH neurons show a different regulation. This suggests that estradiol differentially regulates synaptic plasticity depending on the specific function of each neuronal circuit (Fig. 4.3).

As we have seen in previous chapters, cell adhesion molecules are important participants in plastic brain remodeling. These molecules may also participate in the estrogenic regulation of the interactions between glial processes, neuronal perikarya, and synapses. In early studies we examined plasma membrane composition of arcuate neurons using freeze-fracture techniques. The freeze-fracture method detects the presence of particles in the cellular membranes

---

monkeys treated with vehicle (E) show increased glial coverage (GL) and decreased inhibitory axosomatic synaptic contacts (ST) than ovariectomized monkeys treated with estradiol (F) (based on Naftolin et al., 1993; and Zsarnovszky et al., 2001). Since non-GnRH infundibular/arcuate neurons of monkeys are functionally homologous to arcuate neurons in rats, these findings suggest that the direction of the plastic changes elicited by the regulatory action of ovarian hormones depends on the function of the neuronal circuit.

that are thought to represent membrane proteins. These particles, known as intramembrane particles (IMPs), are of a different size, probably reflecting the heterogeneous protein populations present in cellular membranes. Using this method, we detected that the organization of arcuate neuronal plasma membrane is sexually dimorphic (see Chapter 6). Sex differences in arcuate neuronal plasma membrane composition are irreversibly abolished in adult female rats as they go into constant vaginal estrus as a result of estradiol valerate administration (Garcia-Segura et al., 1992; Olmos et al., 1987). Under these conditions, there is a remodeling of arcuate axosomatic synapses, which is linked to modifications in the glial wrapping of arcuate neurons (Garcia-Segura et al., 1986; Olmos et al., 1987). A similar permanent change in membrane phenotype ensues in aged female rats as they reach senescent constant estrus (Garcia-Segura et al., 1991a). Membrane modifications in aged females may be generated by estradiol, since aging female rats are exposed to increasing amounts of the hormone as they approach reproductive senescence. In contrast to these permanent membrane changes associated with loss of ovarian function, reversible remodeling of neuronal plasma organization is observed in adult female rats following the fluctuation in plasma estradiol levels during the ovarian cycle (Garcia-Segura et al., 1988a). We detected significant changes in the number of IMPs in the plasma membranes of arcuate neurons. The highest IMP density in neuronal perikaryal membranes was reached on diestrus and then decreased during proestrus and estrus. These changes were due to a massive decrease in the number of small IMPs, which was partly balanced by a moderate increase in the number of large IMPs. These changes in the number of IMPs in proestrus were associated with an increased number of exoendocytotic images in the neuronal perikarya, suggestive of an increased remodeling of membranes. Similar changes were observed in the perikaryal plasma membrane of arcuate neurons of ovariectomized rats after the injection of high physiological doses of estradiol (Perez et al., 1993a). Under these conditions, the number of small IMPs was decreased while the number of large IMPs was increased in rats killed 24 hours after the injection of the hormone. These membrane changes were associated with a decrease in the number of axosomatic synapses and an increase in the proportion of arcuate neuronal soma membrane covered by glia. When the number of axosomatic synapses and the amount of glial wrapping of arcuate neuronal perikarya returned to control values by 48 hours after the estradiol injection, the number of IMPs returned also to baseline conditions. Furthermore, blockage by progesterone of the synaptic and glial changes induced by estradiol was also accompanied by an inhibition of the effects of this hormone on neuronal membranes (Perez et al., 1993a). Further evidence for a link between the membrane, synaptic and glial changes that occur in arcuate neurons were obtained in studies assessing the effect of the protein synthesis inhibitor cycloheximide. Modifications in the content of IMPs in arcuate neuronal membranes that follow the inhibition of hypothalamic protein synthesis by cycloheximide resulted in increased glial wrapping of arcuate neuronal perikarya and a decreased number of axo-somatic synapses (Perez et al., 1993b).

The coordinated changes in the number of synaptic inputs, amount of glial ensheathing and ultrastructure of the membrane of neuronal perikarya during the estrus cycle, and the finding of similar IMP changes in arcuate neurons in all experimental paradigms where there is remodeling of the synaptic and glial contacts suggests a causal relationship. One possibility is that membrane changes may precede and cause synaptic changes. IMPs may represent, in part, membrane molecules involved in the control of cell adhesion (Garcia-Segura et al., 1989a), and their changes may alter the interactions of the plasma membranes of postsynaptic neurons with the membranes of their presynaptic inputs or with the membranes of astrocytes. To test this hypothesis, the possible involvement of membrane-mediated cell-to-cell interactions in the plastic effects of estradiol was assessed using serum-free mixed neuronal–glial primary rat hypothalamic cultures. The proportion of process-bearing astrocytes in these cultures was increased by treatment with estradiol (Fig. 4.4). This effect was detected as early as 30 minutes after the addition of the hormone to the cultures, was dose dependent and reversible, and was blocked by the selective estrogen receptor modulator tamoxifen (Garcia-Segura et al., 1989b; Torres-Aleman et al., 1992). One important feature of the effect of estradiol on astroglia in these studies was that direct contact between neurons and glial cells was necessary for their manifestation. In glial cultures, when neurons were absent, the proportion of process-bearing astrocytes was neither modified by estradiol nor by a medium conditioned by estradiol-treated mixed cultures. Furthermore, a preexisting membrane contact between neurons and astrocytes appears to be needed for the initiation of estradiol-induced changes in glial shape. These results suggest that neuron cell surface molecules may be involved in the hormone-induced changes in the interaction between neuronal and glial membranes.

Brain regions such as the hypothalamo-neurohypophysial system, the arcuate nucleus, and the median eminence express high levels of a polysialic acid (PSA)–rich form of neural cell adhesion molecule (N-CAM) (Bonfanti et al., 1992; Theodosis et al., 1991; see also Fig. 4.5). This PSA-rich form of N-CAM (PSA-N-CAM) reduces cell adhesion and allows cellular morphological plasticity (see also Chapters 2 and 3). High immunoreactivity for PSA-N-CAM has also been detected in the region of the GnRH pulse generator of the monkey (Perera et al., 1993), a hypothalamic zone that also shows changes in the number of axosomatic synapses in response to varying gonadal steroid levels (Perera and Plant, 1997; Witkin et al., 1991). A role for PSA-N-CAM in neuroglial plasticity that is under the influence of estrogen was suggested by in vitro studies on hypothalamic monolayer cultures. Immunostaining of these cultures with an antibody that specifically recognizes PSA-N-CAM resulted in prominent labeling of neuronal membranes. As it has been mentioned before, estradiol also induces prominent changes in the shape of astrocytes

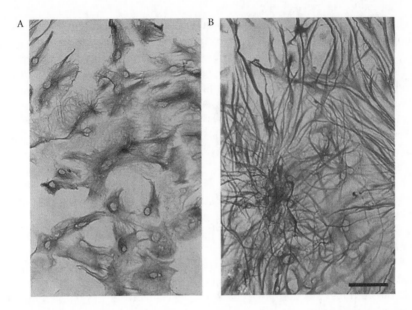

Figure 4.4. Estradiol increases the proportion of process-bearing astrocytes in serum-free mixed neuronal–glial primary rat hypothalamic cultures. (A) Glial fibrillary acidic protein (GFAP) immunoreactive cells in a control culture treated with vehicle. (B) GFAP immunoreactive cells in a culture treated with estradiol. This effect of estradiol is detected as early as 30 minutes after the addition of the hormone to the cultures, and is reversible. Estradiol did not induce changes in the morphology of astrocytes in pure glial cultures or in mixed neuronal–glial cultures in which polysialic acid (PSA) was removed from PSA-neural cell adhesion molecules expressed in neuronal membranes (see Garcia-Segura et al., 1989b, 1995; and Torres-Aleman et al., 1992). These findings suggest that neurons mediate the estradiol-induced glial changes. Scale bar 60 μm. (Microphotographs from the author.)

in these cultures. Interestingly, the effect of estradiol on the morphology of astrocytes was blocked when polysialic acid was removed from PSA-N-CAM by using a bacterial endoneuraminidase that specifically removes polysialic acid from the cell surface (Garcia-Segura et al., 1995a). While these results suggested that PSA-N-CAM may be crucial for estrogen-induced neuroglial plasticity, the direct proof came from studies carried out by Zsófia Hoyk in the laboratory of Dionysia Theodosis in Bordeaux and in the laboratory of Arpad Parducz in Szeged (Hoyk et al., 2001). To asses the role of PSA on synaptic remodeling induced by estradiol in the rat arcuate nucleus in vivo, Hoyk intracerebroventricularly infused antibodies raised against PSA, or microinjected endoneuraminidase-N over the arcuate nucleus in ovariectomized animals injected with estradiol. Both treatments blocked the plastic remodeling

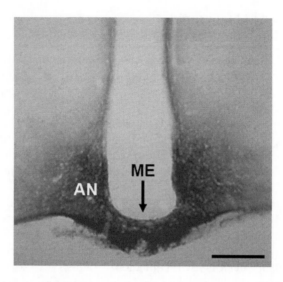

Figure 4.5. Immunoreactivity for the polysialic acid-neural cell adhesion molecule (PSA-NCAM) in the hypothalamus. High levels of PSA-NCAM immunoreactivity are observed in the arcuate nucleus (ME) and the median eminence (AN), brain regions that show a high degree of neuroglial plasticity. Antibody provided by Dr. G. Rougon. Scale bar, 0.5 mm. (Microphotograph from the author.)

of arcuate synapses induced by estradiol, indicating that PSA is a necessary prerequisite for estrogen-induced remodeling of synapses in the adult female arcuate nucleus.

In addition to PSA-N-CAM, other adhesion molecules may be important for the hormonally driven neuroglial plasticity in the arcuate nucleus. Indeed, immunoreactivity for several cell adhesion molecules, such as F3/contactin and its ligand, the matrix glycoprotein tenascin-C, has been detected in the adult hypothalamus. It remains to be determined what role these molecules play in the plastic remodeling induced by estrogen in the adult brain. Ezrin, a membrane cytoskeletal-linking protein involved in the control of adhesion that interacts with the L1 cell adhesion molecule (Sakurai et al., 2008), may also play a role in the estrogenic regulation of the growth and retraction of glial and neuronal processes in the arcuate nucleus (Naftolin et al., 2007). Another factor that may be involved in the regulation of neuroglial plasticity by estradiol is apolipoprotein E (ApoE) (Struble et al., 2007). Estradiol enhances ApoE expression by astroglia and microglia (Stone et al., 1997), and ApoE levels fluctuate in different brain regions during the estrus cycle (Struble et al., 2003). ApoE may regulate the growth of glial and neuronal processes, and is involved in the effects of estradiol on axonal growth in vitro (Nathan et al., 2004).

REGULATION BY ESTRADIOL AND PROGESTERONE OF SYNAPTIC
REMODELING IN THE VENTROMEDIAL HYPOTHALAMIC NUCLEUS

As is the case for arcuate nucleus, the ventromedial hypothalamic nucleus is a key center for the regulation of reproduction and feeding. In female rats, the ventrolateral subdivision of the ventromedial hypothalamic nucleus contains a high proportion of neurons expressing estrogen (DonCarlos et al., 1991; Pfaff and Keiner, 1973; Simerly et al., 1990) and progesterone (DonCarlos et al., 1989) receptors and plays a prominent role in the coordination of fertility with lordosis, the mating postural reflex that allows for copulation. As for many other aspects of the actions of sex hormones in the brain, the work of Donald W. Pfaff at Rockefeller University has been essential for the clarification of the neuronal network that regulates lordosis and for the identification of the cellular and molecular actions of estradiol and progesterone in this network to initiate the lordosis reflex (Pfaff, 1999; see also Pfaus, 2000). Pfaff and his colleagues have provided massive evidence implicating the ventromedial hypothalamic nucleus in the regulation of lordosis (Kow and Pfaff, 1998). Estrogen implants in the ventromedial hypothalamic nucleus activate lordosis, while the inhibition of protein synthesis in this nucleus inhibits lordosis. Furthermore, destruction of the ventromedial hypothalamic nucleus prevents the effect of estradiol on lordosis.

As I have mentioned before in this chapter, Hugo Carrer and Agustín Aoki were the first to report that estrogen affected synaptic connectivity in the ventromedial hypothalamic nucleus, showing, by an electron microscopic quantitative analysis, an increase in the number of synaptic contacts per unit area in ovariectomized rats treated with estrogen compared to ovariectomized controls (Carrer and Aoki, 1982). A few years later, Rochelle S. Cohen at the University of Illinois in Chicago, in collaboration with Donald Pfaff, reported synaptic changes in the midbrain central gray, one of the targets of ventromedial neurons involved in the mediation of estrogen-induced lordosis behavior (Hennessey et al., 1990; Sakuma and Pfaff, 1979). Cohen and her collaborators observed that estradiol administration to ovariectomized rats increases the lordosis response and induces plastic changes in the synaptology of the midbrain central gray, increasing the number of synapses, the number of terminals containing dense-cored vesicles, the length of postsynaptic densities, the number of postsynaptic densities showing perforations, and the number of synapses with positive synaptic curvature (Chung et al., 1988). This study was among the first to demonstrate hormonal-induced synaptic changes associated with a specific behavior.

Given the importance of the actions of estradiol on the ventromedial hypothalamic nucleus for lordosis, Maya Frankfurt, Elizabeth Gould, Catherine S. Woolley, and Bruce S. McEwen examined ventromedial hypothalamic neurons stained with the Golgi method to detect possible morphological correlates of the hormonal action. They found that estradiol or estradiol plus progesterone administration into adult ovariectomized female rats increased the density of dendritic spines on the primary dendrites of ventromedial hypothalamic neurons. Furthermore, the density of dendritic spines was significantly lower at diestrus than proestrus (Frankfurt et al., 1990). Similar effects of estradiol and progesterone on the growth of dendrites in ventromedial neurons was detected by Meisel and Luttrell (1990) in female Syrian hamsters. Treatment of ovariectomized females with estradiol or estradiol plus progesterone increased the total dendritic length of ventromedial nucleus neurons by almost 50% compared with neurons from ovariectomized, oil-treated females. Further analysis by electron microscopy revealed that the increase in dendritic spines induced by estradiol in ovariectomized rats was also accompanied by an increased presynaptic innervation (Frankfurt and McEwen, 1991).

Lyngine H. Calizo and Loretta M. Flanagan-Cato, from the University of Pennsylvania, have explored the effect of estrogen on ventromedial hypothalamic neurons by injecting Lucifer yellow to reveal the entire dendritic morphology. They reported in 2000 the results of an analysis of 53 Lucifer yellow–filled neurons showing that estradiol treatment has a specific regional effect on dendritic spines in the ventromedial hypothalamic nucleus. Estradiol increases the average density of dendritic spines by 46% per neuron per animal, without affecting dendritic length. However, this effect is restricted to the ventral subdivision of the ventromedial hypothalamic nucleus, and the hormone has no effect in neurons located in the dorsal subdivision of the nucleus. Calizo and Flanagan-Cato analyzed the changes in dendritic spines in the longest primary dendrite, the short primary dendrites, and in the secondary dendrites, and they found that estradiol increases spine density on the short primary dendrites, which are randomly oriented in the nucleus, and decreases spine density in the middle portion of the longest primary dendrites, which are ventrolaterally oriented, without affecting spine density on the secondary dendrites (Calizo and Flanagan-Cato, 2000; Flanagan-Cato, 2000). These findings indicate that the remodeling of dendritic spines induced by estradiol in the ventromedial nucleus has a regional specificity and is limited to a specific subset of dendrites and to specific segments within the dendrites. Furthermore, estradiol increases spine density in some dendrites and decreases spine density in other dendrites. Therefore, estradiol is not promoting the growth of dendritic spines in general, but is regulating synaptic plasticity in a very selective manner in specific neuronal circuits. Indeed, the neurons with ventrolaterally oriented dendrites, which show a decrease in dendritic spines after estradiol treatment, project to the midbrain periaquaductal gray (Calizo and Flanagan-Cato, 2002), a region that, as already mentioned, is an essential part of the neuronal circuit that mediates the effect of estradiol on lordosis posture.

REGULATION BY ESTRADIOL AND PROGESTERONE OF SYNAPTIC REMODELING IN THE HIPPOCAMPUS

As I have mentioned at the beginning of this chapter, the pioneering studies of Catherine Woolley, Elizabeth Gould, and their colleagues in Bruce McEwen's laboratory at Rockefeller University, using the Golgi method, revealed a fluctuation in the number of dendritic spines in the CA1 region of the rat hippocampus during the estrus cycle (Woolley et al., 1990a). Since presynaptic excitatory inputs connect to the dendritic spines, their results suggested that synaptic contacts were also fluctuating in the hippocampus during the estrus cycle, as in the arcuate nucleus. The plasticity of presynaptic inputs on CA1 dendritic spines during the estrus cycle was later confirmed by electron microscopy (Woolley et al., 1996; Woolley and McEwen, 1992). In addition, biochemical analyses revealed fluctuations in the mRNA levels of synaptic proteins in the hippocampus during the estrus cycle (Crispino et al., 1999). Woolley and her colleagues also assessed the effect of estradiol and progesterone on hippocampal dendritic spines in rats (Gould et al., 1990a; McEwen and Woolley, 1994; Woolley and McEwen, 1993). By that time, it was known from previous electrophysiological studies by Teyler and collaborators (Teyler et al., 1980), who examined field potentials in CA1 pyramidal neurons, that estradiol rapidly increases the amplitude of population spikes in male and female animals, suggesting an increased presynaptic input. Woolley and her colleagues found that an ovariectomy results in a gradual decline in the number of dendritic spines in CA1 hippocampal pyramidal cells. This decline is reversed by estradiol administration to ovariectomized animals. Similar findings have been obtained in female monkeys (Hao et al., 2003; Leranth et al., 2002). As observed for the transient effects of estradiol on axosomatic synapses in the arcuate nucleus, Woolley and colleagues found that the hormone also induces a reversible modification of hippocampal dendritic spines in rats: the number of dendritic spines increases within 48 hours after estradiol administration, are at their peak by 72 hours and stay elevated for an additional day, and then gradually decreases (Fig. 4.6). Progesterone, in contrast, has a biphasic effect on dendritic spines in CA1 pyramidal neurons. Progesterone treatment following estradiol initially increases spine density for a period of 2 to 6 hours, but then the number of dendritic spines shows a stronger decrease in the animals treated with estradiol and progesterone than in those treated with estradiol alone. These findings suggest that estradiol drives the rapid increase in dendritic spines and that progesterone is important for producing the rapid decline of dendritic spines during the estrus cycle. Then, Woolley assessed the possible mechanisms involved in the effects of estradiol on dendritic spines. After testing the effects of a variety of neurotransmitter receptor antagonists, she found that N-methyl-D-aspartate (NMDA) receptor antagonists blocked the action of estradiol on dendritic spines of CA1 pyramidal neurons. Therefore, Woolley and McEwen concluded that estradiol exerts its effect on hippocampal dendritic spine density via a mechanism requiring the activation of NMDA receptors (Woolley and McEwen, 1994).

After moving to the Department of Neurological Surgery at the University of Washington, Woolley and her colleagues performed electrophysiological studies on hippocampal slices to further characterize the mechanisms of synaptic plasticity induced by estradiol. They recoded CA1 pyramidal neurons

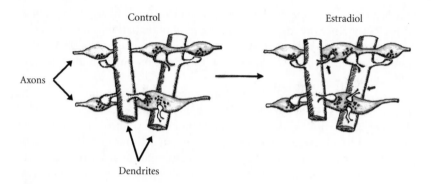

Figure 4.6. Estradiol induces an increase of spine synapses in the apical dendrites of CA1 pyramidal neurons mainly by promoting the formation of new synaptic contacts by preexisting presynaptic boutons and increasing the mean number of synapses per multiple synaptic bouton. A high proportion of these multiple-synaptic boutons form their additional synapses on different CA1 postsynaptic cells (arrows). (Courtesy of Dr. Catherine Woolley. Based on Woolley et al., 1996 and Yankova et al., 2001.)

from ovariectomized rats treated with estradiol or vehicle and then they filled the recorded neurons with biocytin to visualize the spines. Woolley and her collaborators observed that the effects of estradiol on the numbers of dendritic spines are associated with differences in both the intrinsic and synaptic properties of CA1 pyramidal neurons. The increase in the number of dendritic spines induced by estradiol was correlated with a decrease in cellular input resistance and with an increase in the sensitivity of CA1 pyramidal cells to NMDA receptor–mediated synaptic input. Furthermore, analyzing glutamate binding by autoradiography, they noticed an increased binding to the NMDA but not the AMPA subtype of glutamate receptor after estradiol treatment (Woolley, 1998; Woolley et al., 1997).

Changes in the number of dendritic spines and in NMDA receptor transmission may be related to the effects of estradiol on long-term potentiation in CA1. Indeed, the changes in the number of dendritic spines in the hippocampus during the estrus cycle are accompanied by modifications in synaptic long-term potentiation. Females during proestrus, the phase during which CA1 dendritic spines reach the highest values, also show the greatest degree of potentiation (Good et al., 1999; Warren et al., 1995). In contrast, the induction of paired-pulse long-term depression is severely attenuated during proestrus (Good et al., 1999). Furthermore, estradiol administration to ovariectomized rats exerts short- and long-term effects on neuronal excitability and synaptic function in the hippocampus (Wong and Moss, 1992) and increases long-term potentiation in CA1 in vivo (Cordoba Montoya and Carrer, 1997). Estradiol also increases long-term potentiation in hippocampal slices (Foy et al., 1999; Kim et al., 2002). The changes in dendritic spines and in long-term potentiation may be part of the same mechanism elicited by estrogen in regulating synaptic plasticity, since the magnitude of long-term potentiation is increased only when spine density is elevated, together with an increase in NMDA receptor transmission relative to AMPA receptor transmission (Smith and McMahon, 2005, 2006).

The involvement of NMDA receptors in the effect of estradiol on dendritic spines was also detected by Diane D. Murphy, from the National Institute of Neurological Disorders and Stroke, and Menahem Segal, from the Weizmann Institute in Israel, using dissociated hippocampal neurons in culture. The use of such cultures was an important step forward in the pharmacological identification of the mechanism involved in the effects of estradiol on dendritic spines. Murphy and Segal observed an increase in the numerical density of dendritic spines in cultured hippocampal neurons treated with estradiol that peaked within 2–3 days after the onset of hormonal exposure. The hormone increased spine density from 8.91 ± 0.57 to 20.44 ± 0.92 spines per 50 μm dendritic segment (mean $\pm$ SEM in ovariectomized rats treated with vehicle or estradiol, respectively). Murphy and Segal also observed that the increase in the number of dendritic spines caused by estradiol was completely reversed by the NMDA antagonist 2-APV. In contrast, AMPA/kainate antagonist DNQX had only a negligible effect on estradiol-induced spine formation. These data indicate that the effects of estradiol on dendritic spines are mediated by the activation of NMDA receptors (Murphy and Segal, 1996).

Another aspect examined by Murphy and Segal was the role of estrogen receptors in the hormonal induction of dendritic spine formation. They found that the effect of estradiol on hippocampal neurons in culture was stereoselective, since it was observed after incubation with 17β-estradiol but not after incubation with 17α-estradiol. Furthermore, the selective estrogen receptor modulator tamoxifen, which acts as an estrogen receptor antagonist in many situations, blocked the effect of estradiol. This suggested that the effect of estradiol on CA1 dendritic spines was mediated by the activation of classical estrogen receptors. However, it should be noted that other studies have found that the isomer 17α-estradiol is also able to induce the formation of dendritic spines in CA1 in vivo (MacLusky et al., 2005), suggesting that other forms of estrogen receptors (Toran-Allerand et al., 2005) may also be involved in the hormonal action. Murphy and Segal explored the signaling mechanisms involved in the formation of new dendritic spines in response to estradiol as well, and identified the cAMP response element binding protein (CREB) as a mediator of the hormonal effect. They found that estradiol, via the activation of cAMP-dependent protein kinase A, increases the phosphorylation of CREB, and that the CREB response leads to the increase in dendritic spine density (Murphy and Segal, 1997). Therefore, transcriptional regulation by CREB of the proteins involved in the formation of dendritic spines could mediate the effect of estradiol. Furthermore, they found that progesterone, which inhibits the effect of estradiol on the formation of dendritic spines, blocks the phosphorylation of CREB induced by estradiol. The effect of progesterone is probably exerted through its reduced metabolite tetrahydroprogesterone, which enhances spontaneous GABAergic activity and may counteract the effect of estradiol on neuronal excitability (Murphy and Segal, 2000).

Murphy and her collaborators identified brain-derived neurotrophic factor (BDNF) as one of the molecules involved in the effect of estradiol on dendritic spines in CA1 pyramidal neurons. They found that the hormone downregulates BDNF in the hippocampal cultures and that the treatment of these cultures with BDNF blocks the increase in dendritic spines induced by estradiol. In contrast, the effects of estradiol are mimicked by the blockade of BDNF actions with BDNF antibodies or by the inhibition of BDNF synthesis with a selective antisense oligonucleotide. Therefore, the effect of estradiol on the levels of BDNF may lead to the increase in dendritic spine density (Murphy et al., 1998a). The effect of estradiol on BDNF in the hippocampal cultures was associated with a decrease in inhibition and an increased excitatory tone in pyramidal neurons, suggesting that BDNF regulates GABAergic interneurons.

Murphy and her collaborators also examined the hypothesis that estradiol indirectly causes the formation of dendritic spines by reducing GABA inhibition, based on the observation that estrogen receptors are expressed by aspiny inhibitory hippocampal interneurons. They found that estradiol caused a marked decrease in the expression of glutamic acid decarboxylase and number of glutamic acid decarboxylase immunoreactive neurons in the cultures. In addition, estradiol decreased the size and frequency of GABAergic miniature inhibitory postsynaptic currents, and increased the frequency of miniature excitatory postsynaptic currents. Furthermore, the inhibition of the synthesis of GABA in the cultures, using mercaptopropionic acid, induced a significant increase in dendritic spine density, similar in magnitude to that induced by estradiol (Murphy et al., 1998b). These findings suggested that the increase in the density of dendritic spines induced by estradiol could be the consequence of a disinhibition of CA1 pyramidal neurons. Therefore, according to Murphy and Segal, the effect of estrogen on the growth of dendritic spines in CA1 pyramidal neurons in vitro would involve the activation of estrogen receptors on interneurons, causing decreased BDNF levels and glutamic acid decarboxylase expression. This will result in a reduction in inhibitory tone in the culture, leading to an increase in excitatory tone in CA1 pyramidal neurons. Within the postsynaptic CA1 pyramidal cell, excitation will cause an increase in free intracellular calcium concentration and CREB phosphorylation, leading to transcriptional activation to increase the synthesis of proteins necessary for the building of new dendritic spines (Segal and Murphy, 2001).

Evidence for such a mechanism was also obtained in vivo by Catherine Woolley and Charles N. Rudick at Northwestern University. They used c-Fos immunohistochemistry to assess the activation of pyramidal cells after estradiol administration. They observed that estradiol induces two sequential waves of c-Fos immunoreactivity: one at 2 hours and another at 24 hours (Rudick and Woolley, 2000). The first phase of activation of CA1 pyramidal cells by estradiol probably involves rapid nongenomic effects. In contrast, the second phase of activation is probably mediated by the activation of classical estrogen receptors, since it is blocked by tamoxifen (Rudick and Woolley, 2003). Using immunohistochemistry for the 65-kDa isoform of glutamic acid decarboxylase and a whole-cell voltage-clamp recording of GABAergic inhibitory postsynaptic currents, Rudick and Woolley detected that the second wave of pyramidal cell activation, at 24 hours, coincides with a transient suppression of GABAergic inhibition, as reflected by a reduction of GABAergic postsynaptic currents in pyramidal cells and suppression of glutamic acid decarboxylase immunoreactivity in the dendritic layers of CA1 (Rudick and Woolley, 2001). These findings suggested that the second phase of activation of CA1 pyramidal cells by estradiol could be mediated by an indirect suppression of GABAergic inhibitory inputs. Interestingly, the disinhibition of CA1 pyramidal cells after estrogen treatment precedes the increase in dendritic spines, further suggesting that a decrease in GABAergic transmission may be the cause of spine formation.

In addition to depending on local GABAergic neurons, estrogen-induced disinhibition is partially dependent on basal forebrain cholinergic neurons (Rudick et al., 2003). Csaba Leranth at Yale University and his collaborators have examined the role of hippocampal afferents on the plastic changes induced by estradiol on CA1 dendritic spines. They tested the idea that subcortical structures that express estrogen receptors and that are known to regulate hippocampal activity may play a role in the synaptic changes. To eliminate most subcortical afferents to the hippocampus, they performed, in ovariectomized rats, a unilateral transection of the fimbria/fornix. They then evaluated the number of spine synapses in CA1 using electron microscopy. The transection of the fimbria/fornix per se did not significantly affect the number of CA1 spines; however, the number of spines in estrogen-treated rats was higher in the hippocampus contralateral to the lesion than in the ipsilateral hippocampus. This finding suggested that, in addition to local effects of estradiol in the hippocampus, hormonal effects on subcortical afferents contribute to the induction of spine formation in CA1 (Leranth et al., 2000). To directly test this hypothesis, Leranth and Shanabrough (2001) analyzed the effect of local administration of estradiol in one of the brain regions that project to the hippocampus: the supramammillary area. Using retrograde tracer techniques, they first detected the expression of estrogen receptors in a large population of supramammillary neurons that project to the hippocampus. They then implanted cannulae filled with 17β-estradiol unilaterally into the supramammillary area of ovariectomized rats. Estradiol administration in the supramammillary area resulted in a significant increase in the number of spine synapses in CA1 compared to control animals in which cannulae filled with cholesterol were implanted in supramammillary area. Animals receiving estradiol in the supramammillary area also showed a higher number of spine synapses in CA1 than control animals that were implanted with estradiol-filled cannulae in the caudate nucleus. Similar results were obtained by the administration of estradiol in the medial septum/diagonal band of

Broca, a brain region that contains cholinergic neurons that express estrogen receptors and project to the hippocampus. Administration of estradiol in the medial septum/diagonal band induced a significant increase in CA1 spine synapse density (Lam and Leranth, 2003a). Interestingly, this increase was not detected when cholinergic neurons in the medial septum/diagonal band were killed by the infusion of 192 IgG-saporin, a ribosome inactivating protein. Another brain region that participates in the formation of dendritic spines in the hippocampus in response to estradiol is the median raphe. Implantation of estrogen-filled cannulae into the median raphe results in a significant increase in spine density in the hippocampus that is paralleled by a decrease in the density of serotonergic innervation of the strata lacunosum-moleculare and radiatum of the CA1 region (Prange-Kiel et al., 2004; Prange-Kiel and Rune, 2006). These findings indicate that subcortical afferents to the hippocampus are involved in the effects of estrogen on CA1 spine formation.

More recently, Catherine Woolley and Veronica A. Ledoux have examined the possible mechanisms for the estrogen-induced disinhibition of hippocampal CA1 pyramidal cells. They considered two not excluding possibilities: a decrease in the number of inhibitory boutons in synaptic contact with pyramidal cells and/or a decrease in GABA release at individual synapses. To analyze the first possibility, Ledoux and Woolley injected ovariectomized rats with estradiol benzoate or vehicle and reconstructed, from 60–80 serial electron micrographs, patches of CA1 pyramidal cell body membrane. The reconstruction of a structure by electron microscopy from such a large number of serial sections is an extremely time-consuming task reserved for people with exceptional technical skills. The results obtained, however, paid for the effort. Their hypothesis, based on the reported effects of estradiol in the hypothalamic arcuate nucleus, was that the hormone would induce axosomatic bouton displacement and glial hypertrophy. Therefore, they reconstructed the glial processes and the inhibitory boutons apposed to the patches of CA1 neuronal perikarya and quantified the percentage of somatic surface apposed by glia, the density of axosomatic boutons, and the distance from each inhibitory synaptic density to the nearest glial profile. However, none of these parameters was significantly affected by estradiol, indicating that estrogen-induced disinhibition of CA1 pyramidal cells was not mediated by plastic remodeling of axosomatic inhibitory synapses. This was a very important finding that further emphasizes that, rather than to promote identical plastic modifications in all brain structures, estradiol facilitates the onset of a variety of mechanisms of synaptic plasticity with regional specificity, depending on the function of the synaptic circuit involved.

Since estradiol was not affecting the number of inhibitory synapses, Ledoux and Woolley investigated whether the presynaptic boutons showed morphological changes that could be correlated with a decreased GABA release. Therefore, they assessed the volume of presynaptic boutons, the area of presynaptic densities, and the number, density, and distribution of synaptic vesicles in the presynaptic boutons to identify potential morphological correlates of a decreased GABA release. Interestingly, only one of these parameters was affected by estradiol: the location of synaptic vesicles within the presynaptic terminal. Indeed, estradiol induced a significant decrease in the number of synaptic vesicles adjacent to the presynaptic density, suggesting that the hormone induces disinhibition by decreasing the number of synaptic vesicles available for neurotransmitter release (Ledoux and Woolley, 2005). However, further studies using serial-section electron microscopic immunocytochemistry and immunofluorescence have revealed clusters of vesicles immunoreactive for the estrogen receptor α in inhibitory boutons in the hippocampal CA1 cell body layer. These vesicle clusters were detected in approximately one-third of perisomatic GABAergic boutons, but only in a specific neurochemical subpopulation of inhibitory presynaptic terminals. Interestingly, estradiol treatment shifts the location of these vesicles toward synapses (Hart et al., 2007). Therefore, estradiol may selectively affect the activity of specific subpopulations of inhibitory synapses by the regulation of the subcellular localization of a distinct subset of estrogen-responsive synaptic vesicles.

Woolley and her collaborators have also reexamined the presynaptic component involved in the plastic remodeling of dendritic spines. She and her colleagues reconstructed 410 complete presynaptic boutons from serial electron microscope sections from the CA1 stratum radiatum. They observed that estradiol increases the number of presynaptic boutons that form multiple synaptic contacts with dendritic spines, and increases the mean number of synapses per multiple synaptic bouton (Fig. 4.6). These multiple synaptic boutons have a more irregular morphology than single synaptic boutons, suggesting that they suffer shape modifications as they accumulate new synapses. The findings of Woolley and colleagues indicate that estradiol induces an increase of spine synapses mainly by promoting the formation of new postsynaptic contacts by preexisting presynaptic boutons (Woolley et al., 1996). In addition, a very high proportion of these multiple synaptic boutons form their additional synapses on different postsynaptic cells, indicating that estradiol increases the divergence of input from individual presynaptic boutons to multiple postsynaptic CA1 pyramidal cells (Yankova et al., 2001).

REGULATION BY ESTRADIOL AND PROGESTERONE OF GLIAL REMODELING IN THE HIPPOCAMPUS

As in the arcuate nucleus, estradiol and progesterone induce plastic remodeling of astrocytes in the hippocampus. In 1987, with my students Pedro Tranque and Gabriel Olmos, and collaborating with Isabel Suarez from Alcala University and Benjamin Fernandez from the Complutense University of Madrid, we examined the possible effect of estradiol on astrocytes. We found that estradiol administration to ovariectomized rats increases the surface density of GFAP immunoreactive astrocytes, but not the number of GFAP astrocytes, in the dentate gyrus of the hippocampus. The surface density of GFAP immunoreactive cells was assessed using stereological techniques as a measure of the space occupied by GFAP immunoreactive perikarya and processes in the dentate gyrus. Since the number of GFAP immunoreactive perikarya did not change after estradiol treatment, our result suggested that the hormone promotes the growth of astrocytes, probably increasing the growth and/or branching of astrocytic processes (Tranque et al., 1987). Some years later, Sonia Luquin examined the effects of estradiol and progesterone on hippocampal astrocytes and assessed whether astrocytes in this brain region showed plastic changes during the estrus cycle. She did not detect significant effects with an ovariectomy, estrogen treatment, progesterone treatment, or phase of the estrus cycle in the number of GFAP immunoreactive astrocytes in the hilus of the dentate gyrus. However, their surface density showed significant changes—it was increased in the afternoon of proestrus and on the morning of estrus compared to the morning of proestrus, diestrus, and metestrus. Furthermore, the surface density of GFAP immunoreactive astrocytes was decreased after an ovariectomy, and showed a dose-dependent increase in ovariectomized rats injected with 17β-estradiol (1, 10, or 300 μg/rat), alone or in combination with progesterone (500 μg/rat). In contrast, it was not affected by the administration of 17α-estradiol (Luquin et al., 1993).

An interesting finding was that the time-course of estradiol on astrocytes was affected by progesterone. The surface density of GFAP immunoreactive cells was significantly increased over control values by 5 hours after the injection of 17β-estradiol, and as early as 1 hour after the administration of progesterone. In addition, the separate injection of either 17β-estradiol or progesterone had smaller effects on the surface density of immunoreactive cells than did the administration of both hormones together. The surface density of GFAP immunoreactive cells reached maximal values by 24 hours after the combined administration of 17β-estradiol and progesterone and returned to control levels by 48 hours later. In contrast, in the rats injected with only one of the two hormones, the surface density of immunoreactive cells remained over control values for at least 9 days (Luquin et al., 1993). This indicates that, in contrast with the arcuate nucleus where progesterone blocks the effects of estradiol on astrocytes, in the dentate gyrus both progesterone and estradiol promote astroglia remodeling. In addition, both hormones interact to produce the termination of the effect. It is interesting to note that Gould and Woolley detected similar interactions of estradiol and progesterone in the regulation of the number of dendritic spines in CA1 pyramids (Gould et al., 1990a). As mentioned earlier in this chapter, progesterone treatment following estradiol initially increases spine density for a period of 2 to 6 hours but then induces a stronger decrease in spine density that estradiol alone. These findings suggest that the interaction of estradiol and progesterone is important in producing rapid modifications in growth and retraction of glial processes and dendritic spines during the estrus cycle.

The effects of estradiol and progesterone on hippocampal astrocytes may be mediated by direct effects on neurons and glia in the hippocampus or by actions on hippocampal afferents. Indeed, Lam and Leranth (2003b) have reported that estradiol infusion in the medial septum/diagonal band of Broca of adult ovariectomized rats reduces the density of GFAP acidic protein immunoreactive processes in the hippocampal CA1 and CA3 subfields. This effect is not detected in the dentate gyrus and is not mediated by changes in the number of GFAP immunoreactive cells. Therefore, estradiol acting on hippocampal afferents may exert a down-regulation of astroglia cell processes in specific regions of the hippocampus. It is interesting to note that the administration of estradiol in the medial septum/diagonal band of Broca also induces a significant increase in CA1 spine synapse density (Lam and Leranth, 2003a). Parallel changes in dendritic spines and GFAP immunoreactive processes have also been detected after administration of estradiol in another hippocampal afferent, the medial raphe. Local application of estradiol in this structure results in a 47% increase in spine synapse density and a 16% decrease in the density of GFAP immunoreactive processes in the stratum radiatum of the CA1 region (Prange-Kiel et al., 2004). Although the hormonal effects on astrocytes and dendritic spine synapses in the hippocampus have a similar time-course, so far there is no direct evidence for a causal relationship. Indeed, as I have mentioned before, Ledoux and Woolley did not detect any significant changes in the glial processes associated with CA1 pyramidal perikarya associated with the decrease in GABAergic neurotransmission (Ledoux and Woolley, 2005).

REGULATION BY ESTRADIOL AND PROGESTERONE OF ADULT NEUROGENESIS

Another important aspect of adult hippocampal plasticity modulated by estradiol and progesterone is the neurogenesis that occurs in the subgranular zone of the dentate gyrus. Two papers in 1999 demonstrated that cell proliferation in the adult dentate gyrus is affected by gonadal hormones. Liisa A. M. Galea and Bruce S. McEwen reported that cell proliferation, measured by the incorporation of [3H]thymidine, was different in the hippocampus of female wild meadow voles captured in the breeding season than in females captured during the nonbreeding season. Nonbreeding female meadow voles showed a higher number of [3H]thymidine-labeled cells than breeding females. The seasonal change in hippocampal proliferation was correlated with the seasonal change in the levels of adrenal steroids and gonadal steroids in female meadow voles. In particular, high levels of corticosterone and estradiol were correlated with a decreased cell proliferation (Galea and McEwen, 1999). In the same year, a publication from Patima Tanapat, Nicholas B. Hastings, Alison J. Reeves, and Elizabeth Gould from Princeton University reported that estradiol induces a transient increase in neurogenesis in the dentate gyrus of adult female rats. These authors, using the thymidine analog bromodeoxyuridine (BrdU) to assess cell proliferation, found that ovariectomy decreased the number of BrdU-labeled cells, while estradiol increased the number of BrdU-labeled cells in ovariectomized rats. Furthermore, the number of BrdU-labeled cells varied during the estrus cycle, and higher numbers were observed during proestrus compared with estrus and diestrus. Using immunohistochemistry and colocalization of BrdU with neuronal markers, they found that many of the BrdU-labeled cells were immature neurons. Another important observation was that the newly generated neurons showed a relatively short survival time (Tanapat et al., 1999).

The findings of Galea and McEwen showing estrogen regulation of hippocampal neurogenesis seem to be in contradiction with those of Tanapat and collaborators, since high estradiol levels were associated with an increased cell proliferation in rats, while high estradiol levels were associated with decreased proliferation in meadow voles. The differences probably reflect something more than species differences, since other studies have shown that the effect of estradiol on neurogenesis in the adult hippocampus depend on the dose, the duration of the hormonal exposure, and the duration of the previous hormonal deprivation. The effect of estradiol on hippocampal neurogenesis is dose-dependent, and high supraphysiological doses of the hormone do not affect cell proliferation (Tanapat et al., 2005). In addition, estradiol enhances proliferation after an acute administration (Banasr et al., 2001; Ormerod and Galea, 2001; Tanapat et al., 1999), but chronic administration of the hormone does not affect cell proliferation in the dentate gyrus (Perez-Martin et al., 2003; Tanapat et al., 2005). Furthermore, the acute administration of estradiol has a biphasic effect on cell proliferation: it first enhances proliferation in the dente gyrus within 4 hours of the hormonal administration (Banasr et al., 2001; Ormerod and Galea, 2001; Tanapat et al., 1999) and then, after 24–48 hours, it suppresses cell proliferation (Ormerod and Galea, 2001; Ormerod et al., 2003). Long-term ovarian hormone deprivation by ovariectomy also prevents the effect of estradiol on cell proliferation in the dentate gyrus (Perez-Martin et al., 2003). Therefore, the effect of estradiol on hippocampal neurogenesis may be considered an example of metaplasticity (see Chapter 1) in which the hormone, rather than promoting or inhibiting neurogenesis, adapts this plastic modification to changing homeodynamic needs. Progesterone is also involved in the metaplastic regulation, and the interaction of estradiol and progesterone effects may be highly relevant for the physiological fluctuation of neurogenesis, since progesterone reduces the enhancing effects of estradiol on cell proliferation in the dentate gyrus of adult female rats (Galea et al., 2006; Tanapat et al., 2005). Finally, it should be noted that estradiol may have independent effects on cell proliferation and survival. Thus, the work from the laboratory of Liisa Galea at the University of British Columbia, Canada, has shown that estradiol increases cell survival independent of its effects on cell proliferation in male and female meadow voles (Galea et al., 2006; Ormerod et al., 2004).

The effects of estradiol on neurogenesis in the adult hippocampus appear to be mediated by estrogen receptors. Studies from the laboratory of Liisa Galea have shown that the estrogen receptor antagonist ICI 182780 partially blocks the effect of estradiol, and that selective agonists for both estrogen receptor α and estrogen receptor β imitate the effect of estradiol. However, none of the agonists of estrogen receptors enhanced cell proliferation to the same extent as estradiol, and the estrogen receptor antagonist did not completely suppress the proliferative effect of estradiol, suggesting that other mechanisms, independent of classical estrogen receptors, may be involved in the promotion of neurogenesis by estradiol (Galea et al., 2006; Mazzucco et al., 2006). These may include membrane-associated estrogen receptors (Brailoiu et al., 2007), activation of signaling of growth factors such as granulins (Chiba et al., 2007), or the interaction with other neural or hormonal systems. For instance, serotonin innervation seems to be necessary for the acute induction of cell proliferation by estradiol, since the hormonal effect is blocked by a serotonin antagonist (Banasr et al., 2001). In contrast, the suppressive effect of estradiol on cell proliferation appears to be dependent on adrenal steroids (Ormerod et al., 2003). High adrenal steroid levels may also explain the lack of effect on hippocampal neurogenesis of chronic estradiol treatments (Perez-Martin et al., 2003).

In addition to the regulation of hippocampal neurogenesis, estradiol may also affect neuronal replacement in the olfactory bulb. As mentioned in Chapter 1, new neurons are generated in the subventricular zone of adult rodents. These newly generated neurons migrate rostrally and are incorporated in neuronal circuits in the olfactory bulb. Zsófia Hoyk and collaborators in Szeged, Hungary, have examined the effects of estradiol on the survival rate of newly integrated interneurons in the olfactory bulb of adult ovariectomized rats (Hoyk et al., 2006). The hormone was injected for six consecutive days, and on day 6 the animals were injected with BrdU every 2 hours for 8 hours. Twenty-one days after the administration of BrdU, the animals were killed and the number of BrdU cells was analyzed in the olfactory bulb (Fig. 4.7). Hoyk and collaborators detected a significant decrease in the number of BrdU cells in the granule cell layer and in the glomerular layer of the accessory olfactory bulb in the animals treated with estradiol compared to ovariectomized rats treated with a vehicle. In contrast, estradiol did not affect the number of BrdU cells in the main olfactory bulb (Hoyk et al., 2006). These findings suggest that estradiol regulates neuronal replacement in the accessory olfactory bulb, a region involved in the regulation of behavior by pheromones. Several mechanisms may be involved in the effect of estradiol on the number of BrdU immunoreactive cells in the accessory olfactory bulb. The hormone may regulate neurogenesis in the subventricular zone, the migration of newly generated neurons to the accessory olfactory bulb, and/or the survival of newly incorporated neurons in the accessory olfactory bulb. Concerning the first possibility, estradiol is known to regulate the generation of new neurons in the ventricular and subventricular zone of the embryonic neocortex (Martinez-Cerdeno et al., 2006), and in the adult rodent brain, the hormone stimulates the rate of neurogenesis in the subventricular zone in an animal model of experimental diabetes (Saravia et al., 2004) and a model of stroke (Suzuki et al., 2007b). Estradiol also regulates the integration of new neurons in brain regions controlling song in songbirds (Hidalgo et al., 1995; Johnson

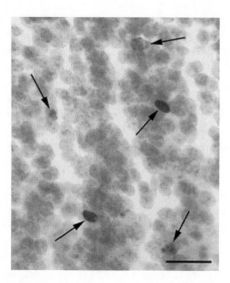

Figure 4.7. Methylene blue–stained section of an olfactory bulb showing BrdU-immunoreactive nuclei (arrows) in the granule cell layer of the main olfactory bulb of an ovariectomized rat. Scale bar = 50 μm. (Microphotograph courtesy of Dr. Arpad Parducz.)

and Bottjer, 1995; Nordeen and Nordeen, 1989), enhances cell proliferation in the hippocampus and the subventricular zone after brain injury in birds (Lee et al., 2007), and reduces glial proliferation after traumatic brain injury in rodents (Garcia-Estrada, 1993; see also Chapter 9). Progesterone and the progesterone metabolites dihydroprogesterone and tetrahydroprogesterone are also involved in the regulation of cell replacement in the adult rodent brain. Dihydroprogesterone and tetrahydroprogesterone have been shown to reduce cell proliferation in the subependymal layer of adult male rats (Giachino et al., 2003, 2004), and progesterone down-regulates glial proliferation after brain injury (Garcia-Estrada, 1993).

ROLE OF BRAIN ESTRADIOL SYNTHESIS IN THE REGULATION OF SYNAPTIC PLASTICITY AND NEURONAL REPLACEMENT

An important question that has recently emerged is the role of local estrogen synthesis by neural tissue in the regulation of synaptic plasticity. Testosterone and other C19 steroids are converted to estradiol by aromatase, an enzyme that consists of two components: a cytochrome P450 (P450arom), the product of the cyp19 gene, and the ubiquitous flavoprotein NADPH (reduced nicotinamide adenine dinucleotide phosphate)–cytochrome P450 reductase (Kamat et al., 2002; Simpson and Davis, 2001). Aromatase activity in the brain was

first detected by Frederick Naftolin and collaborators in the fetal human limbic system and in the rat hypothalamus (Naftolin et al., 1971a, b, 1972a; Ryan
et al., 1972). After these pioneering findings, numerous studies have shown
the expression, activity, and distribution of aromatase in the central nervous system of several species of vertebrates (Flores et al., 1973; Jakab et al.,
1993; Naftolin et al., 1975; Roselli et al., 1985; Schumacher and Balthazart,
1987; Shinoda et al., 1994) including humans (Ishunina et al., 2005; Sasano
et al., 1998; Steckelbroeck et al., 1999; Stoffel-Wagner et al., 1998, 1999; Yague
et al., 2006). Brain aromatase is thought to be involved in regulatory effects
of androgens, via conversion to estrogens, on reproductive neuroendocrine
development. Thus, by the regulation of local estrogen levels, aromatase
activity participates in the sexual differentiation of brain regions involved in
the control of gonadotropin secretion and sexual behavior (see Chapter 6).
During adult life, brain aromatase activity also controls local estrogen levels
within brain regions involved in the regulation of reproduction (Hutchison,
1991; Lephart, 1996; MacLusky and Naftolin, 1981; Naftolin, 1994). In addition to these classical reproductive roles of brain aromatase, its activity may
also modulate mood and affective status (Fink et al., 1999). Thus, aromatase
knockout (ArKO) female mice (Dalla et al., 2004)—but not ArKO male mice
(Dalla et al., 2005)—show increased depressive-like behaviors; polymorphisms
in the cyp19 gene are associated with depressive symptoms in women (Kravitz
et al., 2006). Furthermore, ArKO male mice develop compulsive behaviors,
such as excessive barbering, grooming, and wheel-running (Hill et al., 2007).
Modifications in brain aromatase activity may also play an important role in
the regulation of aggressive behavior (Soma, 2006; Trainor et al., 2006), and in
its modulation by social experiences (Trainor et al., 2006). Some clinical and
experimental studies suggest that aromatase activity also impacts cognitive
function. Two randomized, placebo-controlled clinical trials have assessed
the effect of aromatase inhibition on cognition. In one of these studies, the
aromatase inhibitor letrozole did not affect the improvements in visual and
verbal memory caused by testosterone administration on postmenopausal
women (Shah et al., 2006). In contrast, another clinical trial has shown that
aromatase inhibition in healthy older men prevents the improvement in verbal
memory produced by testosterone (Cherrier et al., 2005). Other studies suggest that aromatase inhibitors used as a treatment for breast cancer may impair
verbal and visual learning in women (Bender et al., 2007; Jenkins et al., 2002).
Studies in animals also suggest that aromatase activity may interfere with
cognitive processing. Local aromatization of testosterone to estradiol within
the brain of songbirds enhances hippocampal function, including spatial
memory performance (Oberlander et al., 2004). In contrast, in male rats, inhibition of brain aromatase counteracts spatial learning impairment induced by
the injection of testosterone into the hippocampus (Moradpour et al., 2006),
and the systemic administration of an aromatase inhibitor facilitates working memory acquisition (Alejandre-Gomez et al., 2007). Aromatase activity
may therefore improve or impair specific cognitive modalities, probably by

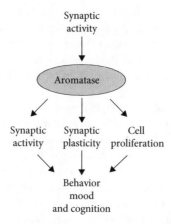

Figure 4.8. Estrogen synthesized in the brain by the enzyme aromatase is a regulator of synaptic plasticity and cellular replacement. Aromatase activity in neurons is rapidly regulated by synaptic activity. In turn, aromatase regulates synaptic function, synaptic plasticity, and neurogenesis. Brain aromatase, conceivably via its actions on synapses and neurogenesis, affects behavior, mood, and cognition.

the fine regulation of estradiol levels at precise moments and in specific brain regions, since estradiol exerts dose, time, and region-specific actions on cognition (Holmes et al., 2002; Sinopoli et al., 2006; Wide et al., 2004).

The role of aromatase on cognition may be related to its regulatory actions on brain plasticity (Fig. 4.8). Gabriele M. Rune from the University of Hamburg and her collaborators have provided solid evidence indicating that local estradiol synthesis in the hippocampus by the enzyme aromatase induces dendritic spine synapses in CA1 pyramidal hippocampal neurons. They have shown that the pharmacological inhibition of aromatase activity in hippocampal slices decreases the number of synapses and the expression of spinophilin, a marker of dendritic spines, and synaptophysin, a protein of presynaptic vesicles (Kretz et al., 2004; Prange-Kiel et al., 2006; Prange-Kiel and Rune, 2006; Rune and Frotscher, 2005). Therefore, at least in vitro, estradiol synthesized by hippocampal cells is an endogenous regulator of synaptic plasticity (see below for in vivo studies using aromatase inhibitors). Studies from Suguru Kawato and his collaborators at the University of Tokyo have shown that, in contrast to what is observed in females, estradiol rapidly enhances long-term synaptic depression in CA1, CA3, and dentate gyrus in hippocampal slices from male rats (Mukai et al., 2007). This suggests that locally formed estradiol in the hippocampus of male rats may exert a different regulation of functional synaptic plasticity than hormonal estradiol in females. However, as in females, estradiol increases the number of dendritic spines in CA1 pyramidal neurons in hippocampal slices from male rats by a mechanism involving the mitogen-activated protein kinase and the estrogen receptor α (Mukai et al., 2007; Ogiue-Ikeda et al., 2008). The enzyme may also influence synaptic development and plasticity in other nonreproductive regions of the central nervous system, since cerebellar Purkinje cells in ArKO mice show decreased dendritic growth and decreased formation of dendritic spines and synapses (Sasahara et al., 2007).

The effects of aromatase on behavior and brain plasticity suggest that the enzyme may affect synaptic function and information processing through neuronal circuits. Interestingly, studies by Jacques Balthazart from the University of Liège and Gregory F. Ball from Johns Hopkins University and their collaborators have demonstrated that brain aromatase is rapidly modulated by afferent synaptic inputs (including glutamatergic afferents) by a mechanism potentially mediated by increased intracellular Ca^{2+} levels, and Ca^{2+}-dependent phosphorylation that could be mimicked by K^+-induced depolarization (Balthazart and Ball, 2006; Balthazart et al., 2006a, b; Cornil et al., 2006). These studies have shown that brain estrogen levels can be regulated within minutes by changes in aromatase activity. The rapid modulation of aromatase activity by synaptic inputs has implications for the processing of information by neuronal circuits. Thus, acute inhibition of aromatase activity in the dorsal horn of the spinal cord in quail results in a rapid (within 1 minute) reduction in the response to a thermal painful stimulus (Evrard, 2006; Evrard and Balthazart, 2004). Therefore, estradiol produced by local aromatase activity exerts rapid effects on neuronal physiology, probably by nongenomic mechanisms of action. This role of aromatase as an acute modulator of neuronal information processing also has implications for behavior. Indeed, Balthazart and colleagues have shown that rapid modulation of aromatase activity and the consequent rapid fluctuations in brain estrogen concentrations are followed within minutes by changes in male sexual behavior (Balthazart and Ball, 2006; Balthazart et al., 2006a, b; Cornil et al., 2006; Taziaux et al., 2007). Therefore, synaptic activity may quickly regulate brain aromatase activity and, consequently, local estrogen formation by aromatase may quickly regulate synaptic function and behavior (Fig. 4.8). In addition, Rune and collaborators have shown that the aromatase inhibitor fadrozole decreases GABA synthesis in hippocampal cultures, while bicuculline, a $GABA_A$ receptor blocker that induces overexcitation of hippocampal neurons, decreases both the number of dendritic spines and the synthesis of estradiol in hippocampal slices, suggesting that aromatase may play an important role in brain function by linking neuronal activity and synaptic plasticity (Zhou et al., 2007). Since testosterone may be synthesized from endogenous cholesterol in the rat hippocampus (Hojo et al., 2004; Mukai et al., 2006), the neuromodulatory role of aromatase may at least in part be independent of exogenous testosterone. However, brain aromatase may be subjected to endocrine regulation, and a recent study from Prange-Kiel, Rune, and collaborators indicate that GnRH regulates estradiol synthesis and spine synaptic density in a dose-dependent manner in hippocampal cells by a mechanism mediated by aromatase (Prange-Kiel et al., 2008). Therefore, the neuromodulatory and neuroplastic actions of brain aromatase may play an important role by coupling neuronal and hormonal signaling with behavior and cognition.

The subcellular localization of aromatase within the brain suggests that its neuromodulatory function may be exerted, at least in part, directly on synapses. In the brain of birds and mammals, aromatase immunoreactivity is located in the cytoplasm of neuronal perikarya and neuronal processes (Hojo et al., 2004; Ishunina et al., 2005; Jakab et al., 1993; Shinoda et al., 1994; Yague et al., 2006). In addition, aromatase is present in presynaptic terminals. The localization of aromatase on synapses was indicated by early studies showing aromatase activity in synaptosomal preparations (Schlinger and Arnold, 1992; Schlinger and Callard, 1989). Immunohistochemical localization of aromatase in brain sections from quails, rats, monkeys, and humans, as well as studies by immunoelectron microscopy, have confirmed that the enzyme is located in presynaptic terminals (Horvath et al., 1997c; Naftolin et al., 1996b; Peterson et al., 2005; Saldanha et al., 2000; Yague et al., 2006). Therefore, estrogen formed on presynaptic terminals may potentially be released to activate estrogen receptors located in postsynaptic structures (Milner et al., 2005; Towart et al., 2003) or may also potentially act within the presynaptic terminals, targeting synaptic vesicles expressing estrogen receptors (Hart et al., 2007; Woolley, 2007) to regulate neurotransmitter release and synaptic plasticity.

Local synthesis of estradiol in the hippocampus is also involved in the regulation of adult neurogenesis. The laboratory of Gabriele Rune in Hamburg has shown that the treatment of hippocampal dispersion cultures with letrozole, a specific aromatase inhibitor, decreases the number of proliferative cells and increases the number of apoptotic cells. Similar effects were observed after the inhibition of steroidogenesis in cultures using siRNA against the steroidogenic acute regulatory protein (StAR). StAR is one of the proteins involved in the transport of cholesterol through the hydrophilic space between the outer and inner mitochondrial membranes to allow cholesterol to reach the cytochrome P450 side-chain cleavage (P450scc), the first enzyme in the steroidogenic pathway, in which converts cholesterol to pregnenolone (Hauet et al., 2005; Stocco, 2001; see also Chapter 9). Application of estradiol to the medium had no effect on proliferation and apoptosis, whereas the antiproliferative and proapoptotic effects of StAR knock-down and letrozole treatment were restored by the treatment of the cultures with estradiol (Fester et al., 2006). These findings suggest that local estradiol formed within the rodent hippocampus may regulate neurogenesis, at least under certain conditions (Fig. 4.8). Locally formed estradiol has also been shown to promote cell proliferation in the hippocampus and the subventricular zone in the zebra finch brain after injury (Lee et al., 2007). Furthermore, other steroids locally synthesized in the hippocampus may also act as modulators of adult neurogenesis. One of these steroids is pregnenolone which is synthesized from cholesterol and is the precursor of progesterone, testosterone, and estradiol. Willy Mayo and his

collaborators at INSERM in Bordeaux, France, analyzed the effect of pregnenolone sulfate on adult hippocampal neurogenesis and found that its administration to young adult or aged male rats increases the number of cells that
incorporate BrdU in the dentate gyrus, and the expression of PSA-N-CAM
(Mayo et al., 2005), which is also a marker of neurogenesis (Bonfanti, 2006).

ANDROGENS, SYNAPTIC PLASTICITY, AND CELLULAR REPLACEMENT IN THE SONG SYSTEM OF SONGBIRDS

In 1980, Fernando Nottebohm from Rockefeller University provided one
of the first and more striking evidence linking androgen-induced neuronal
plasticity in adult animals and the generation of a new specific behavior. He
showed that the treatment of adult ovariectomized female canaries with testosterone increased the volume of two sexually dimorphic regions of the telencephalon, the hyperstriatum ventrale pars caudale (HVC, the caudal nucleus
of the ventral neostriatum, subsequently renamed High Vocal Center and
then HVC as a proper noun; Reiner et al., 2004), and the nucleus robustus
archistriatalis (now robustus arcopallialis or RA) (Nottebohm, 1980). These
telencephalic regions are involved in male song behavior and are larger in
males than in females (see Chapter 6). Interestingly, the hormonal treatment
of adult females resulted in the generation of male-like song behavior, suggesting that the morphological mutability of the HVC and the nucleus RA
induced by testosterone in adult animals was casually linked to the generation
of a new behavior. Further studies demonstrated that physiological seasonal
variation in circulating androgens also induced changes in male song behavior and in the volume of the telencephalic nuclei controlling such behavior
(Kirn et al., 1994; Nottebohm, 1981). Logically, the question arises on how
these testosterone-induced changes in the volume of specific brain structures
are generated. To assess whether testosterone could induce the incorporation
of new neurons, Fernando Nottebohm and Steven A. Goldman identified
proliferating cells using radiolabeled thymidine and autoradiography. They
found a relatively high number of neurons that incorporate [3H]thymidine in
the HVC of adult intact female canaries, even in the absence of testosterone
treatment. This indicated that new neurons were incorporated into this brain
structure, but that this process was not regulated by testosterone (Goldman
and Nottebohm, 1983).

The analysis by electron microscopy of newly generated, [3H]thymidine-
labeled neurons revealed that these neurons, inserted into existing neural
networks, were contacted in the cell body and proximal dendrites by several types of synaptic terminals, with symmetrical or asymmetrical synaptic
junctions (Burd and Nottebohm, 1985). In addition, many newly generated
neurons grow long axons to the nucleus RA and become part of the efferent pathway for song control (Alvarez-Buylla et al., 1990; Kirn et al., 1991).
Therefore, the newly generated neurons are integrated into functional synaptic circuits, and the plasticity in the song system of song birds represents an

example of hormonally regulated cellular replacement within specific neuronal circuits (see also Chapter 8).

Goldman and Nottebohm identified the origin of the new neurons in the ventricular zone overlying the HVC (where stem cells proliferate). They also reported that although testosterone did not induce this process of neurogenesis, the hormone increased glial and endothelial proliferation (Goldman and Nottebohm, 1983). More recent studies have demonstrated that although neurogenesis is not initiated by testosterone, both testosterone and its metabolite estradiol modulate the integration and survival of new neurons in the HVC (Hidalgo et al., 1995; Johnson and Bottjer, 1995; Nordeen and Nordeen, 1989; Rasika et al., 1994). In addition, Abner Louissaint, Sudha Rao, Caroline Leventhal, and Steven A. Goldman have shown that the recruitment of new neurons in the HVC is influenced by previous hormonal effects on endothelial proliferation. Testosterone induces the production of vascular endothelial growth factor and its receptor, VEGFR-2/Quek1/KDR, in the HVC. In turn, vascular endothelial growth factor, but not gonadal steroids, induces endothelial cell proliferation. Then, testosterone induces the production of BDNF (brain-derived neurotrophic factor) by endothelial cells, and this factor promotes the migration and recruitment of neurons from the ventricular zone to the HVC (Louissaint et al., 2002).

To further characterize the morphological cellular changes induced by testosterone and to assess whether the hormone regulates synaptic connectivity in the telencephalic regions controlling singing, Fernando Nottebohm and Timothy J. DeVoogd, using a quantitative analysis on Golgi-stained preparations, examined the effect of hormonal treatments on the dendritic arbor in neurons from the nucleus RA. They found that physiological doses of testosterone, estradiol, or dihydrotestosterone increased dendritic length. In addition, dendrites from ovariectomized females treated with testosterone had more branches than the dendrites from animals treated with estradiol or dihydrotestosterone, and had a morphological appearance that resembled the dendrites of adult males (DeVoogd and Nottebohm, 1981). A further step forward in the characterization of the plastic changes induced by testosterone was the demonstration, together with Barbara Nixdorf, that the number of synapses formed on neurons of the nucleus RA were also affected by the hormonal treatment (DeVoogd et al., 1985). Systemic testosterone treatment of adult female canaries produced a 51% increase in the number of synapses formed on RA neurons, an increase in the number of synaptic vesicles per synapse, and larger synapses. In addition, housing in spring-like conditions was also associated with larger synapses and more vesicles per synapse than housing in fall-like conditions. Plastic changes induced by testosterone have also been observed in the HVC, where singing female canaries implanted with testosterone propionate have an increased number of neuronal soma-somatic gap junctions compared with the untreated singing females. The hormonal effect on gap junctions is accompanied by the development of a male-like song, suggesting that modifications in the electric coupling between neurons of the HVC could be important for the testosterone-dependent changes of the song pattern of canaries (Gahr and Garcia-Segura, 1996).

ANDROGENS AND SYNAPTIC PLASTICITY IN MOTONEURONS

Another region of the central nervous system showing androgen-induced plasticity related to a specific behavior is the spinal cord. In 1986, the laboratory of Arthur P. Arnold reported that castration of adult rats produced a marked decrease in the dendritic length and soma size of androgen-sensitive motoneurons of the spinal nucleus of the bulbocavernosus, and that these plastic changes were reversed by androgen replacement (Kurz et al., 1986). Six years earlier, S. Marc Breedlove and Arthur P. Arnold had reported that the spinal nucleus of the bulbocavernosus is smaller in females than in males, and that both motoneurons in this nucleus and the muscles they innervate express androgen receptors (Breedlove and Arnold, 1980). Furthermore, Breedlove and Arnold found that the size of the individual spinal nucleus of bulbocavernosus neurons was increased in the presence of androgen (Breedlove and Arnold, 1981). Motoneurons of the spinal nucleus of the bulbocavernosus innervate perineal muscles (bulbocavernosus and levator ani) are involved in penile reflexes and mediate male copulatory functions. Thus, the morphological effects in neuronal perikarya and dendrites induced by androgens in these motoneurons (Fargo and Sengelaub, 2004; Kurz et al., 1991) further support a link between androgen-induced neuronal plasticity and a specific behavior.

Further studies showed that testosterone increases the number of synaptic inputs on these neurons (Leedy et al., 1987; Matsumoto, 1997; Matsumoto et al., 1988) and that androgens delay the development-related loss of the multiple innervations to muscle fibers of the levator ani muscle (Jordan et al., 1989). Neuronal size, dendritic length, and size of levator ani and bulbocavernosus muscles are also reduced in the spinal nucleus of the bulbocavernosus in castrated male mice (Zuloaga et al., 2007). Androgens also control synaptic inputs on the dorsolateral nucleus of the rat lumbar spinal cord, increasing dendritic length in motoneurons from this nucleus (Kurz et al., 1991).

Motoneurons of the spinal nucleus of the bulbocavernosus are a good example of how synaptic targets may affect plasticity in presynaptic neurons, since the effect of androgens on the motoneurons is related with an action on the target muscles. Indeed, androgens increase the size of the bulbocavernosus and levator ani muscles, and in turn, muscle size regulates the dendritic size of the motoneurons of the spinal nucleus of the bulbocavernosus. Evidence for this was obtained by Rand and Breedlove (1995), who administered testosterone or an androgen receptor antagonist in the target muscles and observed the effect on dendrites in the spinal nucleus of the bulbocavernosus. They found that motoneurons innervating androgen-deprived muscles had dendritic arbors which were reduced by 44% overall relative to those of motoneurons innervating androgen-stimulated muscles, and significant reductions in dendrite lengths. More recent studies suggest that testosterone may promote the release of trophic factors by muscle cells or interact with trophic factors produced by these cells to induce dendritic growth in motoneurons. Yang et al. (2004) have shown that BDNF administered in the muscle increases dendritic growth in motoneurons from the spinal nucleus of the bulbocavernosus, and that the join treatment with BDNF and testosterone results in longer dendrites than BDNF or testosterone alone.

Androgen effects were also detected in motoneurons that control the syrinx in songbirds. Clower et al. (1989) reported that synapse density was lower in testosterone-treated canaries than in control canaries in the caudal portion of the hypoglossal nucleus, which contains the motoneurons that control the syrinx. In addition, the number of synapses was lower in the fall than in spring, suggesting that the synaptic changes induced by testosterone may be related to the seasonal control of vocalization.

More evidence for the effects of androgens on synaptic inputs on motoneurons was obtained in the laboratory of Kathryn J. Jones at Loyola University Chicago. For many years Jones has been studying the effects of androgens on synaptic inputs on hamster motoneurons after an axotomy. Her work has shown that androgens prevent the synaptic loss of presynaptic inputs on motoneurons that occurs after axotomy (Jones et al., 1997a; see also Chapter 9). Testosterone has been also shown to decrease synaptic loss on motoneurons of the spinal nucleus of the bulbocavernosus muscle after exposure to chronic stress (Matsumoto, 2005).

ANDROGENS, SYNAPTIC PLASTICITY, AND CELLULAR REPLACEMENT IN THE MAMMALIAN BRAIN

The effects of androgens on synaptic plasticity were also detected in regions of the mammalian brain related to neuroendocrine regulation and sexual behavior. The research team of Michael J. Baum at the Department of Biology at Boston University studied the dendrites of a sexually dimorphic group of cells at the dorsal border of the preoptic/anterior hypothalamic area of ferrets, using the Golgi-Cox impregnation method. Tridimensional reconstruction of 78 multipolar neurons from 12 ferrets revealed significant sex differences in the somal area and dendritic morphology, including total length, number of branches, and total dendritic surface area. In addition, testosterone administration increased dendritic arborization in both sexes (Cherry et al., 1992).

Another brain region in which androgens regulate the somal sizeand dendritic length is the medial amygdala, a brain region involved in the control of sexual behavior. Gomez and Newman (1991), using the Golgi method, detected in male Syrian hamsters a decline in dendritic length and branching and a decline in the volume of neuronal perikarya of the posterior medial amygdala. Testosterone and estradiol prevent the effect of castration on the length and branching of dendrites in the posterior medial amygdala. In contrast, the nonaromatizable testosterone metabolite 5α-dihydrotestosterone, which acts on androgen receptors, did not prevent the effect of castration (Gomez and Newman, 1991). This suggests that the effect of testosterone is mediated through the conversion to estradiol by the enzyme aromatase and the consequent activation of estrogen receptors. Bradley M. Cooke, S. Marc Breedlove, and their collaborators have also demonstrated that circulating androgen regulates the volume of the posterodorsal subnucleus of the medial amygdala. These effects of androgens are in part mediated by an increase in the volume of neurons in this brain area. In addition, it is probable that changes in the growth of dendrites and glial processes may also influence the total volume of the nucleus. Testosterone increases the size of neuronal perikarya and the regional volume of the posterodorsal subnucleus of the medial amygdala in castrated male rats. Interestingly, administration of dihydrotestosterone and estradiol reverses the effect of castration, suggesting that the activation of both androgen and estrogen receptors is involved in the action of androgens on neuronal size. In contrast, only estrogen receptors appear to mediate the effects of testosterone on the regional volume of the posterodorsal subnucleus of the medial amygdala (Cooke et al., 1999, 2003). Furthermore, the volume of the posterodorsal subnucleus of the medial amygdala increases significantly during puberty in male Syrian hamsters (Romeo and Sisk, 2001; see also Chapter 7), and seasonal variation in androgen is correlated with morphologic plasticity in this nucleus in the Siberian hamster (Cooke et al., 2002a, b). Furthermore, Christie D. Fowler, Marc E. Freeman, and Zuoxin Wang from Florida State University in Tallahassee have shown that testosterone increases the incorporation of newly generated cells in the amygdala of adult male meadow voles (Fowler et al., 2003). Treatment of castrated animals with testosterone propionate and estradiol benzoate resulted in a significant increase in the density of cells that were labeled with the cell proliferation marker BrdU in the amygdala. In contrast, dihydrotestosterone did not affect the number of BrdU-labeled cells, suggesting that the effect of testosterone may be mediated by its aromatization to estradiol. It is probable that the androgen-induced morphological changes in the medial amygdala are associated with the role of this nucleus in the actions of androgens on sexual behavior (Cooke, 2006).

In addition to their role in the regulation of reproduction and sexual and aggressive behaviors (Bancroft, 2005; Christiansen, 2001; Soma, 2006; Wilson, 2001), androgens exert analgesic and anxiolytic effects (Edinger and Frye, 2005) and modulate mood and cognition (Cherrier, 2005; Christiansen, 2001; Janowsky, 2006). Therefore, neuroplastic actions of androgens in brain regions not involved in the control of reproduction may affect affection, learning, and memory. The effects of androgens on neurogenesis in the adult hippocampus have not been explored in detail, and the results are in some aspects contradictory. Some studies have shown no effect, other studies suggest that androgens promote neurogenesis or survival of newly generated neurons, and there is also evidence that some androgens may reduce neurogenesis (Galea et al., 2006). For instance, DHEA increases cell proliferation and cell survival in the dentate gyrus of adult male rats (Karishma and Herbert, 2002), while 19-nortestosterone reduces the number of BrdU-labeled cells in the dentate gyrus of adult male and female rats (Brannvall et al., 2005). We have more information on the effects of androgens on synaptic plasticity in the hippocampus. This is relatively recent information, since in contrast to the numerous studies that have analyzed the effect of estradiol on synaptic plasticity in the hippocampus, the possible influence of androgens on synaptic plasticity in this brain region was largely ignored. Electrophysiological studies suggested that testosterone reduces long-term potentiation in CA1 in castrated males (Harley et al., 2000), in contrast to the induction of long-term potentiation by estrogen in females. However, the effects of androgens on dendritic spines were not assessed. The situation changed when Csaba Leranth and his collaborators at Yale University, together with Neil J. MacLusky then at Columbia University, New York , demonstrated that castration and testosterone replacement affected the number of synapses on CA1 dendritic spines in male rats (Leranth et al., 2003).

Using unbiased morphometric techniques applied to electron microscopy, Leranth and his collaborators detected that castrated males had a reduction of about 50% in the number of dendritic spine synapses in the stratum radiatum of the CA1 subfield of the hippocampal formation (Leranth et al., 2003). Given that the hippocampus expresses aromatase, the enzyme that catalyzes the conversion of androgens to estrogens, Leranth and his collaborators considered as possible the effect of an orchidectomy might be due to decreased hippocampal estrogen biosynthesis, resulting from the loss of circulating testosterone. To test this idea, rats were orchidectomized and then given replacement treatments with testosterone, dihydrotestosterone, or estradiol. The expectation was that if the effects of orchidectomy were due to the loss of testicular androgen as a substrate for intracerebral estrogen biosynthesis, then these effects should be reversed by treatment with testosterone or estradiol, but not by dihydrotestosterone, a metabolite of testosterone that cannot be aromatized into estradiol (MacLusky et al., 2006b). As expected, the testosterone replacement recovered the number of dendritic spine synapses to control values. These findings indicated that dendritic spine synapses in the hippocampus of male rats are also under the control of gonadal hormones, as in females. However, a crucial and unexpected observation was that dihydrotestosterone had similar effects to that of testosterone, and increased the dendritic spine synapse numbers of castrated males to control levels. This was an important discovery, since it clearly showed that androgens per se, without conversion to estrogens, are able to affect synaptic formation or stability in the hippocampus of adult animals. Furthermore, estradiol treatment did not affect the number of spine synapses in castrated males, further indicating that the effect of testosterone was not mediated by its conversion into estradiol (Leranth et al., 2003).

Subsequent studies by Csaba Leranth and his co-workers lead to another important finding: androgens also regulate spine synapses in the hippocampus of females. It should be noted that testosterone is produced by the rat ovary, and that circulating levels of testosterone in female rats are higher than that of estradiol (Rush and Blake, 1982). Therefore, it was conceivable that testosterone could also affect spine synapses in the hippocampus of female rats. Indeed, Leranth and his collaborators discovered that pyramidal cell spine synapse density was significantly higher in the CA1 stratum radiatum of ovariectomized females treated with testosterone propionate or dihydrotestosterone than that of ovariectomized females treated with vehicle in the same hippocampal region. This finding indicated that androgens also regulate synapse plasticity of CA1 hippocampal dendritic spines in females. An interesting observation was that although both testosterone propionate and dihydrotestosterone increased the number of spine synapses, the effect of testosterone was more potent than that of dihydrotestosterone. This suggested that part of the effect of testosterone propionate in the female hippocampus was due to its conversion into estradiol. Leranth and his collaborators then assessed the effect of an inhibitor of aromatase, the enzyme that catalyzes the conversion of testosterone into estradiol. Treatment of ovariectomized females with the aromatase inhibitor letrozole did not affect the basal number of spine synapses; however, letrozole significantly reduced the effect of testosterone propionate on the number of CA1 spine synapses, confirming that part of the effect of testosterone on CA1 synapses was mediated by estrogen biosynthesis. As expected, the aromatase inhibitor did not affect the response of synapses to the nonaromatizable androgen dihydrotestosterone (Leranth et al., 2004).

These findings suggest that, in male brains, androgens exert a direct effect on the number of CA1 spine synapses, while in females, this effect is in part direct and in part mediated by estrogen. Further studies that assessed the effect of the adrenal androgen DHEA have confirmed this point. Leranth and his collaborators observed that the number of CA1 spine synapses was increased in adult castrated male rats and in adult ovariectomized females after the administration of DHEA. However, the pretreatment with the aromatase inhibitor letrozole abolished the induction of CA1 spine synapses by DHEA in females, but did not significantly affect the response to DHEA in castrated males (Hajszan et al., 2004; MacLusky et al., 2004). Therefore, DHEA may exert its effect on spine synapses in females after consecutive metabolism to testosterone and estradiol, while in males, DHEA does not need to be converted into estradiol to exert its effect.

The mechanisms of action of androgens in regulating spine synapses in the hippocampus have not yet been completely elucidated. In particular, the role of androgen receptors is unclear. DHEA, testosterone, and dihydrotestosterone induced a similar number on synapses, although their potency as androgen receptor agonists is very different. In addition, the androgen receptor antagonist flutamide not only was unable to block the increase in synapses induced by DHEA and dihydrotestosterone, but unexpectedly, also further increased the effects of androgens, and by itself, increased the number of synapses (MacLusky et al., 2004, 2006b). Furthermore, androgen receptor–deficient Tfm male rats exhibit increases in CA1 spine synapse density in response to dihydrotestosterone that are indistinguishable from the effects observed in normal wild-type males (MacLusky et al., 2006a). All these findings suggest that the effects of androgens on CA1 spine synapses are not mediated by classical androgen receptor transcriptional mechanisms. Several possible alternative mechanisms may be postulated, including androgen activation of kinases involved in membrane signaling. In this regard, it is important to mention that androgen receptors have been detected in extranuclear sites in the brain, including dendrites, axons, synaptic terminals, and glial processes (DonCarlos et al., 2003, 2006; Lorenz et al., 2005; Sarkey et al., 2008). Alternatively, androgens may be converted into metabolites capable of interacting with the GABA receptor (Melcangi et al., 2001) or with the estrogen receptor β (Handa et al., 2008). Finally, the possible relation of the changes induced by androgens in the number of dendritic spines with functional modifications in synaptic plasticity remains to be explored.

Chapter 5

Hormonal Influences on Brain Plasticity: III. Peptide Hormones

INTRODUCTION: PEPTIDE HORMONES AS REGULATORS OF BRAIN REMODELING

In the two previous chapters I have examined neuroplastic effects of nonpeptide hormones in the adult central nervous system. In this chapter I will analyze the role of peptide hormones in the regulation of neural mutability and the involved cellular and molecular mechanisms. I will first consider the effects of vasopressin and oxytocin, hormones released in the neurohypophysis. Vasopressin and oxytocin act both as hormones and as neuromodulators. For instance, in addition to being released as a hormone by magnocellular vasopressin neurons, several parvocellular neurons located in the paraventricular and suprachiasmatic nuclei of the hypothalamus, the bed nucleus of the stria terminalis, and the medial amygdala send vasopressinergic innervation to other brain regions. The neuroplastic actions of oxytocin, which is involved in the promotion of synaptic plasticity on magnocellular oxytocinergic neurons in the hypothalamus, may also represent an autocrine or paracrine action rather than a hormonal one, since oxytocin is locally released in the brain in addition to being released in the neurohypophysis.

This duality of hormonal and autocrine/paracrine actions will be a common consideration regarding the effects of peptide hormones on neural remodeling. This will also be the case for the hypothalamic corticotropin-releasing hormone (CRH) and the pituitary hormone prolactin. CRH (also known as corticotropin-releasing factor) regulates synaptic plasticity in different brain regions, including the neuronal networks involved with control of the stress response. CRH, together with several related peptides (the urocortins), is an important mediator for the cognitive and emotional effects of stress. Another peptide hormone, prolactin, affects the activity of specific neurons in the brain (including magnocellular oxytocinergic neurons), and regulates neurogenesis in the subventricular zone of the adult brain.

Gonadotropin-releasing hormone (GnRH) plays an important role in the regulation of synaptic plasticity via the modulation of local estradiol synthesis within the brain. Particular attention will be devoted in this chapter to insulin, since there is abundant information on the neuroplastic alterations caused by insufficient hormonal insulin levels or by decreased responsiveness to the hormone. Insulin is transported through the blood–brain barrier, and may play a prominent role in the regulation of morphological and functional synaptic plasticity and cell replacement in the adult brain. Another protein hormone that is known to regulate brain plasticity is growth hormone. As is the case for insulin and for other peptide hormones, growth hormone crosses the blood–brain barrier, and may act directly on growth hormone receptors expressed in the brain and spinal cord. In addition, growth hormone may indirectly regulate neural mutability via the regulation of the levels of insulin-like growth factor-I (IGF-I), which exerts a variety of morphological and functional plastic effects in the central nervous system. I will analyze with some detail the plastic actions of IGF-I, since they have been relatively well studied.

Less characterized are the neuroplastic effects of erythropoietin, although there is good evidence indicating that this hormone regulates neurogenesis in the adult brain, in particular under pathological conditions. Circulating angiotensin II, as well as angiotensin peptides locally formed in the brain from angiotensin II, regulates functional synaptic plasticity in the hippocampal formation and in the lateral nucleus of the amygdala. Finally, I will consider the effects of feeding hormones leptin and ghrelin on neural plasticity. These hormones exert important plastic actions on the organization of neuronal circuits involved in the control of food intake and energy balance, but also promote, as other peptide hormones do, plastic remodeling of cognitive brain areas. Indeed, influences on cognition are a common consequence of the plastic actions of peptide hormones in the adult brain.

VASOPRESSIN AND OXYTOCIN

In addition to their classical peripheral effects, arginine vasopressin and oxytocin in mammals, and arginine vasotocin, their homologous hormone in nonmammalian vertebrates, also act in the brain and are involved in the regulation of affiliative behavior, matting, maternal and parenting behavior, and social bonding (Bielsky and Young, 2004; Goodson and Bass, 2001; Lim and Young, 2006; Storm and Tecott, 2005). These hormones are also involved in affective disorders (see Chapter 9). Vasopressin acts on vasopressin 1A and 1B receptors expressed in brain and spinal cord regions involved in cardiovascular and temperature regulation, memory, cognition, fear and anxiety-related behavior, sexual behavior, social behavior, aggression, affiliation, pair-bond formation, and social recognition (Bartz and Hollander, 2006; Caldwell et al., 2008; Lim and Young, 2006; Raggenbass, 2008). Vasopressin is also involved in the neuroendocrine response to stress, as well as in affective disorders (Hammock and Young, 2006; Surget and Belzung, 2008). The neuromodulatory actions of vasopressin include the enhancement of inhibitory inputs in some neuronal populations, and the promotion of excitation in other neurons (Raggenbass, 2008; Urban, 1998). Vasopressin promotes neuroplastic modifications during development and in the adult brain, regulating the outgrowth of neuronal processes and neuritic branching in several regions, including the cerebral cortex (Brinton and Gruener, 1987; Chen et al., 2000). An absence of vasopressin in Brattleboro rats is associated with modifications in the branching of basal dendrites of pyramidal cells in the occipital cortex (Greer et al., 1982). The hormone has also been shown to regulate functional synaptic plasticity in the lateral septum (van den Hooff et al., 1989) and the hippocampal formation (Chen et al., 1993; Dubrovsky et al., 2003; Wang et al., 2001); vasopressin 1B receptors are involved in the regulation of adult neurogenesis in the dentate gyrus (Alonso et al., 2004).

In addition to its classical hormonal actions in the regulation of uterine contraction, milk ejection, and other peripheral effects, oxytocin is also involved in matting, maternal behavior, and social memory (Bielsky and Young, 2004; Crawley et al., 2007; Goodson and Bass, 2001; Lim and Young, 2006; Storm and Tecott, 2005). Oxytocin neurons play an important role in coordinating brain plasticity in preparation for maternity. Pregnancy, parturition, and lactation are associated with marked neuroglial modifications in the oxytocin system (see Chapter 2). In addition, oxytocin has been shown to promote glial and synaptic changes on oxytocin magnocellular neurons in the hypothalamus. Since oxytocin is locally released centrally in the brain, the neuronal and glial plastic effects of oxytocin may reflect a paracrine or autocrine action, rather than a hormonal effect. As we have seen in Chapter 2, the stimulation of oxytocin hormone release during different physiological conditions, such as parturition, lactation, and osmotic stimulation, is associated with a transient plastic reorganization of glial processes and synaptic connections on oxytocin neurons in the hypothalamus. Stimulation of oxytocin release is accompanied by the retraction of astrocytic processes around oxytocin neurons in the supraoptic and paraventricular nucleus, allowing the direct juxtaposing of plasma membranes from adjacent neuronal perikarya and adjacent dendrites. The retraction of glial cells processes allows an increased formation of GABAergic and glutamatergic synapses on the soma and dendrites of oxytocin neurons. Dionysia Theodosis and her collaborators have shown that oxytocin participates in the neuroglial and synaptic remodeling associated with an increased oxytocin hormonal release (Theodosis et al., 2006a). Infusion of oxytocin in the third cerebral ventricle produces the same neuroglial remodeling that dehydration, parturition, or lactation does: an increased juxtaposition of neuronal membranes and formation of new synapses associated with a retraction of the glial processes. Oxytocin-induced neuroglial plasticity affects oxytocin neurons exclusively; oxytocin does not induce synaptic changes on vasopressin neurons and does not alter the interaction of these neurons with glial cells.

Theodosis and collaborators have also used acute hypothalamic slices in vitro to assess the effect of oxytocin on synaptic plasticity. Oxytocin facilitates the expression of plastic changes on glial processes and synapses in hypothalamic slices that are identical to those observed in vivo. Once more, the changes are specific for oxytocin neurons. The in vitro studies have allowed the analysis of the time-course of plastic changes. The glial changes in response to oxytocin are rapid (within one hour after the exposure of the hypothalamic slices to the hormone) and transient, since the extension of glial processes return to basal conditions two hours after washing out oxytocin from the incubation medium. The effect of oxytocin on synapses is also rapid and transient. Oxytocin facilitates synapse formation in vitro one hour after the addition to the incubation medium; the new synapses retract two hours after removing oxytocin from the medium (Theodosis et al., 2006b). As observed in vivo, the majority of synapses that undergo in vitro remodeling are GABAergic. The morphological plastic changes facilitated by oxytocin on synapses are associated with an increase in the frequency of miniature inhibitory postsynaptic currents, likely reflecting the increase in the number of GABAergic synaptic inputs. The facilitatory action of oxytocin on GABAergic transmission appears to represent a paracrine mechanism by which oxytocin neurons coordinate their activity to optimize hormonal release (Israel et al., 2008; Oliet et al., 2007). These findings indicate that oxytocin is a key factor for the regulation of morphological and functional neuroglial plasticity in oxytocin neurons. Interestingly, 17β-estradiol facilitates (or even mimics) the effect of oxytocin on synaptic and glial plasticity, both in vivo and in vitro, suggesting that estradiol and oxytocin may activate the same cellular and molecular mechanisms to promote plasticity (Theodosis et al., 2006b). However, the precise mechanisms for the interaction of estradiol and oxytocin on synaptic plasticity have not yet been explored in detail.

Oxytocin may also affect functional synaptic plasticity in the hippocampus. Kazuhito Tomizawa and collaborators have found that one-train tetanus stimulation induces long-lasting, long-term synaptic potentiation and cyclic AMP-responsive element binding protein (CREB) phosphorylation in hippocampal slices perfused with oxytocin. The effect of oxytocin on hippocampal synaptic plasticity is highly relevant for plastic modifications associated with the maternal experience (see Chapter 8). Indeed, multiparous female mice show an increased long-term synaptic potentiation and CREB phosphorylation induced by one-train tetanus compared to virgin mice. Interestingly, the administration of an oxytocin antagonist significantly inhibited the improved spatial memory, long-term synaptic potentiation, and CREB phosphorylation of multiparous females (Tomizawa et al., 2003). These findings indicate that oxytocin is a regulator of synaptic plasticity in the hippocampus of adult female rats, and suggest that the hormone plays an important role in the synaptic and functional modifications associated with motherhood.

CORTICOTROPIN-RELEASING HORMONE AND UROCORTINS

An important mediator for the cognitive and emotional effects of stress is CRH, a highly conserved peptide comprising 41 amino acid residues. CRH is synthesized in the hypothalamus and regulates the release of adrenocorticotropic hormone (ACTH) from the anterior pituitary, which in turn is responsible for the release of adrenocortical steroids, initiating many of the endocrine, autonomic, immunological, and behavioral responses to stress. Thus, part of the effects of CRH on neural plasticity may be mediated by ACTH and gluco-corticoids. In addition, CRH is locally produced by several neuronal systems as an endogenous neuromodulator, and many neurons express CRH recep-tors (type 1 and 2) which are transmembrane G-protein-coupled cell surface receptors (De Souza, 1987; Potter et al., 1994). Furthermore, three paralogs of CRH have been found in bony fish, amphibians, birds, and mammals. These peptides, named urocortin/urotensin 1, urocortin 2, and urocortin 3 are also expressed throughout the central nervous system. CRH and urocortins acti-vate the central sympathetic and serotonergic systems, and act on neuronal circuits that stimulate locomotor activity and other behavioral responses dur-ing stress.

It has been reported that the CRH 1 receptor antagonist SSR125543A reverses the impairment induced by chronic mild stress on dentate gyrus neurogenesis in adult mice (Alonso et al., 2004), suggesting that CRH is a physiological regulator of cellular replacement in the hippocampus. In addi-tion, several studies indicate that locally produced CRH and urocortins reg-ulate synaptic plasticity. An example of this is CRH produced by the neurons of the inferior olivary nucleus. The inferior olivary neurons are the origin of climbing fibers, a potent excitatory input to Purkinje neurons. CRH may act on climbing fibers and Purkinje cells, since both structures express CRH receptors (Swinny et al., 2003). Although climbing fibers are excitatory, their activity triggers long-term depression of parallel fiber synapses, the other major excitatory input to Purkinje neurons, which originates in cerebellar granule cells. Joint stimulation of climbing and parallel fibers in cerebellar slices results in long-term depression of parallel fiber synapses, an effect that is likely highly relevant for the mechanism of codification of information by Purkinje cells. Long-term depression of parallel fiber synapses may also be obtained in cerebellar slices by a combination of stimulation of paral-lel fibers with the injection of depolarizing current pulses in Purkinje cells. Studies from the laboratory of Masao Ito in Japan have demonstrated that CRH released by climbing fibers is essential for the induction of long-term depression in parallel fiber synapses. They show that long-term depression of parallel fiber synapses induced by their conjunctive activation with the stim-ulation of climbing fibers is blocked by the antagonists of CRH receptors. Furthermore, the long-term depression of parallel fiber synapses induced by a combination of stimulation of parallel fibers with the injection of depolar-izing current pulses in Purkinje cells is not observed in animals in which climbing fibers have been eliminated, demonstrating that climbing fibers are required for the induction of long-term depression in the synapses of parallel fibers. Finally, the administration of CRH to cerebellar slices from animals deprived of climbing fibers restored long-term depression in parallel fiber synapses (Miyata et al., 1999).

Several laboratories have shown that local CRH and urocortin actions are also important for the function and synaptic plasticity of the amygdala.

The amygdala is a major extrahypothalamic source of CRH-containing neurons; amygdala neurons express both CRH type 1 and 2 receptors. CRH is released into the amygdala during stress, which activates local CRH receptors. The local actions of CRH and urocortins in the amygdala seem to be involved in modifications of affective behavior, and also in the synaptic plastic changes that occur in this brain region in response to stress. Thus, it has been shown that CRH and urocortins induce the excitation of basolateral amygdala neuronal circuits, and this effect is involved in the generation of long-term potentiation of basolateral amygdala synapses by stress (Matys et al., 2004; Rainnie et al., 2004; Shekhar et al., 2005). In contrast, in the central nucleus of the amygdala, CRH depresses excitatory glutamatergic transmission through type 1 receptors, whereas urocortin 1 facilitates synaptic responses through type 2 receptors (Liu et al., 2004). Therefore, within the amygdala, the synaptic changes regulated by CRH and urocortins seem to have a clear regional specificity.

CRH and urocortins also act with regional specificity to regulate synaptic plasticity in other brain structures related to the stress response. For instance, in the mediolateral nucleus of the lateral septum, CRH and urocortin 1 have opposing effects to those exerted in the central nucleus of the amygdala. CRH facilitates glutamatergic transmission in the mediolateral nucleus of the lateral septum via type 1 receptors, while urocortin 1 depresses transmission via type 2 receptors (Liu et al., 2004). In the bed nucleus of the stria terminalis, a brain region that regulates the hypothalamic–pituitary–adrenal axis and reward circuits, CRH and urocortin enhance, via type 1 receptors, GABAergic transmission (Kash and Winder, 2006). Another region responsive to CRH that is important for the acute stress response is the locus coeruleus. CRH enhances neuronal activity and stimulates the growth and arborization of neuronal processes in the locus coeruleus (acting on type 1 receptors), while urocortin 2 inhibits the outgrowth of neuronal processes (acting on the same receptor, but by the activation of a different intracellular signaling pathway). Protein kinase A, mitogen-activated protein kinase (MAPK), and Rac1 (a member of the Rho family of GTPases that regulates the cytoskeleton) are involved in the plastic changes induced by CRH, while protein kinase C and RhoA mediate the effects of urocortin 2 (Swinny et al., 2006). CRH also regulates synaptic plasticity in the hippocampus, and its injection into the dentate gyrus results in a dose-dependent and long-lasting enhancement of synaptic efficacy (Wang et al., 1998).

CRH and urocortins may also regulate synaptic plastic changes in hypothalamic circuits involved in the stress response. Luis de Lecea and his collaborators (Winsky-Sommerer et al., 2004) have shown that CRH affects the activity of hypocretin neurons in the lateral hypothalamus. Hypocretin-1 (also known as orexin-A) and hypocretin-2 (orexin-B) are two neuropeptides involved in the regulation of vigilance and arousal. They are produced from a common precursor and act via two G-protein-coupled receptors. Hypocretin-expressing neurons are located in the perifornical region of the lateral hypothalamus, and innervate many brain regions, including the hypothalamus, thalamus, and brainstem, as well as the peripheral autonomic nervous system. By means of an elegant and meticulous electron microscopy analysis, Lecea and his colleagues have detected CRH-immunoreactive synaptic boutons in direct contact with hypocretin-expressing neurons in the lateral hypothalamus. They also found numerous hypocretin immunoreactive neurons expressing CRH receptors type 1 and 2, and they show that the application of CRH to hypothalamic slices increases the firing rate of hypocretinergic cells, an effect that was mediated by type 1 receptors. These results suggest that CRH may regulate arousal in response to stress by acting on the hypocretinergic system.

PROLACTIN

Prolactin is a protein hormone secreted by the lactotrophs of the anterior pituitary that stimulates mammary gland development and milk production. In addition, prolactin has many other important effects for maternal physiological functions, including actions in the immune system and the brain. There is little information on neuroplastic effects of prolactin. In the rodent uterine myometrium, prolactin has been shown to reverse the suppression of neuritogenesis induced by estrogen, which induces a rapid and extensive decrease in uterine sympathetic neuritic growth (Krizsan-Agbas and Smith, 2002). It is unknown whether prolactin antagonizes in a similar way the effects of estrogen on synaptic plasticity in the central nervous system. However, it is known that prolactin may affect the activity of specific neuronal populations in the brain, including magnocellular oxytocinergic neurons. By extracellular recording of single neuron activity in identified oxytocin and vasopressin neurons of anesthetized nonpregnant rats, Kokay et al. (2006) have detected that prolactin induces a significant decrease in firing rates of oxytocin neurons. In contrast, prolactin does not affect the activity of vasopressin neurons. The different effects of prolactin on the activity of oxytocin and vasopressin neurons are in agreement with the different expression of prolactin receptors in both populations of magnocellular neurons. In the supraoptic neurons, the majority of magnocellular neurons expressing prolactin receptors are oxytocin neurons, while less than 10% of vasopressin neurons express prolactin receptors. Prolactin receptors are also predominantly expressed by oxytocin neurons in the paraventricular nucleus. In addition, the proportion of oxytocin neurons expressing prolactin receptors increases significantly during pregnancy and lactation (Kokay et al., 2006).

   Another plastic effect of prolactin in the central nervous system is the promotion of remyelination. Remyelination is enhanced in the maternal murine central nervous system and prolactin seems to be involved in this effect, promoting the generation of myelin-forming oligodendrocytes and enhancing remyelination of white matter lesions (Gregg et al., 2007). Prolactin may also affect brain remodeling by promoting astroglia proliferation (DeVito et al.,

1992). However, one of the most dramatic neuroplastic effects of prolactin in the central nervous system is the regulation of adult neurogenesis in the subventricular zone of the brain. New neurons are generated in this brain region, and the newly generated neurons migrate to the olfactory bulb and differentiate in olfactory bulb granule neurons. Tetsuro Shingo and colleagues in the laboratory of Samuel Weiss at the University of Calgary reported that prolactin affects the generation of new neurons in the subventricular zone of the brain (Shingo et al., 2003). They found that the production of new progenitor cells in the subventricular zone of the mouse brain is increased in pregnant females compared to virgins. The rate of neurogenesis peaks on the seventh day of the mouse's 21-day gestation period, and again after delivery. Shingo and colleagues have provided solid evidence indicating that the effect was mediated by prolactin. Furthermore, they have tracked the new neurons and detected that they migrate and become interneurons in the olfactory bulb. Increased neurogenesis was also observed in females that mate with sterile males. It is interesting to note that mating is also associated with an increase in prolactin. Therefore, the findings of Shingo and colleagues suggest that prolactin during pregnancy and/or mating increases the production of new neurons for the olfactory bulb. Given the importance of olfaction and olfactory discrimination for mating, offspring recognition, and rearing, the effect of prolactin may be highly relevant for the regulation of reproduction and maternal behavior (see also Chapter 8).

GONADOTROPIN-RELEASING HORMONE

GnRH regulates the release of gonadotropins and the function of the gonads. It also acts within the central nervous system to modulate synaptic activity (Wong et al., 1990; Yang et al., 1999). Recent studies from the laboratory of Gabriele Rune in Hamburg indicate that GnRH regulates the formation of spine synapses in the CA1 region of hippocampal slices (Prange-Kiel et al., 2008). The effect of GnRH depends on the dose—increasing spine formation at low concentrations and decreasing it at high concentrations. Interestingly, the mechanism involves the regulation of the local production of estradiol in the slices. GnRH increases estradiol synthesis and spine synapses; the inhibition of aromatase, the enzyme that synthesizes estradiol, blocks the effect of GnRH on synapses (Prange-Kiel et al., 2008). In addition, local hippocampal estradiol decreases the expression of GnRH receptors in the hippocampus; this may represent a negative feedback mechanism to regulate adequate amounts of estradiol synthesis within the hippocampus (Prange-Kiel et al., 2008). These findings suggest that the fluctuation in the number of spines synapses observed in the hippocampus during the estrus cycle (see Chapter 8) may, at least in part, be regulated by the fluctuation of GnRH levels via the modulation of local estradiol synthesis within the hippocampus (see also Chapter 4 for the role of local brain estradiol synthesis in the regulation of synaptic plasticity and neurogenesis).

INSULIN

Insulin is one of the best studied hormones, given its implication in the regulation of glucose homeostasis and the serious pathological consequences that insufficient hormonal insulin levels or decreased responsiveness to the hormone have for an organism. However, in contrast to the detailed knowledge of insulin effects in many tissues (accumulated for decades since its discovery), hormonal actions in neural tissue have been poorly studied. The main reason for this situation is due to the fact that, for much too long, the central nervous system was considered to be insensitive to insulin, since it was assumed that the hormone was unable to cross the blood–brain barrier (or that it did in insignificant amounts). A challenge to this idea was the identification of insulin receptors in the nervous system, and the results of several studies showing insulin transport through the blood–brain barrier. Indeed, we know today that insulin is transferred across the blood–brain barrier by a saturable transporter (Woods and Porte, 1977) and acts within the brain on insulin receptors, which are widely distributed in the central nervous system (Havrankova et al., 1978). In addition, insulin at high concentrations may bind and activate IGF-I receptors, which are also broadly distributed in the brain. Thus, insulin seems to be important for brain function. The deleterious effects of diabetes mellitus on brain function are indicative of the role that insulin has in the maintenance of neuronal activity, synaptic plasticity, and cognition, either by direct hormonal effects in the central nervous system, by peripheral effects, or by the control of glycemia (Gispen and Biessels, 2000). It is obvious that from the analysis of the effects of diabetes we cannot infer what the direct effects of insulin on neural plasticity are. Among many other reasons, this is because diabetes has many peripheral effects that may indirectly affect brain plasticity, and because it affects the plasma levels of other hormones (such as IGF-I and gonadal steroids) that are known to regulate neuronal and glial plasticity. However, diabetes gives a general picture of the neural plastic alterations caused by insulin insufficiency or decreased insulin responsiveness in the whole organism. From this picture we may infer the importance that insulin has, acting by direct or indirect mechanisms, for brain function and plasticity under physiological conditions.

It is well known that the peripheral nervous system is affected by diabetes; alterations in peripheral nerves are a common complication of this pathology. In addition, there is also clinical evidence of alterations in the central nervous system as a consequence of diabetes. Small deficits in attention, processing speed, long-term memory, and executive skills have been detected in some children with type 1 diabetes. Type 2 diabetes mellitus, which is not necessarily associated with hypoinsulinemia, also affects brain function. Indeed, electrophysiological studies have detected reduced amplitudes and prolonged latencies of evoked potential components in the brain of adults with both type 1 and type 2 diabetes (Di Mario et al., 1995; Suzuki et al., 2000). Some studies have revealed an association of diabetes with cognitive decline in middle-aged people. In addition, impairments in memory, attention, abstract reasoning, and execution of visual-motor tasks are also frequent in diabetic older people; apparently the negative effects of diabetes on brain function worsen with age. Other studies suggest that diabetes may also increase the risk of vascular dementia, depression, and Alzheimer's disease in older people (Trudeau et al., 2004).

Animal studies have confirmed that diabetes may be associated with different degrees of brain dysfunction. Many of these studies have used systemic administration of the glucosamine-nitrosourea compound streptozotocin to induce diabetes in rodents. This is a well accepted experimental method to induce diabetes, since the insulin-producing β cells of the islets of Langerhans in the pancreas are particularly vulnerable to streptozotocin toxicity (Schnedl et al., 1994). Using this experimental approach, it has been detected that diabetic rodents exhibit impairments in memory processes, such as during shock avoidance and spatial water maze learning (Biessels et al., 1996). The hippocampus is involved in these memory processes impaired by diabetes. Interestingly, the expression and phosphorylation of insulin receptors are increased in the hippocampus of normal rats after training in the water maze tests, suggesting that insulin signaling in the hippocampus is involved in water maze learning (Zhao et al., 1999).

Since the hippocampus seems to be involved in the cognitive impairments associated with diabetes, several laboratories have analyzed this brain region in streptozotocin-injected animals in search of possible alterations in synaptic plasticity. Ana María Magariños and Bruce S. McEwen from Rockefeller University have analyzed the effect of diabetes on morphological synaptic parameters in the hippocampus (Magariños and McEwen, 2000). They found that rats with streptozotocin-induced diabetes have a retraction and reduced number of branch points of apical dendrites of CA3 pyramidal neurons. Diabetes also results in a depletion of synaptic vesicles of mossy fiber terminals that form excitatory synaptic contacts with the proximal CA3 apical dendrites. These morphological changes are similar to those produced by chronic stress (see also Chapters 3 and 8).

Interestingly, Magariños and McEwen detected an interaction between diabetes and chronic stress on dendritic atrophy, since one week of repeated stress (which per se does not affect dendritic morphology in nondiabetic animals) induced a stronger dendritic atrophy in diabetic rats compared to non-stressed diabetic animals. Changes in the expression of synaptic markers also suggest morphological plasticity of synaptic circuits in diabetic animals. For instance, streptozotocin-induced diabetes increases synaptophysin expression in CA1, CA3, and the dentate gyrus in rats (Grillo et al., 2005). Morphological changes in dendrites induced by diabetes are not restricted to the hippocampus; for instance, diabetes also results in dendritic alterations in the retina. Indeed, diabetic retinopathy is a frequent complication of diabetes in humans and a major cause of visual loss and blindness in adults. In rats, streptozotocin-induced diabetes results in a significant loss of retinal ganglion cells. The surviving retinal ganglion cells show an enlargement of their dendritic field, which has been interpreted as a compensatory response to the overall loss of retinal ganglion cells with diabetes (Qin et al., 2006).

In addition to alterations in dendritic morphology, diabetes also induces glial remodeling. In many regions, such as the hippocampus and retina, diabetes increases the expression of glial cell markers associated with reactive gliosis (Baydas et al., 2003; Lieth et al., 1998; Mizutani et al., 1998; Saravia et al., 2006). However, Julie Chowen and her collaborators have recently reported that diabetes reduces the extension of glial fibrillary acidic protein (GFAP)-immueactive astrocytic processes, decreases astroglial proliferation, and increases astroglial cell death in the hypothalamus and cerebellum (Lechuga-Sancho et al., 2006a, b). The glial changes induced by diabetes may have a direct impact on synaptic plasticity, since astrocytes are involved in many plastic changes in the hypothalamus and other brain areas. Furthermore, the glial plastic changes may be associated with a modification in glutamate metabolism, which in turn may affect synaptic plasticity; this has been studied with detail in the retina. Müller glial cells in the retina are important regulators of glucose metabolism, retinal blood flow, and the formation and maintenance of the blood–retinal barrier. Diabetes induces reactive activation of Müller glia (Lieth et al., 1998; Mizutani et al., 1998), which is associated with an accumulation of GABA and decreased activity of glutamine synthetase and the glutamate/aspartate transporter (GLAST) in these cells (Ishikawa et al., 1996; Li and Puro, 2002; Lieth et al., 1998).

The effects of diabetes on functional alterations in synaptic plasticity have been analyzed in the hippocampus. Willem Hendrik Gispen and collaborators in Utrecht were the first to characterize the effects of diabetes in long-term synaptic potentiation in the CA1 region of the hippocampus. They found that streptozotocin-diabetic rats have deficits in learning (assessed in the Morris water maze) and also present deficits in CA1 hippocampal long-term synaptic potentiation (Biessels et al., 1996). Insulin treatment, commenced at the onset of diabetes, prevented these impairments. However, insulin was unable to reverse established deficits in maze learning and restored long-term potentiation only partially (Biessels et al., 1998). Further characterization of the synaptic plastic changes induced by diabetes revealed that the expression of N-methyl-D-aspartate (NMDA) receptor-dependent long-term synaptic potentiation was impaired in the CA1 field and dentate gyrus in hippocampal slices of streptozotocin-diabetic rats. In addition, NMDA receptor-independent long-term synaptic potentiation was impaired in the CA3 field. In contrast, diabetes facilitates the expression of long-term depression in Schaffer collateral synapses in hippocampal CA1 slices (Artola et al., 2005; Kamal et al., 1999).

The alterations in hippocampal synaptic plasticity induced by diabetes develop progressively (Kamal et al., 2005), may involve both metabolic and vascular changes related to chronic hyperglycemia, and may also be the consequence of a lack of direct insulin action in the brain (Gispen and Biessels,

2000). It is difficult to determine the relative weight of each one of these factors in the final effects of diabetes on synaptic plasticity. However, it has been reported that in hippocampal slices from diabetic rats, the addition of pyruvate or incubation of the slices with insulin allows for the recovery of induction of long-term potentiation. Furthermore, incubation with high extracellular glucose levels (30 mmol/L) does not alter the long-term potentiation in slices from healthy animals (Izumi et al., 2003). These results suggest that acute hyperglycemia is likely not the cause of the synaptic impairment. However, these findings do not exclude the possibility that chronic hyperglycemia may have an effect, per se, on synaptic plasticity. Nevertheless, the data supports that impaired energy utilization from insulin deficiency may be one important factor involved in the deficit in synaptic plasticity. Indeed, repeated periods of hypoglycemia causes deficits in long-term synaptic potentiation in the hippocampus (Yamada et al., 2004). Furthermore, long-term potentiation in CA1 and spatial learning are not altered in hyperglycemic Zucker diabetic fatty rats, a model of type 2 diabetes (Belanger et al., 2004). This further suggests that hyperglycemia is not the cause of the alterations of functional synaptic plasticity in the hippocampus. However, hyperglycemic Zucker diabetic fatty rats have high plasma levels of insulin; it is therefore possible that insulin exerts a protective effect against high glucose levels in these animals.

Studies of nondiabetic animals or with nondiabetic models have provided complementary and more direct evidence of the effects on insulin on synaptic plasticity. For instance, it has been detected that insulin, acting on the insulin receptor, induces a rapid potentiation of responses to NMDA in Xenopus oocytes expressing NMDA receptors (Chen and Leonard, 1996; Liao and Leonard, 1999; Liu et al., 1995). In CA1 hippocampal neurons in culture, insulin has been shown to induce long-term synaptic depression or long-term synaptic potentiation, depending on the frequency of stimulation, an effect that involves NMDA receptors; this may be mediated by the activation of the phosphatidylinositol 3-kinase (PI3K)/protein kinase B/Akt signaling pathway associated with insulin receptors (Huang et al., 2004; van der Heide et al., 2005). The effects of diabetes and insulin on hippocampal synaptic plasticity may be mediated by a plastic restructuring of neurotransmitter synaptic receptors, including the reorganization of its subcellular distribution. Early phases of diabetes are associated with an increase of glutamate receptor binding in several brain regions (Valastro et al., 2002); however, chronic diabetes results in a down-regulation of glutamate receptors. Both the expression and phosphorylation of NMDA receptors are decreased in the brain of chronic diabetic rats; this is associated with an alteration of NMDA currents in hippocampal pyramidal neurons monitored by intracellular recording (Di Luca et al., 1999; Gardoni et al., 2002). In contrast, incubation of rat hippocampal slices with insulin results in an increased tyrosine phosphorylation of the NR2A and 2B subunits of NMDA receptors (Christie et al., 1999). In addition, streptozotocin-induced diabetes results in a decrease of [3H]AMPA binding in different brain regions such as the striatum, the cerebral cortex, and the hippocampus. The reduced [3H]AMPA binding in the brain of diabetic rats may be the consequence of changes in the properties of the glutamate receptor subunit GluR1, which is essential for the expression of long-term potentiation in CA1 (Gagné et al., 1997). This alteration may be the consequence of a deficit in the up-regulation of AMPA receptors by phospholipase A2 in the diabetic rat hippocampus (Chabot et al., 1997). Interestingly, insulin may facilitate clathrin-dependent internalization of AMPA receptors, leading to long-term depression of AMPA receptor-mediated synaptic transmission in hippocampal pyramidal neurons (Huang et al., 2003, 2004; Man et al., 2000). Insulin may also enhance NMDA channel activities by recruiting NMDA receptors to the membrane surface (Skeberdis et al., 2001), and may recruit functional GABA$_A$ receptors onto the postsynaptic and dendritic membranes (Wan et al., 1997).

Diabetes may also affect adult neurogenesis. Streptozotocin-induced diabetes is associated with a decrease in cell proliferation in the dentate gyrus of adult rats (Jackson-Guilford et al., 2000) and mice (Saravia et al., 2004), and also causes a decrease in neurogenesis in the subventricular zone of adult mice (Saravia et al., 2004). The mechanisms involved in neurogenesis reduction by diabetes have not been analyzed in detail yet. Potentially, the reduction in neurogenesis may be the direct consequence of a reduction in insulin signaling on neuronal precursors, or may involve the alteration by diabetes of other factors that are involved in the regulation of neurogenesis, such as growth hormone and IGF-I. Interestingly, the group headed by Alejandro De Nicola in Buenos Aires has demonstrated that estradiol therapy may prevent the alterations in neurogenesis induced by diabetes, as well as the alterations in the expression of glial markers (Saravia et al., 2004, 2006). Estradiol is known to regulate neurogenesis and exert neuroprotective effects (see also Chapters 4 and 9); the effects of estradiol on diabetic animals are a good example of the protective actions of the ovarian hormone.

Finally, it should be emphasized that the consequences of neural remodeling induced by diabetes are not limited to cognitive aspects. I have already mentioned that diabetes may induce plastic changes in neurons and glial cells in the retina, which may have an impact on vision. Diabetes-induced synaptic remodeling may also occur in other regions of the central nervous system, including the spinal cord. Indeed, synaptic reorganization in superficial dorsal horn neurons induced by diabetes may be involved in diabetic neuropathic pain. Dorsal horn neurons in the spinal cord receive the input from primary pain afferents, and are involved in pain processing and transmission to higher brain levels. There is evidence that glutamatergic input from primary afferents to dorsal horn neurons is increased in diabetic neuropathic pain in rats (Wang et al., 2007). In addition, GABA$_B$ receptor function at the primary afferent terminals appears to decline under these conditions; this may contribute to increased glutamatergic input, since GABA$_B$ receptors at the glutamatergic terminals can limit synaptic glutamate release in the spinal cord. Therefore, diabetes may cause presynaptic remodeling of pain afferents to dorsal horn neurons, which may result in an anomalous hyperactivity of these neurons that may be linked to an alteration in pain information processing and the development of diabetic neuropathic pain.

GROWTH HORMONE/INSULIN-LIKE GROWTH FACTOR-I

Growth hormone is an important modulator of brain function and plasticity. The amount and pattern of growth hormone release show important changes during life. Growth hormone levels are high in early childhood; the peaks of frequency and amplitude of growth hormone secretion increase during the period of pubertal growth. Then the growth hormone basal levels, and the frequency and amplitude of secretion peaks, decrease progressively in adulthood. Growth hormone crosses the blood–brain barrier and acts within the brain on growth hormone receptors, which is expressed by neurons, astrocytes, oligodendrocytes, and the choroid plexus (Lai et al., 1991; Lobie et al., 1993). High levels of growth hormone receptor expression have been detected in the hypothalamus and the hippocampus, among other brain regions.

Growth hormone deficiency in humans is associated with moderate changes in memory, processing speed, and attention (Falleti et al., 2006; Maruff and Falleti, 2005; van Dam, 2005) and growth hormone therapy has been shown to improve cognitive function in growth hormone deficient patients (Arwert et al., 2006; Maruff and Falleti, 2005; Sathiavageeswaran et al., 2007). The decline of growth hormone levels in plasma with aging may contribute to the development of age-related cognitive deficits in animals and humans. Growth hormone therapy ameliorates cognitive function in elderly patients with adult-onset growth hormone deficiency (Sathiavageeswaran et al., 2007); chronic treatment with growth hormone (or with growth-hormone-releasing hormone, which increases the growth hormone pulse amplitude) have been shown to exert cognitive benefits in aging rats (Ramsey et al., 2004; Thornton et al., 2000), improving the performance in the Morris water maze test to levels similar to those of young animals. These effects may be mediated by an increase in plasmatic levels of IGF-I. In addition, growth hormone administration increases the levels of IGF-I in the brain in an anatomically specific manner (Frago et al., 2002; Lopez-Fernandez et al., 1996). Therefore, it is difficult to differentiate whether the effects of growth hormone in the brain are direct or mediated by IGF-I. For this reason (and since many effects of growth hormone in other target tissues are mediated by IGF-I), I will consider both molecules together. In addition, the nervous tissue is also able to produce growth hormone; there is evidence that this local production may affect brain plasticity and promotes adult neurogenesis in the hippocampus of growth-hormone-deficient animals (Sun et al., 2005a, b; see also Chapter 10). Therefore, growth hormone receptors in the brain may be targeted by growth hormone from both a systemic and local origin.

Since the hippocampus may be involved in the cognitive effects of growth hormone, this brain region has been particularly studied to detect possible hormonal effects on functional synaptic plasticity. For instance, William E. Sonntag and his collaborators have assessed the effect of growth hormone on hippocampal short-term synaptic plasticity in aged rats using an extracellular paired-pulse protocol. The responses to the second stimulus (conditioned response) and to the first stimulus (test response) were compared using the paired-pulse ratio (PPR) calculation. Both facilitatory and inhibitory mechanisms modulate the conditioned response in pyramidal cells. In particular, the amplitude of the conditioned response in pyramidal cells may be reduced compared with the test response due to activation of GABAergic interneurons by the test stimulus. Using this method, Sonntag and his colleagues detected that aged rats have increased paired-pulse ratios compared with adult rats, suggesting an alteration in the balance between excitatory and inhibitory synaptic inputs with aging. However, aged rats that were treated for six months with growth hormone had paired-pulse ratio values comparable to those observed in adult controls (Ramsey et al., 2004). These functional synaptic changes may be mediated by modifications in the subunit composition of $GABA_A$ receptors (in particular, by an increase in the subunit α1) with growth hormone treatment. Thus, growth hormone may affect short-term synaptic plasticity in the hippocampus, and the decline in growth hormone levels with aging may result in an impairment of synaptic plasticity.

Unfortunately, there is limited information concerning the possible effects of growth hormone on morphological plasticity in the brain. As mentioned before, one important problem is to differentiate direct growth hormone actions from effects mediated by IGF-I. Nevertheless, some studies suggest that growth hormone, directly or indirectly, may exert important brain structure remodeling. For instance, in aged rats, administration of growth hormone for 28 days was found to increase the growth of small arterioles on the cortical surface (Sonntag et al., 1997), suggesting that growth hormone plays a role in the maintenance of brain microvasculature. Given the important role of brain microvasculature for neuronal and glial function, this effect of growth hormone is highly relevant. The hormonal effect may reflect a direct action of growth hormone on the microvasculature of the brain, or be secondary to a hormonally induced increase in neuronal activity. Once more, the effect may be mediated by IGF-I, since high levels of IGF-I expression are detected in cerebral cortex microvessels (Sonntag et al., 2000b). There is also evidence that growth hormone may control dendritic morphology. For instance, cortical pyramidal neurons have a decreased dendritic branching in growth hormone receptor null mice, but also in null mice for suppressor of cytokine signaling-2 (SOCS2), an intracellular inhibitor of growth hormone signaling (Ransome et al., 2004). This suggests that adequate levels of growth hormone signaling, neither too low nor too high, are necessary for the maintenance of a normal dendritic morphology. However, the deficits observed in dendritic branching in these animals may reflect a developmental effect of growth hormone rather than a plastic effect in adults, and are accompanied by changes in cortical, neuronal, and glial density that may also reflect a developmental alteration.

Insulin-Like Growth Factor-I and Synaptic Plasticity

The actions of IGF-I on central nervous system plasticity are relatively well documented in comparison with the limited available information for the effects of growth hormone. The main origin of IGF-I in plasma is the liver, where it is produced in response to growth hormone action. In addition, growth hormone induces IGF-I synthesis in target tissues. Therefore, IGF-I acts as a hormonal signal and a paracrine or autocrine factor. This is also the situation in the brain, where IGF-I is locally produced by neurons, glial cells, ependymal cells, endothelial cells, and the choroid plexus of the adult brain (Garcia-Segura et al., 1991b; Werther et al., 1990). IGF-I receptor, a tyrosine–kinase membrane receptor, is also widely expressed in the brain, which also expresses IGF binding proteins. IGF-I receptors are expressed by neurons, glial cells, endothelial cells, the choroid plexus, and meninges in the adult central nervous system (Aguado et al., 1993; Bondy and Cheng, 2004; Garcia-Segura et al., 1997; Werther et al., 1989, 1990). As in other tissues, IGF-I receptors in the brain signal through two major pathways, the MAPK and the PI3K (Bondy and Cheng, 2004; Cardona-Gomez et al., 2002a). In adult rats, the expression of IGF-I is dramatically reduced in many brain areas compared to fetal and postnatal ages (Andersson et al., 1988; Garcia-Segura et al., 1991b; Rotwein et al., 1988), excluding the hypothalamus and the median eminence where IGF-I levels increase with puberty (Daftary and Gore, 2003; Dueñas et al., 1994; Garcia-Segura et al., 1996; Miller and Gore, 2001). In contrast to the decrease in local IGF-I production, the expression of IGF-I receptor is maintained in neurons and glia in the adult rat brain (Garcia-Segura et al., 1997). This suggests that peripheral, rather than locally formed IGF-I, is acting on brain IGF-I receptors in most brain areas during adult life, at least under physiological conditions. Indeed, the importance of peripheral IGF-I in the regulation of synaptic plasticity and neurogenesis has been well documented by the group of Ignacio Torres-Aleman, at the Instituto Cajal in Madrid (Carro et al., 2000, 2001; Torres-Aleman, 1999; Trejo et al., 2001, 2007).

Manuel Castro-Alamancos and Ignacio Torres-Aleman were the first to show that IGF-I may induce plastic functional alterations of synapses. Exploring the effects of IGF-I in the olivocerebellar system, these authors found that IGF-I produces a long-lasting depression of GABA release by cerebellar Purkinje cells in response to glutamate (Castro-Alamancos and Torres-Aleman, 1993). The effect of IGF-I was dose-dependent and mimicked by the electrical stimulation of inferior olivary neurons, the origin of climbing fibers to the cerebellum. Climbing fibers, a potent excitatory input to Purkinje cells, transport IGF-I from the inferior olive to the cerebellum, and are responsible for about half of the IGF-I content of the cerebellum (Nieto-Bona et al., 1993; Torres-Aleman et al., 1991). Interestingly, the electrical stimulation of climbing fibers results in the release of IGF-I in the cerebellar cortex (Castro-Alamancos and Torres-Aleman, 1993). These findings suggested that IGF-I released in the cerebellar cortex after climbing fiber stimulation interacts with Purkinje neurons to modulate their response to glutamate. In addition, these results opened up the possibility of IGF-I involvement in the learning-related phenomenon of cerebellar long-term depression, which is characterized as a protracted inhibition of the glutamatergic synapse between parallel fiber afferents and Purkinje cell dendrites, subsequent to concurrent stimulation of climbing fiber and parallel fiber terminals (Ito, 2002). For this reason, Castro-Alamancos and Torres-Aleman decided to investigate whether IGF-I released by climbing fibers was implicated in the learning or in the retention of the classical conditioning of the eye-blink response, where inferior olive and long-term depression was postulated to be involved. They delivered an antisense oligonucleotide to an inferior olivary nucleus in order to inhibit the synthesis of IGF-I and the consequent release of IGF-I by climbing fibers. As expected, this treatment resulted in a transient depletion of cerebellar IGF-I levels. In addition, the treatment markedly and reversibly impaired the acquisition of the conditioned eye-blink response without affecting its retention once it was learned (Castro-Alamancos and Torres-Aleman, 1994). These findings supported the possible involvement of IGF-I in the long-term depression of the parallel fiber–Purkinje cell dendrite synapse in the acquisition of the conditioned eye-blink response, and provided the first evidence for a causal link between the effects of IGF-I on synaptic plasticity and its effects on a learning task.

Further characterization of the mechanisms involved on the effects of IGF-I on long-term depression of glutamate-induced GABA release revealed a role for protein kinase C and nitric oxide. Short-term inhibition of glutamate-induced GABA release by IGF-I appears to be mediated either by protein kinase C or nitric oxide signaling. In contrast, the long-term depression of glutamate-induced GABA release by IGF-I appears to be mediated by the simultaneous activation of both protein kinase C and nitric oxide signaling (Castro-Alamancos et al., 1996). The functional synaptic plasticity induced in Purkinje cells by IGF-I released from climbing fibers also has a morphological counterpart, since the injection of an IGF-I antisense oligonucleotide in the inferior olivary nucleus of adult rats resulted in a significant reduction in the size and numerical density of Purkinje cell dendritic spines (Nieto-Bona et al., 1997) assessed by electron microscopy. These findings suggest that IGF-I released by climbing fibers participates in the regulation of the formation of Purkinje cell dendritic spines. Finally, it should be mentioned that the regulation of Purkinje cell plasticity by IGF-I released by climbing fibers also has important consequences for the pathophysiology of the olivocerebellar circuit. IGF-I maintains the normal function of this circuit, and there is a correlation between alterations in serum IGF-I levels and pathological alterations of the olivocerebellar system (Busiguina et al., 2000). Loss of IGF-I input to Purkinje cells may result in ataxia; ataxia induced by climbing fiber destruction can be compensated for by the administration of IGF-I (Fernandez et al., 1998, 1999, 2005; see also Chapter 9).

While the plastic effects of IGF-I on the cerebellum are relevant for motor learning and proper motor control, the regulation of synaptic plasticity by

IGF-I in other brain regions may be highly relevant for cognition. William E. Sonntag and collaborators have examined the cognitive effects of IGF-I in male aged rats, and have found that a 28-day intracerebroventricular infusion of IGF-I improves working memory and reference memory, attenuating age-related cognitive deficits (Markowska et al., 1998). These cognitive actions may be related to the effects of IGF-I on hippocampal plasticity. A decrease in CA1 synapses is observed in aged rats; this synaptic change may be associated with the cognitive decline with aging. Although IGF-I infusion is not able to restore aging-associated an decline in CA1 synapses (Shi et al., 2005), it regulates the expression of NMDA receptor subtypes in the hippocampus and reverses the age-related decline in subunits 2A and 2B (Sonntag et al., 2000a). IGF-I infusion also increases local cerebral glucose utilization in the CA1 region of the hippocampus and in the cingulate cortex of aged rats (Lynch et al., 2001). Furthermore, intracerebroventricular infusion of IGF-I increases postsynaptic density length in CA1 synapses of aged rats (Shi et al., 2005). This change may represent a morphological correlate of an increased synaptic function, since both NMDA and AMPA subtypes of glutamate receptors are clustered in the postsynaptic density. In addition, infusion of IGF-I to aged rats increases the number of synaptic profiles in multiple spine button complexes in CA1 synapses (Shi et al., 2005). Multiple spine button complexes originate from preexisting simple synapses and are a morphological correlate of long-term synaptic potentiation. This may therefore reflect and enhance synaptic efficacy related to the cognitive improvement caused by IGF-I treatment. The functional acute effect of IGF-I on CA1 synapses has been assessed on hippocampal slices of young rats (Ramsey et al., 2005). Treatment of the slices for 15 minutes with des-IGF-I, an active fragment of the IGF-I molecule, resulted in a concentration-dependent increase in the slope of CA1 field excitatory postsynaptic potentials. The potentiation was initiated within five minutes of the start of des-IGF-I application, and partially recovered during a 15-minute washout period. This action of des-IGF-I was due to a postsynaptic mechanism involving AMPA but not NMDA receptors, and was mediated by PI3K activation. Therefore, IGF-I may increase AMPA receptor-mediated synaptic transmission, and this effect may be involved in the cognitive actions of the hormone.

Insulin-Like Growth Factor-I and Adult Neurogenesis

Adult neurogenesis is another important plastic modification regulated by IGF-I in the hippocampus. Maria A. I. Åberg and her collaborators at Göteborg University explored the effect of IGF-I on adult hippocampal neurogenesis using bromodeoxyuridine labeling to identify newly generated cells. They observed an increased cellular proliferation and increased neurogenesis in the dentate subgranular proliferative zone after peripheral IGF-I administration (Åberg et al., 2000). This plastic effect of IGF-I may have a strong impact on hippocampal function and cognition. Neurogenesis in the subgranular layer of the hippocampus progressively and significantly decreases with aging—both the number of newly generated cells and their differentiation. Some evidence suggests that there is a link between decreased neurogenesis and cognitive impairment in aged rats. Interestingly, the intracerebroventricular infusion of IGF-I to senescent rats significantly restored neurogenesis through an approximately three-fold increase in the production of new neurons (Lichtenwalner et al., 2001). IGF-I also partially restores neurogenesis and learning performance in the water maze task in aged rats submitted to stress during the prenatal period (Darnaudery et al., 2006). Furthermore, peripheral IGF-I mediates the effects of physical exercise on hippocampal neurogenesis.

The influence of the body on psychological functions was known by early civilizations and postulated by early philosophers; the classic Roman aphorism, *mens sana in corpore sano* (a sound mind in a sound body), is a good example of this. The scientific foundation for this assertion is relatively modern. The idea that a healthy body helps to maintain healthy brain function has received substantial scientific support in recent times by a series of studies showing the importance of physical exercise and a healthy diet for cognitive function. Physical activity enhances learning and memory skills in young and older animals and humans, and appears to reduce the risk of cognitive decline and dementia in later life (Fordyce and Wehner, 1993; Kramer et al., 1999, 2006; Laurin et al., 2001; Lautenschlager and Almeida, 2006). Physical exercise may promote different forms of neural plasticity in the hippocampus: facilitating long-term potentiation of synaptic transmission, increasing the length and complexity of dendrites, and promoting the formation of dendritic spines (Eadie et al., 2005; Farmer et al., 2004). One of the plastic events regulated by physical exercise in the brain is adult hippocampal neurogenesis. Voluntary running in rodents increases cell proliferation and neurogenesis in the adult dentate gyrus (van Praag et al., 1999). IGF-I seems to mediate at least part of these plastic effects of exercise in the brain. Torres-Aleman and his collaborators have detected an increased uptake of circulating IGF-I by cells of different brain regions (including the hippocampus) after physical exercise, and have proposed that this increased uptake of circulating IGF-I by brain cells is involved in the effects of exercise on brain function (Carro et al., 2001). In addition, José Luis Trejo, Eva Carro, and Ignacio Torres-Aleman have shown that peripheral IGF-I mediates the effects of exercise in adult neurogenesis in the hippocampus. To determine the role of peripheral IGF-I on neurogenesis induced by physical exercise, they prevented the entrance of circulating IGF-I into the brain by subcutaneous infusion of a blocking IGF-I antiserum. When the entrance of peripheral IGF-I in the brain of rats undergoing exercise was prevented with this method, a complete inhibition of exercise-induced increases in the number of new neurons in the hippocampus was observed (Trejo et al., 2001). Local IGF-I synthesis in the hippocampus may also be involved in the effects of exercise on synaptic plasticity. Fernando Gomez-Pinilla's group at UCLA has shown that exercise increases IGF-I mRNA levels in the hippocampus, an effect that is mediated by IGF-I receptors. This suggests that exercise may increase IGF-I levels in the brain by increasing IGF-I uptake and by increasing IGF-I local synthesis. Since an

IGF-I receptor blockade (using a specific IGF-I receptor-binding antibody) abolishes the effect of exercise on IGF-I mRNA levels in the hippocampus, it is plausible that peripheral IGF-I acting on brain IGF-I receptors would induce the local synthesis of IGF-I. Furthermore, the blockade of hippocampal IGF-I receptors during a five-day voluntary exercise period prevented the exercise-induced enhancement in memory recall in the Morris water maze task. In contrast, the blockade of IGF-I receptors did not affect the recall abilities of sedentary animals, and did not affect the ability of exercise to enhance learning acquisition (Ding et al., 2006). This finding suggests that IGF-I receptors are specifically involved in mediating the effect of exercise on memory. Gomez-Pinilla and his colleagues have also proposed that an IGF-I receptor blockade may interfere with the effects of exercise in cognition by affecting the expression of brain-derived neurotrophic factor (BDNF), a potent modulator of hippocampal plasticity (Lo, 1995). Indeed, physical activity increases the expression of BDNF in the hippocampus (Gomez-Pinilla et al., 2002; Neeper et al, 1996; Vaynman et al., 2003), as well as the expression of the synaptic protein synapsin I (Ding et al., 2006), which is regulated by BDNF and is involved in presynaptic structure formation and maintenance, and in axonal elongation. Therefore, it has been postulated that BDNF may mediate the effects of exercise on hippocampal plasticity and cognition. In agreement with this proposal, the laboratory of Torres-Aleman has shown that IGF-I increases the expression of BDNF in the hippocampus (Carro et al., 2001). Furthermore, IGF-I receptor blockade abrogates the exercise-induced increase in mRNA and protein levels of BDNF and its precursor (pro-BDNF), and also blocks the effect of exercise on the expression of synapsin I (Ding et al., 2006). Therefore, IGF-I receptors in the hippocampus appear to mediate the effects of exercise on BDNF expression, synaptic molecules, and memory recall.

BDNF is likely not the only mediator of the plastic effects of IGF-I in the central nervous system. As in other organs, the actions of IGF-I in the brain may be affected by the interaction with other molecules. These include neurotransmitters, neuromodulators, cytokines, hormones, and other growth factors. Neurotransmitters, such as glutamate, may affect the actions of IGF-I in the brain by interfering with the signaling of IGF-I receptors. Indeed, the group of Torres-Aleman has shown that glutamate (at high concentrations) induces a loss of sensitivity to IGF-I by phosphorylating the IGF-I receptor docking protein IRS-1 (insulin receptor substrate-1) in serine 307 through a pathway involving the activation of protein kinases A and C (Garcia-Galloway et al., 2003). The proinflammatory cytokine tumor necrosis factor-α also induces IGF-I resistance in neurons by altering IGF-I receptor phosphorylation of IRS-2 (insulin receptor substrate-2) (Venters et al., 1999), and leukemia inhibitory factor has been shown to regulate IGF-I levels in peripheral nerves (de Pablo et al., 2000), where the PI3K/Akt/glycogen synthase kinase 3β (GSK3β) pathway seems to underlay a synergism of nerve growth factor and IGF-I on axonal growth (Jones et al., 2003).

Interactions of Insulin-Like Growth Factor-I and Estradiol in the
Regulation of Brain Plasticity

Among the factors that affect IGF-I action in the nervous system, one of
the best characterized is the ovarian hormone estradiol. IGF-I may regulate
the transcriptional activity of estrogen receptors, and estradiol may rapidly
activate in the brain the two main signal transduction cascades coupled to
the IGF-I receptor: the PI3K and MAPK signaling pathways (see Mendez
et al., 2006, for review). The interaction of estradiol and IGF-I (or estrogen receptors and IGF-I receptors) in the brain during development and
under pathological conditions are reviewed in other chapters in this book
(see Chapters 6 and 9). Here I will mention some studies showing that: (i)
estrogen receptors are involved in the actions of IGF-I to promote adult neurogenesis in the hippocampus, and (ii) estradiol and IGF-I interact to promote synaptic plasticity in the hypothalamus. However, I will first examine
some basic molecular aspects of the interaction between estrogen and IGF-I
receptors in the brain.

IGF-I may affect the hormonal actions of estradiol by modulating estrogen
receptor transcriptional activity. There is now persuasive evidence indicating
that, in addition to the classical activation of estrogen receptors by estradiol
binding, estrogen-receptor-mediated transcriptional activity can be regulated
by ligand-independent mechanisms. Intracellular kinase signaling pathways,
activated by extracellular growth or trophic factors, regulate the ability of
estrogen receptors to promote changes in gene expression. IGF-I is one of the
extracellular regulators of these kinase pathways that have been shown to promote estrogen-receptor-dependent transcription. IGF-I regulation of estrogen
receptor transcriptional activity has been extensively studied in nonneuronal
tissues and cell lines (Klotz et al., 2002; Martin et al., 2000). These studies have
shown that, by phosphorylating estrogen receptors and some transcriptional
cofactors, the intracellular kinases regulated by IGF-I positively regulate
estrogen-receptor-mediated gene expression (Font de Mora and Brown, 2000;
Martin et al., 2000). Several components of the IGF-I intracellular signaling
system have been shown to affect estrogen receptor activity in neuronal cells.
Studies from the laboratory of Adriana Maggi at the University of Milan have
determined that insulin/IGF-I signaling can activate the unliganded estrogen
receptor α in neuronal cells via the Ras-MAPK pathway (Agrati et al., 1997;
Patrone et al., 1996) and that this activation involved the N-terminal activation function 1 (AF-1) domain of the receptor (Patrone et al., 1998). Estradiol-
independent estrogen receptor activation in the brain in vivo is suggested
by studies on an estrogen receptor transgenic strain of mouse with a lucifer-
ase transgene driven by a promoter containing estrogen response elements.
Estrogen-receptor-dependent transgene expression is observed in the brain of
these animals when plasma estrogen levels are low and when brain aromatase
is inhibited, suggesting that estrogen receptors can be activated by estrogen-independent mechanisms (Ciana et al., 2002). This ligand-independent

activation of a hormonal nuclear receptor is not a peculiarity of estrogen receptors. For instance, dopamine and other molecular signals activate the unoccupied progesterone receptors in the brain to regulate sexual receptivity (Auger, 2001; Blaustein, 2004; Mani, 2001).

Although IGF-I promotes ligand-independent estrogen receptor transcriptional activity, it has a different effect in the presence of estradiol. In the absence of estradiol, IGF-I increases estrogen receptor α activity in N2a cells, as in other neuroblastoma cells. In contrast, IGF-I negatively regulates, through activation of the PI3K pathway, the estradiol-induced activation of estrogen receptor α transcriptional activity in this cell type (Mendez and Garcia-Segura, 2006). This effect of IGF-I in N2a cells depends on its ability to regulate GSK3β through the PI3K pathway. In contrast, MAPK blockade has no effect in the regulation by IGF-I of estradiol-induced transcriptional activity of estrogen receptor α (Mendez and Garcia-Segura, 2006). Thus, by using different components of its signaling system, IGF-I may regulate ligand-independent and dependent estrogen receptor transcriptional activity in neuronal cells, and by this mechanism regulate the hormonal actions of estradiol via estrogen receptors.

In addition to the actions of IGF-I on the activity of estrogen receptors in neural cells, we should also consider that estradiol in turn regulates the activity of IGF-I receptor signaling pathways. In vitro and in vivo studies have shown that in the brain, estradiol may rapidly activate the two main signal transduction cascades coupled to the IGF-I receptor: the PI3K and MAPK signaling pathways. In primary cultures of astroglia, primary neuronal cultures, and explants of cerebral cortex and hippocampus, estradiol induces a rapid activation of ERK, in the range of minutes (Toran-Allerand et al., 1999). Estradiol-induced activation of ERK in the brain may also be detected in vivo after systemic administration of the hormone and during cyclic fluctuations of estrogen levels in the estrus cycle (Bi et al., 2001; Cardona-Gomez et al., 2002a, b). ERK activation may be involved in the induction of synaptic plasticity and neurite arborization by estradiol (Bi et al., 2001; Dominguez et al., 2004). Estradiol also induces rapid phosphorylation of Akt (one of the main effectors of the PI3K pathway) in dissociated neurons from the rat cerebral cortex and the hippocampus, in cerebral cortical explants and in the adult rat brain in vivo (Cardona-Gomez et al., 2002b; Ivanova et al., 2002; Wilson et al., 2002; Znamensky et al., 2003). Furthermore, IGF-I and estradiol act synergistically to increase Akt activity in the rat brain (Cardona-Gomez et al., 2002b). Activation of Akt may regulate estradiol-induced synaptic plasticity (Znamensky et al., 2003) and this effect may be mediated by the modulation of GSK3β activity (Cardona-Gomez et al., 2004).

The reciprocal effects of IGF-I on estrogen receptor activity and estradiol on IGF-I receptor signaling may be, at least in part, the consequence of an interaction of the estrogen receptor α and IGF-I receptor in a macromolecular complex associated with components of the PI3K signaling pathway. Immunohistochemical analyses have shown that estrogen receptors and IGF-I

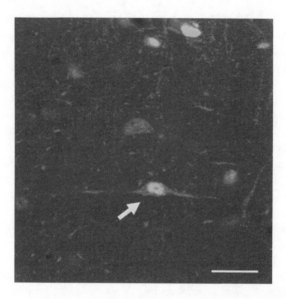

Figure 5.1. Localization of estrogen receptor α and IGF-I receptor immunoreactivities in the arcuate nucleus of the rat hypothalamus. Estrogen receptor α immunoreactivity is observed in neuronal cell nuclei (green) and IGF-I receptor immunoreactivity in the soma and cell processes (red) in the same neurons (arrow). Scale bar, 20 μm. (Microphotograph courtesy of Dr. Gloria Patricia Cardona-Gomez).

receptors are coexpressed by different neuronal and glial populations in the rat central nervous system in vivo (Cardona-Gomez et al., 2000b; Garcia-Segura et al., 2000; see Fig. 5.1). In addition, the administration of estradiol to adult ovariectomized rats results in a transient increase in the association between the IGF-I receptor and estrogen receptor α in the brain, detected by immunoprecipitation studies (Mendez et al., 2003). The maximal association is observed between one and three hours after the hormone administration; however, it should be mentioned that shorter time periods (less than one hour) have not been examined, and therefore the kinetics of the interaction is largely unknown. The association returns to control levels 24 hours after hormone treatment. The interaction is specific for the subtype α of estrogen receptors and is coincidental in time with the increase in tyrosine phosphorylation of the IGF-I receptor, suggesting a possible causal relationship. Estradiol also increases the interaction between the PI3K subunit p85 and insulin receptor substrate-1, one of the first events in the signal transduction of the IGF-I receptor, further suggesting that the increase in IGF-I receptor phosphorylation induced by estradiol reflects a functional activation of this receptor. In addition, estrogen receptor α interacts with other components of the IGF-I receptor signaling pathway in the brain, such as p85, Akt, GSK3β, β-catenin, and tau (Cardona-Gomez et al., 2004; Mendez et al., 2003). Interestingly, the interaction between estrogen and IGF-I systems in the hypothalamus seems to be reciprocal, since the intracerebroventricular administration of IGF-I also resulted in an increase in the levels of association between the estrogen receptor α and IGF-I receptor (Mendez et al., 2003). These findings suggest that the interaction of estrogen receptor α with IGF-I receptor is part of the mechanisms involved in the signaling of both IGF-I and estradiol in the brain. This may explain why estrogen receptor α inhibition blocks IGF-I effects on adult neurogenesis in the hippocampus, and why the inhibition of IGF-I receptors blocks the action of estradiol on synaptic plasticity in the hypothalamus.

Together with my collaborators Margarita Perez-Martin, Iñigo Azcoitia, Jose Luis Trejo, and Amanda Sierra, we examined the role of estrogen receptors on the effect of IGF-I on adult hippocampal neurogenesis (Perez-Martin et al., 2003). We used ovariectomized rats to which either a silastic capsule filled with a mixture of cholesterol and estradiol, or estradiol alone, was inserted subcutaneously. In addition, an osmotic minipump filled with saline, IGF-I, the estrogen receptor antagonist ICI 182780, or a mixture of IGF-I and the estrogen receptor antagonist, was subcutaneously implanted. Minipumps were attached to a brain infusion cannula that was implanted into the right lateral cerebral ventricle. All animals received six daily intraperitoneal injections of 5-bromo-2-deoxyuridine (BrdU) to label proliferating cells. Cells incorporating BrdU were found in the hilus of the dentate gyrus of the hippocampus, in the subgranular zone, and in the inner part of the granule cell layer. Treatment with IGF-I increased the number of total BrdU-positive cells. Interestingly, the estrogen receptor antagonist ICI 182780 blocked the effect of IGF-I, independent of whether the animals were treated or not with estradiol. ICI 182780 by itself did not affect the number of BrdU-positive cells. A study using confocal microscopy to determine the number of BrdU cells labeled with neuronal marker βIII-tubulin revealed that the total number of BrdU-labeled neurons was significantly higher in animals treated either with IGF-I alone or with IGF-I and estradiol, compared to control rats. Interestingly, rats treated with IGF-I and estradiol showed a higher number of BrdU-positive neurons than rats treated with IGF-I alone, and the antiestrogen ICI 182780 blocked the effect of IGF-I on the number of BrdU neurons. Therefore, it seems that estrogen receptors are involved in the effect of IGF-I on hippocampal neurogenesis. It is important to note that the blockade of IGF-I-induced neurogenesis by the estrogen receptor antagonist ICI 182780 was observed in ovariectomized rats in absence of estradiol replacement, indicating that the implication of estrogen receptors in the neurogenic effects of IGF-I is independent of ovarian estradiol. As I have mentioned before, studies on neuroblastoma cells indicate that IGF-I receptor signaling is able to regulate the transcriptional activity of estrogen receptors. Therefore, the effects of IGF-I on adult hippocampal neurogenesis may be, in part, mediated by the regulation by IGF-I of the activity of estrogen receptors. Estrogen receptors may then affect adult hippocampal IGF-I-induced neurogenesis by participating as a component of IGF-I receptor signaling. This interaction of IGF-I with estrogen receptors may occur directly in the proliferating cells, since they express receptors for both IGF-I and estrogen (Isgor and Watson, 2005; Perez-Martin et al., 2003). In addition, the activity of estrogen receptors may be necessary to maintain an adequate expression of IGF-I receptors in the hippocampus in order to sustain the effects of IGF-I on neurogenesis (Cardona-Gomez et al., 2001).

We have also found interactions of estrogen and IGF-I, or estrogen receptors and IGF-I receptors, on synaptic plasticity in the hypothalamic arcuate nucleus, a key center for neuroendocrine regulation of the growth and reproductive axes, and for the control of food intake and energy balance. As it has been already mentioned in Chapter 4, this nucleus shows estrogen-induced and estrus-cycle-related plastic changes in synaptic connectivity and glial–neuronal interactions in female rodents. During the preovulatory and ovulatory phases of the estrus cycle, there is a transient disconnection of axosomatic GABAergic synapses on the arcuate neuronal perikarya of adult female rats and a transient increase in excitatory synaptic inputs on dendritic spines. The synaptic remodeling is induced by estradiol and is linked to plastic modifications in astroglial processes and to modifications in the frequency of neuronal firing of arcuate neurons. The estrogen-induced synaptic and glial remodeling in the arcuate nucleus may participate in the regulation of secretion of parvocellular hypothalamic hormones, such as growth-hormone-releasing hormone, somatostatin, and gonadotropin-releasing hormone (see also Chapters 4 and 8). Peripheral IGF-I produced in the liver and other tissues may reach the brain and may affect neuroendocrine regulation by the hypothalamus. IGF-I may regulate pituitary growth hormone secretion by actions on growth-hormone-releasing hormone and somatostatin neurons in the arcuate nucleus. In addition, IGF-I may also affect pituitary gonadotropins by actions in the arcuate nucleus and the median eminence; IGF-I from a peripheral origin also appears to be one of the signals related to the initiation of puberty. IGF-I levels increase dramatically in the rat arcuate nucleus with the onset of female puberty, and fluctuate during the estrus cycle in parallel to the release of gonadotropins (Dueñas et al., 1994). High levels of IGF-I immunoreactivity in glial cells (mainly in tanycytes) are detected in the afternoon of proestrus and the morning of estrus in the arcuate nucleus of cycling female rats, then IGF-I immunoreactivity declines in the morning of metestrus. Therefore, IGF-I immunoreactivity follows the changes in plasma levels of estradiol and progesterone during the estrus cycle. Indeed, estradiol and progesterone regulate IGF-I immunoreactivity in arcuate glial cells. IGF-l immunoreactivity is low in glial cells of ovariectomized rats and increases in a dose-dependent manner when ovariectomized rats are injected with estradiol, an effect blocked by the simultaneous administration of progesterone. Therefore, IGF-I levels fluctuate in the rat hypothalamic arcuate nucleus during the estrus cycle in parallel with the remodeling of synaptic contacts and the fluctuation of ovarian hormones in plasma. Furthermore, the administration of estradiol to ovariectomized rats results in a significant increase in IGF-I levels in the arcuate in parallel with a decrease in the number of axosomatic synapses. These findings suggest that IGF-I is involved in the effects of estradiol on synapses (Dueñas et al., 1994; Garcia-Segura et al., 1994a). The fluctuation of IGF-I levels in arcuate glia may be in part medi-ated by the over-expression of insulin-like growth factor binding protein-2 by hypothalamic tanycytes (Cardona-Gomez et al., 2000a). Tanycytes are spe-cialized glial cells located in the arcuate nucleus and the median eminence (Rodriguez et al., 2005; see also Chapter 2) that express IGF-I receptors and accumulate IGF-I from the cerebrospinal fluid (Fernandez-Galaz et al., 1996). This accumulation of IGF-I by tanycytes is mediated by IGF-I receptors, and shows marked differences during the estrus cycle. Therefore, tanycytes may regulate IGF-I incorporation in the arcuate nucleus, determining the local availability of this modulator of synaptic plasticity.

Results from in vivo experiments using intracerebroventricular infusion of specific receptor antagonists have shown that both estrogen receptors and IGF-I receptors are involved in the induction of synaptic and glial plastic modifications in the arcuate nucleus during the estrus cycle (Cardona-Gomez et al., 2000a, c; Fernandez-Galaz et al., 1997, 1999a). Under control conditions, the number of synaptic inputs on arcuate neuronal perikarya of cycling female rats decreases between the morning and afternoon of proestrus, remains low in estrus, and recovers the following day; these changes are accompanied by the remodeling of astroglial processes. To explore whether IGF-I may affect this plasticity, Carmen Fernandez-Galaz infused an IGF-I receptor antagonist into the lateral cerebral ventricle of cycling female rats to neutralize the local action of IGF-I in the brain. The intracerebroventricular administration of the IGF-I receptor antagonist JB1 resulted in the blockage of the phasic remodel-ing of synapses and glial processes observed in the arcuate nucleus during the estrus cycle (Fernandez-Galaz et al., 1999a). In contrast, JB1 did not affect the number of synapses in proestrus rats, suggesting that IGF-I receptor activa-tion is necessary for the estrus-cycle-associated synaptic plastic changes but not for the normal maintenance of synaptic inputs.

The decrease in the number of synapses on the day of proestrus can be mimicked by the injection of estradiol to ovariectomized rats. The intrac-erebroventricular administration of ICI 182780, an antagonist of estrogen receptors, or JB1, an antagonist of IGF-I receptors, did not affect the basal number of axosomatic synapses in ovariectomized rats injected with oil. Even the simultaneous administration of both receptor antagonists did not affect the number of axosomatic synapses in rats injected with oil, indicating that the activation of estrogen receptors and IGF-I receptors are not necessary for the maintenance of the synaptic inputs on arcuate neuronal perikarya. In contrast, the infusion in the lateral cerebral ventricle of the estrogen receptor antagonist ICI 182780 prevented the decrease in axosomatic synapses after the administration of estradiol to ovariectomized rats. This finding indicates that estrogen-induced synaptic plasticity in the arcuate nucleus is mediated by the activation of estrogen receptors. In addition, the estrogen-induced decrease in the number of axosomatic synapses is also prevented by the administration of the IGF-I receptor antagonist JB1, either alone or in combination with the estrogen receptor antagonist, indicating that the estradiol-induced decrease in the number of axosomatic synapses in the arcuate nucleus of ovariectomized rats is dependent on IGF-I receptors (Cardona-Gomez et al., 2000c). Therefore, it seems that both estrogen and IGF-I receptors are involved in the induction of synaptic plasticity in the hypothalamus of intact rats during the estrus cycle.

Arcuate neurons express estrogen and IGF-I receptors (Garcia-Segura et al., 1997; Shughrue et al., 1997) and may therefore be a direct target for both estradiol and IGF-I. IGF-I may affect pre- and/or postsynaptic mechanisms, since ultrastructural studies have shown that the IGF-I receptor is present both in axosomatic presynaptic terminals as well as in neuronal perikarya of the rat arcuate nucleus (Garcia-Segura et al., 1997). In addition, arcuate astrocytes are also a target for IGF-I, since they also express IGF-I receptors (Garcia-Segura et al., 1997). Arcuate astrocytes appear to be directly involved in the regulation of synaptic inputs to arcuate neurons, since synaptic disconnection of arcuate neurons in estrus females is accompanied by an increased extension of GFAP immunoreactive astrocytic processes (detected by light microscopy), and by an increase in the ensheathment of neuronal surfaces by astrocytic processes (detected by electron microscopic analysis). Interestingly, studies on hypothalamic tissue fragments from ovariectomized rats have shown that IGF-I receptor activation is needed for the induction of GFAP changes by estrogen in the arcuate nucleus (Fernandez-Galaz et al., 1997). In addition, tanycytes may play an important role in the interaction of estradiol and IGF-I for the regulation of synaptic plasticity, regulating the levels of IGF-I in the arcuate nucleus (Dueñas et al., 1994; Fernandez-Galaz et al., 1996, 1997). Indeed, the administration of the IGF-I receptor antagonist JB1 in the rat lateral cerebral ventricle is able to block both the accumulation of IGF-I by arcuate nucleus tanycytes and estrogen-induced synaptic plasticity (Fernandez-Galaz et al., 1996, 1997; Garcia-Segura et al., 1999a). The interaction of IGF-I and estradiol in the plastic events on the arcuate nucleus during the estrus cycle may participate in the control of gonadotropin secretion and reproduction. However, as we will see later on in this chapter, plastic reorganization of synapses in the arcuate nucleus is also involved in the hormonal control of feeding.

ERYTHROPOIETIN

The glycoprotein erythropoietin (Jelkmann, 2007), the major regulator of erythropoiesis, is a relative newcomer among the hormones that have been shown to regulate neural plasticity. During fetal life, erythropoietin is mainly produced in the liver; in adults it is mainly synthesized in the kidney, and to a lesser extent in liver hepatocytes (Jelkmann, 1992; Krantz, 1991). The expression of erythropoietin in mammals is increased to enhance blood red cell production when oxygen levels are low. In addition to its key function in erythropoiesis, erythropoietin may also target several tissues, including the brain.

The actions of erythropoietin in the brain were unexpected, and were first detected in studies using stimulus-related evoked potentials and neuropsychological tests in hemodialysis patients. These studies revealed an improvement of brain function, cognition, and sensory processing in those patients treated with erythropoietin to increase blood red cell levels compared to hemodialysis patients that were not treated with erythropoietin (Grimm et al., 1990; Marsh et al., 1991; Nissenson, 1992; Sagales et al., 1993). The cognitive effects of erythropoietin in these patients may in part be the consequence of better oxygen delivery to the brain as a result of the increase in blood red cell levels. However, further studies suggested that erythropoietin may also directly affect the central nervous system. In fact, we know today that erythropoietin is able to cross the blood–brain barrier (Brines et al., 2000), and then it may act on erythropoietin receptors, members of the cytokine receptor superfamily (Youssoufian et al., 1993), which are expressed by neurons (Morishita et al., 1997) and brain capillary endothelial cells (Yamaji et al., 1996) from several brain regions, including the cerebral cortex, the hippocampus, the capsula interna, and the midbrain (Digicaylioglu et al., 1995; Morishita et al., 1997). In addition, as is the case for many other hormones, erythropoietin is also locally produced by the nervous tissue. Thus, erythropoietin mRNA has been detected in biopsies from the human hippocampus, amygdala, and temporal cortex, and in various regions of the brain of monkeys and mice (Marti et al., 1996). Astrocytes and neurons are among the cells that synthesize erythropoietin in the adult central nervous system (Bernaudin et al., 1999, 2000; Marti et al., 1996).

Erythropoietin decreases microglia activation, cytokine production, nitric oxide formation, and inflammation; it promotes the expression of BDNF, decreases excitotoxicity, and inhibits neuronal apoptosis, protecting neurons from a variety of pathological insults, including ischemia (see Chapter 9). These neuroprotective actions of erythropoietin are accompanied by plastic remodeling of neuronal connectivity. For instance, the infusion of erythropoietin into the lateral cerebral ventricles of gerbils rescue hippocampal CA1 neurons from ischemic damage, and at the same time increases the number of synapses on CA1 pyramidal neurons (Sakanaka et al., 1998). There is also evidence suggesting that erythropoietin may increase adult neurogenesis in the dentate gyrus after a traumatic brain injury in rats (Lu et al., 2005). Another plastic action of erythropoietin in the rodent adult brain is the promotion of neurogenesis in the subventricular germinal zone, where erythropoietin receptors are expressed (Shingo et al., 2001). In vitro studies have shown that modest hypoxia increases the production of neurons from cultured neural stem cells. This effect of hypoxia is accompanied by an induction of erythropoietin gene expression. Incubation of neural stem cells with erythropoietin also results in an increased production of neurons, while an erythropoietin neutralizing antibody blocks the induction of neuronal production by hypoxia.

These findings suggest that hypoxia induces the expression of erythropoietin in neural stem cells, and erythropoietin then promotes the differentiation of neural stem cells in neuronal progenitors (Shingo et al., 2001). Similar results have been obtained after the infusion of erythropoietin into the lateral cerebral ventricles of young adult mice. Erythropoietin increases the number of newly generated cells migrating to the olfactory bulb in parallel to a decrease in the number of neural stem cells in the subventricular zone. The newly generated cells are incorporated in the olfactory bulb, resulting in an increase in the number of new olfactory bulb interneurons. The infusion of anti-erythropoietin antibodies in the lateral cerebral ventricles increases the number of neural stem cells in the subventricular zone and decreases the generation of new olfactory bulb interneurons. These findings indicate that erythropoietin is a regulator of the production of neuronal progenitor cells by neural stem cells in adult mammals, although erythropoietin regulation of adult neurogenesis may be mediated by an autocrine and/or paracrine mechanism, rather than by a hormonal action (Shingo et al., 2001). In addition, using conditional erythropoietin receptor knock-down mice, Tsai et al. (2006) have demonstrated that the erythropoietin receptor is involved in cell proliferation in the subventricular zone and in poststroke neurogenesis, by mediating migration of neuroblasts to the peri-infarct cortex.

ANGIOTENSIN

The brain renin-angiotensin system (RAS) regulates blood pressure, sodium, and water balance; additionally, the RAS affects the secretion of other hormones. The brain is a target for circulating angiotensin II. Circulating angiotensin I is transformed within the brain into angiotensin II and in turn, angiotensin II may be transformed into angiotensin III. In addition, circulating angiotensin II may directly act on angiotensin II receptors within the brain. The brain expresses both the subtypes 1 and 2 of the angiotensin II receptor, and angiotensin II and III have a similar affinity for both receptor subtypes. Angiotensin II and III promote the release of vasopressin by magnocellular vasopressinergic hypothalamic neurons, increasing blood pressure. Angiotensin II is also involved in the brain response to stress (Saavedra and Benicky, 2007). In addition, the brain expresses the angiotensin IV receptor, which appears to be involved in effects of angiotensin peptides on the regulation of blood flow, exploratory behavior, and cognition. The angiotensin IV receptor interacts with brain matrix metalloproteinases, inducing the modification of extracellular matrix molecules involved in synaptic remodeling (Wright et al., 2002; Wright and Harding, 2004).

Angiotensin II has been shown to regulate functional synaptic plasticity, blocking long-term synaptic potentiation in the hippocampus (Armstrong et al., 1996; Denny et al., 1991; Wayner et al., 1993, 1996) and suppressing both long-term synaptic potentiation and long-term synaptic depression in the lateral nucleus of the amygdala (Tchekalarova and Albrecht, 2007; von Bohlen und Halbach and Albrecht, 1998). Angiotensin III also blocks long-term synaptic potentiation in the hippocampus, but is 40- to 50-fold less potent than angiotensin II (Denny et al., 1991). Angiotensin II also appears to regulate hippocampal neurogenesis, since it has been shown that an antagonist of angiotensin II type 1 receptors significantly reduced running-enhanced neurogenesis in the adult rat hippocampus (Mukuda and Sugiyama, 2007). Besides angiotensin II and III, other angiotensin peptides, such as angiotensin IV and angiotensin-(1–7) may also have important regulatory effects on brain plasticity. Thus, angiotensin IV analogues promote long-term synaptic potentiation in the hippocampus (Kramár et al., 2001; Wayner et al., 2001), while angiotensin-(1–7) increases long-term synaptic potentiation in the hippocampus (Hellner et al., 2005) and in the lateral nucleus of the amygdala (Albrecht, 2007).

Feeding Hormones: Leptin, Ghrelin and Glucagon-Like Peptide-1

Food and feeding affect brain plasticity and cognition. The deleterious cognitive effects of undernutrition at early ages are well-known; diet in adult life may also affect cognition and brain plasticity. Dietary restriction has been reported to enhance neurogenesis in the hippocampus of adult mice (Lee et al., 2002), and a high fat diet suppresses neurogenesis in adult rats (Lindqvist et al., 2006). Food texture and mastication (Aoki et al., 2005; Mitome et al., 2005) also affect neurogenesis in the hippocampus of rodents. In addition, modifications of neurogenesis in the hypothalamic circuits regulating feeding may be an important component in the control of food intake and energy balance (Kokoeva et al., 2005). Several hormonal factors regulate feeding and energy balance, and may have an impact on neural plasticity. Here I will review recent data indicating that actions of leptin, ghrelin, and glucagon-like peptide-1, three major hormonal regulators of feeding, involve brain remodeling.

One of the most surprising findings in the last few decades is the control exerted by adipocytes on the brain. These modest cells, whose function appeared in the past to be limited to fat accumulation, do indeed regulate the function of the most complex organ of the body. Fat cells regulate our impulses to eat and therefore our behavior. This is a good lesson of humility. In my view, the discovery of leptin, the hormone released by fat cells that control feeding behavior, has as many philosophical as scientific implications. Ghrelin, another hormone regulating feeding, appears to also have an impact on cognition. These hormonal effects are associated with plastic changes in the circuits controlling feeding, and in brain cognitive areas such as the hippocampus.

Leptin, which is mainly (but not exclusively) produced by adipocytes, is a 167-amino acid protein encoded by the obese (ob) gene (Zhang et al., 1994). Leptin regulates feeding and energy balance, at least in part by modulating the activity of neuropeptide Y and proopiomelanocortin neurons in the hypothalamic arcuate nucleus (Fig. 5.2). Tamas L. Horvath and his collaborators at Yale University and other institutions have shown the influence

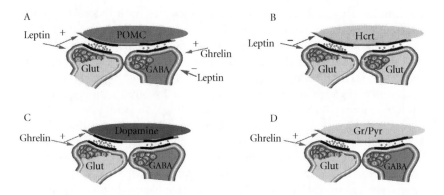

Figure 5.2. Metabolic hormones regulate glutamatergic (Glut) and GABAergic (GABA) synaptic plasticity in different brain regions. In the arcuate nucleus (A), both leptin and ghrelin alter the synaptology of proopiomelanocortin (POMC) neurons in support of either satiety (leptin) or hunger (ghrelin). In the lateral hypothalamus (B), leptin-dependent reorganization of excitatory inputs and miniature excitatory postsynaptic currents were observed on hypocretin (Hcrt) neurons in response to fasting in a manner that promotes increased arousal. In the ventral tegmentum (C), dopamine neurons showed rapid changes in the GABAergic and glutamatergic inputs in response to ghrelin in association with increased dopamine neuronal activity and feeding. Ghrelin also altered synaptic spine density in granular/pyramidal cells of the hippocampus (D) in parallel with increased propagation of long-term synaptic potentiation and enhanced performance of animals in various behavioral tasks. (Courtesy of Dr. Tamas Horvath).

of leptin on hypothalamic synaptic plasticity (Horvath, 2005, 2006). They have shown that leptin-deficient (ob/ob) mice differ from wild-type mice in the number of excitatory and inhibitory synapses. and postsynaptic currents onto neuropeptide Y and proopiomelanocortin neurons (Pinto et al., 2004). When leptin was delivered to ob/ob mice, the synaptic density and synaptic currents were modified toward control wild-type values. This effect was detectable several hours before the effect of leptin on food intake. Therefore, the work of Horvath and his collaborators demonstrates that leptin induces structural and functional synaptic remodeling in the hypothalamic circuits regulating food intake. The time course of these changes, preceding the behavioral effect, is compatible with a causal relationship. These observations also raised the possibility that synaptic rewiring is an inherent and mandatory characteristic of hypothalamic circuits for adequate regulation of energy balance (Horvath and Diano, 2004). Indeed, the laboratory of Tamas Horvath has provided evidence that other neuronal circuits associated with feeding control are also plastic (Fig. 5.2). This is the case with hypocretin/orexin hypothalamic neurons. As I have mentioned before, hypocretin, also called orexin, is a hypothalamic peptide involved in the regulation of feeding and arousal. Hypocretin/orexin neurons are located in the lateral hypothalamus and project to many regions of the brain and spinal cord, forming a circuitry that may synchronize various autonomic, endocrine, and metabolic events (de Lecea et al., 1998; Sakurai et al., 1998; Sutcliffe and de Lecea, 2002). Hypocretin/orexin neurons express leptin receptors (Håkansson et al., 1999; Horvath et al., 1999a) and may be involved with the effects of leptin on arousal. Tamas Horvath and Xiao-Bing Gao examined the afferent inputs to hypocretin/orexin neurons using patch-clamp recordings in lateral hypothalamic slice preparations from transgenic mice in which hypocretin/orexin neurons are visualized by green fluorescence protein. In addition, they assessed the number of synapses on the perikarya of hypocretin/orexin neurons by electron microscopy. They found that overnight food deprivation promoted the formation of more asymmetric, putatively excitatory synapses on hypocretin/orexin perikarya, and increased miniature excitatory post-synaptic currents onto hypocretin/orexin cells. These synaptic changes were not observed when the animals were treated with leptin (Horvath and Gao, 2005). Thus, it appears that leptin may control synaptic plasticity in multiple synaptic circuits related to feeding.

The effects of leptin on synaptic plasticity are not limited to brain regions directly involved in the control of feeding and energy balance. Leptin receptors are expressed in many brain regions such as the cerebral cortex, cerebellum, brainstem, basal ganglia, and hippocampus (Elmquist et al., 1998).Therefore, leptin may have many other actions in the brain, including the modulation of cognition. Lynne J. Shanley, Andrew J. Irving, and Jenni Harvey from the Universities of Dundee and Aberdeen in the UK, reported in 2001 that leptin affects synaptic plasticity in the hippocampus. They used a modest primed burst stimulation of the Schaffer collateral commissural pathway in rat hippocampal slices to induce short-term potentiation of synaptic transmission, which returned to baseline after 30–35 minutes. Incubation with leptin at concentrations comparable with those circulating in plasma and immediately before the stimulation paradigm resulted in the conversion of short-term potentiation into robust long-term potentiation lasting up to 60 minutes. This effect was mediated by a facilitation of NMDA receptor-mediated synaptic transmission. In hippocampal cultures, leptin rapidly enhanced NMDA-induced increases in intracellular Ca^{2+} levels, and this effect was blocked by inhibitors of the PI3K, MAPK, and Src tyrosine kinases (Harvey et al., 2006; Shanley et al., 2001).

Further evidence of the effects of leptin on synaptic plasticity in the hippocampus was provided by the analysis of hippocampal long-term potentiation and long-term depression of excitatory CA1 synapses in two leptin-receptor-deficient rodents: Zucker rats and db/db mice. These animals showed an impaired spatial memory (assessed in the Morris water maze test); in both cases, an impairment of long-term potentiation and long-term depression was observed in hippocampal slices. As expected, due to the lack of receptors, leptin did not affect synaptic plasticity in these animals (Li et al., 2002).

It has also been reported that under conditions of enhanced excitability, evoked in an Mg^{2+}-free medium or following the blockade of $GABA_A$ receptors, leptin induces long-term depression in the CA1 area of the hippocampus (Durakoglugil et al., 2005). This form of long-term synaptic depression in CA1 excitatory synapses induced by leptin is only observed under conditions of enhanced excitability, it seems to be dependent on the activation of NMDA receptors, and is enhanced by the inhibition of PI3K or protein phosphatases 1 and 2A.

Plastic effects of leptin in the hippocampus have also been detected in vivo (Wayner et al., 2004). Administration of leptin in the dentate gyrus of anesthetized rats either enhances or decreases long-term synaptic potentiation in medial perforant path dentate granule cell synapses, depending on the dose. Thus, at a 1.0 micromolar concentration leptin enhances long-term potentiation, while both lower and higher doses of leptin inhibit long-term potentiation. Leptin also has dose-dependent effects on behavioral performance in the Morris water maze test, and on long-term potentiation induced in hippocampal slices (Oomura et al., 2006). The effects of leptin on hippocampal plasticity may be partly direct, and partly related to the synaptic plastic changes induced by leptin in the hypothalamic hypocretin/orexin neurons that I have analyzed before. The lateral hypothalamus is a brain region that facilitates learning and memory; hypocretin/orexin neurons (which project their axons widely in the brain, including the hippocampus) may be involved in these cognitive effects (Jaeger et al., 2002; Telegdy and Adamik, 2002). Hypocretin/orexin neurons may affect hippocampal synaptic plasticity indirectly via the activation of the locus coeruleus noradrenergic system (Horvath et al., 1999b). Noradrenergic projections from the locus coeruleus innervate the hippocampus (in particular, the dentate gyrus), and the activation of these noradrenergic inputs may produce a long-lasting potentiation of the glutamatergic perforant path input to the dentate gyrus (Neuman and Harley, 1983). Indeed, the infusion of hypocretin/orexin into the locus coeruleus of anesthetized rats produces a robust long-lasting potentiation of the perforant path-evoked dentate gyrus population spike (Walling et al., 2004). In addition, hippocampal neurons express hypocretin/orexin receptors, and hypocretin/orexin immunoreactive axon terminals have been detected in the hippocampus. Therefore, leptin may affect hippocampal plasticity via direct hypocretin/orexin projections to the hippocampus. Indeed, hypocretin/orexin infusion into the dentate gyrus of anesthetized rats enhances long-term synaptic potentiation in medial perforant path dentate granule cell synapses (Wayner et al., 2004). Furthermore, hypocretin/orexin receptors in the CA1 hippocampal region of rats are involved in acquisition, consolidation, and retrieval tasks in the Morris water maze (Akbari et al., 2006).

Ghrelin is a 28-amino-acid peptide secreted by oxyntic glands of the stomach, which are located in the gastric mucosa and contain epithelial cells that secrete gastric acid. Ghrelin is also produced by other tissues, including the small intestine, the kidney, or the placenta. Ghrelin stimulates growth hormone release (Kojima et al., 1999) and has other functions, including the regulation of sleep, anxiety, feeding behavior, and energy metabolism (Seoane et al., 2004). Acting on the hypothalamus, ghrelin up-regulates food intake by a mechanism involving the regulation of the neuropeptide Y (NPY) and proopiomelanocortin (POMC) neurons (Cowley et al., 2003; Nakazato et al., 2001). Ghrelin may also regulate food intake acting in other brain regions. For instance, application of ghrelin into the dorsal vagal complex stimulates food intake (Faulconbridge et al., 2003). These hormonal actions of ghrelin in the control of feeding are associated with a remarkable plastic remodeling, including modifications in neurogenesis and synaptic plasticity.

Weizhen Zhang, Michael W. Mulholland, and their colleagues at the University of Michigan were the first to demonstrate that ghrelin stimulates neurogenesis. They analyzed the effect of systemic administration of ghrelin on the incorporation of the thymidine analogue BrdU in the dorsal motor nucleus of the vagus of adult male rats. They found that ghrelin stimulates vagotomy-induced BrdU incorporation in neuronal precursors in this brain structure. Furthermore, ghrelin increased the incorporation of BrdU in neurons from the dorsal motor nucleus of the vagus in culture (Zhang et al., 2004). Similar results were obtained in the nucleus of the solitary tract. Systemic administration of ghrelin significantly increased BrdU incorporation in this nucleus in adult rats with a cervical vagotomy; Ghrelin also increased the incorporation of BrdU in neurons from the nucleus of the solitary tract in culture (Zhang et al., 2004). The effects of ghrelin on neurogenesis, both in the dorsal motor nucleus of the vagus and in the nucleus of the solitary tract, appear to be mediated by the activation of L-type calcium channels.

In addition to regulating neurogenesis, ghrelin also affects synaptic plasticity in different brain regions (Fig. 5.2). For instance, ghrelin regulates feeding and increases dopamine release in the nucleus accumbens by a rapid modulation of synaptic plasticity on ventral tegmental area neurons (Abizaid et al., 2006). Ghrelin also regulates synaptic plasticity in the hippocampus, inducing the formation of synapses on dendritic spines and the generation of long-term synaptic potentiation. These neuroplastic actions are accompanied by enhancing effects of ghrelin on spatial learning and memory (Diano et al., 2006). These findings suggest that ghrelin may have other functions in the brain in addition to the regulation of energy balance.

In addition to leptin and ghrelin, other hormonal signals regulate feeding and energy balance. Furthermore, hormonal signals that regulate feeding may interact in specific brain neuronal circuits with other hormonal signals to integrate different endocrine inputs and coordinate endocrine and behavioral responses. Therefore, it should be expected that different hormones may interact with ghrelin and leptin in the regulation of synaptic plasticity. The laboratory of Tamas L. Horvath has provided evidence for such interactions in the hypothalamus. I have already mentioned that estradiol affects synaptic plasticity in the hypothalamic arcuate nucleus. The plastic changes induced by estradiol in this brain region have been interpreted in relation to the hormonal regulation of gonadotropins. However, as we have seen, the arcuate nucleus is a key center for the regulation of feeding. In addition, estradiol has anorexigenic effects. Therefore, the orexigenic hormone ghrelin and the anorexigenic hormone estradiol may have different effects on synaptic plasticity in the arcuate nucleus. Horvath and his team have analyzed this question using leptin-deficient (ob/ob), leptin receptor-deficient (db/db), and wild-type mice. They found that ghrelin rearranges synapses in wild-type animals to support the suppressed proopiomelanocortin tone, whereas estradiol increases the number of excitatory, glutamate inputs on the perikaryon of proopiomelanocortin neurons, while decreasing food intake and body weight. The neuroplastic effect of estradiol was detected in both wild-type, leptin-deficient (ob/ob), and leptin receptor-deficient (db/db) mice, indicating that it is not mediated by leptin (Gao et al., 2007; Horvath, 2006). These important findings indicate that different hormonal signals that regulate feeding and energy balance may integrate their effects by the selective modulation of synaptic plasticity in specific hypothalamic circuits.

Another hormone involved in the control of feeding that has been shown to regulate synaptic plasticity is glucagon-like peptide-1 (GLP-1), a 37-amino -acid peptide produced by intestinal cells and released into the blood in response to food ingestion. GLP-1 regulates glucose homeostasis by stimulating the insulin synthesis and release from pancreatic β cells, and also has direct effects on the hypothalamus to regulate food intake (Christophe, 1998; Perry and Greig, 2003). GLP-1 and GLP-1 receptors are expressed in several hypothalamic nuclei and in the hippocampus, among other brain regions (Alvarez et al., 2005; Chowen et al., 1999; Rodriguez de Fonseca et al., 2000). In addition to regulating food intake and glucose metabolism acting on the hypothalamus, GLP-1 promotes learning and memory (During et al., 2003), facilitates synaptic transmission, and enhances long-term synaptic potentiation in the hippocampus (Gault and Hölscher, 2008).

HORMONAL INFLUENCES ON BRAIN PLASTICITY: RECAPITULATION OF CHAPTERS 3, 4 AND 5

In this chapter (and the two previous chapters) I have examined the regulatory actions exerted by a variety of hormones on brain plasticity. Although I have examined the neuroplastic actions of each hormone separately in these three chapters, it is obvious that all hormonal actions are integrated in the organism. It is important to consider that different hormones may reciprocally interact in the regulation of their plasma or brain levels. Thus the neuroplastic actions of a given hormone may be mediated by the modification in the levels of other hormones. For instance some actions of growth hormone may be mediated by IGF-I and the actions of some peptide hormones may be mediated by hormonal steroids. In addition, we have seen that several hormones regulate plasticity in the same brain region. For instance, oxytocin, estradiol, and prolactin regulate synaptic and glial plasticity in oxytocin neurons; melatonin, thyroid hormones, estradiol, progesterone, androgens, stress hormones, vasopressin,

GnRH, erythropoietin, IGF-I, ghrelin, GLP-1, and angiotensin regulate synaptic plasticity in pyramidal cells in the hippocampus; ghrelin, leptin, IGF-I, and estradiol regulate synaptic plasticity in the arcuate nucleus; and several hormones regulate neurogenesis in the hippocampus and the subventricular zone. Therefore, the plastic events on oxytocin neurons, CA1 pyramids, and arcuate neurons, and the rate of neurogenesis in the hippocampus and the subventricular zone (among other brain regions) are modulated at every moment by the interaction of many different hormonal signals. We have also seen some examples of the outcome of these hormonal interactions on plasticity, including the interaction of melatonin and gonadal hormones for seasonal brain plasticity in songbirds; the interaction of estradiol and progesterone in the regulation of synaptic and glial plasticity in several brain regions of rodents; the interactions of androgens and estrogens in androgen-regulated synaptic plasticity; the interaction of estradiol and oxytocin on synaptic and glial plasticity associated with oxytocin neurons; or the interaction of leptin and estradiol in the regulation of synaptic plasticity in the arcuate nucleus.

For some hormonal interactions on brain plasticity, we have considerable information regarding the cellular and molecular mechanisms involved. Thus, I have examined with some detail the mechanisms of the interaction of estradiol, progesterone, and IGF-I on synaptic plasticity in the arcuate nucleus. In addition, we have seen that the effects of different hormones on a single neuroplastic event may be exerted via the same intracellular signaling pathways, or via a common intermediary molecule, such as BDNF. Moreover, the neuroplastic response to a given hormone integrates actions on different mechanisms of plasticity and at different brain regions. Thus, we have also seen that a given hormone does not target a single regulatory molecular mechanism or a single neuroplastic event. In fact, the same hormone may have different effects on the same molecular mechanism in different brain regions, and may regulate different mechanisms of plasticity in different cells within the same (or different) brain regions. Therefore, the brain responds to the same hormone by coordinated and, in some cases, opposite changes in functional and morphological synaptic plasticity in different regions. The convergent interaction of multiple hormonal signals on the regulation of single neuroplastic events, together with the divergent action of each hormone on multiple neuroplastic events, opens up the possibility for an integrated metaplastic hormonal regulation of plasticity in adaptation to changing homeodynamic conditions and previous life events (see Fig. 3.1). Therefore, the brain may potentially integrate, under the form of metaplasticity, the consecutive physiological variations in the levels of multiple hormones. As an approximation to the study of the metaplastic regulation exerted by hormones, in the following chapters I will examine integrated multiple hormonal actions within the context of different life stages.

Chapter 6

Life Stages, Hormones, and Brain Remodeling: Early Hormonal Influences on Brain Mutability

INTRODUCTION: HORMONAL IMPRINTING OF THE NERVOUS SYSTEM

As mentioned in Chapter 1, there is no doubt that the phase of maximal mutability of the nervous system corresponds to the developmental period. The developmental organization of the brain and spinal cord from the primitive neural epithelium is not a linear process of growth. Proliferation, differentiation, and maturation of neural cells are also accompanied by cell death, cellular elimination, and tissue remodeling. The adult organization of neural cells in cortical layers and nuclei in the grey matter are the result of several intermediate stages in which consecutive groups of cells, by radial or tangential migration from distant sites, are incorporated into each structure, in some cases transiently. Neuronal connectivity is developed in multiple transitory steps, and the first connections established between neurons will be soon replaced by new ones or reorganized to reach its mature state. Axonal growth cones and dendritic filopodia develop while exploring their environment in a complex process of consecutive advancements and retractions in which they are guided by multiple permissive, attractive, repulsive, and directional signals in the search for their targets. Axons grow for considerable distances in some cases, often following highly intricate trajectories. In parallel, neurons extend their dendritic processes as well, which establish transient connections with incoming axonal terminals. A first phase of developmental exuberance of neuronal synaptic connections is followed by a process of selection of axonal branches, dendrites, and synapses. Then, dendrites and axonal terminals suffer different phases of structural and functional remodeling until the establishment of the final functional pattern of synaptic connectivity.

Glial cells are also highly active during the developmental period. Radial glial cells will act as progenitors for intermediate progenitors, neurons, and other glial cells, and will establish transitory scaffoldings for neuronal migration. Then, in higher vertebrates, radial glial cells will be transformed into astrocytes, which will migrate to new central nervous system regions and change its cellular form and shape in adaptation to the new cellular milieu. Microglial cells participate in the permanent developmental remodeling of neural structures and synaptic connections, removing transitory cellular elements. Oligodendroglial cells, mainly during the early postnatal period, will elaborate myelin and transform unmyelinated regions of the white matter into fully functional myelinated structures. In addition, we should add to the picture the growth of blood vessels and the establishment of anatomical, functional, and metabolic interactions of astrocytes with capillaries and neurons. Thus, the development of the central nervous system represents a process of radical cellular and tissue reorganization. Although the brain and spinal cord will keep a considerable degree of mutability after the end of the developmental period and the plastic responses of neural tissue will be incremented in the case of an injury or under degenerative processes, the central nervous system will never again show such a high degree of plasticity.

Hormonal signaling is essential for the coordinated development of different regions of the body. The developmental maturation of the endocrine system during prenatal and early postnatal life occurs in parallel to the building of the central nervous system, and there is a continuous and progressive interaction between the organizational events in both systems. Early hormonal secretions from endocrine glands affect many aspects of neural development, including the building of the functional organization of the neuroendocrine hypothalamus, which in turn will impact the activity of endocrine glands. Hormones have an important impact on brain development—acting as permissive or organizational factors and exerting an early imprinting in the central nervous system that will affect future neuroendocrine, neuroimmune, behavioral, affective, and cognitive functions. Hormonal imprinting is one of the most important physiological and adaptive influences for the future plasticity of the nervous system (Fig. 6.1). Hormonal modifications of the pattern of neural differentiation during fetal and early postnatal development will have a strong impact on adult life. Fetal life is indeed a very sensitive period for the programming of future individual development in adaptation to maternal and environmental conditions. In addition to hormones, many other factors during fetal life may have permanent organizational effects in the brain.

One highly influential theory elaborated by David J. Barker and colleagues working at the University of Southampton proposed that nourishment before birth and during infancy programs future development and the appearance of risk factors for adult diseases, such as raised blood pressure, fibrinogen concentration, or glucose intolerance. In its original form, the prediction was that poor nutrition early in life increases susceptibility to the effects of an affluent diet (Barker and Osmond, 1986). According to this theory, which has been elaborated on and disseminated in several papers and books, many adult diseases originate through the adaptation that the fetus makes when it is undernourished (Barker, 2004; Hales and Barker, 2001). In agreement with this theory, studies with identical twins have shown that intrauterine environmental factors have a strong impact on the risk of disease in later life (Iliadou et al., 2004). Undernourishment is only one of the multiple influences that may affect development. These include modifications in the temperature and other parameters in the physical environment, modifications in social interactions,

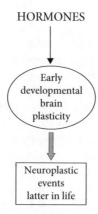

Figure 6.1. Hormonal regulation of brain developmental plasticity is an example of metaplastic regulation, since it predetermines future neuroplastic responses later in life.

infections, and genetic or chromosomal alterations. For instance, since the early works of Marian C. Diamond, Mark R. Rosenzweig, David H. Hubel, Torsten N. Wiesel, and Facundo Valverde and their collaborators, we know that sensory deprivation during development alters neural plasticity in different brain regions of the mammalian brain (Grubb and Thompson, 2004; Hubel and Wiesel, 1965; Ruiz-Marcos and Valverde, 1969; Valverde, 1967, 1968; Walsh, 1980, 1981; Wiesel and Hubel, 1963), while exposure to a physically and socially enriched environment during early postnatal life in mammals promotes an enriched structure and functionality of the adult brain, including increased numbers of glial cells, enhanced adult neurogenesis, enhanced complexity of dendritic trees, and increased numbers of dendritic spines and synaptic contacts (Diamond et al., 1964, 1966; Nithianantharajah and Hannan, 2006; Rosenzweig et al., 1962). Environmental conditions during development also impact on adult brain plasticity in nonmammalian vertebrates (Coss and Globus, 1979; Kihslinger et al., 2006; Kihslinger and Nevitt, 2006; Lema et al., 2005; Zeutzius et al. 1984). Due to its high degree of organizational plasticity during prenatal and early postnatal life, the central nervous system is more sensitive to the influence of environmental and endogenous factors during these periods than at later stages. Environmental factors during prenatal and early postnatal life may interfere with the development of the anatomical and functional structure of the brain and spinal cord, affecting the organization of the pattern of synaptic connectivity and determining future plastic responses of the neural tissue during later periods of life. The plastic response of the developing central nervous system to environmental factors is, in part, adaptive in order to prepare the adult brain for life in a precise environment. However, in extreme conditions, such as undernutrition or infection, the prenatal influences may result in a permanent malfunction of the nervous system.

The influence of environmental factors may be transmitted from the mother to the fetus through hormonal signals. As I have already mentioned, hormones are actively involved in the programming and regulation of neural developmental mutability, coordinating the development of the nervous system with the development of other organs, including the endocrine glands. Therefore, inadequate levels of hormones during fetal or early postnatal life may have dramatic and permanent consequences for the functional organization of the brain and spinal cord. Environmental factors may affect the levels of hormones in the mother and/or fetus, and may result in an altered developmental pattern. For instance, low levels of iodine in the environment results in a decreased synthesis of thyroid hormones, which are essential for regulating the development of the nervous system. The hypothyroid status during prenatal and early postnatal life will cause a deficient developmental organization of the brain, with devastating consequences for its function during postnatal and adult life. Undernutrition may alter the developmental actions of leptin and other hormones on the organization of feeding regulatory centers in the hypothalamus. This will result in alterations in the future plastic functional regulatory activity of the hypothalamic control of feeding and energy balance. Adverse social or physical environment and infections may cause alterations in the levels of stress hormones in the mother that may impact the developmental program of the nervous system of the fetus.

Since the pioneering work conducted by Thompson (Thompson, 1957) and by Levine (Levine, 1967). we know that maternal stress or infantile experience could affect stress response later in life. Stress during prenatal and early postnatal life affects the capacity of the hypothalamic–pituitary–adrenal system to adequately adapt to stress conditions in adult life and during aging. As a result of this maladaptation, the stress response is exacerbated and causes alterations in the function of the adult nervous system, including modifications in synaptic plasticity, adult neurogenesis, learning, affection, and cognition. Therefore, stress during the developmental period may be the cause of future malfunction of the nervous system in adult life, increasing the risk of affective and neurological alterations. In addition, altered levels of stress hormones during development may affect the organizational action of other hormones on the nervous system. For instance, altered levels of stress hormones may affect the organizational actions of leptin in the feeding centers of the hypothalamus, resulting in future malregulation of energy balance and body weight. Stress hormones may also affect the developmental actions of sex hormones, resulting in a distorted sexual differentiation of the brain and the spinal cord. However, the prominent capacity for plasticity of the brain also allows interventions during early postnatal life or even at later life stages to compensate for the deficits caused by an altered prenatal development. For instance, exposure to an enriched environment promotes functional recovery after brain damage and may compensate for neural developmental deficits induced by genetic or chromosomal alterations (Dierssen et al., 2003; Martinez-Cue et al., 2005; Nithianantharajah and Hannan, 2006; Rampon et al., 2000; van Dellen et al., 2000) or by extrinsic factors, including the effect of prenatal stress on adult cognition, neurogenesis, and adult synaptic plasticity (Cui et al., 2006; Koo et al., 2003; Yang et al., 2007).

Therefore, the final organization of the central nervous system after the developmental period is the result of a process of tissue remodeling that is influenced by a variety of intrinsic and extrinsic, prenatal and postnatal factors. Hormones play a central role in this process, generating an emergent homeodynamic equilibrium in the developing organism. I will examine in this chapter the prominent role that hormones have in defining the timing and regional specificity of the plastic developmental changes in the central nervous system and how they coordinate neural maturation with the maturation of other body systems. In addition, I will analyze the consequences that physiological, experimental, and pathological alterations in hormonal levels during the developmental period have for the future plastic responses of the central nervous system in response to the changing external and internal environment.

HORMONAL ORCHESTRATION OF NEURAL DEVELOPMENT DURING PRENATAL LIFE

Thyroid Hormones

Among the hormones that are known to influence neural development, the major role falls to the thyroid hormones, which are essential for the developmental organization of the nervous system of vertebrates. The influence of the thyroid gland on brain development has been recognized since the last decades of the nineteenth century (Ord, 1888) when a committee of the Clinical Society of London associated mental retardation with cretinism. Today we know that thyroid hormones play a major role in the regulation of early fetal development and in the postnatal maturation of the nervous system. We may distinguish three periods in the actions of thyroid hormones on brain development (Porterfield and Hendrich, 1993). Phase II is the period of neural development that precedes the maturation of the fetal thyroid function and the synthesis of fetal thyroid hormones; phase II is the period between the maturation of the fetal thyroid gland and birth; and phase III is the postnatal period. Phase I takes place at approximately the first 17.5–18 days of gestation in rats and the first 10–12 weeks of gestation in humans (Morreale de Escobar et al., 2004b; Porterfield and Hendrich, 1993).

The proliferation, differentiation, and migration of neurons and glial cells in several regions of the central nervous system, including the spinal cord, medulla, pons, cerebellum, midbrain, hypothalamus, thalamus, pallidus, striatum, amygdala, olfactory bulb, hippocampal formation, and cerebral cortex, is initiated during phase I (Howdeshell, 2002). For instance, the genesis of the neocortex, which involves radial and tangential migration of neurons from germinal zones to their final destinations in the layered cortical structure, begins by the fifth week of gestation in humans and by embryonic day 11 in rats. Therefore, the genesis of the neocortex begins during phase I, before the maturation of the fetal thyroid gland. However, this does not mean that the thyroid hormones do not affect the early stages of cortical maturation. During this period, thyroid hormones produced in the mother are essential for proper neural development. Indeed, there is now considerable evidence of the importance of maternal thyroid hormones for the adequate development of the fetal nervous system, and iodine deficiency during pregnancy is a major cause of mental retardation in children (Berbel et al., 2007; Morreale de Escobar et al., 1993, 2004a, b). In the past it was considered that in mammals the placenta and embryonic membranes formed an effective barrier that prevented free passage of T4 and T3 from the mother to the fetus. In addition, maternal T4 is in part inactivated in the placenta by the type III iodothyronine deiodinase enzyme, which removes an iodine molecule. However, today we know that thyroid hormones are present in embryonic and fetal tissues well in advance of the onset of fetal thyroid function and that maternal thyroid hormones reach the fetus and are essential for early neural development. In humans, T3 is required by the cerebral cortex before midgestation, when the mother is the only source of its precursor, T4 (Kester et al., 2004). In agreement with this, experiments in rats by the groups of Pere Berbel in Alicante and Gabriella Morreale de Escobar in Madrid have shown that neocortical cell migration is defective in the progeny of severely hypothyroid dams (Berbel et al., 2001; Lucio et al., 1997) and that even a transient and moderate maternal deficiency in thyroxin during fetal development alters the radial and tangential migration of projection neurons in the neocortex, the cytoarchitecture of the neocortex and hippocampus, and the pattern of interhemispheric cortico-cortical connectivity (Auso et al., 2004; Berbel et al., 1994; Cuevas et al., 2005; Lavado-Autric et al., 2003).

During phase II, when the fetal thyroid has matured and produces thyroid hormones, both thyroid hormones from the mother and the fetus may influence brain development and may impact the final maturation of neuronal processes, synaptic connectivity, and glial cells. Effects of thyroid hormones on astroglia maturation and differentiation (Aizenman and de Vellis, 1987; Nicholson and Altman, 1972; Trentin, 2006) during phases I and II may participate in the cytoarchitectonic organization of the cortex. This possibility is supported by findings from the laboratory of Antonio Ruiz-Marcos at the Instituto Cajal and his collaborators at the Instituto de Investigaciones Biomédicas in Madrid, who have shown that hypothyroidism alters the development of radial glial cells in the fetal hippocampus (Martinez-Galan et al., 1997b), and in the term fetal postnatal neocortex of the rat (Martinez-Galan et al., 2004). The altered development of radial astroglia in the developing hippocampus and neocortex may have a strong negative impact on neuronal migration and the final architectonical and functional organization of these cortical regions. Thus, thyroid hormones may promote an adequate neuronal migration in the hippocampus and neocortex by regulating radial glia development during phases I and II. Finally, during phase III, thyroid hormones will affect the development of several brain structures, such as the cerebellum, in which neurogenesis, neuronal migration, and neuronal and glial maturation occurs during the postnatal period. The actions of thyroid hormones on the postnatal brain will be analyzed later in this chapter.

Sex Hormones

While thyroid hormones appear to be indispensable factors for the normal morphological and functional development of all regions of the nervous system, other hormones, such as sex hormones, appear to exert more specific actions, orienting the developmental organization of certain neural structures versus a male or female phenotype. In 1959, William Caldwell Young (1899–1965), one of the founders of behavioral neuroendocrinology and his collaborators Charles H. Phoenix, Robert W. Goy, and Arnie Gerall at the Department of Anatomy at the University of Kansas published a seminal paper showing that prenatal exposure of genetic female guinea pigs to androgens exerts a permanent alteration in their adult sexual behavior. Females prenatally exposed to androgens showed a permanent suppression of their capacity to display feminine sexual behavior (defeminization) and an enhanced display of masculine sexual behavior (masculinization) (Phoenix et al., 1959). These findings suggested that prenatal androgens generate permanent modifications in the brain systems regulating sexual behavior. Since then, many studies have confirmed that gonadal steroids, in particular testosterone and its metabolites estradiol and dihydrotestosterone, affect mammalian neural development, generating sex differences in the structure and function of the central and peripheral nervous system.

Genes of the sex chromosomes determine the generation of sex differences in the gonads. The sexually differentiated production of gonadal hormones by male and female gonads generates, in turn, sex differences in neural structure (Arnold and Gorski, 1984; MacLusky and Naftolin, 1981). However, it should be quickly remarked that there is considerable evidence indicating that the sexual differentiation of the brain is not exclusively the result of hormonal actions from sexually differentiated gonads, and that genes of the sex chromosomes may have direct sex-specific effects on nerve cells (Agate et al., 2003; Arnold, 2004; Reisert and Pilgrim, 1991). Although some sex differences in neural structure are generated as a result of hormonal actions, we should remember that this is not the exclusive mechanism for generation of sex differences in the nervous system of vertebrates. However, the focus of this book is on hormonal actions on the nervous system, therefore, I will not analyze in this chapter the role of the expression of sex-specific genes on the process of brain sexual differentiation. My aim in this chapter is to analyze how sex hormones may affect the developmental organization of the brain and spinal cord, and I do not intent to examine in detail the mechanisms of sexual differentiation of the nervous system.

Metabolism of sex hormones (in particular of testosterone) within the nervous system is part of the mechanism involved in their developmental actions. Testosterone is locally metabolized into estradiol in the central nervous system by the enzyme aromatase. Testosterone may also be locally converted into dihydrotestosterone, by the enzyme 5α-reductase. Both enzymes are present in the developing brain. Estradiol is a ligand of estrogen receptors and dihydrotestosterone a ligand of androgen receptors. Estradiol and dihydrotestosterone, and therefore estrogen and androgen receptors, are involved in the organizational effects of testosterone in the nervous system. In mammals, testosterone exposure organizes neural development to generate a central nervous system that supports male behavior and male neuroendocrine regulation. Absence of testosterone results in the generation of a nervous system that is basically female. Therefore, at difference with thyroid hormones, which are indispensable for neural development, gonadal hormones are not necessary for the developmental organization of a functional nervous system. Its role is to orient the normal process of neural development in the direction of generating specific male or female traits in the structure and function of the brain, spinal cord, and peripheral nervous system.

The organizational effects of testosterone and its metabolites generate male-specific traits in specific regions of the brain and spinal cord, resulting in differences in the morphology, size, and number of neurons and glial cells, the density of neuronal and glial processes in the neuropil, and the number of synapses between males and females. The organizational action of testosterone in the mammalian nervous system appears to be particularly prominent in defined critical periods during development. These critical periods differ between species and correspond with surges in plasma testosterone during development. In rats and mice, the main critical period spans from late gestation to early postnatal development; in guinea pigs, between days 30 and 37 of gestation; in sheep, from 30 to 147 days of pregnancy; and in rhesus monkeys and humans, it is in the first trimester of pregnancy (Robinson, 2006). However, the critical periods may vary between different brain structures, may surpass these limits in some cases and may be multiple. For instance, both an androgen surge on day 18 of gestation and a neonatal peak of testosterone may contribute to the masculinization of the rat brain (Perakis and Stylianopoulou, 1986). In addition, the organizational effect exerted by sex steroids during these early critical periods may be refined and reshaped by further hormonal actions later on, during postnatal development and puberty (see Chapter 7). It is therefore possible to consider the possible existence of expanded or multiple critical periods for the sexual differentiation of different brain structures (Davis et al., 1995; Robinson, 2006). In addition, during adult reproductive life, steroids exert activational effects on the sexually differentiated brain structures, which generate sexually dimorphic behaviors, sexually dimorphic neuroendocrine regulations, and sexually dimorphic plastic events. These actions of gonadal hormones in adult reproductive life are supposed to activate different sexually dimorphic brain regions without affecting their sexual differentiation, which is expected to have been fixed by the hormonal organizational effects. In theory, it should be easy to differentiate between the activation of a sexually dimorphic neuronal circuit and the generation of a sexual dimorphism in such a circuit. However, in practice this is not always the case, since as we have seen in Chapter 4, sex hormones in the adult exert prominent plastic reorganization of neuronal networks (for instance, during the female's estrus cycle). Is this hormonal remodeling of brain structure in adult life an organizational or an activational event? This question has no simple answers. For instance, we may interpret some structural and functional changes in neuronal circuits during the estrus cycle of adult female rodents as representing transient periods of plastic defeminization of such circuits. Therefore, the difference between organizational and activational effects of gonadal hormones in the brain may not be as unambiguous as originally thought. A similar situation occurs when organizational and activational effects on behavior are analyzed (Arnold and Breedlove, 1985). However, with independence of the precise duration, limits, number and biological significance of the different possible critical periods for sexual differentiation of the nervous system, what is well documented is that sex hormones exert important effects in the developmental organization of the fetal and postnatal brain and spinal cord. In this section I will consider the impact of gonadal hormones on the organization of the fetal central nervous system. Later on in this chapter, I will analyze the impact of gonadal hormones on the organization of the postnatal nervous system before puberty.

One of the most obvious effects of fetal actions of testosterone in some mammalian species is the masculinization of the brain neuronal circuits regulating the release of gonadotropins. The adult female neuronal network regulating the activity and secretion of gonadotropin releasing hormone (GnRH) neurons is under a complex regulation of sex steroids and responds to the estrogen-stimulated GnRH surge. In contrast, the male neuronal network has an impaired response to estrogen (Horvath et al., 1997b) and is under the negative regulation by testicular androgens. The action of testosterone in the fetal brain of guinea pigs (Connolly and Resko, 1994), rats (Foecking et al., 2005), mice (Sullivan and Moenter, 2004), pigs (Elsaesser and Parvizi, 1979), sheep (Fabre-Nys and Venier, 1991; Herbosa et al., 1996; Kim et al., 1999; Robinson, 2006), and rhesus monkeys (Dumesic et al., 1997) results in the reprogramming of the neuronal network regulating GnRH, including modifications in the number and function of synaptic inputs to GnRH neurons (Chen et al., 1990; Kim et al., 1999; Sullivan and Moenter, 2004). The resulting GnRH neuronal network in female animals that have been exposed in utero to testosterone shows an impaired, male-like response to the estrogen-stimulated GnRH surge. Therefore, androgen action in the fetal developing brain drives the development of the neuronal GnRH network that will be desensitized to estrogen stimulation in adult life. This is an example of a hormonal action in the fetal brain that predetermines the function of specific neuronal circuit in the adult brain (Fig. 6.1). The hormonal action is not indispensable for the development of the neuronal circuit, but determines whether its functional organization will follow a male or a female pattern.

While the organizational effect of testosterone in the developing GnRH system appears to mainly affect the sexual differentiation of neuronal connectivity, in other cases the organizational actions of testosterone and its metabolites play an important role in determining the final adult size of specific anatomical neural structures. In vitro studies have shown that gonadal hormones promote the survival of fetal neurons from different brain regions, including the hypothalamus (Chowen et al., 1992; Dueñas et al., 1996), amygdala (Arimatsu and Hatanaka, 1986), hippocampus (Sudo et al., 1997), and neocortex (Brinton et al., 1997). The viability of neuronal cultures from these brain regions is significantly enhanced by the addition of estradiol to the culture media. Estradiol also promotes the survival of dorsal root ganglion neurons in culture (Patrone et al., 1999), while androgens enhance the survival of neurons in cultures from the spinal cord (Hauser and Toran-Allerand, 1989). These findings suggest that sex hormones may promote the survival of specific neuronal populations during the development of the nervous system. These hormonal effects may result in the generation of sex differences in neuronal content. In agreement with these in vitro findings, several studies have shown sex differences in the volume of specific anatomical structures in the brain and the spinal cord in vivo.

One well-known example of a sexually dimorphic structure in the brain that shows sex differences in the number of neurons is the sexually dimorphic nucleus of the preoptic area, a brain region involved in male sexual behavior. This nucleus, discovered by the prominent neuroendocrinologist Roger A. Gorski and his collaborators at UCLA, is a neuronal group in the preoptic area of the rat brain that is several-fold larger in volume in males than in females. Historically, the sexually dimorphic nucleus of the preoptic area represents the first solid evidence for a sex-dimorphic structure in the brain of mammals. This nucleus is still today one of the best studied examples of a sexually dimorphic structure in the brain, and is one of the most robust anatomical sex differences in the rodent brain detected so far (Gorski et al., 1978, 1980). The masculinization of the sexual dimorphic nucleus of the preoptic area appears to be initiated during fetal life, since prenatal exposure to testosterone promotes masculinization of the nucleus provided that testosterone can be converted into estradiol (Ito et al., 1986; Lund et al., 2000). This effect may be in part mediated by the prevention by prenatal testosterone of naturally occurring neuronal apoptosis during the postnatal period, which is more abundant in females than in males (Hsu et al., 2001). Prenatal testosterone and its conversion to estradiol are also necessary for the development of the male nucleus of the preoptic/anterior hypothalamic area of ferrets, a neuronal group that is not present in female brains (Cherry et al., 1990; Tobet et al., 1986). It should be noted that the action of prenatal testosterone in the brain does not always induce an increase in the number of neurons. Indeed, prenatal testosterone decreases the number of neurons in several brain regions, such as the anteroventral periventricular nucleus of the preoptic area of the rat (Nishizuka et al., 1993; Sumida et al., 1993). We will see later in this chapter that the postnatal actions of testosterone also have different outputs depending on the brain region or on the specific neuronal subpopulation within a region.

Although the resulting structural sex differences may be not as obvious as those observed in the preoptic area of rats and ferrets, prenatal testosterone may also affect the organization of several other brain structures, including the suprachiasmatic nucleus (Abizaid et al., 2004) and the accessory olfactory system in rodents (Dominguez-Salazar et al., 2002). These hormonal actions may be involved in the generation of sex differences in circadian rhythms and responsiveness to pheromones, respectively. Sex differences in behavior are not limited to reproductive behaviors (for instance, see Hines, 2003). Accordingly, prenatal androgens also interfere with the development of cognitive brain regions, inducing larger CA1 and CA3 pyramidal cell field volumes and soma sizes in the hippocampus of male rats (Isgor and Sengelaub, 1998). Furthermore, local formation of the testosterone metabolite estradiol in the fetal brain may regulate cortical neurogenesis (Martinez-Cerdeno et al., 2006), and testosterone conversion to estradiol participates in the organization of the catecholamine innervation of the frontal cortex in rats (Stewart and Rajabi, 1994).

Prenatal testosterone also results in the generation of sex differences in the spinal cord. A noticeably sexually dimorphic structure is the spinal nucleus of the bulbocavernosus, a group of motoneurons in the lumbar spinal cord of male rats that innervate perineal muscles and that is markedly reduced or absent in normal females. Prenatal testosterone promotes the masculine development of the spinal nucleus of the bulbocavernosus (Goldstein and Sengelaub, 1992) as well as the development of Onuf's nucleus in dogs. Onuf's nucleus is a group of motoneurons located in the sacral spinal cord that innervates perineal muscles involved in copulatory behavior. This nucleus is also present in the spinal cord of cats and primates, including humans, and is sexually dimorphic (Forger and Breedlove, 1986).

Enduring Effects of Prenatal Stress

Another important hormonal influence on the fetal development of the central nervous system (with long-lasting consequences in postnatal life) is the one exerted by stress hormones. Stress during pregnancy may lead to alterations in the developmental pattern of the brain. These stress-induced alterations in brain prenatal development may result in permanent impairments in brain function and plasticity, and may represent a risk factor for the development of psychiatric and cognitive disorders. In particular, prenatal stress may affect the organization program of the neuroendocrine hypothalamic–pituitary–adrenal axis that controls stress hormone levels in postnatal life and may also affect other hormonal systems, including sex hormones and leptin. In addition, prenatal stress affects the plasticity and function of the hippocampus and its responsiveness to stress hormones. Since the hippocampus mediates negative feedback to the hypothalamic–pituitary–adrenal axis, a hippocampal impairment results in further alteration of the axis and its response to stress in adult life. Therefore, prenatally stressed animals show a variety of nonadaptive responses to stress (Barbazanges et al., 1996; Clarke et al., 1994; Henry et al., 1994; Koehl et al., 1999; Maccari et al., 1995, 2003; Morley-Fletcher et al., 2003a, b; Weinstock et al., 1992).

The influence of stress during pregnancy has received increased attention by clinicians and basic scientists in the last few decades. In humans, prenatal stress is considered a risk factor for the development of behavioral alterations, and has been associated with aggression, hyperactivity, anxiety, attention-deficit disorders, and cognitive problems in adolescence and adulthood (Austin et al., 2005; Gutteling et al., 2005; Huizink et al., 2003, 2004; Meijer, 1985; O'Connor et al., 2003; Talge et al., 2007; Wadhwa et al., 2001), including an increase in the risk of schizophrenia, which is considered to have a developmental component (Brixey et al., 1993; Howes et al., 2004). Indeed, there is evidence suggesting an increased occurrence of schizophrenia in subjects whose mothers were exposed to traumatic or stressful experiences during pregnancy (Huttunen et al., 1994; van Os and Selten, 1998). In agreement with human data, prenatal stress in nonhuman primates has also been shown to produce functional disturbances of the central nervous system in postnatal life. These disturbances are reflected in reduced exploratory behavior, attention-deficits, neuromotor impairments, and a variety of other behavioral disorders (Clarke and Schneider, 1993; Schneider, 1992; Schneider et al., 1999). However, it is in laboratory rodents where the effects of prenatal stress on postnatal brain function have been examined with more detail.

Several experimental protocols to produce chronic stress in rat dams have been assessed, and all have given similar results, indicating that prenatally stressed rodents show neurobiological impairments that may be the direct consequence of the dysfunction of the hypothalamic–pituitary–adrenal axis, such as the increased activation of the sympathetic nervous system (Weinstock et al., 1998) and alterations in circadian rhythms and sleep (Dugovic et al., 1999; Koehl et al., 1997, 1999). Furthermore, prenatally stressed rodents may have alterations in maternal (Fride et al., 1985) and sexually differentiated behaviors (Ward and Stehm, 1991), as well as cognitive impairments. For instance, some paradigms of chronic stress during gestation may reduce the ability to filter or discriminate relevant from irrelevant information in adult life. This is one major defect observed in schizophrenic subjects, and is assessed by measuring prepulse inhibition, a parameter that is disrupted both in schizophrenic patients and in prenatally stressed rats (Koenig et al., 2005). Prenatal stress also produces learning and memory deficits in young, adult, and aged rats, such as impairments in spatial memory assessed in the Morris water maze (Darnaudéry et al., 2006; Gué et al., 2004; Lemaire et al.,

2000; Lordi et al., 1997; Smith et al., 1981; Vallée et al., 1999). However, one of the most obvious effects of prenatal stress in rodents is an increase in affective disorders in adult life. Thus, prenatally stressed rodents show enhanced emotional reactivity (Fride et al., 1986; Thompson, 1957; Vallée et al., 1997b; Wakshlak and Weinstock, 1990; Weinstock, 1997), increased anxiety behaviors (Morley-Fletcher et al., 2003b; Poltyrev et al., 1996; Vallée et al., 1997b), enhanced conditioned fear (Griffin et al., 2003), and an increase in depression-like behaviors (Alonso et al., 1991; Louvart et al., 2005; Morley-Fletcher et al., 2003b; Secoli and Teixeira, 1998). Indeed, prenatal stress in rodents is considered a valid experimental model of depression.

The impact of prenatal stress on the developmental organization program of the neuroendocrine hypothalamic–pituitary–adrenal axis also has relevant consequences for the immune system. Clinical studies have shown that immune function is reduced in patients with anxiety disorders, and animal studies also indicate that there is a link between anxiety and immune function (Koh and Lee, 1998; Leonard and Song, 1996; Stein et al., 1988). Therefore, the increased anxiety observed in prenatally stressed animals may play a key role in triggering immune alterations. Indeed, the group of Stefania Maccari at the University of Lille 1, France, has shown an increased proinflammatory status in the offspring of dams that were submitted to repeated short-time daily restraint immobilization from day 11 of pregnancy until delivery (Vanbesien-Mailliot et al., 2007).

The effects of prenatal stress on the postnatal function of the immune system and central nervous system may be in part mediated by the prenatal action of stress hormones. The brain is very sensitive to prenatal programming by glucocorticoids (Seckl, 2004), and several studies assessing the prenatal effects of the synthetic glucocorticoid dexamethasone, which crosses the placenta, suggest that these hormones may indeed mediate the prenatal actions of stress in the brain as in other organs. The brain of rats treated prenatally with dexamethasone shows an altered sensitivity to stress hormones in adult life (Levitt et al., 1996; Welberg et al., 2001). Furthermore, the administration of dexamethasone to pregnant dams during the third week of gestation mimics the effect of prenatal stress on spatial learning (Brabham et al., 2000). Effects of stress hormones on myelin maturation may be involved in cognitive deficits. For instance, it has been reported that prenatal corticosteroid administration delays myelination of the corpus callosum in fetal sheep (Huang et al., 2001) and therefore may affect the functional communication of cortical neurons between the two cerebral hemispheres.

Thus, prenatal glucocorticoids may program the developing brain and permanently impair the functional plasticity of the hypothalamic–pituitary–adrenal axis during postnatal life. Consequently, prenatally stressed rats produce faster, stronger, and/or more prolonged glucocorticoid responses throughout life than the controls when exposed to novel or challenging situations. These altered glucocorticoid responses in postnatal life may in turn have an additional impact on the brain, producing further modifications in the plasticity of the central nervous system. These alterations in brain plastic responsiveness in animals that were prenatally stressed may contribute to—or even be the cause of—their behavioral, affective, and cognitive disturbances. Indeed, the behavioral and cognitive alterations produced by prenatal stress in young, adult, and aged rodents are associated with modifications in brain development and plasticity. Prenatal stress induces a reduction in the number of dendritic spines on layer II/III pyramidal neurons of the dorsal anterior cingulate and orbitofrontal cortex of young prepubertal male and female rats (Murmu et al., 2006). In addition, prenatally stressed males have a decrease in the length and complexity of pyramidal apical dendrites in both cortical regions (Murmu et al., 2006). Synaptic plasticity in adult life is also affected by prenatal stress; both a reduced long-term synaptic potentiation (Son et al., 2006) and decreased number of dendritic spines of pyramidal neurons, reduced number of synapses, and reduced serotonin concentration have been detected in the hippocampus of prenatally stressed rodents (Hayashi et al., 1998; Ishiwata et al., 2005). In addition, prenatal stress causes neurogenesis impairment and a reduced number of granule cells in the dentate gyrus of the hippocampus (Gould and Tanapat, 1999; Lemaire et al., 2000, 2006a; Schmitz et al., 2002; Weinstock, 2001). This is likely not a peculiarity of prenatal stress in rodents, since impaired neurogenesis in the hippocampus as a consequence of maternal stress has also been observed in the dentate gyrus of juvenile rhesus monkeys (Coe et al., 2003).

The action of other hormones in the brain during prenatal development and during postnatal life may interact with the effects of prenatal stress in the modulation of adult brain plasticity (Fig. 6.1). For instance, the effects of prenatal stress on brain plasticity are not identical in male and female offspring (Weinstock, 2007). Thus, postnatal behavior (Gué et al., 2004; Nishio et al., 2001; Szuran et al., 2000), the number of granule neurons in the dentate gyrus of the hippocampus (Schmitz et al., 2002), and the length and complexity of pyramidal apical dendrites in the dorsal anterior cingulate and orbitofrontal cortex (Murmu et al., 2006) are not equally affected by prenatal stress in male and female rodents. These sex differences in the effect of prenatal stress may in part be the consequence of an interaction of stress and sex hormones during brain development or during postnatal life. Other hormones, such as thyroid hormones, IGF-I, or leptin may also interact with stress hormones during fetal and postnatal brain development and during adult life to modulate adult brain plasticity.

Peptide Hormones

Several peptide hormones may affect the development of the brain and spinal cord and may contribute to organize future neural plastic responses in adult life. Gastric hormones, such as ghrelin and the anorexigenic peptide YY, have been shown to participate in the developmental organization of the central nervous system, affecting neural tube development (Yuzuriha et al., 2007). In addition, ghrelin promotes neurogenesis in the rat fetal spinal cord (Sato et al., 2006). Leptin, another hormone involved in food intake and energy balance, also has neurodevelopmental effects—its actions during development may have an important impact on future body functions. This hormone participates in the control of growth and development of the fetus (Christou et al., 2002), and its developmental organizational actions are very important for the future regulation of energy homeodynamics, food intake, and body composition in postnatal and adult life. In addition, the organizational actions of leptin may be important for normal brain development during fetal and postnatal periods, although our knowledge of leptin actions in the developing brain is still quite limited. Nevertheless, leptin deficient (ob/ob) mice have a reduced brain size, defective neuronal and glial maturation, increased apoptosis, and alterations in myelination and synaptic markers (Ahima et al., 1999; Bereiter and Jeanrenaud, 1979; van der Kroon and Speijers, 1979). Leptin treatment during development is able to counteract these brain alterations (Ahima et al., 1999).

Growth hormone is also known to influence neural development (Scheepens et al., 2005). Clear evidence of the participation of growth hormone on the development of the central nervous system is that the size of the brain and spinal cord are reduced in growth hormone deficient humans and animals (Behringer et al., 1990; Noguchi, 1991). In contrast, transgenic mice that overexpress growth hormone have an increased brain and spinal cord weight (Chen et al., 1998). Interestingly, mice that overexpress a growth hormone antagonist have a reduced velocity and magnitude of postnatal brain and spinal cord growth (McIlwain et al., 2004). The neurodevelopmental effects of growth hormone may be related to the promotion of neuronal proliferation and survival. For instance, growth hormone has been shown to promote neuronal survival during the development in the chick retina (Harvey et al., 2006), and promotes proliferation and differentiation of fetal neurons and astrocytes from the cerebral cortex in a primary culture (Ajo et al., 2003). Growth hormone deficiency also results in a decrease of synaptic formation and hypomyelination, suggesting that growth hormone promotes synaptogenesis and myelin formation (Noguchi, 1996). These findings indicate that growth hormone regulates brain development. However, the mechanisms of the action of this developmental effect of growth hormone are still not clarified. Growth hormone may directly act on growth hormone receptors within the brain, or may have an indirect effect via IGF-I (Ajo et al., 2003), which is a potent promoter of neural development. Local production of growth hormone by brain cells (Hojvat et al., 1982) and its action as a paracrine or autocrine factor (Harvey et al., 2003) may also be involved in its neurodevelopmental effects.

Insulin/IGF-I signaling is essential for neural development in vertebrates (Bateman and McNeill, 2006; Hernandez-Sanchez et al., 2006; Varela-Nieto et al., 2004). Insulin may affect brain and spinal cord development either by direct activation of insulin signaling in the central nervous system, or indirectly by controlling glucose levels. Insulin prevents early neural cell death during embryonic mouse retina development (Valenciano et al, 2006) and participates in oligodendrocyte differentiation (Vicario-Abejon et al., 2003). IGF-I has many developmental effects in the brain and spinal cord—it regulates the proliferation, maturation, and differentiation of neural stem cells (Otaegi et al., 2006; Ye and D'Ercole, 2006), promoting the production of neurons (Camarero et al., 2003; Russo et al., 2005; Vicario-Abejon et al., 2003) and oligodendrocytes (Hsieh et al., 2004; Vicario-Abejon et al., 2003; Zeger et al., 2007) during embryonic development. These actions probably reflect the role of IGF-I as a local growth factor and not its role as a hormone, since IGF-I is highly and widely expressed in the fetal and early postnatal central nervous system (Russo et al., 2005).

HORMONAL REGULATION OF BRAIN MUTABILITY DURING EARLY POSTNATAL LIFE

Metamorphosis in Vertebrates

The maturation of the brain and spinal cord in vertebrates still continues after hatching or birth, and the organization of some brain regions is mainly a postnatal event. One extreme example of neural transformations after hatching is provided by metamorphosis in some vertebrates. There is likely no better illustration of the inherent remodeling capacity of the nervous system than the spectacular transformations that occur in the brain, spinal cord, peripheral nervous system, and sensory organs during a typical amphibian metamorphosis, a process that is regulated by thyroid hormone (Brown and Cai, 2007). The metamorphosis of tadpoles to frogs represents an almost complete reorganization of the body in the adaptation process from living in an aquatic environment to a terrestrial life. Tadpoles are fishlike, water-dwelling animals with external gills and a predominantly vegetarian diet. Frogs are land animals, with skin and lung-based respiration, front legs and forelimbs, and are mainly carnivorous. The development of hind limbs and front legs, the resorption of the tail, and the reorganization of the locomotor system from axial-based swimming to limbed propulsion are among the most obvious changes associated with metamorphosis. These changes are accompanied by other important modifications, which also have a considerable impact on the physiology of the organism. These modifications include: (i) the reorganization of the olfactory system, the resorption of gills, and the development of lungs as part of the transition from aquatic to aerial breathing; (ii) the reorganization of the heart from two to three chambers, in adaptation to a lung-based respiration system; (iii) the reorganization of the skin; (iv) the reorganization of the digestive system, remodeling of the mouth, and growth of the tongue in adaptation of the transition from feeding on microscopic aquatic plants to feeding on a carnivorous diet on land; and (v) the migration of the eyes rostrally and dorsally, giving rise to binocular vision, and the transformation of the retina in adaptation to a land environment. These and other changes require important restructuring of the brain and spinal cord centers and circuits involved in motor control, respiratory rhythm, olfaction, vision, audition, vestibular control, pain, autonomic regulation, and many other functions (Burd, 1991; Grant and Keating, 1986; Hoskins, 1990; Kollros and Bovbjerg, 1997; Marsh-Armstrong et al., 1999, 2004; Shi, 1999).

The process of anuran metamorphosis is governed by a steadily increasing concentration of thyroid hormone in tadpoles (Shi, 1999). Thyroid hormone reaches a peak at the climax of metamorphosis, then gradually declines to reach a low level at the end of metamorphosis, when tail resorption occurs (Regard et al., 1978). The action of T4 in the nervous system is controlled in tadpoles by two deiodinase enzymes. The type II iodothyronine deiodinase enzyme synthesizes the active metabolite T3 from T4 and therefore promotes thyroid hormone action on metamorphosis (Cai and Brown, 2004; Huang et al., 2001) by facilitating the activation of thyroid hormone receptors (Schreiber et al., 2001). In contrast, the type III iodothyronine deiodinase enzyme inactivates T3 by removing an iodine molecule and therefore inhibits the action of T3 on metamorphosis (Huang et al., 1999; Marsh-Armstrong et al., 1999).

Thyroid hormone promotes the remodeling and rewiring of specific neuronal circuits in the central nervous system, including visual, auditory, olfactory, and spinal cord circuits (Brown and Cai, 2007; Burd, 1992; Hoskins, 1990; Marsh-Armstrong et al., 1999, 2004). Thyroid hormone also contributes to the reorganization of hypothalamic circuits controlling neuroendocrine secretions during metamorphosis (Kikuyama et al., 1979; Norris and Gern, 1976), which in turn may affect the secretion of other hormones.

Thyroid hormone also regulates metamorphosis in other vertebrates, participating in the regulation of lamprey metamorphosis (Manzon and Youson, 1997; Manzon et al., 2001) and orchestrating metamorphosis in flatfish (flounder and sole) (Inui and Miwa, 1985; Miwa et al., 1988; Schreiber and Specker, 1998). Thyroid hormones regulate the remodeling of the brain during flatfish metamorphosis, where one eye translocates to the opposite side of the head, and the axes of flatfish eyes and horizontal semicircular canals of the inner ear become oriented perpendicular to each other. This reorganization of the eyes and inner ears involves marked associated modifications in the skull and in specific neuronal circuits in the brain (Graf and Baker, 1983, 1990; Meyer et al., 1981).

Although the main regulator of metamorphosis in vertebrates is the thyroid hormone, other hormones may also participate in the process and contribute to the remodeling of the nervous system. In general, prolactin and growth hormone exert antagonistic effects to thyroid hormone on metamorphosis, including the modifications in the nervous system. The induction in the target tissues of the expression of type III iodothyronine deiodinase enzyme (which, as already mentioned, inactivates T3) may be involved in the antimetamorphic effects of prolactin and growth hormone (Shintani et al., 2002). In contrast, corticotropin-releasing hormone (CRH) and corticoids may facilitate the metamorphic effects of thyroid hormones in the brain by enhancing the expression of brain type II deiodinase and the transformation of T4 into T3 (Kuhn et al., 2005). The effects of thyroid hormone, prolactin, and other hormones on central nervous system metamorphosis are exerted in part by the regulation of neurogenesis (Hunt and Jacobson, 1970, 1971; Marsh-Armstrong et al., 1999, 2004), neuronal death and differentiation (Decker, 1976; Hunt and Jacobson, 1971), cell adhesion molecules (Levi et al., 1990), and by the reorganization of dendrites, axons, and synaptic connections (Hauser and Gona, 1984).

In Xenopus laevis, sex hormones influence the development of the nervous system of tadpoles at the end of metamorphosis when gonads differentiate (Kelley, 1986). One example, studied by Darcy Kelley and her collaborators at Columbia University in New York, is the brain regions associated with the generation of song, which are sexually differentiated in frogs. Sexual differences in the song system of frogs are generated gradually during development, starting in tadpoles, in which the number of laryngeal axons showed a marked increase in males between stages 56 and 62. This increase is not observed in females. Then, there is a period of axonal loss between stage 62 and adulthood, in which axonal loss is greater in females than in males (Kelley and Dennison, 1990). The generation of sex differences in the number of laryngeal axons in tadpoles is driven by androgens (Robertson et al., 1994), likely by a direct action on the laryngeal motoneurons, which express androgen receptors (Perez et al., 1996). In addition, as for other aspects of central nervous system development, the androgen-induced generation of sex differences in laryngeal innervation is dependent on the previous actions of thyroid hormones, which define the timing for the sexual differentiation of the song system (Robertson and Kelley, 1996).

Thyroid Hormone Regulation of Postnatal Brain Development in Non-Metamorphic Vertebrates

Thyroid hormones are also key regulators of postnatal brain development in vertebrates that do not exhibit metamorphosis. Early microscopic studies on the effect of hypothyroidism in the brain of developing rats revealed that thyroid hormones are necessary for the normal postnatal development of the neuropil in the cerebral cortex (Eayrs and Taylor, 1951). More recent studies have confirmed that thyroid hormones during early neonatal and juvenile periods are necessary for the fine maturation of dendrites, dendritic spines, and synapses in neurons from different brain regions, including the caudate nucleus (Lu and Brown, 1977), the basal forebrain (Gould and Butcher, 1989), the Purkinje cells of the cerebellum (Legrand, 1979), the granule and pyramidal cells of the hippocampus (Gould et al., 1990b, 1991; Madeira et al., 1992; Madeira and Paula-Barbosa, 1993; Rami et al., 1986; Rami and Rabie, 1990), and the pyramidal neurons of the cerebral cortex (Ipina and Ruiz-Marcos, 1986; Ipina et al., 1987; Ruiz-Marcos et al., 1979, 1994; Ruiz-Marcos and Ipina, 1986; Sanchez-Toscano et al., 1977). Thyroid hormones also regulate neuronal proliferation, migration, and axonal growth in the early postnatal central nervous system. For instance, in contrast to the migration in the cerebral cortex that occurs during the fetal period, migration of granule cells from the external granular layer to their final destination in the internal granular layer in the cerebellar cortex is a process that occurs during the early postnatal age in mammals. Thyroid hormones promote the proliferation of granule cells in the external granular layer, their migration to the internal granular layer, and their differentiation and maturation of their axons, the parallel fibers, which make contact with Purkinje cell dendritic spines (Lauder, 1978; Nicholson and Altman, 1972; Oppenheimer and Schwartz, 1997). Thyroid hormones also promote the generation of new olfactory receptor neurons in postnatal rats (Paternostro and Meisami, 1989).

Glial cell development is also influenced by thyroid hormones and may significantly contribute to the developmental deficits observed in the central nervous system of hypothyroid animals. Thyroid hormones are essential for oligodendrocyte progenitor cell development and proliferation, for oligodendrocyte differentiation and survival (Ahlgren et al., 1997; Almazan et al., 1985; Baas et al., 1997; Barres et al., 1994; Billon et al., 2002; Jones et al., 2003; Muñoz et al., 1991; Rodriguez-Peña, 1999), and for normal brain myelination (Balazs et al., 1969; Berbel et al., 1994; Martinez-Galan et al., 1997a; Schoonover et al., 2004; Valcana et al., 1975; Walters and Morell, 1981), which is essential for proper brain function. Thyroid hormones regulate also several aspects of astroglia maturation and differentiation (Aizenman and de Vellis, 1987; Nicholson and Altman, 1972; Trentin, 2006). Consequently, thyroid hormone deficiency may alter glial maturation in the postnatal brain. Indeed, hypothyroidism alters the development of radial glial cells in the early postnatal neocortex of the rat (Martinez-Galan et al., 2004). Thyroid hormones may also promote Bergmann glia formation in the cerebellar cortex (Seress et al., 1978), which in turn may facilitate the migration of granule neurons from the external granular layer to the internal granular layer, which occurs during the early postnatal period. Microglial cells are also affected by thyroid hormones; its cellular density and the formation of their cellular processes is reduced in the neocortex of hypothyroid neonatal rats (Lima et al., 2000). Microglial cells play an important role in the remodeling of neural tissue during development. Therefore, the effects of thyroid hormones on brain organization during postnatal development may be, in part, mediated by hormonal actions on microglia.

Gonadal Hormones

Gonadal hormones are also important regulators of neural remodeling during postnatal development. As we have seen earlier in this chapter, the organizational effects of testosterone and its metabolites estradiol and dihydrotestosterone on the central nervous system structure and function are initiated during fetal life in mammals. However, the organizational actions of sex steroids in the brain and spinal cord continue during the early postnatal life, infancy, adolescence, and puberty. Even in the adult, gonadal hormones play an important role in modulating the size, morphology, and synaptic density of sex-steroid-responsive structures in the central nervous system. Several brain structures in which the organizational action of sex steroids is initiated in embryonic life are still sensitive to hormonal organizational effects in early postnatal life. I will present here only a few selected examples; the reader is referred to several reviews for a more comprehensive catalogue of neural structures showing hormonally induced sex differences in their organization (Arnold and Gorski, 1984; Cooke et al., 1998; Guillamón and Segovia, 1997; Morris et al., 2004; Segovia and Guillamón, 1993; Segovia et al., 1999; Simerly, 2002).

Let me start with the first reported evidence for a sexually dimorphic structure in the brain. Fernando Nottebohm and Arthur P. Arnold communicated in 1976 the existence of structural sex differences in the neural song system of zebra finch in correlation with sex differences in singing behavior. The communication, published in a memorable paper in the journal *Science* (Nottebohm and Arnold, 1976), promoted the search at many other laboratories of similar structural sex differences in the brain of other species that could be related with sex differences in behavior. The seminal discovery by Nottebohm and Arnold was followed by similar findings in mammals, including the discovery of the sexually dimorphic nucleus of the preoptic area by Roger A. Gorski and his collaborators that I have previously mentioned in this chapter (Gorski et al., 1978) and many other structural brain sex differences. After the publication of the paper by Nottebohm and Arnold, many studies have analyzed the influence of sex hormones in the generation of sex differences in the structure of the brain nuclei controlling song production in songbirds. The song system in songbirds is a very interesting and complex example of a functional network composed of different brain structures whose development is affected by gonadal hormones (Arnold et al., 1986). The neural song system in songbirds, such as the zebra finch, shows a marked sexual dimorphism (Nottebohm and Arnold, 1976) that varies among different species in correlation with species differences in singing behavior. Thus, those species that show pronounced sex differences in singing behavior are also those in which the structural sex differences in the brain song system are more noticeable (Ball and MacDougall-Shackleton, 2001; MacDougall-Shackleton and Ball, 1999). A few exceptions to this rule have however been noted. In zebra finches, the sexual dimorphism in the brain nuclei that control song develops after hatching by neuronal atrophy and death in the female brain, as well as from an increase in cell-body size and afferent terminals in the male (Konishi and Akutagawa, 1985). Neurodevelopmental actions of estradiol affect the neural song system and produces sex differences in cell size and number. Although the administration of testosterone and estradiol to female chicks results in the development of a more masculine structure in song nuclei, such as the nucleus robustus archistriatalis (Gurney, 1981; now nucleus robustus arcopallialis or RA; Reiner et al., 2004), the sexual differentiation of the neural song system appears to correlate with estrogenic actions during postnatal development (Adkins-Regan et al.,

1994; Konishi and Akutagawa, 1987, 1988). It should be noted, however, that although exogenous administration of estrogen may masculinize the neural song system in female zebra finches, it is unclear to what extent gonadal hormones are really involved in the generation of sex dimorphism in the neural song system under normal conditions. Indeed, the song system is not dependent on gonadally derived steroids for many of its organizational and activational events (Schlinger, 1998). Arthur P. Arnold and his collaborators have proposed that the generation of sex differences in the neural song system is regulated by factors intrinsic to the brain, likely by the expression of sex chromosome genes. According to this hypothesis, these genes may influence local synthesis of estradiol within the brain and/or the responses of brain tissue to estradiol (Wade and Arnold, 2004). In fact, the laboratory of Barney Schlinger has provided convincing evidence for local steroid synthesis in the developing songbird brain (London et al., 2006; London and Schlinger, 2007). Therefore, sex differences in the neural song system may, in fact, be the consequence of autocrine and paracrine actions of steroids within the brain, and not mediated by hormonal effects.

In mammals, one brain structure sensitive to the organizational effects of testosterone after birth is the sexually dimorphic nucleus of the preoptic area. The structural sex difference in this nucleus in rats is at least partially due to neonatal androgens, which promote, after their conversion to estrogens, the survival of a specific population of neurons (Davis et al., 1996; Dodson et al., 1988; Jacobson et al., 1981). Postnatal action of androgens and its conversion to estrogens is also necessary for the generation of a male structure in the sexually dimorphic nucleus in the preoptic area of ferrets. However, in this case the regulation of cell death does not seem to be involved in the hormonal action (Park et al., 1998).

Another well characterized sexually dimorphic neural structure that is generated during postnatal development is the spinal nucleus of the bulbocavernosus, discovered in rats by S. Marc Breedlove and Arthur P. Arnold at UCLA (Breedlove and Arnold, 1980, 1981, 1983). This nucleus is formed by a group of motoneurons, located in the dorsomedial portion of the ventral horn in the lower lumbar spinal cord, which innervate the bulbocavernosus and levator ani muscles. Males have more and larger neurons in the spinal nucleus of the bulbocavernosus than females. The structural sex difference is generated because androgens prevent normally occurring death of motoneurons during the postnatal development. This hormonal effect seems to be indirect, by preventing the loss of target muscles (Nordeen et al., 1985; Sengelaub and Arnold, 1989; Sengelaub et al., 1989a, b).

Some sex differences in neuronal numbers are not as obvious anatomically as those generated by gonadal hormones in the sexually dimorphic nucleus of the preoptic area and the spinal nucleus of the bulbocavernosus. Nevertheless, these more subtle sex differences may also have a considerable functional impact. For instance, one physiological function that is sexually dimorphic is that of somatic growth. After the onset of puberty, male rats grow significantly faster than females, and this is now known to be the result, at least in part, of differing growth hormone secretory patterns. It is well established that sex steroids are intimately involved in this process, and exert both organizational and activational effects on this system. The pulsatile release of growth hormone is under the reciprocal control of hypothalamic growth-hormone-releasing hormone (GHRH) and somatostatin neurons, suggesting that the sexual dimorphism in this system is at least partially mediated at the level of the hypothalamus. Julie Ann Chowen has significantly contributed to clarifying the basis for this hypothalamic functional sex dimorphism, showing that adult male rats have significantly more GHRH neurons in the hypothalamus than adult females. This sex difference in neuronal numbers is the result of exposure to testosterone during the neonatal period (Chowen et al., 1993). In this case, is still unclear whether testosterone enhances the survival of GHRH neurons or the differentiation to a GHRH expressing phenotype.

I have already mentioned that the role of androgens and its metabolites on the sexual differentiation of central nervous system in fetal life is not always in the direction of increasing neuronal survival; this is also true for the hormonal effects on postnatal life. Gonadal hormones promote neuronal survival or neuronal death with high cellular and regional selectivity during postnatal central nervous system development. An example of opposite effects of gonadal steroids on neuronal survival was provided by Antonio Guillamón and his collaborators at the Universidad Nacional de Educación a Distancia in Madrid. They demonstrated that within the bed nucleus of the stria terminalis of the rat, gonadal steroids have opposite effects in different anatomical regions. Within the medial posterior division of the bed nucleus of the stria terminalis, males have a greater number of neurons than females; however, in the anterior region of the lateral division of this same nucleus, females have significantly more neurons than males. These differences can be obliterated by modulating the neonatal steroid environment of the animal (Guillamón et al., 1988), indicating that gonadal hormones are exerting regional specific effects on neuronal survival. Another interesting example of opposite effects of gonadal hormones on neuronal survival is the anteroventral periventricular nucleus of rats and mice, which is involved in the regulation of the female estrus cycle, and is larger in females than in males (Bleier et al., 1982). Richard B. Simerly and his collaborators at the Oregon National Primate Research Center have studied the process of sexual differentiation of this nucleus, finding that androgens, after conversion to estrogen and activation of estrogen receptors, induce apoptosis, resulting in a smaller number of dopaminergic neurons in males (Simerly, 2002; Simerly et al., 1997). Interestingly, Simerly and his colleagues have found that within the anteroventral periventricular nucleus, different neuronal populations show opposite sex differences. While dopaminergic neurons are more abundant in females, other peptide neuronal populations are more abundant in males. Hence, gonadal steroids may either increase or decrease the number of specific neuronal populations within the same neural region. This selective effect of gonadal hormones on neuronal survival and death results in a specific modulation of the number of cells with different phenotypes sending out processes, which in turn may generate sex differences in the volume and composition of the neuropil and synaptic connectivity.

The number of neurons within a specific anatomical region is one important factor determining the availability of suitable postsynaptic neuronal membrane for the formation and support of synaptic contacts with incoming axons. Differences in axonal and dendritic growth and in dendritic branching also contribute to the specification of the final number of synaptic contacts. Therefore, it is not surprising that the generation of sex differences in neuronal content, neuritic growth, and glial differentiation by gonadal hormones is accompanied by sexual dimorphisms in synaptic connectivity. The possible influence of gonadal hormones (in particular, testosterone) on the connectivity of the developing brain was suggested in 1970 by the prominent British endocrinologist Geoffrey Wingfield Harris (1913–1971). Harris predicted that if testosterone acted in an inductive way to develop a male neural mechanism in the anterior hypothalamic-preoptic region, then this differentiation might be reflected in anatomical or ultrastructural modifications (Harris, 1970). A few years later, in 1973, the first evidence for a role of gonadal hormones in determining the differentiation of the neuropil was published by Geoffrey Raisman and Pauline M. Field from the department of human anatomy at Oxford University, who detected an influence of androgens during early postnatal life on synapses in the preoptic area of the rat brain (Raisman and Field, 1973). As a consequence of the hormonal effect, males have more axosomatic synapses and fewer dendritic spine synapses than females. Then, in 1976, Dominique Toran-Allerand reported that estradiol promoted the growth of neural processes in explant organotypic cultures of the hypothalamus and preoptic area of newborn mice, suggesting that this hormonal effect could be involved in the generation of sex differences in the neuropil. Testosterone was also able to induce neuritogenesis, although after its transformation to estradiol (Toran-Allerand, 1976, 1980). Further studies showed sex differences in the dendritic patterns in the preoptic area of hamsters (Greenough et al., 1977), and androgen regulation of dendritic growth and retraction during the development of the spinal nucleus of the bulbocavernosus (Goldstein et al., 1990). In addition, in vitro studies demonstrated that estradiol increases axonal and dendritic length and neurite branches per cell in hypothalamic neurons in explant cultures (Diaz et al., 1992; Dueñas et al., 1996; Ferreira and Caceres, 1991; Toran-Allerand, 1976; Toran-Allerand et al., 1983). These studies showed that gonadal hormones are intimately involved in determining dendritic and axonal length, as well as in the modulation of dendritic branching in specific areas of the central nervous system.

Today we know that gonadal hormones influence dendritic development, the growth of dendritic spines, and the formation of the pattern of synaptic connectivity in many regions of the central nervous system, including diencephalic and telencephalic structures that control reproductive behaviors, such as the ventromedial hypothalamic nucleus (Matsumoto, 1991; Matsumoto and Arai, 1986), lateral septum (DeVries et al., 1983, 1984), amygdala (Cooke et al., 2007; Nishizuka and Arai, 1981a, b), and the sexually dimorphic nucleus of the preoptic area in the rat (Hammer and Jacobson, 1984) and in the neuroendocrine diencephalic regions that control the release of pituitary hormones, such as the hypothalamic arcuate nucleus (Garcia-Segura et al., 1994a; Matsumoto and Arai, 1980, 1986; Mong et al., 2001; Perez et al., 1990) and the preoptic area (Chen et al., 1990; Lariva-Sahd, 1991; Raisman and Field, 1973; Watson et al., 1986). Sex differences in wiring pattern have been also detected in the hypothalamic suprachiasmatic nucleus, the brain's endogenous clock that, amongst other functions, orchestrates neuroendocrine rhythms (Güldner, 1982). Furthermore, in addition to those areas directly involved with reproduction or other endocrine functions, postnatal development of dendritic arbors and synaptic connectivity is also under the influence of gonadal hormones in other brain regions, such as the cerebellar cortex (Sakamoto et al., 2003; Tsutsui et al., 2004), the cerebral cortex (Juraska, 1991; Medosch and Diamond, 1982; Muñoz-Cueto et al., 1990, 1991; Stewart and Kolb, 1994) and hippocampal formation (Gould et al., 1990b, 1991; Juraska, 1991; Madeira et al., 1991; Parducz and Garcia-Segura, 1993). Early postnatal influence of sex hormones, generating sex differences in dendritic arbors and synapses, may affect the plastic responses of hippocampal neurons to environmental enrichment (Juraska et al., 1985, 1988) and may result in different synaptic plastic responses to hormonal actions in adult life (Fig. 6.1). For instance, estrogen induction of the formation of dendritic spines in the ventromedial hypothalamic nucleus and in the CA1 region of the adult rat hippocampus is influenced by the organizational effects of gonadal steroids (Lewis et al., 1995). Similar influences of the organizational effects of sex hormones on adult plastic responses have been detected in the neocortex. An ovariectomy in adulthood increases apical dendritic spine density and the dendritic arbor of layer II/III pyramidal neurons of the rat parietal cortex. However, this effect is not observed in rats treated neonatally with testosterone (Stewart and Kolb, 1994). Therefore, the organizational action of testosterone during the postnatal period precludes the generation of plastic changes in the cerebral cortex after ovarian hormone deprivation in adulthood (Fig. 6.1). Organizational action of testosterone in the development of the hypothalamic arcuate nucleus synaptic connectivity may also be the cause of the lack of manifestation of synaptic plasticity in response to estradiol in this hypothalamic region of adult male rats (Horvath et al., 1997b).

Gonadal hormones may promote sex differences in synaptic connectivity by regulating microtubule assembly in neuronal processes, one of the key events involved in neurite elongation. Microtubule-associated proteins are known to promote tubulin polymerization or microtubule stability during active process extension. Interestingly, the effects of estradiol on the growth of neurites in vitro are paralleled by an increase in the expression of microtubule-associated proteins, such as tau or microtubule-associated protein 2

(Ferreira and Caceres, 1991; Lorenzo et al., 1992). In addition, estradiol and progesterone regulate the expression of microtubule-associated protein 2 in the brain in vivo (Reyna-Neyra et al., 2002), and testosterone (Papasozomenos and Shanavas, 2002), estradiol (Alvarez-de-la-Rosa et al., 2005; Cardona-Gomez et al., 2004), and progesterone (Guerra-Araiza et al., 2007) regulate tau phosphorylation, which is essential for its association with axonal microtubules and the regulation of axonal growth. Estradiol also regulates the interaction of tau with neurotransmitter receptors (Cardona-Gomez et al., 2006). All these hormonal effects may be involved in the regulation of neuritic growth and synaptic plasticity. In addition, gonadal hormonal regulation and sex differences in the expression of focal adhesion kinase and paxillin in the arcuate nucleus suggest that these two important regulators of neuronal process formation are involved in the generation of sex differences in synaptic connectivity in this brain region (Speert et al., 2007).

Hormonal actions on glial cells may also be highly relevant for the sexual differentiation of neuronal connectivity. This is substantiated by the findings of several laboratories indicating that the morphology, immunoreactivity, enzymatic activity, and gene expression of astroglia are sexually dimorphic in several brain areas, and can be modified by the postnatal actions of sex hormones (Chowen et al., 1995; Conejo et al., 2005; Garcia-Segura et al., 1988c; Mong et al., 1999). Furthermore, glial cells express receptors for gonadal hormones, and participate in steroid metabolism and in the synthesis of endogenous steroids by the nervous system (see Garcia-Segura and Melcangi, 2006, for a review). Considering the close morphological and functional relationship between glial cells and neurons, it is obvious that hormonal effects on glia during the development of the nervous system may have important functional consequences. Several steps during the genesis of sexually dimorphic neuronal networks could conceivably be regulated by glial cells, including the proliferation, survival, migration, and functional maturation of neurons. Hormonal modulation of glial cell morphology may be involved in the establishment of the sexually dimorphic pattern of neuronal connectivity seen in various brain nuclei. In support of this concept, the laboratory of Margaret McCarthy at the University of Maryland and our own laboratory have provided evidence for a parallel maturation of astroglia and synaptic connectivity in the rat hypothalamic arcuate nucleus. The development of sex differences in the number of axosomatic synapses in this nucleus occur in parallel to the development of sex differences in: (i) the levels of glial fibrillary acidic protein (GFAP), a component of the cytoskeleton of astrocytes; (ii) the morphological differentiation of astrocytes; and (iii) the amount of neuronal membrane surface covered by astroglial cell processes (Chowen et al., 1995; Garcia-Segura et al., 1995b; Mong and Blutstein, 2006; Perez et al., 1990). These sex differences are induced by the perinatal secretion of testosterone in male rats (Fig. 6.2). This hormone induces the stellation of astrocytes, an increased expression of GFAP, and an increased coverage of neuronal membranes by astrocytic processes. Coincident with these changes in astrocytic morphology is a strong reduction

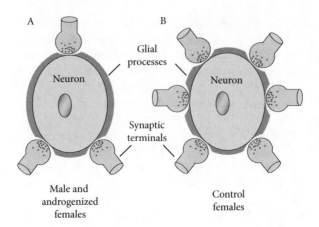

Figure 6.2. Action of androgens during early postnatal life in rats predetermines the synaptic connectivity in adult arcuate neurons. Neonatal administration of testosterone to female pups (androgenized females) or endogenous action of testosterone in neonatal males results in a decreased number of axosomatic synaptic contacts and an increased glial coverage of arcuate neuronal somas in adults (A) compared to normal female rats (B).

in the density of dendritic spines and axosomatic synapses on arcuate neurons (Garcia-Segura et al., 1995b; Mong et al., 1996, 1999; Mong and McCarthy, 1999). The effect of testosterone on astrocytes and synapses is likely mediated by its conversion into estradiol. Although these findings suggest that astrocytes are involved in the hormonal modulation of synaptogenesis, it is still a matter of debate as to whether glial cells play an active role in the generation of sex differences in synaptic connectivity (Garcia-Segura and McCarthy, 2004). Jessica Mong and her colleagues have provided evidence that neurons, via the neurotransmitter GABA, play a critical role in the sexual differentiation of astrocytes in the arcuate nucleus (Mong et al., 2002). In addition, estradiol increases the glial expression of glutamine synthetase, which facilitates the conversion of glutamate into glutamine. Glutamine may then be used by neurons for glutamate synthesis, which in turn may affect neuronal and glial function (Blutstein et al., 2006; Mong and Blutstein, 2006).

The coordinated modification in the extension of glial processes covering neuronal membranes and the formation of synapses may be the consequence of a modification in the adhesion and recognition properties of neuronal membranes. We have postulated that hormonal modifications in the organization of the neuronal plasma membrane may precede, and be the cause of, the synaptic and glial changes in the arcuate nucleus, and perhaps in other brain regions as well. It is important to note that the generation of sex differences in the number of axosomatic synapses in the rat hypothalamic arcuate nucleus takes place between postnatal day 10 and postnatal day 20; that is, several days after the perinatal androgen peak in males, and when testosterone levels in plasma and the hypothalamus have reached low values (Perez et al., 1990). This observation raises the question as to what mechanisms underlie this delay in the manifestation of gonadal steroid-induced sex differences in the number of synapses. Androgens, or its metabolite estradiol, should exert some effect in the arcuate nucleus that causes the generation of sex differences in synapses several days later. Our hypothesis is that hormonal modifications in the recognition properties of neuronal membranes and cell adhesion molecules may result in increased or decreased affinity for glial membranes, and consequently in an increased or decreased glial coverage (Garcia-Segura et al., 1995b; Naftolin et al., 1996a).

The involvement of neuronal membrane molecules in the induction of neuroglial plasticity by gonadal steroids is supported by freeze-fracture studies on arcuate neurons which demonstrate gender differences in the structure of their plasma membrane. Neuronal plasma membranes from male and female rats differ in their content of intramembrane particles (IMPs), structures thought to represent proteins embedded in the membrane bilayer. Plasma membranes from developing females have a higher numerical density of small IMPs (< 10 nm), while neuronal membranes from developing males have a modest excess of large IMPs (> 10 nm) (Garcia-Segura et al., 1985; Perez et al., 1990). Small IMPs in the plasma membranes of arcuate neuronal somas bind concanavalin A (Fig. 6.3) and may, therefore, represent membrane glycoproteins involved in cellular recognition (Garcia-Segura et al., 1989a). This sexually dimorphic membrane phenotype is changed by neonatal sex steroid exposure; the number of small IMPs falls, while the number of large IMPs increases to male levels after the administration of testosterone to newborn females. The number of concanavalin A binding sites is also reduced to male levels in androgenized females (Fig. 6.3). These findings suggest that gender differences in arcuate neuronal plasma membrane composition may be induced by the fetal burst of androgen production by males. Hormone-induced changes in the number of IMPs appear to be linked to modifications in the exoendocytotic activity of arcuate neuronal membranes (Garcia-Segura et al., 1987b, 1988b). Changes in the number of exoendocytotic images accompany the sexual differentiation of IMP content in arcuate neuronal membranes and precede the generation of sex differences in synapses and glia. Exoendocytotic images are higher in newborn and 10-day-old males than in females of the same ages, before the appearance of sex differences in the number of axosomatic synapses. The increased exoendocytosis in male membranes likely reflects an active membrane remodeling that may be the cause of the different IMP composition in male and female membranes. Exoendocytotic activity in male membranes declines after postnatal day 10 to reach female levels by postnatal day 20, when sex differences in synapses are already established. Androgenization of females with a single injection of testosterone propionate on the day of birth results in a significant increase in the endocytotic activity

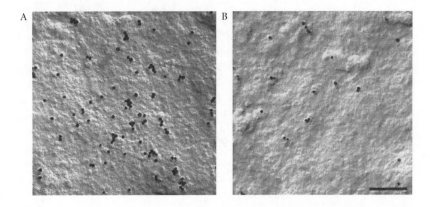

Figure 6.3. Concanavalin A binding to intramembrane protein particles in the plasma membrane of arcuate neurons. Concanavalin A, which binds to glycoproteins, is recognized by colloidal gold labeling (black dots); (A) from a control adult female rat, (B) from an adult female rat that was injected with testosterone on the day of birth. Developmental actions of testosterone cause a permanent modification in the phenotype of the plasma membrane of arcuate neurons. Scale bar, 0.25 μm. (Microphotographs from the author. Based on Garcia-Segura et al., 1989a.)

in the arcuate membranes to levels similar to those observed in male animals (Garcia-Segura et al., 1988b).

As it is probably the case for the sexual differentiation of the number of axosomatic synapses in the arcuate nucleus, the effect of testosterone on arcuate membranes may be mediated by its conversion to estradiol in the hypothalamus, where high levels of aromatase enzyme have been found. Indeed, an increase in the number of exoendocytotic images is observed after the administration of high doses of estradiol to adult female rats, a treatment that also abolishes the sex differences in IMP content (Olmos et al., 1987). Estradiol also induces a rapid increase in exoendocytotic images in the plasma membrane of cortical neurons in monolayer cultures; this increase precedes changes in IMP numbers (Garcia-Segura et al., 1989c). Thus, the modulation of exoendocytotic activity could be involved in the mechanism by which estradiol affects the number of IMPs in neuronal membranes. The increase in the number of exoendocytotic images appears to be, at least in part, related to increased membrane internalization, since estradiol induces a rapid increase in the endocytosis of extracellular markers in arcuate tissue slices perfused with physiological levels of this hormone (Garcia-Segura et al., 1987b). The effect of estradiol on exoendocytotic images is dose dependent, reversible, and is elicited within one minute after the perfusion of hypothalamic slices has begun (Garcia-Segura et al., 1987b). The rapidness of this hormonal response suggests a nongenomic effect of estradiol on neuronal membranes. Such rapid hormonal membrane effects may modulate the insertion or the endocytotic removal of IMPs from the plasma membrane of arcuate neurons and this, in turn, could change the intercellular affinities, allowing synaptic and neuroglial plasticity. The marked hormonally induced sex differences in the content of IMPs in arcuate neuronal perikarya plasma membranes suggest that the postsynaptic membrane composition could be involved in the genesis of synaptic differences. The sex differences in the neuronal plasma membrane that already exist in the newborn rat (Garcia-Segura et al., 1985) could be directing the formation of the synaptic pattern that occurs later in development and up to several days after the perinatal peak of testosterone. According to this hypothesis, the effect of gonadal steroids on the neuronal plasma membrane may result in a sexual differentiation of synaptic connectivity, either because growth cones will find a different postsynaptic membrane organization in males than in females, or because neuronal membranes have an increased gliophilic structure in males, resulting in an increased astrocytic ensheathing of neurons and, therefore, a decreased number of available postsynaptic sites for the growing axons.

Stress Hormones

Stress hormones also have an impact on the developmental organization of the brain during postnatal life. We have seen earlier in this chapter that stress during pregnancy may have a permanent impact on brain plasticity and function. Glucocorticoids may program the fetal brain, altering its future plasticity and function during adult life. It should be noted, however, that dams subjected to stress during pregnancy may show an altered maternal care and this may contribute to the behavioral deficits of their offspring (Champagne and Meaney, 2006). Therefore, it is not always easy to separate gestational effects of stress from early postnatal effects, which also have an important impact on adult life.

As prenatal stress does, early postnatal stress also profoundly influences brain plasticity, cognitive function, behavior, and emotions in adult life (Fig. 6.1). Stress and stress hormones may exert organizational effects in the postnatal developing brain that will persist throughout adulthood. In humans, early adverse experiences in postnatal life are a developmental risk factor for the appearance of psychopathological alterations in adulthood (Brunson et al., 2005; Sanchez et al., 2001; Welberg et al., 2001). For instance, maltreated children or children exposed to traumatic or stressful events have an increased probability of developing major depression, posttraumatic stress disorder, and attention deficit/hyperactivity (Gutman and Nemeroff, 2003; Heim et al., 2004). The affective alterations caused by early life stress in humans are associated with functional modifications in the adult brain. For instance, positron emission tomography studies have revealed that women with histories of childhood sexual abuse (which have increased symptoms of depression and anxiety compared to women without a history of childhood abuse [McCauley et al., 1997]), have an increased cerebral blood flow in the anterior paralimbic regions of the brain (Shin et al., 1999). In addition, studies with magnetic resonance imaging have detected decreased hippocampal volumes and abnormal neuronal network function in the brain of children that have suffered physical or sexual abuse, and in adult people that suffered these abuses early in life (Bremner et al., 1997; Chugani et al., 2001; DeBellis et al., 2002; Stein et al., 1997). Furthermore, it has been reported that dopamine release after stress is higher in the striatum of human subjects with low maternal care (Pruessner et al., 2004).

Maternal deprivation, poor maternal care, and post-partum stress and depression are a source of stress in early life that may affect child development and have a permanent impact on brain function and plasticity. In monkeys, maternal or sibling deprivation during rearing results in aggressive behavior, incapacity to cope with stressful situations, heightened fear, and learning and memory deficits later in life (Levine et al., 1993; Ruppenthal et al., 1976; Sanchez et al., 1998). Altered maternal care in rodents is also associated with cognitive impairment in adult life (Brunson et al., 2005). In contrast, enhanced maternal care in rodents and primates is associated with better cognitive skills in adult life (Liu et al., 1997; Sanchez et al., 1998). The quality of maternal care in the offspring predetermines functional and structural brain plastic responses to stress and corticosterone in later life (Champagne et al., 2008), exerting a metaplastic regulation of brain plasticity. An extreme case is the prolonged maternal separation during the early postnatal period in rodents, a stressful situation for both the dam and pups. Adult rats that were separated from their mothers for extended periods in early postnatal life have an altered responsiveness of their hypothalamic–pituitary–adrenal axis after exposure to stressful experiences, showing prolonged increases in CRH, adrenocorticotropic hormone (ACTH), and corticosterone in response to stress (Plotsky and Meaney, 1993). As previously mentioned regarding prenatal stress, early postnatal stress also results in permanent behavioral alterations and cognitive effects. Thus, rats submitted to early postnatal prolonged maternal separation have increased measures of anxiety (Huot et al., 2001) and depression (MacQueen et al., 2003), and impairments in fear conditioning (Kosten et al., 2006), spatial learning, and recognition memory (Brunson et al., 2005; Huot et al., 2002). Interestingly, maternal separation affects maternal care in adulthood (Lovic et al., 2001), an alteration also produced with prenatal stress. In addition, as mentioned earlier regarding the effect of prenatal stress, postnatal stress in rats caused by early maternal separation may produce a disruption in the prepulse inhibition (Ellenbroek and Cools, 1998; Ellenbroek et al., 1998), an attention deficit characteristic of schizophrenic patients. However, the effect of early postnatal stress on prepulse inhibition depends on the genetic background of the animals, having been observed in Wistar rats but not in other strains (Fumagalli et al., 2007). This suggests an interaction between postnatal stress and genetic factors.

As mentioned for prenatal stress, the behavioral and cognitive alterations produced in adult animals by early postnatal stress are also associated with remodeling of hippocampal circuits, including abnormal synaptic physiology in CA3, remodeling of excitatory mossy fiber innervation, and impairment of long-term potentiation in CA3 and CA1 (Brunson et al., 2005; Champagne et al., 2008; Huot et al., 2002). In contrast, long-term potentiation is enhanced in the hippocampal dentate gyrus by postnatal stress. Kehoe and Bronzino (1999) have studied a model of repeated infant isolation stress, in which rats were isolated from their mothers for one hour per day during postnatal days two through nine. This early postnatal stress results in a long-lasting enhancement of the induction of long-term potentiation in the dentate gyrus. In addition, early postnatal stress caused by prolonged bouts of separation from the mother, in this case three hours each day between postnatal day 1 and postnatal day 14, also causes a long-lasting suppression of adult neurogenesis and diminished plastic responses in neurogenesis after exposure to stress in adult life (Mirescu et al., 2004). Maternal separation for 24 hours causes a significant decrease in the number of granule cells in the hippocampus (Fabricius et al., 2008), and the administration of high levels of corticosterone to postpartum dams results in a decreased postnatal cell proliferation in the dentate gyrus of the male, but not female, offspring (Brummelte et al., 2006), suggesting an interaction with gonadal hormones.

The effects of early life stress on adult hippocampal plasticity may be mediated by hormonal alterations during hippocampal development. Stress in neonatal rats may activate the hypothalamic–pituitary–adrenal axis, causing the release of CRH from neurons of the hypothalamic paraventricular nucleus. CRH, in turn, induces the secretion of ACTH from the anterior pituitary gland, and ACTH induces the release of glucocorticoids from the adrenal glands. The hippocampus and other brain areas are sensitive to glucocorticoids and express glucocorticoid receptors; these hormones may affect neuronal development and synaptogenesis in the hippocampus. Therefore, permanent alteration of hippocampal function by early life stress may be the result of an unbalanced release of CRH during hippocampal development. Indeed, the administration of CRH in the cerebral ventricles of immature rats results in deficits in the hippocampal function in adult life, and these deficits have the same characteristics of those caused by early life stress (Brunson et al., 2001).

Peptide Hormones

In addition to CRH, other peptide hormones are also involved in the regulation of brain mutability during early postnatal life. Insulin appears to modulate developmental synaptic plasticity, since it has been shown that the addition of insulin accelerates the decline in silent glutamatergic synapses and the concomitant increase in functional synapses during the development of the thalamocortical projection in vitro (Plitzko et al., 2001). In contrast, repetitive insulin-induced hypoglycemia in young rats results in neuronal loss in the neocortex and impaired long-term potentiation of synapses in the hippocampus (Yamada et al., 2004). IGF-I also promotes the membrane expansion of nerve growth cones (Laurino et al., 2005) and axon outgrowth

(Ozdinler and Macklis, 2006), and may regulate neuronal migration (Jiang et al., 1998), synaptogenesis (O'Kusky et al., 2003), and other aspects of the postnatal development of the central nervous system, including the process of myelination by preventing the apoptotic death of oligodendrocytes during postnatal life (Popken et al., 2004). Furthermore, IGF-I may interact with gonadal hormones in the regulation of developmental plasticity of the nervous system. I have analyzed in Chapter 5 the importance of the cross talk between estradiol and IGF-I for the regulation of synaptic plasticity in the adult brain. Such cross talk is also highly relevant for the developmental plasticity of the central nervous system. Indeed, an interaction between these two factors may contribute to the generation of structural sex differences in the central nervous system by the regulation of the survival and differentiation of developing neurons in specific regions of the brain and spinal cord involved in the regulation of neuroendocrine events and reproduction (Carrer and Cambiasso, 2002). The first evidence of such an interaction was obtained by Dominique Toran-Allerand, Leland Ellis, and Karl H. Pfenninger at Columbia University, who in 1988 reported a synergic effect of estrogen and insulin on neuritic growth in fetal rat and mouse brain explants (Toran-Allerand et al., 1988). Although IGF-I was not directly tested in this seminal study, Toran-Allerand and her collaborators convincingly proposed that the effect of insulin could be mediated by the activation of IGF-I receptors, since insulin, at the concentrations used in their experiments, could have activated the IGF-I receptors. Support of this interpretation arrived almost one decade later from Europe. The laboratory of Adriana Maggi at the University of Milan (Ma et al., 1994) reported that insulin and insulin growth factors promoted the elongation of neuronal processes, and induced the growth arrest of a neuroblastoma cell line, but only when these cells were transfected with estrogen receptor α (the only known estrogen receptor at that time; therefore, in the original paper it was not labeled yet with the Greek character α). Furthermore, Maggi and her collaborators showed that IGF-I was able to activate estrogen receptor-α-mediated-transcription in neuroblastoma cells (Ma et al., 1994; Patrone et al., 1996). This finding was of extraordinary importance—the implication is that IGF-I could exert part of its developmental actions in neurons by regulating the activity of estrogen receptors. Since then, several studies have demonstrated that estradiol may also regulate IGF-I signaling in the developing central nervous system, and that there is an interdependence of estrogen receptors and IGF-I receptors in the promotion of neuronal survival and differentiation in primary cultures of developing hypothalamic neurons (Cambiasso et al., 2000; Carrer and Cambiasso, 2002; Dueñas et al., 1996).

After the highly interesting report by Adriana Maggi's group (Ma et al., 1994) showing that estrogen receptor α was indispensable for the effects of IGF-I on neuritic extension in neuroblastoma cells, we decided in our laboratory to examine the possible interaction of IGF-I and estrogen receptors on the differentiation and survival of primary neurons (Dueñas et al., 1996). Both estradiol and IGF-I promoted neuronal survival and differentiation in primary neuronal cultures grown in a defined medium deprived of serum and hormones. In these cultures, the induction of neuronal survival and differentiation by IGF-I was prevented by inhibiting the synthesis of estrogen receptor α, using a specific antisense oligonucleotide. The effect of IGF-I was also prevented by the estrogen receptor antagonist ICI 182780. In turn, the promotion of neuronal survival and differentiation by estradiol was prevented by blocking the synthesis of IGF-I in the cultures using a specific IGF-I antisense oligonucleotide, as well as by the pharmacological blockade of the MAPK and PI3K signaling pathways, both activated by the IGF-I receptor (Dueñas et al., 1996; Garcia-Segura et al., 2000). Therefore, estrogen receptor α mediates the effects of IGF-I, and IGF-I receptor mediates the effects of estradiol on hypothalamic neurons. Similar results have been obtained in neuroblastoma PC12 cells in the laboratory of Anne M. Etgen at the Albert Einstein College of Medicine. Topalli and Etgen demonstrated that both estradiol and IGF-I increases neuritic growth in PC12 cells transfected with the estrogen receptor α, and that antagonists of estrogen receptors and IGF-I receptors block the effect of both factors, indicating that estrogen receptor α mediates the effects of IGF-I, and IGF-I receptor mediates the effects of estradiol on neuritic growth in PC12 cells (Topalli and Etgen, 2004). A role for IGF-I receptors in neuronal development has also been detected in the laboratory of Hugo F. Carrer at the University of Córdoba, Argentina (Cambiasso et al., 2000; Carrer and Cambiasso, 2002). Carrer and his collaborators have shown that estradiol induces an increase in axonal growth and in the expression of TrkB and IGF-I receptors in ventromedial hypothalamic neurons derived from male rats. However, this effect is only detected when neurons are cultured in the presence of conditioned media from glial cells removed from target regions. This suggests that growth factors released by glia are involved in the neuritogenic effect of estradiol, and that IGF-I receptors are involved in this effect. Therefore, estradiol, IGF-I and its respective receptors may interact via diverse mechanisms in the regulation of neural development.

Another peptide hormone that influences postnatal brain development is leptin. Developmental actions of leptin may participate in the maturation of the neuronal circuits that control feeding and energy homeodynamics. Therefore, factors that influence fetal leptin levels may alter this maturation, with long-lasting consequences for metabolism. In addition, leptin may have an impact on the development of other central nervous system structures, including brain cognitive regions which express high levels of leptin receptors. Leptin may also interact with the developmental actions of other hormones, such as glucocorticoids. Plasma levels of leptin are high in human neonates (Gomez et al., 1999) and early postnatal rodents (Ahima et al., 1998; Rayner et al., 1997), and are inversely related to basal corticosterone secretion (Walker CD et al., 2004b). During this developmental period, leptin may have an important effect on the organization of neuronal circuits regulating stress responses. For instance, during early postnatal life, leptin increases the efficiency of the response to glucocorticoid inhibitory feedback and inhibits responses to stress (Proulx et al., 2001; Walker CD et al., 2004b). This effect may be in part mediated by an increase in the expression of glucocorticoid receptors in the hippocampus and in the hypothalamic paraventricular hypothalamic nucleus, brain structures that are involved in mediating the glucocorticoid feedback onto the hypothalamic–pituitary–adrenal axis. Leptin may also decrease responses to stress in the pups by the actions of maternal behavior (Oates et al., 2000). In turn, one of the main sources of circulating leptin during this period is likely to be maternal milk (Walker CD et al., 2004a).

EARLY HORMONAL INFLUENCES ON BRAIN MUTABILITY: RECAPITULATION

We have seen in this chapter that a variety of hormonal signals are involved in the regulation of the developmental plasticity of the central nervous system during fetal and early postnatal life. Some hormones, such as thyroid hormones, appear to play the role of master regulators of neural development, and are indispensable for the coordinated morphological and functional maturation of all regions of the central nervous system. Other hormones, such as growth hormone and IGF-I, are important for determining the final number of neurons and glial cells. Several hormones, such as gonadal steroids and stress hormones, exert more specific organizational actions in the proliferation and differentiation of neurons and glial cells, and the organization of neuronal circuits in specific brain regions. However, all the hormonal signals that regulate the developmental mutability of the central nervous system act in concert. We have seen that several hormones affect similar developmental processes. Thus, thyroid hormones, insulin, growth hormone, and IGF-I regulate the formation of myelin. All these hormones and stress hormones regulate neurogenesis; many hormones affect the functional organization of neuronal circuits. Therefore, several hormones may interact in the regulation of the same plastic event during brain development, and influence the action of other hormones. For instance, neuroplastic developmental actions of stress hormones are influenced by sex hormones, and have different outcomes in males and females. In turn, leptin and sex hormones affect the developmental actions of stress hormones, while prolactin and growth hormone exert antagonistic effects to thyroid hormone on brain metamorphosis in amphibians. In contrast, CRH and corticoids facilitate the metamorphic effects of thyroid hormones in the brain. In consequence, the organizational effects of a given hormone on the developing central nervous system depend on the general hormonal context.

Hormonal regulation of developmental brain mutability predetermines the future brain plastic responses during adult life (Fig. 6.1). On one hand, the developmental action of a given hormone influences future plastic responses in the neuronal circuits governing its own hormonal secretion or governing other hormonal systems. Thus, for example, the developmental actions of thyroid hormones are essential for the general maturation of the neuronal circuits that regulate hypothalamic hormonal secretions. On the other hand, other hormones exert more specific effects. For instance, sex hormones determine a sexually dimorphic maturation of the hypothalamic neuronal systems regulating their own secretions and those of other hormones, such as growth hormone. Furthermore, the developmental actions of a given hormone determine future neuroplastic responses of the brain to the same hormone and to other hormonal signals during adult life. For instance, the developmental actions of sex hormones may predetermine sex dimorphic neuroplastic responses and a sex-dimorphic regulation of brain plasticity by sex hormones or other hormones in adult life, while developmental actions of stress hormones influence future neuroplastic responses to stress, leptin, and sex hormones. Moreover, early hormonal regulation of brain development is determinant for the future responses of the nervous system to other exteroceptive and interoceptive regulators of brain plasticity. Thus, inadequate hormonal levels during the developmental period may cause permanent impairments in the adaptation of brain plasticity and behavior to the physical and social environment. In conclusion, we may consider that hormonal actions on brain development regulate metaplasticity, since they predetermine the future neuroplastic responses during adult life.

Chapter 7

Life Stages, Hormones, and Brain Remodeling: The Transition from Childhood to Adulthood

INTRODUCTION: PREPUBERTAL MATURATION, PUBERTY, AND ADOLESCENCE

The transition from childhood to adulthood is a critical period of transformation in the life cycle. Although mature gonadal function in vertebrates is reached at puberty, the full process of transition from childhood to adulthood involves a progressive maturation that is initiated before puberty, and not entirely completed by the time of puberty. Puberty is the moment of initiation of adolescence, which will end when full adult body characteristics are attained. Accordingly, the transition from a juvenile to the adult stage may be divided into three periods: prepubertal maturation, puberty, and adolescence. Although I will follow this division in this chapter, it is important to pay attention to the fact that the prepubertal and postpubertal periods of maturation have a different duration among species, and that some authors consider adolescence as the gradual period of transition from childhood to adulthood, including pubertal maturation. For simplification, I will also use in this chapter the term *peripubertal maturation* to include the three periods of transition from childhood to adulthood: prepubertal maturation, puberty, and adolescence.

The transition from the juvenile to adult stage is accompanied by a considerable degree of anatomical and functional body remodeling, including a remarkable readjustment in the activity of endocrine glands. The central nervous system, which plays an essential role in the generation of the hormonal changes associated with peripubertal maturation, also undergoes an important structural and functional transformation during this phase of life. The functional reorganization of the endocrine glands and the nervous system during the prepubertal period, puberty, and adolescence are interrelated. From one side, brain remodeling results in new patterns of neural regulation of hormonal secretion, and contributes to the initiation of puberty and to the hormonal changes associated with puberty and adolescence. In turn, new patterns of endocrine secretions generated during prepubertal maturation, puberty, and adolescence will regulate new morphological and functional plastic modifications in the brain and spinal cord, and will activate specific behaviors and additional neuroendocrine regulations. Thus, during the peri-pubertal period, the cross talk between the brain and the endocrine glands is readjusted to reach a new status of homeodynamic equilibrium in adulthood.

Given the complexity of the cross talk between the brain and the endocrine glands, it is not always evident as to whether a specific brain plastic modification observed during the prepubertal period, puberty, and adolescence is the cause or the consequence of the hormonal changes, or whether it represents an independent phenomenon. Having this consideration in mind and being aware of this limitation, I may now proceed to analyze the hormonal influences on brain plasticity during the prepubertal period, puberty, and adolescence. Our approach will be first to describe some examples of brain plastic changes associated with this life stage; then I will consider how hormones may affect these neuroplastic modifications; and finally, I will analyze the impact of brain remodeling during prepubertal maturation, puberty, and adolescence on the activity of endocrine glands.

BRAIN REMODELING DURING THE TRANSITION FROM CHILDHOOD TO ADULTHOOD

We are only beginning to appreciate the importance of the structural and functional modifications that occur in the brain during the transformation from childhood to adult life. This developmental transition is a phase of considerable modifications in cognition, mood, arousal, motivation, sleeping patterns, personality, social interactions, behavior, and affection in humans (Blakemore, 2008; Spear, 2000; Steinberg, 2005). The brain then undergoes radical functional alterations that are associated with a high degree of plastic structural remodeling. Imaging techniques have allowed for the assessment of these brain changes in humans, revealing important nonlinear modifications in brain growth during childhood, puberty, and adolescence. Different brain regions have different peaks of maturation, and the changes include modifications in the volume of gray and white matter. Gray matter matures first in the primary sensorimotor cortices along with the frontal and occipital poles. Then the rest of the cerebral cortex matures in a parietal-to-frontal direction. In some cortical regions containing association areas that integrate information from different sensory modalities (such as the temporal lobes), gray matter volume does not reach an adult steady state until the early to mid-twenties (Giedd et al., 1999; Gogtay et al., 2004). Both volume and myelination of the white matter increase progressively, in a region-specific fashion, during childhood and adolescence (Paus et al., 2001). However, striking nonlinear changes occur in white matter volume during the process of myelination of cortical and subcortical axons and the maturation of cortical connections (Thompson et al., 2000). In general, pubertal maturation represents a period in which brain growth is first increased, and then decreased and stabilized. Gray matter volume increases in the prepubertal period and decreases after puberty (Giedd et al., 1999; Gogtay et al., 2004; Jernigan et al., 1991; Paus,

2005; Pfefferbaum et al., 1994; Shaw et al., 2006; Sowell et al., 1999). Growth rates in fibers innervating association and language cortices are also attenuated after puberty (Thompson et al., 2000).

Animal studies have also revealed marked changes in brain structure during the transition from childhood to adulthood. These studies have detected synaptic and dendritic remodeling in different regions of the central nervous system during prepubertal maturation, puberty, and adolescence. In general, studies in animals are in agreement with the observations in humans, indicating that there is a reduction in the overall connectivity in the gray matter after puberty, which suggests a possible reshaping of synaptic circuits during this life stage. Axons, dendrites, synapses, and synaptic receptors are modified in several brain regions between puberty and adulthood (Sisk and Zehr, 2005). One of the first piece of evidence was obtained by Gundela Meyer and her collaborators at the University of La Laguna in the Canary Islands. They studied the morphology of hippocampal CA1 neurons in male rats using the Golgi method, and discovered that the density of dendritic spines increases at puberty onset and then decreases after puberty (Meyer et al., 1978). More recent studies, using spinophilin immunoreactivity to label dendritic spines, have detected a 46% decrease in the number of dendritic spines in the stratum radiatum of area CA1 in postpubertal female rats (postnatal day 49) compared to peripubertal (postnatal day 35) and prepubertal (postnatal day 22) females (Yildirim et al., 2008).

Loss of dendritic spines associated with pubertal maturation has also been detected in the cerebral cortex—analysis with the Golgi method of layer III pyramidal neurons in areas 9 and 46 of male and female rhesus monkey prefrontal cortex has revealed an increase in spine density on both basal and apical dendrites during the first two postnatal months, followed by a plateau through 1.5 years of age, then a decrease at peripubertal age (Anderson et al., 1995). Similar changes have been observed in the density of parvalbumin-immunoreactive axon terminals of the chandelier cortical interneurons (Anderson et al., 1995).

Another example of dendritic plasticity at puberty is provided by the spinal nucleus of the bulbocavernosus, a sexually dimorphic group of motoneurons whose development and maintenance are under androgenic control (see Chapter 6). Dendrites reach maximum lengths in male animals by the fourth postnatal week, then retract to adult lengths by seven weeks of age (Goldstein et al., 1990). Similarly, in the hypothalamic ventromedial nucleus of female rats, spine density of dendrites and somas is significantly higher in juvenile versus peripubertal ages (Segarra and McEwen, 1991). In the preoptic area, the number of dendritic spines increases during prepubertal maturation, although the timing of the plastic changes shows some regional differences. In neurons located in the posterior inferior quadrant of the preoptic area, there is an increase in dendritic spines prior to vaginal opening. Then, dendritic spines increase in number in neurons located in the anterior superior and posterior superior portions of the preoptic area at the age of vaginal opening. The plastic modification is transient—the entire posterior preoptic area maintains an increased number of dendritic spines for several days; however, by 75 days of age the number of dendritic spines is dramatically decreased (Anderson, 1982).

More recently, Cheryl L. Sisk from Michigan State University and her collaborators analyzed the changes in the posterodorsal medial amygdala in male Syrian hamsters during puberty (Zehr et al., 2006). This brain region is involved in several behaviors that mature during puberty, such as aggressive, risk-taking, fear-related, parental, and mating behaviors. Sisk and her collaborators detected a significant pruning in the number of dendrites emanating from the cell body, and in the density of dendritic spines with puberty. Another important modification during puberty is the cellular position of the origin of axons in medial amygdala neurons. Approximately half of all posterodorsal medial amygdala neurons had an axon emanating from a dendrite rather than the cell body, and during puberty there is a shift in the origin of axons from higher-order dendritic segments to primary-order dendrites. The morphological remodeling is accompanied by significant modifications in the expression of synaptic proteins, such as spinophilin and synaptophysin (Zehr et al., 2006).

All these findings indicate that the transition from childhood to adulthood is accompanied by a reorganization of synaptic connectivity, a decrease in the number of dendritic spines, and the pruning of dendrites in several regions of the mammalian central nervous system. These neuroplastic modifications may represent a process of refinement of the neuronal circuits, which may be associated with new behavioral performances. Indeed, there is evidence suggesting that plastic modifications in dendrites, dendritic spines, and synapses during the transition to adulthood in songbirds are involved in song learning.

Barbara Nixdorf-Bergweiler and her collaborators analyzed the dendrites of spiny neurons in the lateral magnocellular nucleus of the anterior neostriatum (now renamed nidopallium; see Reiner et al., 2004) of male zebra finches before, during, and after song learning, using the Golgi method. They found that the number of dendritic spines increase during development between three and five weeks of age, then decline. The number of spines in the middle dendritic segments decreases by 14% between five and seven weeks of age, then decreases further by 48% between 7 weeks and adulthood. In addition, second-order dendrites have a decreased branching, and third-order dendrites are shorter in adults than in younger birds (Nixdorf-Bergweiler et al., 1995). Furthermore, subsequent electron microscopic analysis revealed that the decrease in the number of dendritic spines in the lateral magnocellular nucleus of the anterior neostriatum is associated with a decrease in both the density and total number of synaptic inputs. However, the length of the post-synaptic density increases between juvenile birds and adulthood, suggesting that the dendritic and synaptic pruning likely reflects a process of synaptic selection (Nixdorf-Bergweiler, 2001). The plastic dendritic and synaptic changes from juvenile to adult birds in the lateral magnocellular nucleus of the anterior neostriatum are observed in males and not females, and are most likely associated with a plastic reorganization of the neuronal circuits involved in song learning, since they occur when males are learning songs and coincide with a massive decrease in the afferent projections from the medial portion of the dorsolateral nucleus of the anterior thalamus, which are necessary for song learning (Johnson and Bottjer, 1992). In addition, the reduction in the number of dendritic spines is not observed in males that are raised in colonies without adult males, that is, in the absence of a live tutor for song learning. In contrast, the presence of adult males in the colony, and therefore the exposure to songs, results in the normal decrease in the number of dendritic spines in the transition to adult life (Wallhausser-Franke et al., 1995).

Studies by electron microscopy have also confirmed that synaptic connectivity decreases in parallel to dendritic pruning during the transition from childhood to adult life in other species and brain regions. Several studies have detected an overproduction of synapses in infancy followed by their elimination during adolescence. For instance, Zecevic and Rakic (1991) detected this change in the somatosensory cortex of rhesus monkeys. The number of synapses increases steadily throughout the late fetal ages and early infancy. In late infancy, there is a moderate decrease in the number of synapses, and during puberty the synaptic pruning accelerates. The decline is specific for certain types of synapses. It mainly affects asymmetrical junctions located on dendritic spines, while symmetrical synapses on dendritic shafts and cell bodies remain relatively constant during postnatal life. In coincidence with the structural synaptic pruning after puberty, biochemical analyses have revealed similar modifications in the expression of synaptic receptors. Thus, D1 and D2 dopamine receptors are overproduced prior to puberty in the rat striatum, and pruned back to adult levels thereafter (Teicher et al., 1995). This apparent reduction in dendrites, synapses, and neurotransmitter receptors may represent a refinement of connectivity. Indeed, during prepubertal maturation there is a maturation of the interactions between dopamine D1 receptors and NMDA receptors in the prefrontal cortex that may be critical for developing mature cognitive abilities (Tseng and O'Donnell, 2005).

The neuronal number is also modified during puberty and adolescence in some brain regions. An increased cell death has been detected in the visual cortex of female rats during adolescence. The laboratory of Janice M. Juraska at the University of Illinois at Urbana–Champaign has detected an increased cell death in the visual cortex of female rats during adolescence (Nunez et al., 2001). In addition, the total neuron number in the ventral portion of the medial prefrontal cortex decreased between days 35 and 90 in both male and female rats, the change being more pronounced in females (Markham et al., 2007). The capacity to generate new neurons also appears to be modified in the mammalian brain during the transition from childhood to adulthood. Thus, the neuron number increases in the vasopressin and oxytocin-containing nucleus of the pig hypothalamus during adolescence, apparently due to an increase in postnatal neurogenesis (Rankin et al., 2003). In addition, He and Crews (2007) have reported much higher levels of neurogenesis in the subgranular layer of the hippocampal dentate gyrus and in the forebrain subventricular zone of prepubertal mice than in adult mice. This suggests that the rate of neurogenesis in these brain regions suffers a decline after puberty in mice. The decline in dentate gyrus neurogenesis after puberty seems to also occur in primates (Eckenhoff and Rakic, 1988). In contrast, the capacity for adult neurogenesis does not decline in adult reproductive life in songbirds in which new neurons are incorporated into avian song nuclei during adolescence (Nordeen and Nordeen, 1989), in association with the maturation of the song brain system and song behavior.

HORMONES AS REGULATORS OF BRAIN PLASTICITY DURING PREPUBERTAL MATURATION, PUBERTY, AND ADOLESCENCE

The complex hormonal changes that occur during the transition from childhood to adulthood contribute to the regulation of the structural and physiological remodeling of the brain associated with this period of life. Most likely, the gonadal hormones are one of the main regulators of neuroplastic modifications during the peripubertal period in which sex differences in brain maturation are observed (De Bellis et al., 2001; Giedd, 2004; Giedd et al., 1997; Markham et al., 2007; Nunez et al., 2001). Puberty is the period when the functional consequences of early developmental actions of sex hormones in the brain are manifested, with the apparition of sexually differentiated behaviors and sexually differentiated neuroendocrine regulation (Fig. 7.1). Numerous structural sex differences in the brain are manifested by the time of puberty, although not all of them appear to be dependent on gonadal hormones. In humans, the rates of brain growth show sex differences in some brain regions, such as the cerebral cortex, the hippocampus, the amygdala, the bed nucleus of the stria terminalis, and the corpus callosum (De Bellis et al., 2001; Giedd et al., 1997). Thus, in general, the age of peak cortical gray matter thickness occurs earlier in girls than in boys accordingly, with the earlier puberty onset in girls (De Bellis et al., 2001; Giedd, 2004). In contrast, boys had more prominent age-related white matter volume and corpus callosal area increases compared with girls (De Bellis et al., 2001). Furthermore, some sex differences in brain structure are generated during pubertal maturation, such as the differences in volume and number of neurons in the bed nucleus of the stria terminalis, which is larger in men (Chung et al., 2002). Sex differences in the volume and number of neurons of specific brain regions may be the consequence of a different rate of neuronal death during the transition from childhood to adulthood. For instance, in rats there is a sexually dimorphic increase in cell death in the visual cortex during adolescence (Nunez et al., 2001), resulting in adult male rats having 19% more neurons than female rats in the binocular region, and 18% more in the monocular region of the primary visual cortex (Reid and Juraska, 1992). The volume and number of neurons of

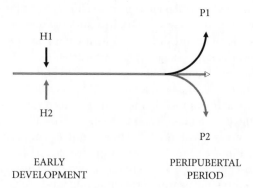

Figure 7.1. Early hormonal regulation of developmental brain plasticity (hormones H1 and H2, such as sex hormones or stress hormones) predetermine future brain plastic responses (P1, P2) during the peripubertal period. Therefore, early hormonal effects influence brain metaplasticity during the transition from childhood to adulthood. In addition, early hormonal effects also predetermine the future regulation of brain metaplasticity by new hormonal signals acting during the peripubertal period and during postpubertal life.

the ventral portion of the prefrontal cortex are also reduced in female rats, but not males between day 35 and day 90 (Markham et al., 2007).

The appearance of sex differences in brain structure by the time of puberty suggests that gonadal hormones may regulate neural plasticity during the peripubertal period. Indeed, neuroplastic actions of gonadal hormones during the transition from childhood to adulthood have been detected in cortical regions of the brain. For instance, testicular hormones are responsible for both the increase in the density of dendritic spines in hippocampal neurons of male rats during puberty, and for their decrease after puberty, since these plastic modifications are prevented by castration before puberty (Meyer et al., 1978). Testicular hormones are also associated with functional modifications in synaptic plasticity in the hippocampus during puberty. Thus, Hebbard and colleagues (2003) have shown that male rats that were gonadectomized at the onset of puberty and treated with testosterone during puberty showed a shift from long-term synaptic potentiation toward long-term synaptic depression in the CA1 region of the hippocampus, and a reduction of social memory. Testosterone also regulates dendritic formation and dendritic pruning in the spinal nucleus of the bulbocavernosus (Goldstein et al., 1990), promoting the initial growth of dendrites. Furthermore, the increase of testicular hormones with puberty appears to prevent further dendritic retraction, stabilizing dendritic length at adult levels (Goldstein et al., 1990). Estradiol is also involved in the regulation of brain plasticity during the transition from childhood to adulthood. For instance, estradiol increases dendritic and soma spine density in the hypothalamic ventromedial nucleus in juvenile and peripubertal male and female rats (Segarra and McEwen, 1991). In addition, the decrease in neuronal numbers in the visual cortex of female rats during puberty is prevented by a prepubertal ovariectomy, suggesting that ovarian hormones are the main regulators of this developmental change in the cerebral cortex (Nunez et al., 2002). A modification in the regulation of IGF-I receptor signaling by estradiol during pubertal maturation in the prefrontal cortex of female rats may be involved with the plastic modifications occurring in this brain region (Sanz et al., 2008). The actions of gonadal hormones during the peripubertal period are also involved in the differentiation of the pattern of axonal connectivity of neurokinin-B-expressing neurons in the rat hypothalamic arcuate nucleus. Neurokinin-B-expressing neurons project their ventral axons to capillary vessels in males, and to the neuropil in females. This sexually dimorphic pattern of axonal projections is apparently regulated by a masculinizing action of testosterone via androgen receptors, and a feminizing action of estradiol at puberty (Ciofi et al., 2007). Ovarian hormones during the peripubertal period are also involved in the regulation of the connectivity between the two brain hemispheres, since an ovariectomy on postnatal day 20 results in an increase in the number of myelinated axons in the splenium of the corpus callosum of young adult rats. Ovarian hormones seem to affect the process of myelinization, but the total number of axons is not affected by a prepubertal ovariectomy (Yates and Juraska, 2008).

Some of the neuroplastic modifications exerted by gonadal hormones during the transition from childhood to adulthood are influenced or preprogrammed by early hormonal actions, and may represent an example of metaplastic hormonal effects (Fig. 7.1). Roger Gorsky and his collaborators at the University of California, Los Angeles, showed that the sexual dimorphism in the volume of the anteroventral periventricular nucleus of the rat hypothalamus (which is larger in females than in males) arises between postnatal days 30 and 40. Then, the length of the nucleus becomes sexually dimorphic between days 60 and 80. However, the appearance of this sexual dimorphism is dependent on perinatal levels of androgens, since the castration of male rats on the day of birth sex-reversed the anteroventral periventricular nucleus volume in adulthood, and the anteroventral periventricular nucleus length was sex-reversed by the castration of males five days after birth (Davis et al., 1996). These findings suggest that prenatal and early postnatal regulation of brain mutability by sex hormones may predetermine some of the structural and functional plastic changes that these hormones may regulate later on during the peripubertal period.

Another example has been provided by Antonio Guillamón's group at the Universidad Nacional de Educación a Distancia in Madrid. They have characterized a sex difference in volume of the locus coeruleus of rats that is due to a greater number of neurons in females. The number of neurons progressively increases in the locus coeruleus in both sexes; however, postpubertal females have more neurons in the locus coeruleus than postpubertal males, likely because of a sex difference in neuronal migration or neurogenesis around the time of puberty (Pinos et al., 2001). Interestingly, the sex difference in the number of neurons in the locus coeruleus depends on perinatal levels of androgens; but, as for the anteroventral periventricular nucleus, it is manifested during puberty.

Another important hormonal influence for brain plasticity during the transition from childhood to adulthood is provided by stress hormones. The adolescent brain is highly sensitive to the plastic actions of stress hormones (Ferris, 2000), which exert effects that will be transmitted to adulthood. Physiological and behavioral responses to stress change during puberty, which is the moment when the fully functional maturation of the hypothalamic–pituitary–adrenal axis occurs (DiLuigi et al., 2006; Goel and Bale, 2007; Meaney et al., 1985; Romeo et al., 2004, 2006). This is also a period in which previous stressful experiences during early life may have an impact on brain plasticity and function. For instance, early stress has some effects on synaptic plasticity that are not manifested until adolescence. One example is maternal deprivation, which causes a disruption of prepulse inhibition of synapses in rats that is only detected after puberty (Ellenbroek et al., 1998). Interestingly, alterations in prepulse inhibition also occur in schizophrenia, and the manifestation of the disruption of prepulse inhibition after puberty in maternally deprived rats coincides with the temporal profile for the onset of schizophrenic symptoms in humans. Early stress also interferes with the maturation of interneurons in the medial prefrontal cortex of rodents at around pubescence (Helmeke et al, 2008). In some cases, interactions with developmental and/or peripubertal actions of sex hormones occur. Thus, neonatal handling increases the stress-induced activation of the posterior cingulate cortex of adolescent female rats and not of adolescent males (Park et al., 2003). In contrast, cognitive deficits and behavioral alterations as a consequence of prenatal stress have been detected in adolescent male rats and not in adolescent females (Llorente et al., 2007; Nishio et al., 2001). In addition, stress during adolescence may also have different effects in male and female brains. For instance, stress during adolescence enhances locomotor sensitization to nicotine in adult female rats, but not in adult male rats (McCormick et al., 2004).

Finally, it is important to consider that periods of adjustment in the communication between the brain and the endocrine glands, such as the transition from childhood to adulthood, may increase the vulnerability of the brain to pathological alterations. Indeed, puberty and adolescence are associated with an increased risk of a manifestation of affective disorders (such as major depression), and it is during adolescence that some major neuropsychiatric disorders such as schizophrenia become evident. This is also a period of greater vulnerability for addictive behaviors and drug abuse (Spear, 2000; Witt, 2007), which may be related to an enhanced activity of the brain endocannabinoid system during adolescence (Marco et al., 2007). This increased vulnerability to pathological alterations may be in part the consequence of an inadequate plastic brain remodeling during prepubertal maturation, puberty, and adolescence (Walker EF et al., 2004). For instance, it has been detected that the rates of brain volume reduction during adolescence are significantly higher for patients with childhood-onset schizophrenia than for healthy comparison subjects (Sporn et al., 2003). On the other hand, the high level of plasticity in the adolescent brain allows therapeutic interventions to compensate for the negative impact of early stressful experiences in life. Thus, the exposure to an enriched environment during adolescence is able to compensate or reverse the effect of prenatal stress on cognition, play behavior, depressive behavior, and emotionality in rats (Cui et al., 2006; Laviola et al., 2004; Morley-Fletcher et al., 2003a). The potential contribution to the development of psychiatric disorders of possible alterations in the hormonal regulation of brain plasticity during the transition from childhood to adulthood merits to be adequately explored.

BRAIN REMODELING AS A CAUSE OF HORMONAL CHANGES DURING PUBERTY

The other important aspect of the relation between puberty and brain plasticity is that plastic reorganization of the brain is involved in the initiation of the hormonal modifications associated with puberty. Although several brain structures regulating different hormonal systems may show considerable changes during puberty, including the neuronal networks controlling the hypothalamic-pituitary-adrenal axis (Romeo and McEwen, 2006), the best characterized plastic changes during the peripubertal period are those that occur in the synaptic circuits that govern the neuronal activity that produce gonadotropin releasing hormone (GnRH). These circuits show a plastic functional reorganization during the prepubertal period that dramatically alters the activity of GnRH neurons, generating a gradual increase in the frequency and amplitude of the pulses of GnRH secretion. The new pattern of GnRH secretion activates the secretion of pituitary gonadotropins, which in turn stimulates the production of gonadal hormones.

Several neuronal systems, including GABAergic neurons, preproenkephalinergic neurons, glutamatergic neurons, and kisspeptin-expressing neurons, regulate the activity of GnRH cells at puberty; some of these neuronal systems show plastic modifications during the peripubertal period. GnRH neurons suffer plastic modifications during the peripubertal period that are likely associated with a functional and structural reorganization of their presynaptic inputs. In male mice, the number of spines on dendrites and the cell body of GnRH neurons increases during the peripubertal period. However, the complexity of the dendritic tree is decreased between the prepubertal period and adulthood (Cottrell et al., 2006). These modifications in dendrites and dendritic spines of GnRH neurons are likely related to modifications in the number of excitatory synaptic inputs. Quantitative electron microscopic studies have revealed a significant decrease in the number of synaptic inputs on GnRH neurons during puberty in male rhesus monkeys (Perera and Plant, 1997). In addition to this structural plasticity, the action of synaptic inputs on GnRH neurons may also suffer functional modifications at puberty. For instance, the action of GABAergic inputs on GnRH neurons in mice show a dramatic functional plastic modification, switching from depolarizing to hyperpolarizing actions on GnRH neurons around puberty (Han et al., 2002).

Kisspeptin neurons are one of the neuronal systems that regulate GnRH cells, and show modifications during the peripubertal period. Among the multiple neuronal and glial systems involved in the regulation of GnRH cells, kisspeptin neurons appear to play an indispensable role in the activation of GnRH release during puberty onset. Kisspeptin neurons express sex steroid receptors (Smith, 2008) and therefore may mediate the effects of sex hormones on the activity of GnRH neurons. Kisspeptin, which is encoded by the KiSS1 gene, exerts a potent depolarizing effect on the excitability of GnRH neurons (Han et al., 2005). Its action is mediated by the G-protein-coupled receptor GPR54 (Seminara et al., 2003), which is expressed by GnRH neurons (Han et al., 2005). Therefore, kisspeptin may directly act on GnRH neurons to regulate GnRH release.

The kisspeptin/GPR54 system shows significant changes at puberty—the expression of kisspeptin and GPR54 increases in the hypothalamus at puberty in both male and female rats (Navarro et al., 2004), and in both male and female monkeys (Shahab et al., 2005). Furthermore, the hypothalamic maturation of the kisspeptin/GPR54 system is influenced by metabolic and environmental factors, such as undernutrition, that also affect pubertal maturation (Castellano et al., 2005; Navarro et al., 2007; Tena-Sempere, 2006). Different neuronal populations expressing kisspeptin, such as those present in the anteroventral periventricular nucleus and in the arcuate nucleus (among other locations), show a different response to sex steroids and may have different regulatory effects on GnRH cells (Dungan et al., 2006). For instance, kisspeptin expression is decreased by estradiol and testosterone in the hypothalamic arcuate nucleus, and is increased by these hormones in the anteroventral periventricular nucleus. Therefore, it has been suggested that kisspeptin neurons in the hypothalamic arcuate nucleus participate in the negative feedback regulation of gonadotropin secretion, while those located in the anteroventral periventricular nucleus participate in the generation of the preovulatory gonadotropin surge in the female. In this regard, it is interesting to note that the expression of kisspeptin increases dramatically in the anteroventral periventricular nucleus during the transition from juvenile to adult life in mice (Han et al., 2005).

Astrocytes may also contribute to the maturation of GnRH activity by increasing their release of glutamate and therefore enhancing the excitatory drive to the GnRH neuronal network (Roth et al., 2006). In response to estradiol, astrocytes may also release progesterone, which may act on estrogen-induced progesterone receptors in neurons that control GnRH activity (Micevych and Sinchak, 2008). In addition, astrocytes release different factors, such as transforming growth factor α and neuroregulins (see Chapter 2), which act on other glial cells to promote the release of prostaglandin E2 that, in turn, binds to specific receptors in GnRH neurons and elicits GnRH release (Ma et al., 1997; Ojeda et al., 1992; Ojeda and Ma, 1998). The release of prostaglandin E2 by glial cells may mediate the facilitatory effects of several hormones, such as estradiol (Rage et al., 1997) and oxytocin (Parent et al., 2008) on GnRH release. Furthermore, estradiol and progesterone also facilitate GnRH release by (i) increasing the production of transforming growth factor α by glial cells; (ii) facilitating the action of neuroregulins by increasing the expression of ErbB-2 and ErbB-4 receptors in astrocytes; and (iii) facilitating the action of prostaglandin E2 by increasing the expression of its receptors in GnRH neurons (Ojeda and Ma, 1999). Modifications in the expression of ErbB-2 and ErbB-4 in astrocytes seems to be an important step in the mechanism of initiation of puberty. Its expression increases in astrocytes before the onset of puberty and therefore before the pubertal augmentation in the levels of gonadal steroids (Ma et al., 1999; Ojeda et al., 2000), likely by the mediation of neuron-to-glia glutamatergic signaling (Dziedzic et al., 2003). Then, on the day of the first preovulatory surge of gonadotropins, the expression of ErbB-2 and ErbB-4 receptors is further increased by gonadal hormones (Ma et al., 1999; Ojeda et al., 2000).

Plastic changes during puberty may also affect GnRH neurons at the level of their neurosecretory endings. The retraction of tanycyte cellular processes, which engulf the terminals of GnRH axons in the median eminence, is one of the plastic changes contributing to the release of GnRH in the portal blood at puberty. Gonadal hormones activate the plastic reorganization of tanycytes and GnRH axons at puberty. Tanycytes, which express estrogen receptors (Gudino-Cabrera and Nieto-Sampedro, 1999), may be one of the direct cellular targets of gonadal hormones for the initiation of the plastic changes. As we have seen in Chapter 2, tanycytic processes in the median eminence are closely associated with GnRH axons and GnRH axonal terminals. The retraction of tanycytic processes during puberty allows the apposition of GnRH neurosecretory terminals with portal capillaries and the release of GnRH to portal blood. The laboratory of Sergio Ojeda has characterized different soluble factors, such as transforming growth factor α and transforming growth factor β, and molecules involved in cell-to-cell membrane interactions, such as SynCAM, the short form for the receptor protein for tyrosine phosphatase β, and contactin, which may participate in the remodeling of tanycytic processes and GnRH axons at puberty (see Chapter 2 for details). In addition, several genes, such as Oct2, thyroid transcription factor-1 (TTF-1) and enhanced at puberty-1 (EAP1) may potentially act as upper-echelon genes and coordinate the expression of a hierarchical network of other regulatory genes involved in the initiation of the plastic functional and structural neuroglial reorganization of the median eminence and the hypothalamus associated with GnRH release at puberty (Ojeda et al., 2006).

Tanycytes are also a target for other hormones that may influence the pubertal onset. For instance, tanycytes express receptors for IGF-I, a hormone that may contribute to the initiation of puberty by the activation of GnRH release. IGF-I acts on the regulation of GnRH release both as a hormone and as a local paracrine or autocrine factor. Andrea C. Gore and her collaborators have shown that IGF-I is expressed by GnRH cells, and that the expression of IGF-I in GnRH cells is increased at puberty (Daftary and Gore, 2003, 2004; Miller and Gore, 2001). Furthermore, during the peripubertal period in female rats, IGF-I increases GnRH synthesis in the anterior hypothalamus–preoptic area, where GnRH neuronal somas are located. These findings strongly suggest that IGF-I, produced by GnRH neurons, acts as an autocrine or paracrine factor to enhance GnRH release at puberty (Daftary and Gore, 2005). On the other hand, our own findings indicate that tanycytes uptake peripheral IGF-I by a mechanism regulated by estradiol and progesterone (Cardona-Gomez et al., 2000a; Fernandez-Galaz et al., 1996, 1997; Garcia-Segura et al., 1999a). The uptake of blood-borne IGF-I by tanycytes is highly enhanced at puberty in male and female rats (Dueñas et al., 1994). Peripheral IGF-I may contribute to the regulation of GnRH release at puberty, acting directly on GnRH cells or in the neuronal circuits that control the activity of GnRH neurons (such as those located in the anteroventral periventricular nucleus and the hypothalamic arcuate nucleus). Indeed, IGF-I participates in the structural remodeling of glial cells and synapses induced by estradiol in the hypothalamic arcuate nucleus in association with GnRH release in female rats (see also Chapter 5).

The reorganization of synapses and glia in the arcuate nucleus with pubertal onset in female rats is the result of a gradual and sexually dimorphic process of developmental organization (see Chapter 6). This process, which is characterized by a parallel maturation of neuronal membranes, glial cells, and synaptic inputs during the juvenile and prepubertal maturation period (Chowen et al., 1995; Garcia-Segura et al., 1995b; Matsumoto and Arai, 1976, 1977; Mong and Blutstein, 2006; Perez et al., 1990), generates a sexually dimorphic organization of synapses and glia. The sexually differentiated synaptic circuit is responsive to neuroplastic actions of estradiol after puberty in females (Csakvari et al., 2007; Olmos et al, 1989) and not in males (Horvath et al., 1997b). The arcuate nucleus contains several neuronal populations that are involved in the control of GnRH cells, including a subpopulation of neurons expressing kisspeptin (Dungan et al., 2006), a factor that, as previously mentioned, may be involved in the initiation of puberty (Kauffman et al., 2007; Navarro et al., 2007). In addition, the arcuate nucleus is responsive to other hormonal signals that regulate energy balance, food intake, and pubertal maturation, such as ghrelin and leptin (Blüher and Mantzoros, 2007; Tena-Sempere, 2008), which may also regulate synaptic plasticity in this hypothalamic region (Horvath, 2006; Pinto et al., 2004; see also Chapter 5). Therefore, neuroglial plasticity in the arcuate nucleus may integrate the action of different hormonal signals, including estradiol, leptin, and ghrelin, which may coordinate GnRH release with other physiological changes at the onset of puberty. In addition, as in the median eminence, the structural remodeling of glial cells and synapses in the arcuate nucleus may be regulated by soluble factors, including IGF-I (Fernandez-Galaz et al., 1997; Garcia-Segura et al., 1999a) and adhesion molecules, including PSA-N-CAM (Hoyk et al., 2001). Finally, it is tempting to speculate on the possibility that upper-echelon regulatory genes, such as Oct2, TTF-1 and EAP1 (Ojeda et al., 2006), may coordinate hormonal signals with the plasticity of tanycytes and GnRH axons in the median eminence, the uptake of IGF-I by tanycytes, the plasticity of the hypothalamic neuronal circuits regulating GnRH neurons, and the plasticity and neurosecretory activity of GnRH neurons at puberty.

CHAPTER SUMMARY

The transition from juvenile to adult life is accompanied by prominent structural and functional modifications in the central nervous system, which are associated with modifications in cognition, mood, sleeping patterns, personality, social interactions, behavior, and affection. The peripubertal period is a moment of intense growth, reshaping and maturation of the gray and white matters in the human brain, with marked regional and sex differences. In general, cortical gray matter thickness peaks earlier in females than in males, and some sex differences in brain structure are generated during pubertal maturation. Different studies, using a variety of techniques, lead to a common conclusion: in humans, monkeys, rodents, and other species, there is a decrease in gray matter, neuronal number, dendritic complexity, and synaptic connectivity during adolescence. These changes have been detected in different brain regions, including affective and cognitive areas. However, not all brain regions show the same tendency. The general decrease in synaptic connectivity during adolescence may reflect, at least in part, a process of refinement of the neuronal network in adaptation to the new physiological conditions, and are associated with the maturation of new specific behaviors. However, some modifications, such as the decrease in the generation of new neurons in the hippocampus between puberty and adulthood, suggest a possible reduction in the capacity of the brain to generate some forms of plasticity during adolescence.

Some of the structural and functional plastic changes that occur in the central nervous system during prepubertal maturation, puberty, and adolescence are hormonally regulated. From one side, the functional consequences of many early hormonal effects on brain organization are manifested at puberty. Prenatal and early postnatal neuroplastic regulatory actions of sex and stress hormones may predetermine future metaplastic modifications in several brain regions at puberty and during adolescence. In addition, the adolescent brain is highly sensitive to actions of sex and stress hormones, and likely of other hormones as well. Therefore, hormonal actions during this life stage may cause further and long-term modifications in the pattern of synaptic plasticity, affection, cognition, and behavior.

Finally, the reorganization of the brain that occurs during the transition from childhood to adulthood has an impact on the hormonal changes that accompany the process of sexual maturation and generation of adult behaviors. The hypothalamic circuits that regulate hormonal secretion mature during the prepubertal period. By the pubescence period, the circuits that control the activity and secretion of GnRH neurons, including GABAergic neurons, preproenkephalinergic neurons, glutamatergic neurons, and kiss-peptin expressing neurons, their associated glial cells and the dendrites and axons of GnRH neurons themselves, are ready to suffer a series of plastic modifications that will facilitate the initiation of the adult pattern of GnRH release and the consequent adult pattern of pituitary gonadotropin and sex hormone secretion. This remodeling of the brain during the onset of puberty is a process regulated by a variety of soluble factors and cell adhesion molecules that are likely under the control of several master genes that may coordinate the influence of hormonal signals with the metaplastic reorganization of different hypothalamic regions and the median eminence, and with the structural and functional metaplasticity of GnRH neurons.

Chapter 8

Life Stages, Hormones, and Brain Remodeling: Adult Reproductive Life

INTRODUCTION: HORMONAL REGULATION OF BRAIN PLASTICITY DURING ADULT LIFE

After the substantial plastic reorganization of the nervous system that occurs during the transition from the prepubertal period to adulthood, a new homeodynamic equilibrium is established between the brain and the endocrine glands. This new equilibrium, however, is still sustained by a constant process of neural mutability. Plastic adaptations of the central nervous system during adult life are indispensable for maintaining the adequate physiological responses to the modifications in the physical, biological, and social environment that an adult organism has to confront. Most, if not all, the actions that an adult vertebrate organism performs are accompanied by changes in hormonal levels in plasma and by plastic modifications in different brain and spinal cord regions. In many cases, hormonal and behavioral modifications may likely result in further alterations in neural plasticity. For instance, mating behavior produces alterations in the morphology of dendrites in the ventrolateral subdivision of the hypothalamic ventromedial nucleus in female rats (Flanagan-Cato et al., 2006); exploratory behavior modulates hippocampal synaptic plasticity (Yang et al., 2006) and produces the reorganization of the receptor fields in neurons from the barrel somatosensory cortex in rats (Frostig, 2006); hunting behavior induces plastic modifications in brain sensory maps in the optic tectum of birds (Bergan et al., 2005); a predatory attack provokes functional plasticity in the limbic circuits of mammals (Adamec et al., 2006); food storing behavior is associated with an increased hippocampal neurogenesis in birds (Hoshooley and Sherry, 2007); mastication affects neurogenesis in the hippocampus of rodents (Aoki et al., 2005; Mitome et al., 2005); social interactions cause a variety of plastic modifications in the brain, including changes in the rate of hippocampal neurogenesis (Yap et al., 2006), plastic reorganization of dendrites in hippocampal pyramidal neurons (Kole et al., 2004), and functional modifications in synaptic plasticity in the hippocampus (Artola et al., 2006); physical activity per se induces plastic modifications in the brain, promoting the formation of dendritic spines, enhancing the complexity of dendritic arbors, facilitating long-term potentiation of synaptic transmission in the hippocampus (Eadie et al., 2005; Farmer et al., 2004; van Praag et al., 1999), enhancing hippocampal neurogenesis (van Praag 2008; van

Praag et al., 1999), and causing the remodeling of the innervation of hypothalamic neurons (Higa-Taniguchi et al., 2007).

These are some examples of the studies that have explored the association of brain plastic modifications associated with specific behaviors. The life
events analyzed in these studies, together with many other behavioral, social,
and environmental situations that result in modifications in brain plasticity,
are associated with modifications in plasma hormonal levels. Brain plastic
responses during these conditions may be the consequence of an interaction
between behavior, hormones, and neuronal activity. In turn, the resulting
reorganization of neuronal circuits may influence future behavioral, endocrine, and neural events.

Hormones that influence brain plasticity (see Chapters 3, 4, and 5) participate in the adaptation of the organism to the variable physical environmental conditions during adult life, such as seasonality in external temperature
and food availability. For instance, seasonal hormonal fluctuations have an
impact on brain circuits for adapting metabolic regulation and behavior to
environmental conditions. Evolutionary selection, based on reproductive suc-
cess, has shaped the response of the endocrine and nervous systems to suc-
cessfully confront the environmental changes. Hormones also influence brain
plastic adjustments for social and reproductive interactions, to fight predators,
to explore new environments, or to execute new behavioral tasks. Hormones,
therefore, facilitate the reorganization of different neuronal circuits to adapt
brain function to the variable adult-life circumstances. Stress hormones,
which are involved in the integration of emotions with behavioral responses
and remodeling of neuronal circuits, play a key role in this homeodynamic
adaptation. However, many other hormones are also involved in the interaction of behavior and brain plasticity. In this chapter I will consider a few
selected examples of interactions of hormonal changes with brain plasticity
in adult reproductive life. I will briefly examine hormonal and brain plastic
modifications associated with circadian rhythms, seasonal behaviors, hibernation, reproductive cycles, motherhood, and social interactions.

Circadian changes in glial, neuronal, and synaptic plasticity in the suprachiasmatic nucleus and in other brain regions may be involved in the synchronization of the endogenous circadian clock to the light/dark cycle, and to the
adaptation of hormonal secretion patterns and behavior to seasonal changes
in day length. In turn, several hormones may be involved in the regulation of
circadian brain plasticity, including melatonin, glucocorticoids, sex steroids,
and prolactin. Seasonal alterations in the secretion of these hormones may
contribute to the regulation of metaplastic brain modifications in seasonal
change adaptations. Hormones regulate seasonal plasticity of brain regions
involved in cognitive function, such as the hippocampus, in association
with seasonal changes in specific behaviors, such as food storing behavior.
Hormones also participate in the modulation of seasonal neuroplastic changes
in brain regions involved in the control of reproduction, to adapt mating and
parental behaviors to the seasons. In songbirds, several hormones, including

testosterone and its metabolites, thyroid hormones, and melatonin, participate in the regulation of the seasonal reorganization of brain song system,
which involves metaplastic changes in dendritic structure, the rate of growth
of dendrites and axons, the rate of formation of dendritic spines and synapses,
and the rate of glial, neuronal, and endothelial cellular replacement within the
neuronal networks and brain structures that control song.

Hibernation in mammals, in adaptation to extended periods of low food
supply and extreme cold ambient temperatures, provides another example of
hormonally regulated seasonal brain plasticity. Both the endocrine glands and
the nervous system contribute to the regulation of the physiological modifications during hibernation. Melatonin is a main endocrine regulator of hibernation. Other hormones involved in the regulation of hibernation include
arginine-vasopressin, glucocorticoids, prolactin, thyrotropin-releasing hormone, thyroid-stimulating hormone, thyroid hormones, glucagon, insulin,
leptin, ghrelin, fibroblast growth factor 21, IGF-I, and hibernation-specific
protein complex (HPc). Among other targets tissues, these endocrine signals
act on different brain regions involved in the neural control of hibernation,
and contribute to the regulation of neuronal and glial plasticity during each
torpor-activity cycle during the hibernating period. In turn, plastic reorganization of the brain during hibernation is involved in the generation of physiological and hormonal changes associated with torpor and arousal.

Brain seasonal plasticity is also involved in the regulation of gonadal hormones and reproduction in seasonal breeders. In particular, seasonal modifications in the interactions of GnRH terminals and glial cell processes in
the median eminence appear to regulate the access of GnRH terminals to the
basal lamina of portal capillaries, and the release of GnRH into portal blood.
Seasonal changes in gonadotropin secretion are also accompanied by plastic
reorganization of astrocytic processes and in changes of the number of synaptic terminals contacting GnRH neurons. Seasonal neuroplastic modifications
are also detected in brain regions that control the activity of GnRH neurons.
Several hormones, including thyroid hormone and melatonin, may regulate
seasonal plasticity in GnRH neurons or in the neuronal systems controlling
the activity of GnRH neurons in seasonal breeders.

In nonseasonal breeders, there are also plastic modifications in brain
regions controlling GnRH release. These plastic changes are associated with
reproductive cycles and are regulated by gonadal hormones. In adult female
rodents, brain regions that regulate the activity of GnRH neurons, such as the
rostral preoptic area, the anteroventral periventricular nucleus, and the hypothalamic arcuate nucleus, exhibit repetitive synaptic and glial remodeling that
is regulated by the variations in ovarian hormones during the estrus cycle.
Tanycytic processes in the median eminence also show cycles of extension
and retraction following the changes in ovarian hormones during the estrus
cycle, participating in the regulation of GnRH release in the portal vasculature. In rodents, neuroplastic changes involved in the regulation of GnRH
release are coordinated by plastic modifications in brain regions that regulate

sexual behavior, such as the ventromedial hypothalamic nucleus. In addition, the hippocampus, a cognitive region that integrates different hormonal signals, also shows cyclic changes in glial reorganization, synaptic plasticity, and neurogenesis. All these plastic changes during the ovarian cycle are regulated by gonadal hormones, which facilitate the simultaneous generation of different (or even opposite) forms of synaptic and glial plasticity in different brain regions. This suggests that gonadal hormones may synchronize metaplastic modifications in brain regions that coordinate ovulation with sexual receptivity, lordosis, and hippocampal-dependent behaviors. Gonadal hormones may interact with local factors released by neurons and glial cells, including neurotransmitters, growth factors, and prostaglandin E2, and with other hormones, such as IGF-I, to regulate glial and synaptic plasticity during the estrus cycle.

Another phase in the life of adult females in which there is a noticeable interaction of brain plasticity with hormonal regulation is motherhood. The marked physiological changes during pregnancy, parturition, and the postpartum period are regulated by multiple neural and endocrine homeodynamic mechanisms involving modifications in the plasma levels of numerous hormones, including progesterone, estradiol, prolactin, oxytocin, relaxin, and glucocorticoids. Synaptic and glial plasticity in the magnocellular hypothalamic neurosecretory system is associated with the release of oxytocin during parturition and lactation. Plasticity in the hypothalamus is coordinated with plastic changes in pituicytes in the neurohypophysis, which modify its interactions with neurosecretory axons, regulating the occupation of the basal lamina of capillaries by neurosecretory terminals. Brain regions involved in the regulation of maternal behavior, the interaction with pups, and the response to stress, such as the medial preoptic area, the olfactory bulb, and the medial nucleus of the amygdala, respectively, also suffer marked plastic changes during motherhood. Furthermore, the cerebral cortex in lactating mothers shows plastic modifications as a consequence of the activation of tactile inputs of the nipples by pups. Interaction with pups may also affect morphological and functional synaptic plasticity in the hippocampus, and the cell proliferation rate in the subgranular layer of the dentate gyrus shows dramatic changes after delivery and lactation, which are associated with profound modifications in learning. Different hormones, including prolactin, oxytocin, glucocorticoids, and gonadal steroids, regulate these complex neuroplastic changes during motherhood.

In this chapter I will also analyze the regulation of brain plasticity by hormones within the context of social interactions. Prolactin and luteinizing hormone mediate the enhancement of neurogenesis in the female brain caused by the interaction with dominant males. Stress hormones may control emotional, cognitive, and behavioral responses to the social environment by regulating synaptic plasticity in the hippocampus, the amygdala, the prefrontal cortex, and other brain regions. Oxytocin and vasopressin may control social behavior by regulating synaptic plasticity in mesolimbic dopaminergic circuits of reward and reinforcement. Furthermore, temporal modifications of plasticity in GnRH and arginine vasotocin neurons are associated with seasonal changes in social interactions, territoriality, and parental care in some species. In general, social interactions are associated with transient homeodynamic changes in brain plasticity. However, chronic stress associated with social defeat may result in nonadaptive endocrine and neural responses, and may cause depression and other affective and emotional disturbances. Altered regulation of metaplasticity in some brain regions, such as the nucleus accumbens, the basolateral amygdala, and the hippocampus, may be involved in the behavioral and affective alterations caused by social defeat. Alterations in the regulation of metaplasticity in the amygdala and other brain regions, such as the hippocampus and cerebellum, may also be involved in the psychological consequences of traumatic experiences and in the alterations associated with posttraumatic stress disorder.

HORMONES AND CIRCADIAN BRAIN PLASTICITY

The suprachiasmatic nucleus of the hypothalamus is a key element of the internal circadian timing system. The neurons of the suprachiasmatic nucleus have an endogenous circadian discharge rhythm (Klein et al., 1991) that determines the circadian period (Ralph et al., 1990). In addition, there is a diurnal rhythm in glial and synaptic plasticity in the suprachiasmatic nucleus that likely plays an important role in the synchronization of the endogenous circadian rhythm, and in its adaptation to seasonal changes in day length. The suprachiasmatic nucleus regulates body rhythms via the parasympathetic and sympathetic autonomous nervous system. In addition, the suprachiasmatic nucleus regulates the secretion of melatonin by the pineal gland to adapt circadian and seasonal biological rhythms to environmental lighting. In turn, melatonin and other hormones affected by the circadian clock may regulate plastic events and neuronal activity in the suprachiasmatic nucleus and other brain regions.

The suprachiasmatic nucleus exhibits different forms of morphological and functional plasticity associated with circadian rhythms. High expression levels of the polysialylated form of the neural cell adhesion molecule (PSA-N-CAM) are detected in the suprachiasmatic nucleus (Glass et al., 1994), as in other brain regions with a high degree of structural plasticity. Polysialyc acid residue associated with the N-CAM confers a higher degree of plasticity to the intercellular interactions and its removal; using the enzyme endoneuraminidase, it blocks neuroglial plasticity in other brain regions (Theodosis et al., 1999; see also Chapters 2, 3, 4, and 7). Interestingly, an endoneuraminidase microinjection in the suprachiasmatic nucleus impairs circadian clock function (Shen et al., 1997). In agreement with the high expression of PSA-N-CAM in the suprachiasmatic nucleus and its potential role in the circadian clock function, circadian structural remodeling has been detected in this brain region.

The morphology of astrocytes, immunostained for glial fibrillary acidic protein (GFAP) and the expression of GFAP, show circadian changes in the suprachiasmatic nucleus of Syrian hamsters and rats (Becquet et al., 2008; Glass and Chen, 1999; Lavialle and Serviere, 1993). The astrocytic changes are in synchrony with a rhythm in suprachiasmatic nucleus glucose consumption (Lavialle and Serviere, 1993), and are dependent on light entrainment, suggesting that glial plasticity in this nucleus may be related to the synchronization of the clock to the light/dark cycle (Becquet et al., 2008). In addition, the glial changes may be induced by serotonin in a phase-dependent manner (Glass and Chen, 1999). Interestingly, PSA-N-CAM levels in the suprachiasmatic nucleus are also regulated by serotonin (Brezun and Daszuta, 1999), suggesting a possible causal relation between serotonin activity, PSA-N-CAM expression, and circadian glial remodeling.

Circadian glial changes are accompanied by circadian modifications in synaptic connectivity. At night, the glial coverage of the dendrites of rat suprachiasmatic neurons expressing vasoactive intestinal peptide increases in parallel with a decrease in the coverage by axon terminals of the neuronal perikarya and dendrites. In contrast, the glial coverage of the dendrites of suprachiasmatic neurons expressing arginine vasopressin decreases at night, in parallel to an increase in somal and dendritic membrane appositions between these neurons (Becquet et al., 2008). Therefore, different neuronal populations within the suprachiasmatic nucleus show a different form of daily rhythmic plasticity. Plastic remodeling of synapses has also been detected in the suprachiasmatic nucleus after experimental manipulation of lighting conditions. Prolonged periods of light or prolonged periods of darkness affect the ultrastructure and number of synapses from the retinal axons on suprachiasmatic neurons. Compared to rats exposed to a prolonged period of darkness, animals exposed to a prolonged period of light have larger synaptic buttons and a smaller amount of postsynaptic density material, among other ultrastructural differences. In addition, prolonged darkness reduced the number of Gray type I (asymmetric, presumably excitatory) synaptic junctions and increased the number of Gray type II (symmetric, presumably inhibitory) junctions (Güldner and Ingham, 1979; Güldner et al., 1997), suggesting a readjustment of the balance between excitatory and inhibitory inputs. Furthermore, the suprachiasmatic nucleus exhibits circadian changes in the long-term potentiation of synaptic transmission elicited by optic nerve stimulation (Nishikawa et al., 1995) and a diurnal rhythm of short-term synaptic plasticity of GABAergic synapses (Gompf and Allen, 2004).

Glial and synaptic plasticity in the suprachiasmatic nucleus may be involved in the synchronization of the endogenous circadian rhythm by internal and external signals to the nucleus. Among the external signals, melatonin is one of the identified hormonal regulators of synaptic plasticity in the suprachiasmatic nucleus (Fukunaga et al., 2002). Circadian fluctuation of glucocorticoids (Becquet et al., 2008; Maurel et al., 2000) as well as the activity of synaptic inputs from the optic nerve (Lavialle et al., 2001) or peripheral metabolic information (Yi et al., 2006) may also participate in the circadian glial remodeling in the suprachiasmatic nucleus. Circadian neuroplastic changes in the suprachiasmatic nucleus may also be influenced by gonadal hormones. In female rats, an ovariectomy impairs circadian changes in c-Fos expression (used as a marker of neuronal transcriptional activity) in the dorso-medial suprachiasmatic nucleus. Estradiol administration to ovariectomized rats restores the circadian activity (Peterfi et al., 2004). In contrast, castration in males results only in a moderate rise in c-Fos expression in the ventrolateral suprachiasmatic nucleus during the light period (Peterfi et al., 2004).

Circadian rhythms in neuronal activity and synaptic plasticity are also detected in other brain regions. For instance, diurnal variations in the expression of c-Fos have been detected in several nuclei of the preoptic area and the hypothalamus in rats, in addition to the suprachiasmatic nucleus (Fig 8.1). The median preoptic nucleus and the ventrolateral preoptic nucleus show maximal levels of c-Fos expression during the light period. In contrast, the arcuate nucleus, the anterodorsal preoptic nucleus, and the anteroventral periventricular nucleus show maximal c-Fos expression during the dark period. These

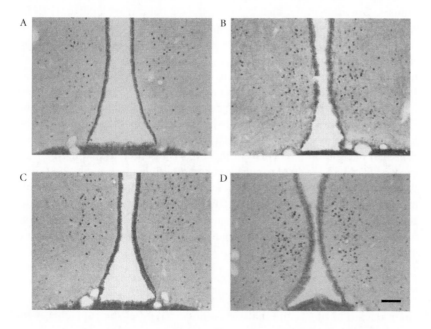

Figure 8.1. c-Fos immunoreactive cells in the anteroventral periventricular nucleus from a female rat killed during light period (A); female rat killed during dark period (B); ovariectomized rat killed during the dark period (C); ovariectomized and 17β-estradiol-treated rat killed during the dark period (D). Scale bar, 100 μm. (Courtesy of Dr. Arpad Parducz. Based on Peterfi et al., 2004).

circadian changes in c-Fos immunoreactivity show sex differences, and are influenced by estradiol in female rats (Peterfi et al., 2004; see Fig. 8.1).

Differences in GFAP immunoreactivity between morning and afternoon have been detected in a region dorsal to the suprachiasmatic nucleus and close to the third ventricle in estrogen-treated, as well as in control, ovariectomized female rats. Estrogen treatment increased the diurnal fluctuation in GFAP immunoreactivity and luteinizing hormone rhythms, suggesting that the region dorsal to the suprachiasmatic nucleus may be involved in coupling the circadian rhythms to the generation of the luteinizing hormone surge (Fernandez-Galaz et al., 1999b). A diurnal rhythm in astrocytic morphology has also been detected in the rostral preoptic area of female rats during proestrus. The cell surface area of astrocytes in close apposition to gonadotropin releasing hormone (GnRH) neurons decreases between 08:00 h and 12:00 h, before the initiation of the luteinizing hormone surge (Cashion et al., 2003). Similar diurnal changes during proestrus in the growth of astrocytic processes occur in the arcuate nucleus of the hypothalamus. The glial plastic modifications in the arcuate nucleus are induced by estradiol and are associated with changes in the number of synaptic inputs (Csakvari et al., 2007; Garcia-Segura et al., 1994a; see below).

Another brain region showing circadian changes in activity is the hippocampus. Growth factors, such as brain derived neurotrophic factor (BDNF), which regulate synaptic plasticity and adult hippocampal neurogenesis, show circadian fluctuations in different brain areas, including the hippocampus (Pollock et al., 2001). The hippocampus shows circadian fluctuations in synaptic excitability and long-term synaptic plasticity (Barnes et al., 1977; Chaudhury et al., 2005; Harris and Teyler, 1983; Raghavan et al., 1999). Circadian rhythms in synaptic plasticity in the hippocampus may represent an endogenous mechanism that may be influenced by melatonin and other hormones (such as glucocorticoids). In this regard, it is noteworthy that the circadian fluctuation of corticosterone levels is essential to maintain a basal expression of PSA-N-CAM in the hippocampus (Rodriguez et al., 1998). Since PSA-N-CAM expression in the hippocampus plays an important role in the maintenance of functional and structural synaptic plasticity and adult neurogenesis, this finding suggests that the circadian fluctuation of corticosterone may play an important role in the regulation of circadian activity and plasticity of hippocampal neurons.

HORMONES AND SEASONAL BRAIN PLASTICITY

The modulation of the internal rhythmical activity of the suprachiasmatic nucleus by seasonal changes in day length allows the physiological adaptation of the organism to seasonal modifications in the environment. Melatonin released by the pineal gland during the dark period of the light-dark cycle is the key hormone in this process. However, its effects may be mediated by seasonal modifications in the levels of other hormones, such as sex steroids.

Melatonin acts on GnRH neurons to regulate GnRH release, and subsequent luteinizing hormone and follicle stimulating hormone release by the pituitary. The resulting seasonal modification in sex steroids may affect neuronal and glial plasticity in sex-steroid-sensitive regions of the brain. Acting on the hypothalamus, melatonin may also affect the levels of other hormones that regulate brain plasticity, such as prolactin. Seasonal changes in glucocorticoid levels may also affect neuronal and glial plasticity in several brain regions, including the hippocampus. The hormonal regulation of seasonal plasticity represents a phenomenon of metaplasticity in which circadian plasticity is modified in adaptation to seasonal changes in lighting (Fig. 8.2).

Several brain regions show seasonal changes in volume that are correlated in some cases with plasma levels of hormonal steroids. Vomeronasal organs, which transmit information to the brain for courtship and mating, show seasonal changes in volume in the red-backed salamander (*Plethodon cinereus*). During the summer, the volume of vomeronasal organs is larger in both sexes than at any other time of the year. In addition, males have significantly larger vomeronasal organs than females at all times of the year (Dawley and Crowder, 1995). In reptiles, seasonal changes in the volume of the preoptic area and amygdala in males and the preoptic area in females have been detected in the brain of free-living tree lizards (*Urosaurus ornatus*) (Kabelik et al., 2006). However, these changes are not correlated with plasma levels of hormonal steroids. In contrast, seasonal variations in the volume of the preoptic area and the ventromedial hypothalamus of female red-sided garter snakes (*Thamnophis sirtalis parietalis*) appear to be facilitated by estradiol. In addition, no seasonal changes in the volume of these brain regions are detected in males (Crews et al., 1993).

Seasonal brain plasticity in birds is also well documented, in particular the plasticity of the song system of songbirds that will be analyzed later in this chapter. However, other brain regions present seasonal modifications as

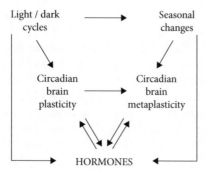

Figure 8.2. Hormonal regulation of circadian brain plasticity in adaptation to seasonal changes in lighting represents an example of metaplasticity.

well. In the Japanese quail (*Coturnix japonica*) the nucleus preopticus medialis, which is involved in the expression of male copulatory behavior, shows seasonal plastic changes. The volume of the nucleus and the size of the soma of a dorsolateral population of neurons within the nucleus are larger when the animals are housed under long day conditions that imitate the spring/summer breeding season than during short day conditions corresponding to fall/ winter. These changes may be regulated by the modifications in testosterone levels in plasma, which are higher during long day conditions and are associated with modifications in sexual behavior (Thompson and Adkins-Regan, 1994). Cognitive brain regions also show seasonal plasticity in birds. The volume of the hippocampus and the rate of hippocampal neurogenesis have been reported to increase in October in wild black-capped chickadees (Barnea and Nottebohn, 1994; Smulders et al., 1995). Since October is the month of maximal activity of food storage by these animals, the plastic modifications have been correlated to food-storing behavior. In support of this interpretation, the volume of the hippocampus does not show seasonal modifications in song sparrows, which are non-food-storing birds (Lee et al., 2001). Several hormones known to regulate adult neurogenesis may be involved in these changes, but the hormonal regulation of seasonal brain plasticity of black-capped chickadees has not been analyzed in detail.

In several mammalian species the volume of the brain shows seasonal changes. In wild-trapped voles and shrews, the weight of several brain regions decreases from summer to fall and increases from winter to spring. The hippocampus is one of the brain regions showing more pronounced seasonal changes, and this is associated with seasonal modifications in hippocampal-related behaviors, including food-storing behavior. Gonadal hormones may play some role in the seasonal modifications in the hippocampus, since males show a greater increase in hippocampal weight during spring than females in both the wild-trapped voles and shrews (Jacobs, 1996; Yaskin, 1984, 1994). The photoperiod has also been shown to affect the volume and plasticity of the hippocampus of male white-footed mice (*Peromyscus leucopus*). When housed for 10 days under short day conditions, male white-footed mice have a decreased brain mass and hippocampal volume compared to animals housed under long days. In addition, short days decrease spine density in the stratum lacunosum-moleculare and increase dendritic spine density in the stratum oriens of the hippocampus, compared to long days. These plastic morphological changes are associated with impaired long-term spatial learning and memory in animals housed under short days (Pyter et al., 2005). The photoperiod also affects the expression of PSA-N-CAM in the hypothalamus of Siberian hamsters, suggesting possible structural seasonal modifications in this brain region (Lee et al., 1995). Another brain structure affected by photoperiod in mammals is the amygdala. The volume of the posterodorsal subdivision of the medial amygdala, which is involved in male mating behavior, is larger in photostimulated male Syrian hamsters compared to photoinhibited males (Romeo and Sisk, 2001). Seasonal variation in androgen is correlated with morphologic plasticity in this nucleus in the Siberian hamster (Cooke et al., 2002a, b). In humans, seasonal plasticity has been described in the suprachiasmatic nucleus. The volume of the human suprachiasmatic nucleus and the number of vasopressin-immunoreactive neurons located in this nucleus show a significant and marked increase in autumn compared to summer (Hofman and Swaab, 1992). Seasonal differences in vasopressin innervation have been detected in other mammals, such as the European hamster (*Cricetus cricetus*). A dense vasopressin innervation is observed in many brain regions in the male hamster during the spring period. In contrast, vasopressin axonal density decreases in some brain regions during spring in females. In autumn, vasopressin fibers show a marked decline in those brain regions that show a sexually dimorphic innervation in spring (Buijs et al., 1986).

Seasonal changes in adult neurogenesis have also been detected in mammals, and may contribute to seasonal changes in behavior. For instance, it has been reported that in hamsters housed under short day conditions, there is an increase in neurogenesis in the dentate gyrus and the subependymal zone compared to animals maintained in long days (Huang et al., 1998). In addition, Galea and McEwen (1999) have shown that female meadow voles captured during the nonbreeding season have a higher rate of cell proliferation in the dentate gyrus than breeding females captured during the breeding season. However, seasonal changes in neurogenesis cannot be generalized to all seasonal mammals, since Lavenex and colleagues (2000) have not detected seasonal differences in the cell proliferation rate or in the total neuron number in the granule cell layer of the dentate gyrus of wild adult eastern grey squirrels (*Sciurus carolinensis*) captured during the fall, winter, and summer. Several hormones that are known to regulate neurogenesis may participate in the seasonal modifications. For instance, in female meadow voles, high levels of corticosterone and estradiol are associated with lower levels of cell proliferation (Galea and McEwen, 1999).

SEASONAL BRAIN PLASTICITY IN THE SONG SYSTEM OF SONGBIRDS

The annual reorganization of the complex brain network that control song in songbirds (Passeriformes: Oscine) is one of the most dramatic examples of seasonal plasticity of the central nervous system in any vertebrate species. Seasonal brain plasticity in the song system of songbirds is a patent example of hormonal regulation of metaplasticity involving both cellular replacement and synaptic plasticity (Fig. 8.3). Seasonal modifications in hormonal levels in songbirds are associated with modifications in the proliferation of endothelial, glial, and neuronal cells in different brain regions. These newly generated cells contribute to the formation of transient neuronal brain structures, which are involved in the seasonal control of song (Fig. 8.3).

Songbirds learn to produce songs and use these songs to attract mates and to defend their breeding territories during the breeding season. Fernando Nottebohm, from Rockefeller University, was the first to detect seasonal

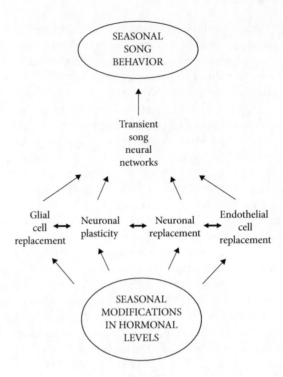

Figure 8.3. Seasonal plasticity of brain centers that control song behavior in song-birds is an example of metaplasticity involving modifications in both cellular plasticity and cellular replacement. Seasonal modifications in hormonal levels result in seasonal metaplastic changes in the hormonal regulation of brain plasticity, modifying the rate of proliferation and migration of glial cells, the rate of incorporation of new neurons to neuronal circuits controlling song, the plasticity of these neuronal circuits, and the rate of blood vessels' growth. These transient modifications in neuronal plasticity and cellular replacement result in the generation of transient neural networks that control seasonal song behavior.

changes in the volume of three telencephalic regions of the brain of adult male canaries. These regions are the hyperstriatum ventrale, pars caudale (caudal nucleus of the ventral neostriatum, also called at some point in time "High Vocal Center" and now renamed HVC as a proper name; Reiner et al. 2004), and the nucleus robustus archistriatalis (now nucleus robustus arcopallialis or RA; Reiner et al. 2004). All regions are important centers for the control of song and their volume is much larger in the spring breeding season, when canaries are producing stable songs, than in the fall, when canaries are learning and incorporating new songs to their repertoire (Nottebohm, 1981; Nottebohm et al., 1987). Canaries keep a considerable capacity for song plasticity in adult life. Male canaries sing a relatively stable repertoire during the breeding season in spring. However, at other times of the year they innovate and practice new syllables that will finally be incorporated into their songs. Thus, at the beginning Nottebohm hypothesized that the plastic seasonal alterations in the song system were related to the stable–executive and unstable–innovative phases in singing. However, later on, it was discovered that seasonal plasticity in the song system also occurs in songbirds that learn most of their entire vocal repertoire during juvenile development. Therefore, the seasonal plasticity in the volume of the song system may be necessary but is not sufficient for song learning. Alternatively, seasonal changes in the song system may be related to the motor control or execution rather than to the learning of songs. Regardless of its biological significance, the seasonal plasticity of the song system, which includes other nuclei, such as the area X (Brenowitz et al., 1998; Brown and Bottjer, 1993; Smith et al., 1997), appears to be a generalized phenomenon in seasonally breeding songbirds (Arai et al., 1989; Brenowitz et al., 1991; Smith, 1996; Smith et al., 1995; Tramontin and Brenowitz, 2000).

Neurogenesis seems to play an essential role in the generation of the adult seasonal plastic modifications in the volume of the HVC. In the avian brain there is an active production of new neurons during adult life (Alvarez-Buylla and Kirn, 1997). New neurons are born in the ventricular zone and migrate to numerous brain regions, including the HVC. Fernando Nottebohm and his collaborators provided clear evidence of seasonal fluctuations in neurogenesis, neuronal migration, and incorporation of new neurons in this nucleus. They observed a correlation between the seasonal variations in the volume of the HVC during adult life and seasonal variations in the incorporation of new neurons (Alvarez-Buylla et al., 1990; Alvarez-Buylla and Kirn, 1997; Kirn et al., 1991). Newly generated neurons incorporated in the HVC (Burd and Nottebohm, 1985) integrate into the neuronal networks controlling song, since their axons grow and reach the nucleus RA, a region involved in the production of song (Alvarez-Buylla et al., 1990; Alvarez-Buylla and Kirn, 1997; Kirn et al., 1991).

In contrast to the HVC, the incorporation of new neurons is apparently not the cause of the seasonal changes in the volume of other nuclei of the song control system, such as the nucleus RA and the area X. The volume of individual neurons, as well as the volume of the interneuronal space, increase in the nucleus RA during the breeding season. Modifications in the interneuronal space reflect plastic changes in the neuropil, including modifications in dendritic length and branching (DeVoogd and Nottebohm, 1981), dendritic spines, and the volume and number of synapses (DeVoogd et al., 1985; Hill and DeVoogd, 1991), including those synapses coming from the HVC. The seasonal growth of the nucleus RA and the area X likely requires the growing innervation from the HVC. Interestingly, each seasonal phase of growth of the song system is followed by a phase of reduction. The addition of new neurons and connections to the song system in the spring breeding season is followed by a phase of neuronal loss and loss of connections in the following months (Alvarez-Buylla and Kirn, 1997; Kirn and Nottebohm, 1993). Therefore, seasonal plasticity in the song system of songbirds represents an example of neuronal replacement (Fig. 8.3), and every year the song system may suffer an almost complete cycle of building and demolition.

Hormonal modifications associated with the day length regulate the seasonal changes in the volume of song nuclei. Blood levels of testosterone start to increase during the lengthening days of late winter and early spring when the growth of the song nuclei occurs in preparation for breeding. There is numerous evidence indicating that testosterone or its active metabolites are the main hormonal influence that facilitates the seasonal changes in the volumes of song nuclei. Physiological seasonal variation in circulating testosterone and its metabolites coincide with the seasonal plasticity of the song system (Bernard and Ball, 1997; Kirn et al., 1994; Meitzen and Thompson, 2008; Nottebohm, 1981; Nottebohm et al., 1987; Smith et al., 1995). In addition, experimental manipulation of testosterone or estradiol levels affects the growth of song nuclei. For instance, castration attenuates the seasonal growth of song nuclei (Bernard et al., 1997; Gulledge and Deviche, 1997; Smith et al., 1997). In contrast, testosterone administration induces the growth of song nuclei in castrated males and nonbreeding males independent of the season (Bernard and Ball, 1997; Johnson and Bottjer, 1993; Nottebohm, 1980; Rasika et al., 1994; Smith et al., 1997). In turn, testosterone withdrawal results in a progressive reduction in the volume of song nuclei. For instance, in adult male white-crowned sparrows the HVC suffers a rapid (12 hours) reduction in volume after testosterone withdrawal (Thompson et al., 2007). This rapid decrease in volume is associated with a decrease in interneuronal space. Over the next four days, the reduction in the volume of the nucleus is associated with a reduction in the volume and number of neurons (Thompson et al., 2007). In the nucleus RA and area X, which in the connectivity pattern are downstream to the HVC, the decrease in volume after testosterone withdrawal occurs more slowly than in the HVC; the volume changes are associated with a reduction in interneuronal space and do not involve changes in the number of neurons (Thompson et al., 2007). In addition to hormonal regulation of songbird brain plasticity by testosterone, paracrine actions of locally produced testosterone and its metabolites may also be involved in the generation of seasonal changes in plasticity (London and Schlinger, 2007) and song structure (Fusani and Gahr, 2006).

As we have seen in Chapter 4, testosterone and its metabolite estradiol modulate the integration and survival of new neurons in the HVC (Hidalgo et al., 1995; Johnson and Bottjer, 1995; Nordeen and Nordeen, 1989; Rasika et al., 1994). Testosterone also promotes glial and endothelial proliferation (Fig. 8.3), which contributes to the increase in nuclear volume (Goldman and Nottebohm, 1983) and increases the number of neuronal soma-somatic gap junctions (Gahr and Garcia-Segura, 1996). The effects of testosterone may be mediated by growth factors, such as BDNF (Rasika et al., 1999). BDNF produced by endothelial cells in response to testosterone promotes the migration and recruitment of neurons from the ventricular zone to the HVC (Louissaint et al., 2002). Testosterone-induced seasonal fluctuations in the expression of reelin, a molecule involved in the determination of the final positioning of migrating neurons, may also contribute to the seasonal changes in the incorporation of new neurons to the HVC (Absil et al., 2003). Finally, in the nucleus RA, testosterone and its metabolites estradiol and dihydrotestosterone increase the differentiation of dendrites (DeVoogd and Nottebohm, 1981), the formation of new synaptic contacts, the number of vesicles per synapse, and the size of synapses (DeVoogd et al., 1985). The effect of testosterone and its metabolites in one region of the brain network that control song may affect the plasticity of other structures within the network. Thus, actions of testosterone and its metabolites in the HVC, via the activation of androgen and estrogen receptors, facilitate plastic modifications in the nucleus RA and changes in song stereotypy (Meitzen et al., 2007).

Furthermore, other hormonal influences may participate in the seasonal plastic changes. Some evidence suggest that thyroid hormones, which affect seasonal changes in testicular activity in birds (Mishra et al., 2004) may also interfere with seasonal neurogenesis in the zebra finch telencephalon (Tekumalla et al., 2002). Another major hormonal influence is melatonin (Bentley, 2001). Melatonin receptors are expressed in the song control system (Aste et al., 2001; Whitfield-Rucker and Cassone, 1996), and exogenous melatonin administration inhibits the seasonal growth of the song system (Bentley et al., 1999). It has been postulated that the effect of melatonin may be mediated by interactions with thyroid hormones. Finally, IGF-I may regulate seasonal plasticity of the song system by promoting the recruitment of new neurons generated in the ventricular region (Jiang et al., 1998). However, this likely reflects a local action of IGF-I rather than a hormonal effect.

EXTREME SEASONAL BRAIN PLASTICITY IN MAMMALS: HIBERNATION

Some mammals hibernate to minimize energy expenditure as a strategy to survive for extended periods with low food supply and adverse cold ambient temperature. During the hibernation period, animals suffer repeated bouts of torpor, each of which can last up to two weeks, interrupted by brief spontaneous arousals of approximately one day in duration. During torpor (the nadir of metabolism), there is a decrease in body and brain temperature (Strumwasser, 1959) as well as in metabolic, heart, and respiratory rates (Buck and Barnes, 2000; Geiser and Kenagy, 1988). During arousals bouts, animals return to euthermic body temperature. The transition from torpor to interbout arousals occurs within hours. Some mammalian species are obligate hibernators. In these animals, hibernation follows an endogenous circannual rhythm and occurs independent of the duration of the photoperiod or food availability. Marmots, ground squirrels, and chipmunks are examples of obligate hibernators. Other species, like Syrian hamsters (*Mesocricetus auratus*), are facultative hibernators. In these animals, hibernation is induced by short photoperiods, and the frequency of torpor is increased by low ambient temperatures and by decreased food availability (Geiser, 2004). Finally, some species such as brown bears, black bears and badgers, are not deep hibernators and their body temperature does not drop below 25°C. In contrast, body temperature in deep hibernating mammals, such as squirrels, may drop to near 0°C.

The physiological changes occurring during hibernation are regulated, at least in part, by the central nervous system. Several neurotransmitters and brain regions, including the preoptic area, the hypothalamus, the hippocampus, the medial septum-diagonal band complex, and nuclei of the autonomic nervous system, are involved in the neural control of hibernation (Drew et al., 2007). In addition, the process of hibernation is regulated by endocrine signals. Several hormones participate in the preparation of the hibernation process, in the induction of hibernation, and in the reactivation of physiological function after hibernation. Melatonin is one of the major endocrine players in the regulation of hibernation, and may participate in the recovery from torpor. The daily rhythm of pineal melatonin production and secretion is abolished during torpor in several hibernating species (Darrow et al., 1986; Florant et al., 1984; Vanecek et al., 1984). In contrast, the daily rhythm of pineal melatonin is restored and melatonin levels in plasma increase during arousal from daily torpor (Florant et al., 1984; Larkin et al., 2003). Melatonin may contribute to activate thermogenesis by direct actions on the brain (Saarela and Reiter, 1994), and may contribute to defining the timing of reactivation of reproduction after hibernation, at least in hedgehogs (Fowler, 1988; Fowler and Racey, 1990). However, it has been reported that continuous intracerebroventricular infusion of melatonin in hibernating ground squirrels prolongs hibernation (Stanton et al., 1987), suggesting that the hormone may contribute to determining the duration of torpor.

The suprachiasmatic nucleus (which, as has been mentioned before, is involved in the control of circadian rhythms and receives direct inputs from the retina), is affected by melatonin and likely plays an important role in the integration of hormonal and metabolic signals and in the control of the autonomic nervous system to regulate hibernation. For instance, arginine-vasopressin secreted by neurons in the suprachiasmatic nucleus may play an important role in the resetting of circadian rhythms after hibernation in European ground squirrels (Hut et al., 2002). The suprachiasmatic nucleus may also affect the activity of the autonomic nervous system and the activity of other brain centers regulating metabolism through neuronal synaptic networks. In turn, the suprachiasmatic nucleus receives synaptic inputs from other brain regions involved in the control of hibernation. In addition, hormonal regulatory signals may be transmitted to the suprachiasmatic nucleus via direct or indirect synaptic inputs. For instance, glucocorticoids, which are important regulators of energy balance and seasonal changes in adrenocortical function (Boonstra et al., 2001; Boswell et al., 1994; Place and Kenagy, 2000; Shivatcheva et al., 1988), may influence the activity of the suprachiasmatic nucleus via the hippocampus. In addition, peptide hormones may act on the suprachiasmatic nucleus via the circumventricular organs.

Other hormones, in addition to melatonin, are involved in the recovery from hibernation. For instance, prolactin is important in defining the timing of reactivation of reproduction after hibernation (Fowler, 1988). Thyrotropin-releasing hormone plays an important role in the recovery from hibernation, accelerating metabolism and contributing to the elevation of body temperature to return to euthermia after torpor (Shintani et al., 2005; Stanton et al., 1992; Tamura et al., 2005). These effects of thyrotropin-releasing hormone are achieved by the direct activation of the sympathetic nervous system, by direct actions on brain regions regulating body brain temperature and energy balance, and through the release of thyroid-stimulating hormone from the pituitary. Changing plasma levels of thyroid hormones participate in the regulation of body energy metabolism during hibernation (Fowler, 1988; Magnus and Henderson, 1988; Nevretdinova et al., 1992; Nicol et al., 2000; Tomasi et al., 1998) while parathyroid hormone may contribute to prevent bone loss in hibernating black bears (Donahue et al., 2006).

Hormones released by the endocrine pancreas likely contribute to the regulation of energy balance during hibernation as well. For instance, glucagon and insulin are elevated during hibernation in the little brown bat (*Myotis lucifugus*) (Bauman, 1990). Leptin and ghrelin, key hormones for the regulation of food intake and metabolism, are also expected to play an important role in the regulation of metabolism in hibernating animals. Indeed, serum leptin levels are reduced in Siberian hamsters undergoing daily torpor, and exogenous administration of leptin for 14 days eliminates torpor (Freeman et al., 2004), suggesting that leptin may contribute to metabolic recovery from hibernation. In contrast, ghrelin, which has opposite effects to leptin in energy balance, induces torpor in fasting mice, an effect that seems to be mediated by neuropeptide Y neurons in the hypothalamic arcuate nucleus (Gluck et al., 2006).

Hormones produced by the liver are also involved in the regulation of hibernation and torpor. The endocrine hormone fibroblast growth factor 21 (FGF21), which is induced in the liver by peroxisome proliferator-activated receptor α in response to fasting, stimulates the use of stored fats as energy and causes torpor in mice (Inagaki et al., 2007). Serum levels of IGF-I, which are mainly the result of liver production of IGF-I, are strongly reduced during hibernation in the golden-mantled ground squirrel (*Spermophilus lateralis*) (Schmidt and Kelley, 2001). IGF-I actions during hibernation may affect a variety of tissues, including the brain. Interestingly, IGF-I receptor signaling appears to be down-regulated in the brain during hibernation (Cai et al., 2004). Furthermore, there is evidence for the existence of a new liver hormone that, acting on the brain, regulates hibernation. Noriaki Kondo and Jun Kondo reported in 1992 the discovery in chipmunks of four proteins that disappeared in the blood during hibernation and reappeared as hibernation ceased (Kondo and Kondo, 1992). These proteins are produced in the liver and secreted to the blood and form a 140-kDa complex, which was named hibernation-specific protein complex (HPc). Three proteins forming the HPc (HP20, HP25, and HP27) form a complex called HP20c. The fourth protein, HP55, is associated with HP20c in the blood, forming the HPc (Takamatsu et al., 1993, 1997). The levels of HP20, HP25, and HP27 increase in the cerebrospinal fluid before the onset of hibernation, reach highest levels at the middle stage of hibernation, then abruptly decrease with the termination of hibernation (Kondo et al., 2006). The proposed hypothesis is that an endogenous circannual rhythm generator will regulate the synthesis of HPc in the liver and its transport to the cerebrospinal fluid, and that the dissociation of the HPc from HP55 in the brain will allow HP20c to exert its actions as a regulator of hibernation (Kondo et al., 2006).

Therefore, a variety of hormonal signals regulate the physiological modifications during the different phases of the hibernation process, and some may regulate the activity of brain regions controlling hibernation. In turn, the physiological metabolic, cardiovascular, and respiratory changes associated with hibernation, as well as the body and brain temperature modifications, have an impact on brain function. The prominent physiological alterations associated with torpor are accompanied by a profound decrease in neural activity (Daan et al., 1991; Krilowicz et al., 1988; Strumwasser, 1959; Walker et al., 1977) and are associated with significant plastic morphological alterations in neuronal structure. For instance, hippocampal pyramidal neurons in Siberian ground squirrels (*Citellus undulatus*) have shorter apical dendrites with fewer branches and fewer dendritic spines during torpor than during phases of spontaneous activity between hibernation bouts (Popov et al., 1992). The plastic modifications are fast: within two hours after arousal from torpor, dendrites recover their morphology. In addition, the plastic remodeling of apical pyramidal hippocampal dendrites occurs during each torpor-activity cycle; that is, several times in each hibernating period. Similar rapid, reversible, and repetitive changes also occur in mossy fiber synapses on CA3 hippocampal neurons in Siberian ground squirrels. During hibernation, there is a reduction in the size and number of dendritic spine infoldings in the mossy fiber synapses. In addition, the number of postsynaptic densities is also decreased. After arousal these parameters are quickly reversed within two hours (Popov and Bocharova, 1992). A gradual regression of mossy fiber synapses and corresponding postsynaptic elements during torpor, associated with the accumulation of the phosphorylated form of the microtubule associated protein tau at postsynaptic sites, has been detected in European ground squirrels (*Spermophilus citellus*) (Arendt et al., 2003). Decreased dendritic complexity and decreased number of dendritic spines under hibernation has been also detected in CA3 pyramidal neurons in golden-mantled ground squirrels (von der Ohe et al., 2006) and in European hamsters (*Cricetus cricetus*) (Magariños et al., 2006). In European hamsters, changes in CA3 dendrites during torpor are associated with a significant reduction in synaptic vesicle density in mossy fiber terminals and in the area of mossy fiber terminals covered by spine profiles. Within two hours after arousal from torpor, dendritic lengths, dendritic branching, number of dendritic spines, synaptic vesicles in mossy fiber terminals, and density of mossy fiber terminal covered by spines return to basal active conditions. Therefore, all these studies indicate that hibernation causes rapid and reversible plastic changes in synaptic connectivity in the hippocampus.

Synaptic plasticity during hibernation is not restricted to the hippocampus. Plastic modifications in dendrites and dendritic spines during hibernation have also been observed in spiny stellate cells from layer 4 of the somatosensory cortex and in ventral posterior thalamic somatosensory relay neurons of golden-mantled ground squirrels (von der Ohe et al., 2006). In addition, reversible plastic alterations in the ultrastructure of asymmetric axospinous synapses have been described during hibernation in layer 2 of the frontal cortex in European ground squirrels (Ruediger et al., 2007). The length of postsynaptic densities and the synaptic apposition length increase during torpor, while the width and surface area of postsynaptic densities decrease. At the beginning of arousal, the width of the postsynaptic densities increases to reach spring values at late arousals. The morphological synaptic plastic modifications during a torpor bout are of a similar magnitude in all brain regions examined and across distinct regions within cells, and are reversible when returning to euthermia (von der Ohe et al., 2006). The synaptic changes during torpor are associated with a dissociation of synaptic proteins from the cytoskeletal active zone and from the postsynaptic density, and it has been proposed that the rapid recovery of synapses at the beginning of arousal may be the consequence of a rapid reassociation of synaptic proteins to the active zone and the postsynaptic density (von der Ohe et al., 2007).

Plastic reorganization of brain tissue during hibernation may in part be the consequence of the associated hormonally induced physiological modifications, such as the decrease in body temperature during torpor (von der Ohe et al., 2006, 2007). However, the brain plastic reorganization during hibernation may also be involved in the generation of the physiological changes associated with torpor and arousal. For instance, as mentioned before, the production of arginine-vasopressin by neurons in the suprachiasmatic nucleus appears to be involved in the reappearance of post-hibernation circadian rhythmicity (Hut et al., 2002). Therefore, hibernation is an excellent illustration of the cross-interaction of hormones and brain plasticity in adult life. Brain plastic modifications, induced in part by hormonal transmission of changes occurring in the external environment, contribute to modify hormonal secretions to adapt the organism (by regulating the metabolic and energetic physiological conditions) to the initiation of hibernation, to torpor, and to the return to normal homeodynamics after hibernation. In turn, hormonal secretions, directly or indirectly, induce plastic modifications in the brain, adapting neural function to the metabolic conditions associated with hibernation.

BRAIN PLASTICITY AND THE CONTROL OF HORMONAL
HOMEODYNAMICS IN SEASONAL BREEDERS

Seasonal plasticity in the neuronal systems that regulate gonadotropin secretion has been detected in several species of birds and mammals. In birds living in the tropics, seasonal breeding and seasonal plastic modifications in the GnRH system can occur in the absence of significant changes in the photoperiod (Moore et al., 2006). In contrast, the photoperiod regulates seasonal reproductive cycles and affects the plasticity of GnRH neurons in many species of birds living in high latitudes. For instance, the photoperiod affects GnRH immunoreactivity, the number of GnRH immunoreactive cells, and GnRH fiber density in the cardueline finch (Pereyra et al., 2005). Photoperiod also affects the interactions of GnRH terminals and glial cell processes in the median eminence of Japanese quails (Yamamura et al., 2004). In animals maintained under short day conditions, glial processes are interposed between GnRH terminals and the basal lamina of portal capillaries in the median eminence. In contrast, GnRH nerve terminals are in close proximity to the basal lamina in animals kept under long day conditions. The seasonal structural remodeling of glial cells and GnRH terminals may be under the control of thyroid hormones, since thyroid hormone receptors are highly expressed in the median eminence of Japanese quails, and triiodothyronin implantation in the mediobasal hypothalamus decreases the interposition of glial processes between GnRH terminals and the basal lamina of portal capillaries (Yamamura et al., 2006).

In mammalian seasonal breeders, seasonal changes in the responsiveness of GnRH neurons to the inhibitory effects of gonadal hormones are accompanied by seasonal changes in the number of synaptic inputs to GnRH neurons (see also Chapter 2). In ewes, preoptic GnRH neurons receive more than twice the mean number of total synaptic inputs per unit of plasma membrane in breeding season than in anestrus animals (Lehman et al., 1997; Xiong et al., 1997). The plastic changes in the number of total synaptic inputs affect both the dendrites and the perikaryon of GnRH neurons. The increase in the number of synaptic inputs on GnRH neurons during the breeding season seems to be due mainly to neuropeptide Y (NPY) terminals (Jansen et al., 2003). This is consistent with the fact that NPY is known to increase luteinizing hormone release in ewes. The increase in NPY synaptic inputs seems to be dependent on an increased production of NPY, since it is associated with an increase in the number of NPY immunoreactive neuronal perikarya (Skinner and Herbison, 1997). GABAergic inputs also increase during the breeding season in a subpopulation of GnRH neurons (Jansen et al., 2003), although the proportion of GnRH neurons contacted by GABAergic inputs decreases (Pompolo et al., 2003). The seasonal synaptic plasticity on GnRH neurons is associated with seasonal plastic remodeling of astroglial processes and in their apposition to neuronal perikarya (Jansen et al., 2003), and are associated with seasonal modifications in the expression of PSA-N-CAM (Viguie et al., 2001), which, as has been mentioned before, is a permissive molecule for structural synaptic plasticity. In addition to the seasonal remodeling of synaptic inputs on GnRH neurons, seasonal synaptic plasticity also occurs on other neuronal populations that control GnRH release, such as the A15 dopaminergic cell group in the retrochiasmatic area, which mediate estrogen negative feedback to GnRH neurons during anestrus. Both the number of synaptic inputs and the length of dendrites increase in these neurons during anestrus (Adams et al., 2006).

Seasonal synaptic plasticity on GnRH neurons does not seem to be dependent on gonadal hormones, since it is observed both in intact ewes and in ovariectomized animals bearing estradiol implants. Other hormonal signals may participate in the regulation of plasticity of neuronal inputs on GnRH neurons and on the associated neuronal networks. It has been proposed that seasonal variation in the duration of melatonin secretion may regulate seasonal plasticity in GnRH neurons in seasonal breeders by a direct action of melatonin on synapses involved in the regulation of GnRH secretion. Melatonin may act on neurons in the arcuate and ventromedial hypothalamic nucleus that, in turn, regulate GnRH neuronal activity, may act on GnRH release at the level of the pars tuberalis, and likely may directly interact with the synaptic inputs on GnRH neurons as well (Kennaway and Rowe, 1995). Thyroid hormones, which are required for the transition from the breeding to anestrus season, may also play a relevant role, since GnRH neurons express thyroid hormone receptors (Lehman et al., 1997). However, a thyroidectomy late in the breeding season does not affect the synaptic input or glial escheatment of GnRH neurons in anestrus. In contrast, a thyroidectomy blocks the above-mentioned increase in dendritic length in the A15 dopaminergic cell group during the anestrus period (Adams et al., 2006), suggesting that thyroid hormones may impact on the circuits controlling the activity of GnRH neurons at different levels.

BRAIN PLASTICITY AND REPRODUCTIVE CYCLES IN NONSEASONAL BREEDERS

Brain Structures Controlling GnRH Neurons

As we have seen in Chapter 4, ovarian hormones induce a variety of plastic modifications in the rodent brain. Some of these brain plastic modifications show a cyclic pattern during the reproductive cycles in rodents in association with the cyclic fluctuation in the circulating levels of ovarian hormones. In adult female rodents, the hypothalamic arcuate nucleus exhibits a natural phasic synaptic remodeling that is linked to hormonal variations during the ovarian cycle (Naftolin et al., 2007; Olmos et al., 1989). The number of axosomatic synapses on arcuate neurons falls between the morning and the afternoon of proestrus, remains low until the morning of estrus, then rises to baseline conditions by the metestrus morning. The fluctuation in the number of axosomatic synaptic profiles cannot be ascribed to changes in the size of the synaptic terminals or to modifications in the perimeter of arcuate neuronal perikarya, but reflects a modification in the number of terminals contacting arcuate perikarya (Fig. 8.4). On the other hand, since the changes in synapses are not accompanied by the appearance of images of degeneration, the reduction in the number of synaptic contacts on the day of proestrus could involve a retraction of the synaptic terminal or a displacement of synapses from the soma to the neurites rather than a degenerative loss. The surge of luteinizing hormone on the afternoon of proestrus is thus coincident with the decrease in

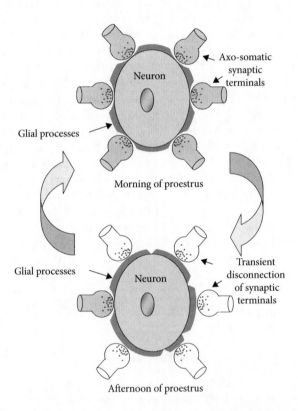

Figure 8.4. Neuroglial remodeling in the arcuate nucleus during the estrus cycle. The number of GABAergic axosomatic synaptic contacts on arcuate neurons of adult female rats falls between the morning and the afternoon of proestrus in each estrus cycle. The cyclic changes in the number of axosomatic synaptic contacts are accompanied by cyclic modifications in the glial wrapping of the neuronal somas. Glial processes are interposed between the presynaptic inputs and the postsynaptic membrane, and the retraction of glial processes in diestrus is accompanied by the reinnervation of arcuate neuronal somas.

the number of axosomatic synapses on arcuate neurons. Since arcuate neurons appear to be involved in the control of GnRH secretion, and hence gonadotropin secretion, it is conceivable that the observed synaptic modifications have an important relationship with the estrogen-induced gonadotropin surge. Indeed, gonadal steroids appear to play a fundamental role in the induction of synaptic remodeling in the arcuate nucleus. Studies in ovariectomized rats showed that the administration of a single dose of 17β-estradiol, resulting in plasma levels of the hormone similar to those detected during proestrus, induced a reversible decline in the number of arcuate axosomatic synapses (Perez et al., 1993a). These results suggest that the synaptic changes detected in arcuate neurons during the estrus cycle are driven by the rise in plasma 17β-estradiol levels that occur during proestrus. Furthermore, the simultaneous administration of progesterone and 17β-estradiol to ovariectomized rats, a treatment known to inhibit the ability of estrogen to evoke luteinizing hormone surges (Banks and Freeman, 1980; Barraclough et al., 1986), inhibits the effect of 17β-estradiol on arcuate synapses (Perez et al., 1993a). This finding further supports the concept that estrogen-induced synaptic changes in the arcuate nucleus are involved in the hypothalamic control of luteinizing hormone release. The synaptic remodeling during the estrus cycle occurs in parallel with changes in luteinizing hormone release, and may reflect a reorganization of part of the synaptic circuits that control GnRH neurons. Therefore, the preovulatory surge of gonadotropins may, at least in part, be induced by the remodeling of synaptic connections in the arcuate nucleus (Horvath et al., 1997a). In addition, at least part of the arcuate neurons involved in the synaptic remodeling project their axons to the median eminence, and are probably neurosecretory neurons that may be involved in the control of prolactin (Csakvari et al., 2008; Parducz et al., 2003). Since the arcuate nucleus is a key neuroendocrine control center that is not only involved in the regulation of reproduction but also in growth, energy balance, and food intake, the changes in arcuate neuronal activity during the estrus cycle may have a broad physiological impact.

Synaptic plasticity associated with the estrus cycle has also been detected in another brain region involved in the control of GnRH neurons, the anteroventral periventricular nucleus. Studies by M. Chris Langub, Bruce E. Maley, and Robert E. Watson have shown that, in contrast to arcuate nucleus, axosomatic synapses increase in the anteroventral periventricular nucleus of cycling female rats between proestrus and estrus, and then decreases in metestrus. Furthermore, an ovariectomy increases the number of axosomatic synapses in the anteroventral periventricular nucleus relative to proestrus and metestrus (Langub et al., 1994). Thus, axosomatic synapses change in opposite directions during the estrus cycle in two different brain regions in the same species, the arcuate nucleus and the anteroventral periventricular nucleus,.

To gain further insight into the physiological significance of the synaptic remodeling associated with the rat ovarian cycle, in collaboration with Arpad Parducz from the Institute of Biophysics of the Hungarian Academy of

Sciences in Szeged we analyzed the influence of gonadal hormone administration on immunocytochemically identified GABAergic synaptic terminals. By that time we already knew from the data of other laboratories that GABAergic axons are abundant in the rat arcuate nucleus and that these axons form axosomatic synapses on estrogen-sensitive cells. In addition, it was already described that a large population of GABAergic neurons in the arcuate nucleus express estrogen and/or progesterone receptors, and that GABA is involved in the control of luteinizing hormone and prolactin release. Furthermore, electrophysiological studies had shown that most arcuate neurons were hyperpolarized by GABA. In addition, both GABA levels and GABA receptors were known to be modulated by gonadal steroids in several brain areas, including the arcuate nucleus. Thus, it was reasonable to suppose that the changes in axosomatic synapses during the estrus cycle may affect GABAergic synaptic terminals. The immunocytochemical characterization of synaptic inputs on arcuate neurons using colloidal gold immunolabeling revealed that the majority of the axosomatic synaptic terminals on arcuate neurons of female rats are GABA-immunoreactive. We first analyzed the effect of the administration of estradiol on the number of axosomatic synapses in ovariectomized rats, and found that the administration of the hormone produced a significant decrease in the number of GABA-immunoreactive axosomatic synapses. In contrast, estradiol administration had no significant effect on the number of nonimmunoreactive axosomatic synapses on these neurons. Likewise, the percentage of perikaryal membrane covered by immunoreactive synapses was significantly reduced by estradiol, while the percentage of perikaryal membrane covered by nonimmunoreactive synapses remained unchanged (Parducz et al., 1993). These results suggest that at least the majority of the axosomatic synapses affected by estradiol during the rat estrus cycle are GABAergic. A transient change in inhibitory GABAergic inputs during the estrus cycle was consistent with the observation that estradiol induces an increase in arcuate neuronal firing that is temporally correlated with the release of luteinizing hormone during the ovarian cycle (Kis et al., 1999; Yeoman and Jenkins, 1989).

Further morphometric analysis of synapses in the arcuate nucleus revealed that the decrease in the number of GABAergic inhibitory synapses induced by estradiol is accompanied by a parallel increase in the number of excitatory synapses in dendritic spines, further indicating that the final effect of estradiol is to decrease inhibition and increase excitation of arcuate neurons. This was corroborated by the use of electrophysiological recordings, which revealed an increased frequency of neuronal firing in a subpopulation of arcuate neurons in response to estradiol (Parducz et al., 2002). GABAergic axosomatic synapses and synapses on dendritic spines also show variations during the estrus cycle. The number of GABAergic axosomatic synapses decreases significantly from proestrus morning to proestrus afternoon, and remains lower on the day of estrus. Then, the number of GABAergic axosomatic synapses increases in metestrus and remained at the same levels in diestrus and in the morning of proestrus. In contrast, the numerical density of non GABAergic axosomatic synapses does not show significant changes during the estrus cycle. This is also the case for both the GABAergic and nonGABAergic synapses on dendritic shafts. In contrast, synapses on dendritic spines show a highly significant increase in number on proestrus afternoon, remain high on estrus day and return to the base level during the next two days (Csakvari et al., 2006).

The decrease in the number of inhibitory GABAergic synapses and the increase in the number of spine synapses during the estrus phase of the estrus cycle in the rat arcuate nucleus are temporally correlated with morphological modifications that indicate a general cellular activation of arcuate neurons. For example, the nuclear volume and number of nuclear pores increase in arcuate neurons after estradiol administration to ovariectomized rats and during the estrus phase of the estrus cycle (Garcia-Segura et al., 1987a; Perez et al., 1991). Furthermore, the expression of histone H1°, a protein involved in the induction and stability of the higher-order structure of chromatin, is negatively and reversibly regulated in arcuate neurons during the estrus cycle by the rise of estradiol in plasma (Garcia-Segura et al., 1993). This suggests that gene transcription and nucleocytoplasmic transport are enhanced in arcuate neurons during the phases of increased neuronal firing and synaptic remodeling. This increased cellular activity may be a consequence of the increased neuronal firing due to the decrease in inhibitory synaptic inputs on perikarya and the increase in excitatory inputs on dendritic spines, although it may also partially reflect transcriptional changes involved in the mechanisms of synaptic plasticity.

The synaptic reorganization in the arcuate nucleus during the estrus cycle is accompanied by a plastic remodeling of astroglia and astroglial processes (Garcia-Segura et al., 1994a, b, 2008; Kohama et al., 1995). GFAP mRNA, the surface density of GFAP-immunoreactive cell perikarya and processes, the number of astroglial profiles in the arcuate neuropil, and the amount of neuronal perikaryal membrane covered by glial processes are increased on the afternoon of proestrus and on the morning of estrus compared to other phases of the estrus cycle or to ovariectomized rats (Fig. 8.5). The increase in the amount of neuronal perikaryal membrane covered by glial processes during proestrus and estrus is associated with a transient displacement of axosomatic terminals. In contrast, glial retraction in diestrus is accompanied by the reinnervation of arcuate neuronal perikarya (Garcia-Segura et al., 1994a, b; Fig. 8.4). Glial remodeling during the estrus cycle is also detected in the rostral preoptic area in rats. There, the surface area of astrocytes and the number of processes per astrocyte decreased from the morning of proestrus, before the initiation of the GnRH induced luteinizing hormone surge, to the afternoon of proestrus. The following day, on estrus, both the surface area of astrocytes and the number of processes per astrocyte return to levels similar to those seen on proestrus morning (Cashion et al., 2003).

The plastic changes in astrocytes during the estrus cycle show interesting differences in the arcuate nucleus and the rostral preoptic area. Astrocytic processes increase in the arcuate nucleus and decrease in the rostral preoptic

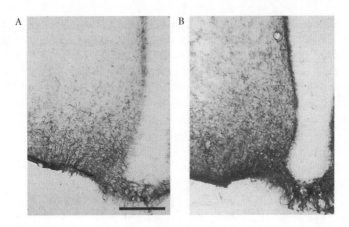

Figure 8.5. Immunoreactivity for the astroglial marker glial fibrillary acidic protein (GFAP) in the arcuate nucleus of female rats. (A) From a rat in the morning of proestrus. (B) From a rat in the morning of estrus. Changes in GFAP immunoreactivity in the rat arcuate nucleus during the estrus cycle are accompanied by modifications in the growth of astrocytic processes, the coverage of arcuate neuronal somas by glial processes, and the interposition of glial processes between presynaptic axosomatic inhibitory synaptic terminals and the arcuate neuronal somas. Scale bar, 0.7 mm. (Microphotographs from the author. Based on Garcia-Segura et al., 1994b).

area in the afternoon of proestrus, in association with the increase in luteinizing hormone release. In the rostral preoptic area, astrocytic processes contact GnRH neurons and, interestingly, the number of synapses on the soma of GnRH neurons (at least in monkeys) increases in association with the peak in luteinizing hormone release (Witkin et al., 1991), while the number of axosomatic synapses decreases in the arcuate nucleus at this moment. Therefore, glial and synaptic plasticity show similar characteristics in the arcuate nucleus and the rostral preoptic area. However, the timing of the plastic changes is different. A similar situation occurs in the median eminence. Changes in the extension of tanycytic processes in the median eminence during the estrus cycle regulate the contacts of GnRH neurosecretory terminals with portal vasculature (see also Chapter 2). In the afternoon of proestrus, tanycytic processes retract, allowing the contact of GnRH neuronal terminals with portal capillaries and the subsequent release of GnRH (King and Letourneau, 1994; Prevot et al., 1999). Thus, in the median eminence (like in the rostral preoptic area) glial processes retract at the same moment in the estrus cycle when glial processes grow in the arcuate nucleus. Furthermore, as mentioned earlier in this chapter, the number of axosomatic synapses increases in the anteroventral periventricular nucleus in proestrus, when axosomatic synapses decrease in the arcuate nucleus. All this suggests that gonadal hormones are facilitating glial and synaptic plasticity in different brain regions during the estrus cycle, but are not promoting a specific direction to the plastic changes. According to this interpretation, gonadal hormones will not induce the growth or the retraction of glial processes, or the connection or the disconnection of synapses. Gonadal hormones will act as permissive factors, allowing coordinated plastic and metaplastic events that may adopt different characteristics in different brain regions (see also Chapter 4).

One of the questions that are still under debate is whether the glial changes that are linked to estradiol-induced synaptic plasticity are the result of direct hormonal effects on glial cells or are neuronally mediated. Astrocytes are influenced by the neuronal environment, either by direct contact via adhesion molecules, such as PSA-N-CAM, or by soluble factors, such as glutamate, released by neurons (see also Chapter 4). Thus, the effect of estradiol on arcuate astroglia may depend, at least in part, on neurons bearing hormone receptors, which are abundant in the arcuate nucleus. Alternatively, it cannot be excluded that the hormone may act directly on arcuate glial cells. Indeed, several laboratories have reported the expression of estrogen receptors in astrocytes (for review, see Garcia-Ovejero et al., 2005). Thus, Langub and Watson (1992) reported the existence of glia immunoreactive for estrogen receptors in the guinea pig hypothalamus, using electron microscope immunocytochemistry, and Gudino-Cabrera and Nieto-Sampedro (1999) detected immunoreactivity for estrogen receptor α in rat tanycytes. On the other hand, there is evidence that soluble factors, such as growth factors and neurotransmitters, may mediate neuron–glia communication in the arcuate nucleus. Thus, Jessica Mong and her collaborators have shown that neurotransmitters (such as GABA) released by arcuate neurons may affect astrocyte morphology (Mong et al., 2002). In addition, estradiol increases the glial expression of glutamine synthetase, which facilitates the conversion of glutamate to glutamine. Glutamine may then be used by neurons for glutamate synthesis, which in turn may affect neuronal and glial function (Blutstein et al., 2006; Mong and Blutstein, 2006). In addition, the laboratory of Sergio Ojeda at the Oregon Regional Primate Research Center has provided detailed information on other soluble factors released by hypothalamic glia that may affect neurons and other glial cells to regulate GnRH release, and may potentially affect glial and neuronal remodeling in the arcuate nucleus and the median eminence (see also Chapters 2 and 7). These include growth factors, such as transforming growth factor α, and the neuregulins, which are produced in hypothalamic astrocytes and act in a paracrine or autocrine way on the same cell types to elicit the production of other soluble factors, such as prostaglandin E2, which stimulates GnRH secretion upon binding to specific receptors on GnRH neurons (Ojeda et al., 2000; Prevot, 2002; Prevot et al., 2007). The activity of Zn^{2+} metalloproteinases (which varies in the median eminence during the estrus cycle, showing high levels of activity in proestrus) may also be involved in the neuroglial remodeling in the median eminence (Estrella et al., 2004; Prevot et al., 2003). Molecules released by endothelial cells in the median eminence, such as Sema3A, a chemotrophic factor (Campagne et al.,

2006), or nitric oxide (De Serrano et al., 2004, 2005; Prevot et al., 2007) may also regulate the retraction and extension of tanycytes during the estrus cycle (see Chapter 2).

IGF-I is another soluble factor that appears to be highly relevant in the communication of glia and neurons for the regulation of synaptic plasticity in the arcuate nucleus (see also Chapter 5). IGF-I receptors mediate (i) estrogen activation of astroglia in hypothalamic arcuate nucleus tissue fragments; (ii) estrogen-induced synaptic plasticity in the arcuate nucleus in vivo; and (iii) synaptic remodeling during the estrus cycle in the arcuate nucleus (Fernandez-Galaz et al., 1996, 1997; Garcia-Segura et al., 1999a). Furthermore, IGF-I levels in the neuroendocrine hypothalamus are regulated by estradiol and progesterone, and IGF-I levels in tanycytes in the arcuate nucleus and the median eminence fluctuate in accordance with the natural variations in plasma levels of ovarian steroids that are associated with the estrus cycle (Fernandez-Galaz et al., 1996, 1997; Garcia-Segura et al., 1999a). Therefore, the final glial–neuronal remodeling in the arcuate nucleus during the estrus cycle may be regulated by a finely orchestrated bidirectional cross talk between neurons and astroglia, mediated by growth factors, prostaglandin E2, and neurotransmitters. In addition, neuroglia interactions may be regulated by direct cell-to-cell communication, mediated by cell adhesion molecules.

The Ventromedial Hypothalamic Nucleus

Synaptic plasticity during the estrus cycle is not limited to brain regions controlling GnRH secretion. Plastic modifications have also been detected in the ventromedial hypothalamic nucleus, which is involved in the control of lordosis behavior; and in the hippocampus, which is involved in cognitive function. The laboratory of Bruce S. McEwen was the first to report that the number of dendritic spines on primary dendrites of ventromedial hypothalamic neurons fluctuated during the estrus cycle in rats. The density of dendritic spines is significantly lower at diestrus than in proestrus (Frankfurt et al., 1990). The fluctuation of dendritic spines across the estrus cycle was confirmed by M. Dulce Madeira, Luís Ferreira-Silva, and Manuel Paula-Barbosa from the University of Porto in Portugal, which in 2001 reported the results of a detailed stereological analysis of the ventromedial hypothalamic nucleus of adult male rats and of intact age-matched females killed on proestrus and diestrus day one (Madeira et al., 2001). They found that males and females have a similar number of neurons in the ventromedial hypothalamic nucleus (55,000), but the total volume of the nucleus and the volume of the neuropil are larger in males than in females. Furthermore, the volume of the nucleus increases in proestrus due to an increase in the volume of neuronal perikarya. They also found that the density of dendritic spines in ventromedial hypothalamic neurons is higher in females than in males. Furthermore, in the neurons located in the ventrolateral part of the nucleus, the density of dendritic spines fluctuate across the estrus cycle, being higher in proestrus than in diestrus, as previously reported by Maya Frankfurt and her colleagues in the laboratory of Bruce

S. McEwen. Morphometric analyses by electron microscopy have shown that the increase in dendritic spines in proestrus is accompanied by an increase in the number of presynaptic terminals. Thus, Susana Sá and M. Dulce Madeira have shown that the neurons located in the ventral subdivision of the ventro-medial hypothalamic nucleus receive around 7,000 synapses during diestrus, and approximately 10,000 synapses during proestrus (Sá and Madeira, 2005).

The Hippocampus

The hippocampus is another brain region in which there are plastic changes associated with the estrus cycle, including modifications in (i) the number of dendritic spines and presynaptic terminals in CA1 pyramidal neurons; (ii) functional synaptic plasticity; (iii) the morphology of astroglia; and (iv) the rate of neurogenesis. In contrast to the plastic modifications in the hypothalamus, which may be associated with the control of GnRH release or sexual behavior, the functional significance of the hippocampal plasticity is still unclear. However, the hippocampus is an important brain region for the integration of different hormonal signals, including stress hormones and sex steroids; in addition to its cognitive functions it contributes to the regulation of hypothalamic hormonal secretions. Therefore, hippocampal plasticity during the estrus cycle may reflect a homeodynamic response to adapt mood and cognition to the changing endocrine environment.

As I have mentioned in Chapter 4, the first description of synaptic plasticity associated with the estrus cycle in the hippocampus was provided by Catherine Woolley and her colleagues in the laboratory of Bruce S. McEwen. Using the Golgi method, Woolley and her collaborators discovered that the number of dendritic spines in the CA1 region of the rat hippocampus fluctuates during the estrus cycle, showing a peak in proestrus (Woolley et al., 1990a). The modification in the number of dendritic spines is associated with plastic changes in the number of presynaptic inputs (Woolley and McEwen, 1992; Woolley et al., 1996) and in the expression of synaptic proteins (Crispino et al., 1999). Functional synaptic plasticity is also modified during the estrus cycle. Long-term synaptic potentiation is increased during proestrus (Good et al., 1999; Warren et al., 1995), while the induction of paired-pulse long-term depression is severely attenuated during proestrus (Good et al., 1999).

Glial cells show also structural remodeling in the rat hippocampus during the estrus cycle. The surface density of GFAP immunoreactive astrocytes increases in the afternoon of proestrus and the morning of estrus compared to the morning of proestrus, diestrus, and metestrus, and these changes are regulated by estradiol and progesterone (Luquin et al., 1993). In contrast to the clear association between glial modifications and synaptic changes in the arcuate nucleus during the estrus cycle, the possible relation between glial remodeling and synaptic plasticity is less obvious in the hippocampus (see Chapter 4). However, considering the multiple metabolic roles of astrocytes and the importance of astrocyte signaling for synaptic function, astroglial plasticity may play an essential role in the coordination of modifications in hippocampal activity during the estrus cycle. Finally, another aspect of hippocampal plasticity that is modified during the estrus cycle is neurogenesis in the dentate gyrus. Neuronal proliferation in the subgranular layer of the dentate gyrus fluctuates during the estrus cycle, showing a peak during proestrus (Tanapat et al., 1999). The coincidence in proestrus of peaks in neurogenesis, in dendritic spine formation in CA1 pyramidal cells, and in the number of synaptic inputs to CA1 dendritic spines, together with an enhanced synaptic long-term potentiation and increased growth of glial processes, suggest that all these plastic modifications may be functionally interrelated.

HORMONES AND BRAIN REMODELING DURING MOTHERHOOD

Motherhood is one of the most complex periods of cross talk between hormones and the brain in adult life. The dramatic physiological changes and behavioral demands associated with motherhood are regulated by multiple neural end endocrine homeodynamic mechanisms (Brunton and Russell, 2008; Russell et al., 2001). Pregnancy, parturition, and the postpartum period, which includes lactation and many other forms of maternal care, are accompanied by extraordinary modifications in the plasma levels of numerous hormones, including progesterone, estradiol, prolactin, oxytocin, relaxin, and glucocorticoids. Brain remodeling during motherhood contributes to the regulation of these various hormonal changes. In turn, the resulting hormonal adjustments have an impact on the manifestation of different forms of brain plasticity during pregnancy, parturition, and lactation. Different exteroceptive and interoceptive signals contribute to modulate the cross talk between the brain and the endocrine glands during motherhood. Among these, the interaction with pups is one of the most important exteroceptive signals that affect hormonal release and neural plasticity in mothers. Neural plastic modifications resulting from the interaction of exteroceptive and interoceptive signals, the endocrine glands, and the brain will finally determine the manifestation of adequate or inadequate maternal behaviors.

The hypothalamus is the main brain region, but not the only one, in which plastic neuronal and glial remodeling is involved in the regulation of hormonal changes during motherhood. Dramatic plastic reorganization of synaptic connectivity and neuroglia interactions occur in magnocellular neurons in paraventricular and supraoptic nuclei during parturition (Hatton et al., 1982; Montagnese et al., 1987; Theodosis and Poulain, 1984a) and lactation (Hatton et al., 1982; Montagnese et al., 1987; Theodosis and Poulain, 1984a; Theodosis et al., 1986a). During parturition and lactation, oxytocin magnocellular neurons hypertrophy, their dendrites retract, and their axons enlarge and ramify. In parallel, there is a retraction of astrocytic processes and an increase in inhibitory and excitatory synaptic inputs on oxytocin neurons (see Chapter 2 for further details). The reorganization of magnocellular neurons and associated astroglial cells in the supraoptic and paraventricular nuclei allow an increased coupling of the activity of neurosecretory cells. In addition, these plastic changes are accompanied by a reorganization of the interaction of pituicytes with neurosecretory axons in the pituitary, allowing an increased occupation of the basal lamina of capillaries by neurosecretory terminals, and presumably an enhanced hormonal release (Tweedle and Hatton, 1982, 1987). The plastic remodeling of the hypothalamic magnocellular system during parturition and lactation allows the adequate release of oxytocin needed for uterine contractions and milk ejections, and is the best example that we have so far to illustrate how brain remodeling control hormonal secretions during motherhood (see also Chapter 2).

The medial preoptic area, which is involved in the regulation of maternal behavior, also shows plastic modifications associated with motherhood. In the California mouse (*Peromyscus californicus*) neuronal soma size in the medial preoptic area increases significantly with motherhood (Gubernick et al., 1993). In the preoptic area of rats, neuronal volume, the number of basal dendritic branches, and cumulative basal dendritic length increase during pregnancy, probably due to the action of ovarian hormones (Gubernick et al., 1993; Keyser-Marcus et al., 2001). Neuronal morphology is also affected by motherhood in the medial nucleus of the amygdala, a brain region involved in endocrine regulation and the response to stress. Multiparous females have more dendritic spines in the anterior portion of the medial nucleus of the amygdala, and fewer in the posterodorsal region compared to virgin females (Rasia-Filho et al., 2004).

Another important brain region involved in behavioral responses during motherhood is the olfactory bulb. Olfactory cues are important exteroceptive signals for the modulation of maternal care and the interactions between the mother and her pups (Levy et al., 2004). In several mammalian species, odors from the pups and the young are essential to elicit maternal care. An important functional plastic reorganization in the regulation of olfaction occurs at parturition, when olfactory cues that inhibit or do not elicit maternal behavior in nonpregnant females become key signals to elicit maternal care in new mothers. The plastic reorganization of the olfaction system is induced by the new homeodynamic conditions at the end of pregnancy and parturition, including marked modifications in plasma levels of estradiol and progesterone (Fleming et al., 1989).

Plasticity in the olfactory bulb during pregnancy is at least in part mediated by the incorporation of new neurons. Tetsuro Shingo and colleagues at the University of Calgary found that pregnancy and lactation increase the generation of new neurons in the subventricular zone of the mouse brain. The new neurons migrate to the periglomerular and granule layers of the olfactory bulb, and integrate in the neuronal circuits. The rate of neurogenesis peaks on the seventh day of pregnancy, and again after delivery (Shingo et al., 2003). Prolactin has been identified as the regulator of neurogenesis during pregnancy and lactation in mice (Shingo et al., 2003). Similar findings have been obtained in rats, although in this case the peak in neurogenesis in the subventricular zone is detected on day 21 of pregnancy, but not on day 7 of pregnancy

(Furuta and Bridges, 2005). Prolactin, which is increased in plasma during late pregnancy in rats, may also be involved in these changes. The effects of prolactin on neurogenesis in postpartum and virgin female mice are mimicked by the exposure to male pheromones, which increase prolactin levels, increase neurogenesis in the subventricular zone, increase the incorporation of new neurons to the olfactory bulb, and induce maternal behavior (Larsen et al., 2008). Prolactin and pregnancy also increase the generation of oligodendrocytes and the number of myelinated axons (Gregg et al., 2007), suggesting that important plastic modifications in neuronal connectivity mediated by myelinated axons may occur in the maternal brain during pregnancy.

The cerebral cortex also suffers plastic remodeling in lactating mothers. During lactation, the activation of tactile inputs of the nipples by pups causes a functional reorganization of the primary somatosensory representation of the ventral trunk in the cerebral cortex. Christian Xerri and his colleagues have found that the primary somatosensory cortical representation of the ventral trunk skin is almost twice as large in lactating rats than in matched postpartum nonlactating or virgin controls (Xerri et al., 1994). The reorganization of cortical neuron receptive fields and the expansion of cortical representation involve the nursing modulation of GABAergic inhibition and NMDA-dependent synaptic efficacy (Rosselet et al., 2006). Plastic modifications in the receptive fields of neurons in the somatosensory cortex may indirectly impact the processing of information in other cortical and subcortical regions, including cognitive areas. Indeed, it is known that motherhood and previous maternal experience induce cognitive modifications in the mother. In 1999, Craig H. Kinsley and collaborators reported that multiparous female rats that had given birth and lactated twice, made significantly more correct choices during the first six days of testing in a radial-arm maze than age-matched virgin females. Furthermore, in the dry-land version of the Morris water maze test, maternal females took significantly less time to recall and locate the food reward than virgin females. These findings were interpreted as a proof that motherhood improves learning and memory (Kinsley et al., 1999).

The effect of maternal experience on hippocampal-dependent memory has been confirmed by other laboratories (Lemaire et al., 2006b; Pawluski et al., 2006a), has been shown to be long-lasting (Gatewood et al., 2005; Love et al., 2005; Pawluski et al., 2006b), and shown to be abolished by stress induced during pregnancy (Lemaire et al., 2006b). Indeed, pregnancy and not only mothering experience appears to affect the hippocampus-dependent learning and memory in the mother. This is emphasized by the results obtained by Jodi L. Pawluski and collaborators in the laboratory of Lisa Galea, using the spatial working/reference version of the radial-arm maze. They have found that primiparous rats make fewer errors compared to multi- and nulliparous rats, and that pregnant-only rats completed the task on significantly fewer days than primiparous, multiparous, and nulliparous rats (Pawluski et al., 2006b). In addition, marked modifications in hippocampal plasticity and function occur during the early postpartum period, probably associated with the decreased plasma levels of estradiol after delivery and the increased levels of glucocorticoids. Early postpartum females show a reduced spatial learning and then an enhanced retention two weeks later compared to virgin rats. These behavioral modifications are associated with a marked decrease in cell proliferation rate in the subgranular layer of the dentate gyrus of the hippocampus after delivery, without significant changes in the survival of newly generated neurons two weeks later (Darnaudery et al., 2007). In addition, Leuner and colleagues (2007) have reported that cell proliferation in the dentate gyrus is suppressed in lactating postpartum females until the time of weaning, an effect that is dependent on the elevated basal glucocorticoid levels associated with lactation. Pups are the cause of both the elevated glucocorticoids levels and the decrease in neurogenesis. Thus, removal of pups shortly after birth prevents the decrease in hippocampal cell proliferation and reduces basal corticosterone levels in postpartum females. Furthermore, the decrease in cell proliferation in postpartum females is prevented by an adrenalectomy and low-dose corticosterone replacement (Leuner et al., 2007). The important and transient changes in spatial learning and neurogenesis after delivery and during lactation emphasize the complexity of the interactions between hormones, brain plasticity, and behavior in the context of the profound homeodynamic adjustments occurring during motherhood.

Additional structural and functional plastic modifications in the hippocampus are associated with maternal experience. For instance, multiparous female mice show increased long-term synaptic potentiation along Schaffer collaterals in the hippocampus compared to virgin mice. This functional plastic modification is facilitated by oxytocin, and is abolished by the administration of an oxytocin antagonist (Tomizawa et al., 2003). Morphological studies using the Golgi-Cox staining method have revealed that both pregnant rats (at day 21 of pregnancy) and lactating rats have an increased density of dendritic spines in apical dendrites of CA1 hippocampal pyramidal neurons compared to virgin cycling females in diestrus, estrus, or proestrus (Kinsley et al., 2006). Other studies with Golgi impregnation have detected a decrease in the number of branch points and dendritic length in CA3 and CA1 pyramidal neurons in primiparous rats compared to multiparous and nulliparous rats. In addition, multiparous rats have greater spine density in the basal region of CA1 pyramidal neurons (Pawluski and Galea, 2006). Gonadal hormones and glucocorticoids, which are known to regulate the number of dendritic spines in CA1 neurons, may regulate these plastic changes in mothers. Interestingly, spine density in the basal region of CA1 pyramidal neurons is correlated with the number of male pups in a litter (Pawluski and Galea, 2006). Higher levels of testosterone in the uterus of the mother with a higher number of male pups and the increased time spent by the mother in anogenital licking of male offspring may be among the factors involved in this neuroplastic effect (Pawluski and Galea, 2006).

SOCIAL INTERACTIONS, HORMONES, AND BRAIN PLASTICITY

Social interactions are an important source of exteroceptive signals for brain plasticity. I have briefly mentioned an interesting example in the previous chapter when analyzing the plastic maturation of the song control system in the brain of songbirds. Male songbirds that mature in the presence of adult males and learn songs from them, show a reduction in synaptic connectivity in the lateral magnocellular nucleus of the anterior neostriatum in parallel to song learning. In contrast, songbirds that mature in colonies without adult males do not learn songs and do not show synaptic plasticity in the song system (Wallhausser-Franke et al., 1995). This is just one of many other examples that may be presented to sustain the influence of social interactions on developmental brain plasticity. In this section of the book I will examine the influence of social interactions on brain plasticity in adulthood.

Social influences interact with hormonal regulatory actions to modulate brain plasticity. In the case of the plasticity in the brain song system, social interactions with adult males interact with regulatory hormonal actions, such as those exerted by gonadal hormones, and with the singing activity by itself (Ball et al., 2004), to modulate neural plasticity in the song system. For instance, the regulatory action of testosterone on singing rate and the volume of the HVC and the nucleus RA is modulated in male canaries by the social interactions, including the presence or absence of other males and females (Boseret et al., 2006). Interaction with males may also cause prominent plastic changes in the female rat brain; these changes are elicited by male pheromones. Exposure to pheromones from dominant, but not from subordinate males, enhances cell proliferation and neurogenesis in the subventricular zone and in the dentate gyrus of adult females. The effect of male pheromones on neurogenesis in the adult female brain is mediated by luteinizing hormone and prolactin. Luteinizing hormone mediates the enhancement of cell proliferation in the dentate gyrus, while prolactin mediates male pheromone-induced cell proliferation in the subventricular zone (Mak et al., 2007). Therefore, two different hormones mediate, with regional specificity, the changes in neurogenesis in the brain of adult female rats as a consequence of their interaction with males. In turn, the plastic changes in neurogenesis regulated by luteinizing hormone and prolactin in the female brain appear to be required for female mate preference (Mak et al., 2007).

Other hormones, such as stress hormones, are also important players in the adaptation of brain plasticity for the generation of homeodynamic behavioral and endocrine responses in a changing social environment. Acute activation of physiological stress systems by social interactions result in transient synaptic plastic changes in the hippocampus, amygdala, prefrontal cortex, and other brain regions. These changes allow the generation of new emotional, cognitive, and behavioral responses. Other hormones, such as vasopressin and oxytocin, are also important for the regulation of social behavior, social affiliation, social recognition, parental nurturing behavior, the formation of selective mother–infant bonds, and the formation and maintenance of pair bonding in monogamous mating species (Keverne and Curley, 2004; Lim and Young, 2006; Wang and Aragona, 2004). Plasticity of mesolimbic dopaminergic circuits of reward and reinforcement may be involved in the actions of oxytocin and vasopressin on social behavior. Actions of corticotropin-releasing hormone in the nucleus accumbens are also important for partner preference and pair bonding (Lim et al., 2007).

In some species, social interactions result in marked plastic reorganization of the brain. In electric fish (*Apteronotus leptorhynchus*), long-term social interaction results in plastic changes in the diencephalic prepacemaker nucleus, which controls chirping, an electrocommunication behavior involved in aggression. Paired fish have an increased number of new cells added to the periventricular zone adjacent to the diencephalic prepacemaker nucleus, and an increased immunoreactivity for vimentin, a marker of radial glia, in the same brain region. The plastic brain changes coincide temporally with the onset of chirping behavior (Dunlap et al., 2006). Similar results were obtained after the administration of cortisol, suggesting that the hormone may be involved in the association of brain plasticity and the onset of chirping behavior. In the halfspotted goby (*Asterropteryx semipunctata*), temporal modifications in the number and size of GnRH and arginine vasotocin neurons in different brain regions are associated with seasonal changes in social interactions, territoriality, and parental care (Maruska et al., 2007), and in several species the activity of GnRH neurons is regulated by social cues (Bakker and Baum, 2000; Rissman, 1996). In the African cichlid fish, *Haplochromis burtoni*, changes in social status, including events such as losing or winning a territorial encounter, result in plastic alterations in the activity of GnRH neurons, in the volume of hypothalamic neurons regulating growth hormone secretion and in the expression of androgen and estrogen receptors and arginine vasotocin in the brain (Burmeister et al., 2007; Greenwood and Fernald, 2004; Greenwood et al., 2008; Hofmann and Fernald, 2000). Different forms of social defeat, such as that experienced by a male that loses a fight against a dominant male for control of territory and females, are associated with prominent plastic changes in the brain, which are regulated by stress hormones. In our society, several forms of emotional abuse and hostile behaviors in the workplace, frequent phenomena popularly known as mobbing or bullying, are also a source of stress. Different aggressive, submissive, and defensive behaviors are displayed in these conflictive situations. These behaviors may have long-term effects on the brain, which in turn will sustain the generation of new behavioral responses. The result of a conflictive social interaction may have very different outcomes in brain plasticity depending on whether one is a "winner" or a "loser." We may assume that winning a social conflict is a form of acute stress that may have "positive" effects for brain function. However, we do not know much regarding the brain changes associated with winners in social conflicts. In contrast, several studies have analyzed the physiological and behavioral effects of social defeat. Social defeat in humans may have serious detrimental consequences for brain function, and may cause depression and other affective and emotional disturbances (Huhman, 2006). Social defeat in rats evokes anhedonia and motivational deficits (Rygula et al., 2005). Several brain regions appear to experience plastic reorganization after social defeat. Expression of BDNF in the nucleus accumbens appears to be required for the development of long-term neural and behavioral plasticity in response to social defeat (Berton et al., 2006). In addition, plastic synaptic modifications in the basolateral amygdala appear to be involved in learning associated with the experience of losing a social conflict (Huhman, 2006). Another brain area affected by social defeat is the hippocampus. Social defeat in rats and mice decreases the ratio between mineralocorticoid and glucocorticoid receptors in the hippocampus, and therefore the response of the hippocampus to stress hormones (Buwalda et al., 2005). Alterations in the hippocampus induced by social defeat include a decrease in cell proliferation in the dentate gyrus (Yap et al., 2006). In addition, both brief and repetitive social defeats induce a reorganization of dendrites in CA3 pyramidal neurons. In both cases there is a decrease in apical dendritic volume, surface area, and length. In addition, brief social defeat produces an increased length, volume, and branch complexity of basal dendrites (Kole et al., 2004). These morphological changes are associated with a long-lasting impairment of long-term synaptic potentiation, which is also observed in the CA1 region of the hippocampus (Artola et al., 2006).

TRAUMATIC EXPERIENCES, HORMONES, AND BRAIN PLASTICITY

One of the most important sources of stress in the wild is predator attack. In the human society context, predator attack has been replaced by different forms of traumatic experiences, including traffic accidents, wars, terrorist attacks, male violence against children and women, and sexual abuse. All these forms of stress may have permanent psychological consequences and lasting changes in affect. In more severe cases, serious alterations may appear in the individuals that have suffered the stress, then the situation is recognized as posttraumatic stress disorder. Traumatic stress may result in plastic remodeling of certain brain regions, such as the amygdala.

Brain imaging studies reveal a hyperexcitability of the right amygdala in the brain of humans exposed to traumatic situations (Rauch and Shin, 1997; Rauch et al., 1997; Shin et al., 2006). The amygdala also shows plastic changes in animals exposed to a fear conditioning paradigm. Fear conditioning is a form of associative Pavlovian learning in which the animals are exposed to a stressful situation, such as en electric shock, that is associated with a sensory stimulus. In this paradigm, the animals learn to associate the sensory stimulus with the traumatic experience. Thus, after learning the association, the sensory stimulus per se may switch on the fear response. Plastic synaptic changes in the amygdala underlie both acquisition and extinction of the enhanced fear response. Fear conditioning induces long-term potentiation of synaptic inputs to the amygdala, and several data support the view that fear conditioning is mediated by changes in synaptic strength at sensory inputs to the lateral nucleus of the amygdala (Blair et al., 2001; Maren, 2005; Maren et al., 1994; Rogan et al., 1997; Schafe et al., 2001; Sigurdsson et al., 2006). Exposure to predators produces a fear response similar to that obtained with the fear conditioning paradigm. The amygdala is also involved in the stress and fear response to the exposure to predator stimuli, and predator stress also leads to changes in long-term synaptic potentiation over several amygdala afferent and efferent pathways involved in the defensive response (Adamec et al., 2006). Stress hormones may be involved in the generation of the plastic synaptic changes elicited in the amygdala by the fear conditioning paradigm and by exposure to a predator. In turn, the synaptic changes may be critical in mediating the hormonal regulation of memory consolidation (Adamec et al., 2006; McGaugh and Roozendaal, 2002; Roozendaal et al., 2006).

Plastic synaptic changes in other brain structures, in addition to the amygdala, appear to be involved in the processing of fear memory. Synaptic plasticity in the medial prefrontal cortex, the hippocampus, and amygdala are likely involved in the extinction of fear memory (Maren and Quirk, 2004; Sotres-Bayon et al., 2006). However, the plastic changes may also affect other forms of memory. As we have seen before, neural cell adhesion molecules may be involved in the synaptic plastic changes associated with stress. Interestingly, Carmen Sandi and her collaborators have reported that both spatial memory and N-CAM levels in the hippocampus are affected by exposing trained rats to a cat. Predator exposure impairs spatial memory and dramatically reduces the levels of the N-CAM-180 isoform in the hippocampus. These authors showed that 30 minutes of cat exposure resulted in a reduction of N-CAM-180 levels in the hippocampus to approximately 60% of control values (Sandi et al., 2005). Another region involved in fear memory is the cerebellum. Saccheti and colleagues (2004) have demonstrated plastic changes in the cerebellum that are linked to the consolidation of fear memory. These authors detected a long-lasting potentiation of the synapse between parallel fibers and Purkinje cells in cerebellar slices at 10 minutes and 24 hours following fear conditioning. The mechanism of parallel fiber long-term potentiation was postsynaptic and mediated by an increased AMPA response. Climbing fiber synapses, in contrast, did not show modifications. In addition, when the parallel fiber long-term synaptic potentiation is blocked, fear conditioning is affected. The discovery that the cerebellum participates in the consolidation of fear conditioning was unexpected, since this brain structure is usually considered a region exclusively involved in motor control. However, some studies have correlated cerebellar lesions with emotional disorders, including depression and schizophrenia (Schutter and van Honk, 2005).

CHAPTER SUMMARY

In this chapter, I have examined the interaction of hormones and brain plasticity during adult reproductive life. With this aim, I have presented some examples of brain mutability and its associated hormonal changes in the context of adult life events. The first examples analyzed the hormonal regulation of circadian and seasonal changes in brain plasticity. We have seen that hormones regulate brain plasticity to synchronize the endogenous circadian clock and regulate brain metaplasticity to adapt circadian plasticity to seasonal changes in day length or external temperature. These neuroplastic modifications are associated with seasonal changes in specific behaviors, including mating, parental behaviors or hibernation. I have also examined the hormonal regulation of brain plasticity associated with reproductive cycles. In this case, hormones may synchronize metaplastic modifications in brain regions that coordinate ovulation with sexual receptivity, lordosis, and hippocampal-dependent behaviors. Hormones also regulate brain plasticity during pregnancy, parturition, and the postpartum period, coordinating metaplastic changes in brain regions involved in the regulation of maternal behavior, the interaction with pups, the response to stress and the hormonal release by the neurohypophysis. I have also examined in this chapter the hormonal regulation of brain plasticity to control emotional, cognitive, and behavioral responses to the social environment. In addition, I have presented some examples to illustrate that altered regulation of metaplasticity by stress hormones as a consequence of chronic stress or traumatic experiences may result in brain pathology. However, the interaction of hormones, brain plasticity, and pathology has many other facets that I must explore with more detail in the next chapter.

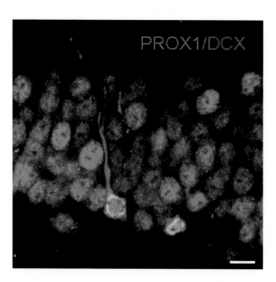

Figure 1.3. Incorporation of new neurons in the granule cell layer of the dentate gyrus of the hippocampus. The figure corresponds to a young adult (4 months old) female mouse. Newly incorporated neurons are immunolabeled in red for doublecortin (DCX), a cytoskeletal maker of immature differentiating neurons. Granule cells are immunolabeled in green for the prospero-related homeobox 1 gene (Prox 1), a granule cell–specific transcription factor. The colocalization of green and red labeling indicates that the newly incorporated neurons are granule cells. Scale bar, 10 μm. (Courtesy of María Llorens-Martín and José Luis Trejo. Based on Llorens-Martín et al., 2007.)

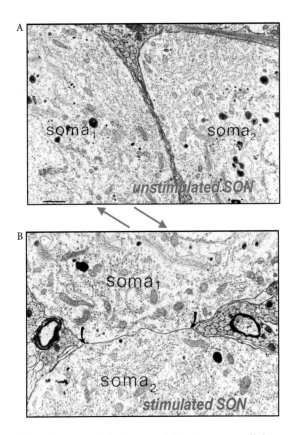

Figure 2.2. Glial and neuronal plastic remodeling in magnocellular neurons associated with the release of oxytocin in the adult supraoptic nucleus (SON). A: Under basal unstimulated conditions, neuronal somas are separated by multiple astrocytic processes. B: Under conditions of high hormonal release, glial processes retract, and the proportion of magnocellular somas in juxtaposition with other somas (black arrows) is increased. These plastic modifications are interpreted as a mechanism to facilitate synchronization of hormonal release by magnocellular neurons. When activity is back to basal conditions (red arrows), astrocytic processes again separate neuronal profiles. (Courtesy of Dr. Dionysia T. Theodosis. Based on Theodosis and Poulain, 1987.)

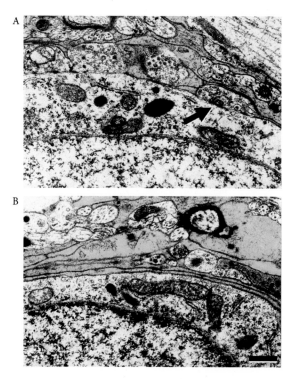

Figure 2.3. Modifications in glial processes (highlighted in yellow) and axosomatic synaptic terminals (arrow) in the rat arcuate nucleus during the estrus cycle. The electron micrographs show two arcuate neuronal somas. (A) In the morning of proestrus, before the peak of estrogen in plasma. (B) In the morning of estrus. The number of axosomatic synaptic inputs decreases from proestrus to estrus. In parallel, there is an increased warping of arcuate neuronal somas by glial processes. Scale bar, 0.5 μm. (Microphotographs from the author.)

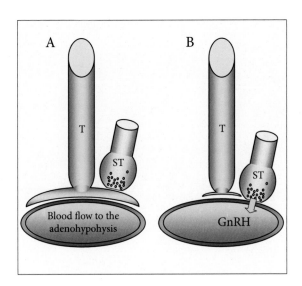

Figure 2.5. Neuroglial plasticity associated with the release of gonadotropin releasing hormone (GnRH) into the blood flow in the median eminence. The cellular processes of tanycytes (T), specialized bipolar glial cells, are closely associated with gonadotropin-releasing hormone fibers in the median eminence. Tanycytic processes extend and retract following hormonal changes during the estrus cycle in rodents. (A) Growth of tanycytic processes results in the ensheathment of gonadotropin-releasing hormone synaptic terminals (ST), preventing gonadotropin-releasing hormone release in the blood flow to the adenohypohysis. (B) Retraction of tanycytic processes during the preovulatory stage of the estrus cycle, allows the contact of gonadotropin-releasing hormone terminals with portal capillaries and the release of gonadotropin-releasing hormone to the blood flow.

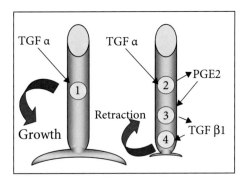

Figure 2.6. Transforming growth factor α (TGFα) regulates the extension and retraction of tanycytic processes in the median eminence in association with the release of gonadotropin-releasing hormone. TGFα first induces the cellular extension of tanycytes and the release of prostaglandin E2 (PGE2). Then, PGE2 induces the release of transforming growth factor β1 (TGFβ1); this factor finally induces the cellular retraction of tanycytes. (A) TGFα released by astrocytes acts on tanycytes (1) and induces the growth of tanycytic processes. (B) Tanycytes also respond to TGFα (2) by releasing PGE2. In turn, PGE2 induces the release of TGFβ1 by tanycytes (3). Then, TGFβ1 induces the retraction of tanycytic processes (4). (Based on Prevot, 2002; Prevot et al., 2003, 2007).

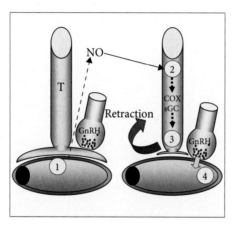

Figure 2.7. Endothelial cells (E) may also play a critical role in regulating the extension and retraction of tanycytic processes in the median eminence in association with the release of gonadotropin-releasing hormone (GnRH). Endothelial cells of the median eminence use nitric oxide (NO) to promote cytoarchitectural changes in tanycytes (T). The stimulatory effect of NO on tanycyte plasticity involves the participation of soluble guanylyl cyclase (sGC) and cyclooxigenase (COX) activities. NO released by endothelial cells (1) acts on tanycytes (2), causes retraction of tanycytic processes (3), which enables GnRH nerve terminals to directly contact the pericapillary space (4). (Courtesy of Dr. Vincent Prevot. Based on De Seranno et al., 2004; Prevot et al., 2007).

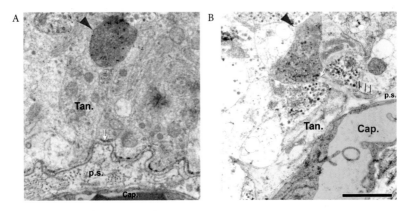

Figure 2.8. Activation of endogenous NO secretion in the media eminence induces structural changes, allowing gonadotropin-releasing hormone (GnRH) nerve terminals to form direct neurovascular junctions. Representative electron micrograph of GnRH-immunoreactive terminals (large arrowhead, green) in the external zone of the median eminence in close proximity of the fenestrated capillaries (Cap, red) of the portal vasculature in absence (A) or presence (B) of L-arginine, the precursor of NO. (A) Under basal unstimulated conditions, GnRH nerve terminals (labeled with 15 nm gold particles) are entirely embedded in tanycytic end feet (Tan, yellow), which prevent them from contacting the pericapillary space (p.s., pink) delineated by the parenchymatous basal lamina (white arrow). (B) GnRH nerve terminals forming neurovascular junctions (i.e., directly contacting the pericapillary space; white arrow) in median eminence explants after incubation for 30 minutes with L-arginine. Very few tanycytic processes (yellow) remain around GnRH nerve endings that have direct access to the pericapillary space (black arrows), suggesting that tanycytic end feet underwent retraction. Scale bar: 0.5 μm. (Courtesy of Dr. Vincent Prevot. Based on De Seranno et al., 2004)

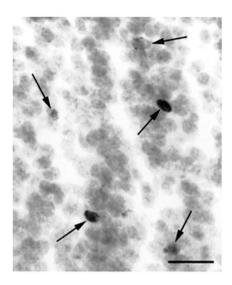

Figure 4.7. Methylene blue–stained section of an olfactory bulb showing BrdU-immunoreactive nuclei (arrows) in the granule cell layer of the main olfactory bulb of an ovariectomized rat. Scale bar = 50 μm. (Microphotograph courtesy of Dr. Arpad Parducz.)

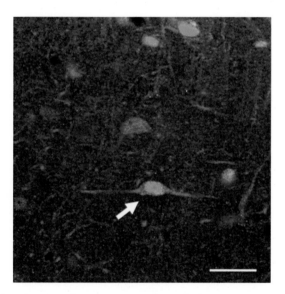

Figure 5.1. Localization of estrogen receptor α and IGF-I receptor immunoreactivities in the arcuate nucleus of the rat hypothalamus. Estrogen receptor α immunoreactivity is observed in neuronal cell nuclei (green) and IGF-I receptor immunoreactivity in the soma and cell processes (red) in the same neurons (arrow). Scale bar, 20 μm. (Microphotograph courtesy of Dr. Gloria Patricia Cardona-Gomez).

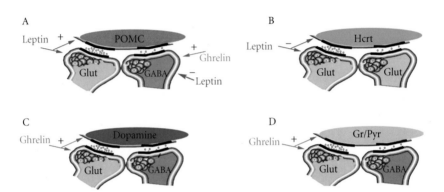

Figure 5.2. Metabolic hormones regulate glutamatergic (Glut) and GABAergic (GABA) synaptic plasticity in different brain regions. In the arcuate nucleus (A), both leptin and ghrelin alter the synaptology of proopiomelanocortin (POMC) neurons in support of either satiety (leptin) or hunger (ghrelin). In the lateral hypothalamus (B), leptin-dependent reorganization of excitatory inputs and miniature excitatory postsynaptic currents were observed on hypocretin (Hcrt) neurons in response to fasting in a manner that promotes increased arousal. In the ventral tegmentum (C), dopamine neurons showed rapid changes in the GABAergic and glutamatergic inputs in response to ghrelin in association with increased dopamine neuronal activity and feeding. Ghrelin also altered synaptic spine density in granular/pyramidal cells of the hippocampus (D) in parallel with increased propagation of long-term synaptic potentiation and enhanced performance of animals in various behavioral tasks. (Courtesy of Dr. Tamas Horvath).

Chapter 9

Life Stages, Hormones, and Brain Remodeling: Disease and Neuroprotection

INTRODUCTION: ALTERED CROSS TALK BETWEEN ENDOCRINE GLANDS AND THE BRAIN UNDER PATHOLOGICAL CONDITIONS

In previous chapters I have analyzed examples of modifications in the cross talk between the brain and the endocrine glands in adaptation to changes in the physical, biological, and social environment during different life stages. I have examined brain plastic modifications associated with complex alterations in endocrine secretions, such as those occurring during fetal and early postnatal development, the transition from childhood to adulthood, circadian rhythms, reproductive cycles, and motherhood; also in adaptation to social interactions or seasonal environmental changes, including brain remodeling during extreme physical conditions (such as is the case of hibernating animals during winter). These and other modifications examined so far regarding the interaction of hormonal secretions and brain plasticity in response to changing life conditions represent examples of adaptive responses aimed at maintaining the homeodynamic equilibrium under physiological circumstances. However, both the regulatory actions that hormones exert on brain plasticity and the regulatory control exerted by brain remodeling on the endocrine glands are altered during pathological conditions. Some examples of these alterations have been introduced in previous chapters. In this chapter I will examine, with more detail and in a broader context, the interaction of hormones and brain plasticity under pathological conditions.

Pathological alterations in the central nervous system result in modifications in the communication of the brain with the endocrine glands, which in turn results in altered hormonal secretions and altered hormonal signaling to the nervous system. Endocrine diseases also result in altered hormonal levels, which have an impact on the brain and may result in impaired regulation of brain plasticity and the development of cognitive and affective disorders. As a consequence of these modifications in the cross talk between the brain and the endocrine glands, a new homeodynamic equilibrium may be reached. However, the system may be unable to adapt to chronic pathology of the brain or endocrine glands, resulting in permanent alterations in neuroendocrine communication, brain plasticity, and endocrine secretions, further enhancing the pathological condition. In this chapter I will examine first the evidence indicating that pathological brain remodeling affects hormonal secretions. Then I will consider how pathological alterations in hormone levels or hormonal signaling, due to endocrine diseases or other causes, affect brain plasticity and function. Finally, I will analyze the influence of specific hormones on the reorganization of nervous tissue after injury or neurodegeneration.

PATHOLOGICAL BRAIN REMODELING AFFECTS HORMONAL SECRETIONS

The genetically programmed brain mutability is also manifested under pathological conditions. The nervous tissue reacts to injury with the generation of an endogenous response that is evolutionary programmed to promote the protection, reorganization, and recuperation of the damaged tissue. Neurodegenerative and affective disorders are accompanied by functional and structural modifications in neuronal connectivity and cellular replacement. Affective disorders are accompanied by changes in the rate of neurogenesis in the hippocampus, by modifications in the branching of dendrites and the growth of dendritic spines, and by alterations in functional synaptic plasticity. Neurodegeneration causes the structural loss of synaptic connections and the functional alteration of the synaptic circuits. The death of a postsynaptic neuron alters the function of the presynaptic cells, and vice versa. The axons and dendrites of surviving neurons show plastic modifications in an attempt to establish new synaptic contacts. Some new synaptic circuits are generated (or some old ones are reinforced) as an adaptive mechanism to compensate for the functional impairment caused by the damaged neuronal networks.

Glial cells are also key players in the reorganization of neural tissue under pathological conditions: microglia, astrocytes, and oligodendrocytes contribute to the remodeling of neural tissue after injury and under neurodegenerative conditions. Astroglia and microglia are activated and recruited to the zones of neurodegeneration, and are involved in the formation of a glial scar in wounds of the brain and spinal cord. Glial activation is accompanied by striking changes in cellular morphology. Microglial cells reduce the branching of their cellular processes, which become thicker or retract, and the activated cells acquire an amoeboid phenotype. Activated astroglial cells show an increased cell volume, and thicker and less branched cellular processes than resting astroglia. Microglial cells participate in the remodeling of the damaged tissue by the phagocytosis of neural or glial debris. Activated astroglia also participate in the structural remodeling of the damaged neuronal circuits. In addition, both astroglia and microglia secrete a variety of factors that regulate neuronal survival and axonal regeneration in the damaged tissue. Oligodendrocytes and oligodendrocyte precursors are involved in the process of remyelination. Neurodegeneration is also accompanied by the remodeling of blood vessels. The plastic reorganization of neural tissue after injury represents, at least in part, an attempt to reach a new homeodynamic equilibrium in the function of the nervous system.

The plastic and regenerative responses of the nervous tissue to injury may affect the neuronal circuits that control pituitary hormone secretions; some brain pathologies are suspected to alter the cross talk between the endocrine organs and the brain. For instance, epilepsy is frequently associated with modifications in the levels of reproductive hormones (Montouris and Morris, 2005), which in turn may affect seizure frequency, hippocampal synaptic plasticity, and hippocampal neurogenesis (Hajszan and MacLusky, 2006). Experimental middle cerebral artery occlusion in rats induces an increase in the levels of erythropoietin to control systemic oxygen homeostasis and erythropoiesis (Gendron et al., 2004). Experimental damage of the hypothalamic arcuate nucleus in neonatal rats alters the secretion of gonadotropin-releasing hormone (GnRH) (Sasaki et al., 1994), gonadotropins (Terentini et al., 1974), growth-hormone-releasing hormone (Bloch et al., 1984; Sasaki et al., 1994), growth hormone (Maiter et al., 1991) and the plasma levels of leptin (Frederich et al., 1995; Morris et al., 1998).

In humans, the best characterized evidence for a link between brain pathology and altered hormonal levels is a traumatic brain injury. The first patient described with hypopituitarism as a result of traumatic brain injury occurred as early as in 1918 (Cyran, 1918), and other cases were soon discovered (Escamilla and Lisser, 1942). However, traumatic brain injury was considered an exceptional cause of hypopituitarism many decades thereafter (Benvenga, 2005). It is only in the last few years that new studies have revealed that pituitary dysfunction is in fact a common consequence of traumatic brain injury (Lorenzo et al., 2005; Popovic, 2005). Traumatic brain injury affects children, adolescents, adults, and the elderly. Traffic accidents and violence-related events are the most common causes of traumatic brain injury. Recent estimations indicate that approximately 25% to 50% of patients with traumatic brain injury will develop some degree of pituitary dysfunction (Aimaretti et al., 2004; Kelly et al., 2000; Tanriverdi et al., 2006). This represents a high number of total patients, since the incidence of traumatic brain injury (which is similar around the world) is approximately 200 cases per 100,000 inhabitants per year (Bondanelli et al., 2005; Bruns and Hauser, 2003; Popovic et al., 2005). In addition, there are other forms of brain injury not included in these figures that have been identified as a cause of pituitary dysfunction and hormonal imbalance. One example is a subarachnoid hemorrhage (Aimaretti et al., 2004; Dimopoulou et al., 2004; Kreitschmann-Andermahr, 2005). Chronic repetitive head trauma associated with contact sports is another source of pituitary dysfunction (Tanriverdi et al., 2007). Therefore, pituitary dysfunction after brain injury represents a major health problem.

Hormonal changes after a traumatic brain injury follow two different phases (Bondanelli et al., 2005). During the first acute phase there is an endocrine modification that may, at least in part, represent a homeodynamic response in adaptation to brain injury. Many hormonal changes during the acute phase are reversible and spontaneously disappear. The second phase corresponds to the permanent hypothalamic–pituitary dysfunction that remains as a consequence of the injury in many individuals. During the acute phase after traumatic brain injury there is, in general, an increase in the plasma levels of adrenocorticotropin and prolactin; cortisol levels are also frequently elevated. In contrast, luteinizing hormone, follicle-stimulating hormone, thyrotropin, and thyroxine levels may either decrease or remain unchanged, while triiodothyronine (T3) levels rapidly decrease after injury. A deficiency in gonadal hormones is a frequent finding during the early post-injury period in both sexes. In general, clinical data suggest an imbalance of the neuroendocrine system controlling growth hormone secretion during the acute phase after traumatic brain injury, and both low and high basal levels of growth hormone have been reported during this phase. Diabetes insipidus also has a relatively high prevalence during the acute phase after injury.

Although the acute hormonal modifications after a traumatic brain injury are in general transitory, a significant proportion of patients are left with permanent hormonal alterations (Bondanelli et al., 2005). This is the second phase of hormonal modifications after traumatic brain injury, which is associated with a permanent hypopituitarism. The development and severity of the permanent post-traumatic hypopituitarism depends on several factors, including the severity of the traumatic brain injury and the secondary cerebral damage. It has been estimated that approximately 75% of the patients with post-traumatic hypopituitarism will develop an isolated hormonal deficit, 21.9% will have multiple hormonal deficits, and 3.4% will suffer from panhypopituitarism. The most common chronic hormonal alterations after traumatic brain injury are growth hormone deficiency and gonadotropin deficiency (Aimaretti et al., 2004; Bondanelli et al., 2005; Tanriverdi et al., 2006). These alterations are observed in approximately 30% of patients with post-traumatic hypopituitarism. Corticotropin deficiency and thyrotropin deficiency are detected in 18.5% of patients that suffer post-traumatic hypopituitarism. Diabetes insipidus, which is a relatively common finding in the acute hormonal response to brain injury, persists as a chronic alteration in only 2.7% of the patients (Bondanelli et al., 2005).

The potential effects of pituitary deficiency during development represent an additional cause of concern when considering traumatic brain injury in children and adolescents. The consequences that brain pathological alterations may have on hormonal secretions during development are largely unexplored. However, it is known that traumatic brain injury in children is a common cause of growth hormone deficiency and growth retardation. Gonadotropin deficiency is also common after a traumatic brain injury in children. In addition, cases of central precocious puberty have also been reported (Acerini et al., 2006; Acerini and Tasker, 2007; Niederland et al., 2007).

In summary, the limited evidence reviewed in this section indicates that the cross talk between brain plasticity and endocrine signals is modified when brain function is affected by pathological alterations. Brain disease, such as a traumatic brain injury, causes modifications in the plasma levels of several hormones. In turn, hormonal alterations under brain disease conditions may have an important impact on body homeodynamics, including the function of the nervous system. Therefore, hormonal alterations after a brain injury may interfere with the process of brain recovery. Some of the hormonal changes, such as those occurring during the acute phase, may in part reflect a homeodynamic adaptation. However, the altered neuroendocrine regulation after a brain injury may result in hormonal levels that are not adapted to homeodynamic needs and may negatively impact the brain, increasing neural damage or preventing recovery. For instance, normal growth hormone secretion may facilitate brain recovery after traumatic injury in humans (Bondanelli et al., 2007). In the following section of this chapter I will analyze this part of the loop in the cross talk between brain plasticity and hormones, addressing the question of how hormones contribute to the plastic reorganization of the pathological brain.

PATHOLOGICAL ALTERATIONS IN HORMONAL LEVELS OR HORMONAL SIGNALING AFFECT BRAIN PLASTICITY

Altered hormonal levels caused by endocrine pathologies or other causes, including traumatic brain injury, may affect brain plasticity and function. It is known that several endocrine pathologies such as hypothyroidism, Cushing's syndrome, diabetes, or growth hormone deficiency are associated with changes in the function of the nervous system, and leads to deficits in cognition (see also Chapters 3, 5, and 6). Therefore, altered hormonal levels or hormonal signaling due to pathological conditions may affect brain function. Impaired regulation of brain plasticity as a conscience of the hormonal deficit may be involved in these effects; a good example is hypothyroidism. Thyroid hormone deficiency during adult life is associated with cognitive impairment and behavioral alterations (Rivas and Naranjo, 2007), indicating that thyroid hormones contribute to maintaining a healthy brain function. Hypothyroidism in nondemented elderly people is associated with impairments in learning, word fluency, visual–spatial abilities, attention, visual scanning, and motor speed (Osterweil et al., 1992). Even subclinical hypothyroidism may have an impact on cognitive function, impairing working memory (Zhu et al., 2006). Hormonal therapy ameliorates at least some of the cognitive impairments of hypothyroidism (Miller et al., 2006), including memory performance and frontal cortex executive functions in individuals with subclinical hypothyroidism (Zhu et al., 2006). The cognitive effects of thyroid hormones may be related to their actions on brain plasticity (see Chapter 3), including the regulation of adult hippocampal neurogenesis. Indeed, adult-onset hypothyroidism causes a decrease in the survival and differentiation of new neurons in the subgranular zone of the dentate gyrus in the hippocampal formation (Ambrogini et al., 2005; Desouza et al., 2005; Montero-Pedrazuela et al., 2006), and hormonal therapy recovers the rate of adult hippocampal neurogenesis (Montero-Pedrazuela et al., 2006). In addition, adult-onset thyroid hormone deficiency decreases the number of dendritic spines in layer V pyramidal neurons of the visual cerebral cortex, and affects functional synaptic plasticity in the hippocampus and cerebral cortex (Alzoubi et al., 2005; Ruiz-Marcos et al., 1988; Sui et al., 2006). Thyroid hormone therapy is able to recover synaptic plasticity to normal conditions (Alzoubi et al., 2005; Montero-Pedrazuela et al., 2006; Ruiz-Marcos et al., 1982a, b, 1994), suggesting that thyroid hormone is exerting a protective role in the adult brain regulating neural plasticity under physiological conditions. Another action of thyroid hormone with relevant clinical implications is its ability to down-regulate the expression of the amyloid-β precursor protein (APP) via a negative thyroid hormone response element in the first exon of the APP gene. Accordingly, APP gene expression is increased in the brain of hypothyroid mice and decreased in the brain of hyperthyroid mice (O'Barr et al., 2006). Therefore, hypothyroidism may represent a risk factor for the development of Alzheimer's disease, and thyroid hormone may be a protective factor against this neurological illness.

Insulin, directly or by the regulation of glucose metabolism (see Chapter 5), is a protective factor for the central and peripheral nervous system. Insulin deficiency and insulin resistance are associated with neurodegeneration, alterations in synaptic plasticity, and cognitive impairment (Artola et al., 2005; Biessels et al., 1996; Grillo et al., 2005; Kamal et al., 2005; Magariños and McEwen, 2000; Qin et al., 2006). Diabetes also produces a reduction in adult neurogenesis in the hippocampus and the subventricular zone (Jackson-Guilford et al., 2000; Saravia et al., 2004), induces neuronal apoptosis (Li et al., 2002), and impairs glial plasticity, promoting gliosis in several brain regions (Baydas et al., 2003; Lieth et al., 1998; Mizutani et al., 1998; Saravia et al., 2006) and decreasing astroglial proliferation and survival in the hypothalamus and cerebellum (Lechuga-Sancho et al., 2006a, b). The effects of insulin deficiency and insulin resistance on synaptic plasticity and hippocampal neurogenesis in rodents may in part be mediated by increased corticosterone levels (Stranahan et al., 2008). This suggests that stress may increase neurological deficits induced by diabetes. In addition, it has been proposed that insulin dysfunction may play a role in the genesis of Alzheimer's disease (Carro and Torres-Aleman, 2004; Gasparini et al., 2002; Gasparini and Xu, 2003; Trudeau et al., 2004; Wickelgren, 1998). Insulin targets two important molecules in Alzheimer's disease: β-amyloid peptides and the microtubule-associated protein tau. Insulin promotes β-amyloid release from neurons, then reduces β-amyloid degradation by an insulin-degrading enzyme, which is a protease that degrades both insulin and β-amyloid (Gasparini et al., 2001). Therefore, insulin decreases intracellular levels and increase extracellular levels of β-amyloid peptides. In addition, insulin also transiently increases and then decreases the phosphorylation of tau (Hong and Lee, 1997; Lesort et al., 1999).

Alterations in the levels of growth hormone and IGF-I may also influence brain plasticity and function. Growth hormone deficiency in humans is associated with moderate changes in cognitive function (Arwert et al., 2006; Falleti et al., 2006; Maruff and Falleti, 2005; Sathiavageeswaran et al., 2007; van Dam, 2005). In addition, different neurodegenerative conditions are associated with modifications in serum IGF-I levels (Busiguina et al., 2000; Carro et al., 2000). Furthermore, mice with low levels of serum IGF-I, as a consequence of specific targeted disruption of the IGF-I gene in the liver, had reduced neurogenesis in the hippocampus together with impaired spatial learning (Trejo et al., 2008). Moreover, the disruption of IGF-I input to the brain promotes amyloidosis, cognitive disturbance, hyperphosphorylated tau deposits, gliosis, and synaptic protein loss (Carro et al., 2006). This finding supports the hypothesis that disrupted IGF-I signaling may be involved in the pathology of Alzheimer's disease. Indeed, systemic IGF-I promotes brain β-amyloid clearance, stimulating the neuronal release of the molecule and the transport into the brain of β-amyloid carrier proteins that will take the molecule out of the brain (Carro et al., 2002; Carro and Torres-Aleman, 2004). Therefore, decreased systemic IGF-I levels may result in an impaired β-amyloid clearance.

Glucocorticoids play a key role in the integration of brain plasticity, emotions, behavior, and body homeodynamics. These hormones mediate effects of acute and chronic stress to the brain, regulating the rate of adult hippocampal neurogenesis (Mirescu and Gould, 2006) and other forms of morphological and functional brain plasticity (see Chapter 3). While acute stress and acute glucocorticoid actions are essential to adapt brain plastic responses to homeodynamic conditions, repeated stress or chronic glucocorticoid administration may result in permanent synaptic alterations, memory disturbances, anxiety, and depression (McEwen and Wingfield, 2003). Chronic stress or chronic glucocorticoid exposure impairs functional synaptic plasticity (Foy et al., 1987; Pavlides et al., 2002; Shors et al., 1989) and induces remodeling of dendrites and synaptic contacts in different brain regions, including the hypertrophy of dendritic trees in pyramidal-like and stellate neurons in the basolateral nucleus of the amygdala (Vyas et al., 2002, 2004), the retraction of the apical dendritic tree of pyramidal neurons in the anterior cingulate and prelimbic cerebral cortex (Cook and Wellman, 2004; Radley et al., 2004; Wellman, 2001), and the retraction of apical dendrites of CA3 pyramidal neurons of the hippocampus (Magariños and McEwen, 1995; Magariños et al., 1997; McKittrick et al., 2000; Sandi et al., 2003; Sousa et al., 2000; Stewart et al., 2005; Watanabe et al., 1992; Woolley et al., 1990b). In addition, an adrenalectomy increases, while corticosterone decreases, adult hippocampal neurogenesis (Mirescu and Gould, 2006). These alterations induced by chronic stress and chronic glucocorticoids may be reversible (Conrad et al., 1999; Radley and Morrison, 2005) and may represent a compensatory response to chronic stress (Conrad, 2006). However, long-term alteration in the regulation of the hypothalamic–pituitary–adrenal axis (such as those produced by prenatal and early postnatal stress, traumatic experiences, or social defeat) may result in permanent impairment of hippocampal plasticity and function, cognitive alterations, and depression (see also Chapters 6 and 8). In addition, chronic glucocorticoid exposure may exacerbate neurological and psychiatric disorders of different etiology. Experimental studies in rats have shown that chronic treatment with corticosterone increases the vulnerability of the hippocampus to neurotoxicity (Conrad et al., 2007). In humans, different disorders associated with elevated plasma glucocorticoids, such as major depression and Cushing's syndrome, may result in a reduction in hippocampal volume (Campbell and MacQueen, 2006; MacMaster et al., 2008; Maller et al., 2007). In addition, there is evidence of glial cell loss in the human brain under conditions of elevated glucocorticoid exposure, such as major depression (Cotter et al., 2001; Rajkowska and Miguel-Hidalgo, 2007). Thus, altered glucocorticoid levels or an altered response to glucocorticoids may represent a risk factor for brain pathological remodeling.

Alterations in the hypothalamo–pituitary–adrenal system caused by stress also result in the activation of arginine-vasopressin and oxytocin neurons in the hypothalamus (Bao et al., 2008). Thus, stress conditions in humans result in elevated plasma concentrations of the hormones arginine-vasopressin and oxytocin. In addition, plasma levels of arginine-vasopressin are elevated in depressed patients (van Londen et al., 1997), and are associated with an increased risk of suicide (Bao et al., 2008). It has also been proposed that alterations in vasopressin and oxytocin may be involved in autism (Hammock and Young, 2006). Angiotensin II, which participates in the brain's response to stress, promotes the release of vasopressin by magnocellular vasopressinergic hypothalamic neurons (Saavedra and Benicky, 2007). Angiotensin II has proinflammatory effects in the brain, and it has been postulated that it may be involved in the physiopathological mechanisms of several brain disorders, such as stroke, bipolar disorder, and schizophrenia. Antagonists of angiotensin II type 1 receptors prevent the hormonal and sympathoadrenal response to isolation stress and the development of stress-induced gastric ulcers (Saavedra, 2005; Saavedra et al., 2005). Angiotensin II–type receptor antagonists also prevent the pathological hypertrophy and inflammation of brain vasculature caused by genetic hypertension, and protect against experimental stroke (Ando et al., 2004; Saavedra, 2005; Zhou et al., 2005). However, angiotensin II also plays an important role in the regulation of physiological brain plasticity (see Chapter 5), and in the control of blood–brain barrier permeability (Wosik et al., 2007). Furthermore, angiotensin II type 2 receptor–deficient mice have morphological alterations in the dendritic spines and cognitive deficits (Maul et al., 2008). Thus, a disbalance in angiotensin II levels or angiotensin II signaling in the brain may be the cause of different pathological disorders.

Experimental studies have shown that gonadal hormone deficiency results in alterations in brain plasticity (see Chapter 4). For instance, ovarian hormone deprivation results in alterations in dendritic and synaptic plasticity in rodents and primates (Hao et al., 2003; Leranth et al., 2002; Witkin et al., 1991), modifications in glial plasticity (Luquin et al., 1993), and impaired neurogenesis in the adult hippocampus of rodents (Perez-Martin et al., 2003; Tanapat et al., 1999). Physiological fluctuations of ovarian hormones during the menstrual cycle in women may affect implicit memory (Maki et al., 2002), and ovarian hormone deprivation by surgical menopause may result in cognitive deficits that primarily affect verbal episodic memory (Henderson and Sherwin, 2007). Furthermore, ovarian hormone deprivation during the climacteric period may cause alterations in mood and behavior and mild cognitive impairments (Genazzani et al., 2007). These changes may be associated with plastic modifications in the human brain. Indeed, studies with proton magnetic resonance spectroscopy suggest that acute ovarian hormone suppression affects neuronal–glial membrane turnover in the dorsolateral prefrontal cortex in young women (Craig et al., 2007). In contrast, estrogen therapy appears to increase neuronal–glial membrane turnover in the brain of postmenopausal women (Robertson et al., 2001) and increase the volume of the hippocampus (Lord et al., 2008). Deprivation of testicular hormones also alter dendritic and synaptic plasticity in different regions of the central nervous system (Gomez and Newman, 1991; Kurz et al., 1986; Leranth et al., 2003); decreased levels of testosterone may result in cognitive deficits (Beauchet, 2006) and may represent a risk factor for the development of affective, cognitive, and neurodegenerative diseases in humans (Bialek et al., 2004; Gold and Voskuhl, 2006; Pike et al., 2006). Furthermore, congenital hypogonadism may cause structural alterations in the human brain, affecting cortical function (Itti et al., 2006).

Pathological alterations in the hormones that regulate energy balance, such as ghrelin (McNay, 2007) and leptin (Harvey, 2007), may also affect brain function and cognition. Animal studies indicate that leptin-deficient obese mice (ob/ob) have a reduced brain size, defective neuronal and glial maturation, increased apoptosis, and alterations in myelination and synaptic markers (Ahima et al., 1999; Bereiter and Jeanrenaud, 1979; van der Kroon and Speijers, 1979). In addition, leptin receptor-deficient rodents have spatial memory deficits (Li XL et al., 2002). Although these brain alterations may in part reflect the role of leptin on brain development, it is possible that leptin deficiency in adulthood may also have a negative impact for brain function. Indeed, leptin deficiency alters synaptic plasticity in the hypothalamus (Pinto et al., 2004).

HORMONES REGULATE PLASTICITY AND EXERT NEUROPROTECTIVE ACTIONS IN THE INJURED BRAIN

There is much evidence indicating that hormones influence the plastic cellular responses of the central nervous system after injury and neurodegeneration. Experimental studies have shown that a variety of hormones promote neuronal survival after injury of the brain or spinal cord. In addition, hormones regulate the growth and reorganization of microvasculature in damaged neural regions. Some hormones also affect the morphological and functional transformation of quiescent glial cells into reactive astroglia and reactive microglia, and the proliferation and migration of astroglia and microglia to the neurodegenerative regions. Hormonal actions on cognition and affective status after brain damage may also involve the regulation of the generation of new neurons in the hippocampus and their incorporation into functional neuronal circuits. In addition, hormones may affect the regeneration of the injured neural tissue by the modulation of the growth of neuronal processes, and the reorganization of neuronal connectivity after brain injury. Hormones may also affect the generation, proliferation, and migration of new oligodendrocytes, and the remyelination of damaged white matter regions. Finally, hormones may regulate the establishment of new functional synaptic connections and the reorganization of neuronal maps. I will now examine specific hormonal actions that may influence the remodeling of the damaged brain and spinal cord, with special emphasis on neuroprotective effects.

Peptide Hormones

Adrenomedullin, a vasodilating hormone that also produces vascular regeneration (Brain and Grant, 2004; Lopez and Martinez, 2002), has been shown to be neuroprotective after brain ischemia. Transgenic mice overproducing adrenomedullin in the liver showed reduced brain edema, neuronal loss and gliosis, an increased vascular regeneration and neurogenesis, and an improved motor function after transient middle cerebral artery occlusion. Exogenous administration of adrenomedullin had similar effects, reducing infarct area, promoting vascular regeneration, and improving neurological function (Miyashita et al., 2006).

Another peptide hormone that affects the remodeling of brain tissue under pathological conditions is corticotropin releasing hormone (CRH). CRH is a hypothalamic hormone that regulates the endocrine, autonomic, immunological, and behavioral responses to stress; actions of CRH are essential to maintain proper functioning of the stress response. In addition, CRH promotes memory and regulates synaptic plasticity in different brain regions (see Chapter 5). The finding of reduced levels of CRH in the brain and cerebrospinal fluid of patients with Alzheimer's disease and a decrease in CRH immunoreactive fibers in the brain of these patients suggests that this hormone may exert some protective effect (Bayatti and Behl, 2005). CRH neurons are also activated in depressed patients (Swaab et al., 2005). There is also evidence suggesting that CRH receptors may be involved in the response of neural tissue to experimental ischemia, although the results are contradictory in many aspects. While some studies have reported that an antagonist of CRH type 1 receptor promotes neuronal survival (Lyons et al., 1991; Strijbos et al., 1994), other studies suggest that the activation of CRH receptors is neuroprotective (Bayatti and Behl, 2005; Bayatti et al., 2003; Fox et al., 1993).

Prolactin may also regulate the response to brain injury. Its expression is increased in the neural tissue of juvenile rats affected by a hypoxic ischemic injury. The expression of prolactin after injury occurs mainly in astroglia and microglia. Administration of prolactin does not reduce neuronal damage, but promotes glial proliferation (Moderscheim et al., 2007). An important action of prolactin is to promote the generation of oligodendrocytes, and remyelination following white matter lesions (Gregg et al., 2007). In addition, effects of prolactin on neurogenesis (Shingo et al., 2003) may potentially contribute to the reparative process of the brain after injury.

Growth hormone is also involved in the regulation of neural plasticity after injury, and exerts neuroprotective actions after a hypoxic-ischemic brain injury (Gustafson et al., 1999; Scheepens et al., 2001; Shin et al., 2004). The administration of hexarelin, a growth hormone secretagogue, to seven-day-old rats that have suffered a hypoxia-ischemia brain lesion, reduces the extent of brain damage (Brywe et al., 2005a). The neuroprotective effect of hexarelin is mediated through the phosphatidylinositol 3-kinase (PI3K)/Akt pathway, via the inhibition of glycogen synthase kinase 3β (GSK3β) (Brywe et al., 2005a). In addition, growth hormone reduces cognitive deficits (Ramsey et al., 2004; Thornton et al., 2000), promotes the growth of brain microvessels (Sonntag et al., 1997), and reduces neuronal loss (Azcoitia et al., 2005) in the aged rat brain. These effects of growth hormone may be exerted directly on growth hormone receptors expressed by brain cells (Scheepens et al., 2001), and may also in part mediated by increasing the levels of IGF-I, a very potent neuroprotective hormone. IGF-I is important for brain development and plasticity (see Chapters 5 and 6), promotes neuronal survival, and inhibits neuronal apoptosis in vitro and in vivo in a variety of experimental models of neurodegeneration (Åberg et al., 2006; Carro et al., 2003; Trejo et al., 2004). In vivo, IGF-I has also been shown to be a neuroprotective factor against a variety of neurodegenerative conditions, including hypoxic-ischemic brain injury (Guan et al., 1993, 2003), excitotoxicity (Azcoitia et al., 1999b; Carro et al., 2001), and cerebellar ataxia (Fernandez et al., 1998, 1999, 2005). Effects of IGF-I on synaptic plasticity, adult hippocampal neurogenesis, and local brain-derived neurotrophic factor (BDNF) formation in the brain (see Chapter 5) may contribute to its neuroprotective activity. IGF-I neuroprotective effects are exerted by the activation of the main intracellular signaling pathways associated with IGF-I receptors, the mitogen-activated protein kinase/extracellular signal-regulated kinases (MAPK/ERK), and the PI3K/Akt pathways (Guan et al., 2003). In particular, the inhibition of GSK3β activity, which is downstream of the PI3K/Akt pathway, seems to be an essential step in the neuroprotective mechanism (Brywe et al., 2005b). In addition, IGF-I may interact with other hormones, such as erythropoietin and estradiol, to promote neuroprotection (Digicaylioglu et al., 2004; Garcia-Segura et al., 2006; Mendez et al., 2006). Besides preventing neuronal death, IGF-I protects white matter and promotes the formation of new oligodendrocytes (Åberg et al., 2007; Chesik et al., 2007; Guan et al., 2003). This is very important in cases of human stroke where the main injury is usually in the white matter, and for other pathologies involving demyelination, such as multiple sclerosis.

An important question to consider is the role of local versus systemic IGF-I in the regulation of brain plasticity under neurodegenerative conditions. As we have seen in Chapter 5, IGF-I is both a growth factor locally produced in the brain, and a hormone produced in the liver in response to growth hormone signaling. Both local and hormonal IGF-I appear to be involved in endogenous neuroprotective mechanisms. The expression of different molecular components of the IGF-I system, including IGF-I, IGFBP-2, and IGFBP-3, increase in the brain after a neurodegenerative stimuli (Beilharz et al., 1998; Chung et al., 2003; Garcia-Estrada et al., 1992; Hwang et al., 2004). This has been interpreted as an endogenous local neuroprotective response of neural tissue. In addition to the neuroprotective actions of locally produced IGF-I, there is extensive evidence indicating that hormonal IGF-I plays a major role in the prevention of neurodegeneration. Indeed, peripheral administration of IGF-I is neuroprotective (Fernandez et al., 1999), indicating that peripheral IGF-I may enter the brain to exert neuroprotection. Furthermore, the work of Eva Carro and her collaborators in the laboratory of Ignacio Torres-Aleman has unquestionably shown that endogenous circulating IGF-I is neuroprotective and mediates the neuroprotective effects of exercise: when the passage of IGF-I into the brain is blocked, exercise is no longer neuroprotective (Carro et al., 2001, 2006). Finally, the importance of serum IGF-I for brain function has also been demonstrated by the studies of Jose Luis Trejo and collaborators, which showed that mice with low-serum IGF-I levels (due to specific, targeted disruption of the IGF-I gene in the liver) presented cognitive deficits, disrupted long-term synaptic potentiation in the hippocampus, and reduced the density of glutamatergic synaptic terminals in the hippocampus. Chronic systemic IGF-I administration to IGF-I–deficient mice ameliorated the cognitive alterations and impaired synaptic plasticity, and restored the density of glutamatergic synapses (Trejo et al., 2008). Therefore, liver-derived circulating IGF-I seems to play a major role in the regulation of brain plasticity; deficits in serum levels of IGF-I may contribute to the development of brain pathological alterations, as we have seen earlier in this chapter.

The hormone erythropoietin, in addition to being involved in the regulation of erythropoiesis, has many neuroprotective actions. These include promoting the survival of septal cholinergic neurons and learning improvement in adult rats which had undergone fimbria-fornix transections (Konishi et al., 1993; Mala et al., 2005; Mogensen et al., 2004). Erythropoietin also plays an important role in the protection of neurons and prevention of cognitive impairment after ischemia (Bernaudin et al., 1999; Catania et al., 2002; Junk et al., 2002; Sadamoto et al., 1998; Sakanaka et al., 1998; Siren et al., 2001), and is an essential mediator of protection in hypoxic-ischemic preconditioning (Malhotra et al., 2006; Prass et al., 2003). Another characterized action of erythropoietin with important clinical implications is its ability to reduce damage in experimental autoimmune encephalomyelitis models in mice (Li et al., 2004; Zhang J et al., 2005). Many other neuroprotective actions of erythropoietin have been described, including the prevention of retinal ganglion cell death after an axotomy (Kilic Ü et al., 2005), the promotion of retinal ganglion cell axonal regeneration (King et al., 2007), the protection of the spinal cord and brain from traumatic injury (Gorio et al., 2002; Siren et al., 2006; Verdonck et al., 2007; Yatsiv et al., 2005), and the reduction of cell death after an experimental intracerebral hemorrhage (Lee et al., 2006). This impressive list of neuroprotective actions suggests that erythropoietin is a promising candidate for neuroprotective therapies. Indeed, recent clinical studies have shown that erythropoietin therapy ameliorates cognition in chronic schizophrenic patients (Ehrenreich et al., 2007). Further clinical trials should determine the extent of the neuroprotective activity of this hormone.

The neuroprotective effects of erythropoietin may be mediated by multiple mechanisms, including (i) the decrease of nitric oxide formation (Calapai et al., 2000; Genc et al., 2006); (ii) the increase of the expression of growth factors, such as BDNF (Viviani et al., 2005; Zhang et al., 2006); (iii) the inhibition of neuronal apoptosis (Celik et al., 2002; Chong et al., 2002, 2003; Digicaylioglu and Lipton, 2001; Siren et al., 2001; Villa et al., 2003; Wen et al., 2002); (iv) the enhancement of neurogenesis (Lu et al., 2005; Shingo et al., 2001); (v) the decrease in excitotoxic glutamate release (Kawakami et al., 2001); and (vi) the down-regulation of microglia activation, cytokine production, and inflammation (Chong et al., 2003; Genc et al., 2006; Villa et al., 2003). Furthermore, the endogenous production of erythropoietin and the expression of erythropoietin receptors are increased in the brain after reduced oxygenation (Bernaudin et al., 1999, 2000; Marti et al., 1996). The induction of the erythropoietin system in the brain after ischemia follows a precise time course with cellular specificity: erythropoietin and its receptor are induced first (within one day) in endothelial cells, then by day three in microglia/macrophage cells, and finally, one week after ischemia, in reactive astrocytes (Bernaudin et al., 1999, 2000). This precise induction of the erythropoietin system in the brain may represent an endogenous mechanism to protect neural tissue from damage after a reduction in blood flow (Bernaudin et al., 1999, 2000; Kilic E et al., 2005).

There is also evidence indicating that hormones involved in the regulation of energy homeodynamics and food intake exert protective actions in the brain against different neurodegenerative stimuli. In mice, leptin has been shown to prevent excitotoxic brain damage in vivo and excitotoxic-induced neuronal loss in vitro (Dicou et al., 2001), and reduces brain infarct volume induced by middle cerebral artery occlusion (Zhang F et al., 2007). In addition, leptin prevents neuronal death induced by oxygen-glucose deprivation in rat primary cultures of the cerebral cortex (Zhang F et al., 2007). Janus kinase/STAT, MAPK, and PI3K/Akt have been identified as signaling molecules involved in the neuroprotective effect of leptin in neuroblastoma cells (Lu et al., 2006; Russo et al., 2004). Ghrelin also exerts protective and antiapoptotic effects in the brain. Chronic systemic treatment of male rats with growth-hormone-releasing peptide-6, an agonist of the ghrelin receptor, increases antiapoptotic signaling and reduces cell death in different brain regions. In addition, growth-hormone-releasing peptide-6 inhibits the activation of caspases and apoptotic cell death in the hypothalamus and cerebellum induced by the administration of monosodium glutamate (Delgado-Rubin de Celix et al., 2006), and reduces apoptosis in the cerebellum of aged rats (Paneda et al., 2003). These protective effects may be, at least in part, mediated by an increase in the brain levels of IGF-I (Frago et al., 2002). The administration of ghrelin has also been shown to be neuroprotective, reducing apoptosis in experimental models of cerebral ischemia (Miao et al., 2007). Glucagon-like peptide-1

(GLP-1), which is involved in the regulation of glucose homeodynamics and food intake, also has neuroprotective properties, preventing neuronal damage induced by excitotoxicity, oxidative stress, and β-amyloid (During et al., 2003; Perry and Greig, 2003; Perry et al., 2003), and GLP-1 agonists reverse the impairment in long-term synaptic potentiation induced in the hippocampus by β-amyloid (Gault and Hölscher, 2008).

Melatonin and Thyroid Hormones

Melatonin has been reported to protect neurons from apoptosis (Cagnoli et al., 1995; Feng et al., 2004), excitotoxicity (Chung and Han, 2003; Espinar et al., 2000; Giusti et al., 1996; Skaper et al., 1998; Vega-Naredo et al., 2005), traumatic brain injury (Mesenge et al., 1998), and transient cerebral ischemia (Lee et al., 2005; Sun et al., 2002), among other brain insults. The hormone also protects white matter from excitotoxicity (Husson et al., 2002), reduces motoneuron death after a sciatic nerve transection (Rogerio et al., 2002), and exerts some protection in experimental models of Parkinson's and Alzheimer's diseases (Feng et al., 2004; Sharma et al., 2006). Melatonin has also been proposed as a potential treatment for amyotrophic lateral sclerosis (Jacob et al., 2002; Weishaupt et al., 2006). The neuroprotective effects of melatonin are accompanied by the prevention of behavioral deficits associated with brain injury. For instance, treatment of male rats with melatonin after a global cerebral ischemia prevents cognitive deficits induced by the ischemic episode. Melatonin ameliorates hippocampal-dependent place learning (assessed in the Morris water maze), and working memory (assessed with the eight-arm Olton radial maze). In addition, melatonin treatment reduces neuronal loss in the hippocampal formation (CA1, CA2, CA3, and the dentate gyrus) induced by ischemia (Letechipia-Vallejo et al., 2007). These neuroprotective effects of melatonin are associated with a plastic remodeling of dendrites and dendritic spines in hippocampal pyramidal neurons (González-Burgos et al., 2007). Actions of melatonin on glial cell remodeling after injury may also be involved in neuroprotective effects. Melatonin enhances the survival of astrocytes after an ischemia induced by the occlusion of the middle cerebral artery (Borlongan et al., 2000), and decreases astrocytic hypertrophy in the spinal cord associated with a motoneuron axotomy (Rogerio et al., 2002). In addition, melatonin inhibits microglia activation in the hippocampus after kainic acid administration (Chung and Han, 2003).

Thyroid hormones also affect brain remodeling after injury. Treatment with triiodothyronine stimulates axonal regeneration in the cerebral cortex and corpus callosum after a stab wound injury, and promotes wound healing (Heinicke, 1977). Furthermore, there is substantial evidence indicating that thyroid hormone promotes axonal regeneration in damaged peripheral nerves (Barakat-Walter, 1999; Barakat-Walter et al., 2007). Another important aspect of thyroid hormone in the regulation of neural remodeling after injury is its essential role in the maturation of oligodendrocytes. This thyroid hormone action suggests that it may contribute to central nervous system remyelination in different pathological conditions, including multiple sclerosis (Calzà et al., 2005; D'Intino et al., 2006). Indeed, experimental evidence indicates that thyroid hormone enhances and accelerates remyelination in experimental models of chronic demyelination (Fernandez et al., 2004b).

Steroid Hormones

Glucocorticoids

As mentioned in Chapter 3, glucocorticoid and mineralocorticoid receptors have opposite roles regarding neuronal survival. While the sustained activation of glucocorticoid receptors may result in brain functional impairment, mineralocorticoid receptors appear to be neuroprotective. Mice overexpressing mineralocorticoid receptors in the forebrain show a reduced neuronal death after a transient cerebral global ischemia, and have better spatial memory retention and reduced anxiety compared to normal mice (Lai et al., 2007). In addition to affecting neurogenesis, neuronal survival, and synaptic plasticity, the effects of glucocorticoids in the damaged brain may in part be related with the regulation of glial plasticity. Glucocorticoids influence the metabolism of glutamate in astrocytes, increasing the expression of both glutamine synthetase and glutamate dehydrogenase in astrocytes (Hardin-Pouzet et al., 1996; Vardimon et al., 1999). Glucocorticoids may also be detrimental to reactive astrocytes by mechanisms involving the depletion of intracellular ATP levels and deterioration of mitochondrial transmembrane potentials (Shin et al., 2001). In addition, glucocorticoids decrease microglia proliferation in response to hippocampal deafferentation (Woods et al., 1999), and cortisol represses the inflammatory induction of nitric oxide production in primary cultured microglia and transformed N9 microglial cells (Drew and Chavis, 2000a). These antiinflammatory actions of glucocorticoids on glial cells may represent a positive protective response and a better functional brain recovery after an acute injury. Therefore, the regulation of glial gene expression and plasticity by glucocorticoids after brain injury in part may represent an adaptive response to restore homeodynamics. Glial responses to glucocorticoids may be involved in the regulation of neuronal apoptosis and adult hippocampal neurogenesis, promoting brain repair after neurodegeneration (Nichols et al., 2005). However, under some circumstances glucocorticoids may have the opposite effects. Thus, stress-induced elevated levels of glucocorticoids activate microglia in vivo and may induce a proinflammatory response in the brain (Nair and Bonneau, 2006). In addition, glucocorticoids decrease the proliferation of oligodendrocyte precursors (Alonso, 2000) and the expression of myelin basic protein in oligodendrocytes (Melcangi et al., 1997); therefore, glucocorticoids may affect the process of myelination and remyelination after brain injury, or in demyelination diseases. The actions of glucocorticoids on glial cells are also important for their effect on peripheral nerve remodeling after injury or degeneration. For instance, glucocorticoids modulate glutamate metabolism and myelin formation by Schwann cells, enhancing the expression of glutamine synthetase and cytosolic aspartate aminotransferase (Grenier et al., 2005), and stimulating the activity of the promoters of peripheral myelin protein-22 (PMP22) and myelin protein zero (P0) genes (Désarnaud et al., 2000).

Dehydroepiandrosterone

The adrenal steroid dehydroepiandrosterone (DHEA) is another hormonal factor that regulates the plastic responses of neural tissue to injury. After transection of a rat sciatic nerve, treatment with DHEA reduces the extent of denervation atrophy (as evaluated by gastrochemius muscle weight), and induced an earlier onset of axonal regeneration (as confirmed by the increase of myelinated axons) of larger average fiber diameter and greater axonal cross-sectional areas in the proximal, middle, and distal sections (Ayhan et al., 2003). Moreover, this hormone is also able to enhance the functional recovery following a crush injury of a rat sciatic nerve. Thus, in this experimental model, DHEA induces a faster return to normal values of sciatic function index (determined by walking track analysis), and an increase in the number of myelinated fibers and fiber diameters (Gudemez et al., 2002). DHEA has also been shown to reduce sciatic nerve functional impairment in diabetic rats (Yorek et al., 2002). In vitro, DHEA protects cells of the clonal mouse hippocampal cell line HT22 against the excitatory amino acid glutamate (Cardounel et al., 1999), as well as primary hippocampal cultured neurons against the neurotoxic actions of AMPA and kainic acid (Kimonides et al., 1998). In vivo, DHEA protects hippocampal pyramidal neurons against unilateral infusions of N-methyl-D-aspartic acid (NMDA) (Kimonides et al., 1998), or systemic administration of kainic acid (Veiga et al., 2003). DHEA and its sulfate derivative have been shown to protect neurons from other degenerative stimuli as well, including neurotoxic effects of corticosterone, oxidative stress, ischemia, and amyloid-β protein toxicity (Bastianetto et al., 1999; Bologa et al., 1987; Cardounel et al., 1999; Kaasik et al., 2001; Kimonides et al., 1999; Lapchak et al., 2000; Li et al., 2001; Tomas-Camardiel et al., 2002). Furthermore, DHEA displays memory-enhancing properties (Flood et al., 1992; Vallée et al., 2001) and increases adult neurogenesis in the hippocampus of rodents (Karishma and Herbert, 2002).

DHEA may exert neuroprotection through different mechanisms. These may include antioxidative effects (Aragno et al., 2000), the modulation of GABA$_A$, NMDA, and sigma-1 receptors (Bergeron et al., 1996; Maurice et al., 2001), the down-regulation of glucocorticoid receptors (Cardounel et al., 1999), and the regulation of protein kinase C signaling (Racchi et al., 2001). In addition, DHEA regulates reactive gliosis, decreasing the formation of reactive astroglia (Garcia-Estrada et al., 1999; Hoyk et al., 2004), and reduces the inflammatory response of reactive astroglia and reactive microglia (Barger et al., 2000; Kipper-Galperin et al., 1999; Tomas-Camardiel et al., 2002; Wang et al., 2001). For instance, DHEA inhibits the production of nitric oxide by microglia (Barger et al., 2000), and the production of tumor necrosis factor α

and interleukin-6 by astrocytes (Kipper-Galperin et al., 1999). DHEA could also act as a precursor of sex steroid hormones and exert neuroprotective actions through these molecules (see below).

Sex Steroids

Sex steroids are potent modulators of neural plasticity under pathological conditions. The brain's response to injury and the incidence of neurodegenerative diseases and affective disorders is different among men and women (Azcoitia et al., 2002; Garcia-Segura et al., 2001; Leung and Chue, 2000; Stein, 2007). Premenopausal women have fewer strokes than men of the same age; however, after menopause, the incidence of stroke increases in women. Pregnancy and childbirth are also associated with an increased risk of stroke. In addition, women have different types of strokes. Subarachnoid hemorrhages occur with higher frequency in women than in men. Sex differences are also observed in neurodegenerative diseases. For instance, gender discrepancies in incidence, symptoms, and medication effects have been detected for Parkinson's disease. The incidence of Alzheimer's disease is higher in postmenopausal women than in men of the same age. Men are less susceptible to multiple sclerosis than women, and the disease activity decreases during late pregnancy. Sex differences in the age of onset and the severity and type of symptoms are also observed for schizophrenia, which generally occurs slightly later in women and, until menopause, has a less severe course in women than in men. Moreover, although the peak age of onset for schizophrenia is generally late adolescence to early adulthood in both men and women, a second cohort of women develop schizophrenia at the onset of menopause. Depression, anxiety, and eating disorders affect many more women than men. In contrast, alcoholism and antisocial personality are more common in men. All these examples suggest that the brain of women and men have different susceptibilities to pathological alterations, and different capacities to cope with these alterations. In agreement with the observations in humans, animal studies have also detected sex differences in the outcome of brain injury. Thus, in several experimental neural lesion models, male animals are more vulnerable than female animals. For instance, female rats have better stroke outcomes after vascular occlusion than males (Alkayed et al., 1998; Zhang et al., 1998), while male rats show stronger memory deficits after entorhinal cortex lesions than females (Roof et al., 1993a). Sex differences have also been observed in striatal dopaminergic neurotoxicity in mice (Miller et al., 1998). Two neurotoxicants tested, 1-methyl-4-phenyl-1,2,3,6-tetrahydropyridine (MPTP) and methamphetamine, resulted in a greater dopamine depletion in males than in females (Miller et al., 1998; Yu and Wagner, 1994). In females, the outcome after a brain injury depends on the hormonal fluctuations during the estrus and menstrual cycle (Azcoitia et al., 1999a; Datla et al., 2003; Hortnagl et al., 1993; Stein, 2007). Sex differences have also been detected in experimental animals in anxiety and emotional learning (Toufexis et al., 2006). Sex differences in the outcome of a brain injury suggest a regulatory role of neural tissue remodeling by gonadal hormones under pathological conditions. Next, is an examination of the neuroplastic actions of gonadal hormones under conditions of neural degeneration and injury.

Progesterone

Protective and regenerative effects of progesterone have been well characterized in experimental models of degeneration occurring after physical injury of peripheral nerves. The possible beneficial effect of progesterone for the treatment of peripheral neuropathy was first suggested by Koenig and colleagues in the laboratory of Étienne Émile Baulieu, who demonstrated that progesterone, when given locally, is able to counteract the decrease of myelin membranes amounts induced by a cryolesion in the sciatic nerve of the mouse (Baulieu and Schumacher, 2000; Koenig et al., 1995). Successive studies in the laboratory of Roberto C. Melcangi in Milan showed that, in an experimental model of sciatic nerve transection, the treatment with progesterone is also able to modulate the expression of the myelin proteins P0 and PMP22. Indeed, the treatment with progesterone or its metabolite 5α-dihydroprogesterone significantly increases the low P0 mRNA levels present in the distal portion from the cut (Melcangi et al, 2000a). These effects have also been detected in rat Schwann cell cultures (Désarnaud et al., 1998; Magnaghi et al., 2001; Melcangi 2000a, b). In the same models, the gene expression of PMP22 is influenced only by 3α,5α-tetrahydroprogesterone, a metabolite of dihydroprogesterone (Melcangi et al., 1999b). Progesterone also stimulates the expression of the transcription factor Krox-20, which plays an important role in the myelination of peripheral nerves, as well as other transcriptions expressed by Schwann cells, such as Krox-24, Egr3, and FosB, that may be involved in the initiation of myelination (Guennoun et al., 2001; Magnaghi et al., 2007; Mercier et al., 2001; Schumacher et al. 2001). Protective and regenerative effects of progesterone have been characterized in several experimental models of peripheral nerve injury (Chavez-Delgado et al., 2005; Leonelli et al., 2006; Melcangi et al., 2003, 2005), and the hormone has been shown to prevent myelin structural and functional abnormalities induced by experimental diabetes in the sciatic nerve of rats (Leonelli et al., 2007; Veiga et al., 2006).

   Progesterone has neuroprotective properties in different experimental models of central nervous system neurodegeneration, including colchicine-induced hippocampal damage (Vongher and Frye, 1999), brain and spinal cord excitotoxicity (Ciriza et al., 2006; Hoffman et al., 2003; Ogata et al., 1993), traumatic brain injury (Asbury et al., 1998; Djebaili et al., 2004, 2005; Grossman et al., 2004; Robertson et al., 2006; Roof et al., 1994, 1996, 1997; Shear et al., 2002; Stein, 2005), cerebral ischemia (Cervantes et al., 2002; Chen et al., 1999; Gibson and Murphy, 2004; Kumon et al., 2000; Morali et al., 2005; Murphy et al., 2002; Sayeed et al., 2007), experimental Parkinson's disease (Callier et al., 2001), spinal cord trauma (Labombarda et al., 2002; Thomas et al., 1999), spinal cord motoneuron disease (Gonzalez Deniselle et al., 2002, 2005), motoneuron axotomy (Yu, 1989), and experimental autoimmune encephalomyelitis (Garay et al., 2007). The mechanisms involved in the neuroprotective effects of progesterone are still not completely understood. However, it is known that the hormone has antioxidant properties (Roof et al., 1997), elicits the activation of intracellular signaling pathways involved in the promotion of cell survival (Nilsen and Brinton, 2002b, 2003b; Singh, 2001, 2005), promotes the expression of growth factors such as BDNF (De Nicola et al., 2006; Gonzalez et al., 2004, 2005; Gonzalez Deniselle et al., 2007), increases the expression of antiapoptotic molecules such as Bcl-2 and Bcl-X$_L$ (Nilsen and Brinton, 2002b; Yao et al., 2005), and reduces the expression of proapoptotic molecules such as BAX, BAD, and caspase-3 (Djebaili et al., 2005; Yao et al., 2005). Glial cells may also be involved in the neuroprotective effects of progesterone. Glial cells express progesterone receptors (Labombarda et al., 2000), and brain injury induces the expression of the membrane-associated progesterone-binding protein 25-Dx in astrocytes (Meffre et al., 2005). Progesterone reduces reactive astrogliosis (Djebaili et al., 2005; Garcia-Estrada et al., 1993, 1999) and the expression of aquaporin-4 by astrocytes (Guo et al., 2006) after a brain injury, and may decrease brain edema acting on astrocytes (Guo et al., 2006; Meffre et al., 2005). Progesterone may also promote neuroprotection by regulating the inflammatory activity of microglia (Drew and Chavis, 2000b). In addition, progesterone increases the density of oligodendrocyte progenitors in the injured spinal cord (De Nicola et al., 2006; Labombarda et al., 2006a), the proliferation of oligodendrocyte precursors in organotypic slice cultures of cerebellum (Ghoumari et al., 2005), and the cellular branching of oligodendrocyte progenitors in primary cultures (Marin-Husstege et al., 2004). Furthermore, the hormone promotes myelination, remyelination, and the expression of myelin proteins in the central nervous system (Garay et al., 2007, 2008; Ghoumari et al., 2003; Jung-Testas et al., 1996; Schumacher et al., 2004, 2007).

Some of the neuroprotective effects of progesterone may be mediated by the activation of classical progestin receptors, which are widely expressed in the brain (Guerra-Araiza et al., 2003). However, the hormone may also exert neuroprotection by mechanisms independent of the classical progestin receptor (VanLandingham et al., 2006) via membrane progestin receptors (Zhu et al., 2003) or by the membrane-associated progesterone-binding protein 25-Dx (Guennoun et al., 2008; Labombarda et al., 2003; Meffre et al., 2005). Furthermore, reduced metabolites of progesterone, such as tetrahydroprogesterone, may exert rapid membrane effects by the modulation of the GABA$_A$ receptor complex (Belelli and Lambert, 2005; Follesa et al., 2001; Lambert et al., 2003). In the central nervous system, progesterone is rapidly metabolized into dihydroprogesterone, which is subsequently further reduced to tetrahydroprogesterone (Mellon et al., 2001; Stoffel-Wagner et al., 1998). These conversions are catalyzed by the enzymes 5α-reductase and 3α-hydroxysteroid dehydrogenase, respectively (Mellon et al., 2001). This latter enzyme can either reduce dihydroprogesterone to tetrahydroprogesterone or oxidize tetrahydroprogesterone back to dihydroprogesterone (Celotti et al.,

1992; Mellon et al., 2001). It has been shown that endogenous regulation of dihydroprogesterone and tetrahydroprogesterone production in the spinal cord is involved in the control of neuronal communication in the nociceptive circuits (Patte-Mensah et al., 2005). Similar regulation of dihydroprogesterone and tetrahydroprogesterone formation may be involved in the control of different brain functions and behavior (Matsumoto et al., 2005; Petralia et al., 2005; Walf et al., 2006). Progesterone metabolism also seems to be involved in the neuroprotective effects of the hormone, since both dihydroprogesterone and tetrahydroprogesterone have been shown to exert similar neuroprotective effects to progesterone (Ciriza et al., 2004a, 2006; Djebaili et al., 2004, 2005; Frank and Sagratella, 2000; Frye, 1995; Frye and Scalise, 2000; He et al., 2004; Lockhart et al., 2002; Rhodes and Frye, 2004; Rhodes et al., 2004; Sayeed et al., 2006), including the down-regulation of reactive gliosis (Ciriza et al., 2004a). In addition, the pharmacological inhibition of progesterone metabolism abolishes the neuroprotective effect of the hormone (Ciriza et al., 2006; Rhodes et al., 2004). The administration of the 5α-reductase inhibitor finasteride reduces the increase in plasma and hippocampal levels of dihydroprogesterone and tetrahydroprogesterone after progesterone administration to ovariectomized rats, and prevents the neuroprotective effect of progesterone in the hippocampus of ovariectomized rats injected with the excitotoxin kainic acid (Ciriza et al., 2006). Furthermore, the inhibitor of 3α-hydroxysteroid dehydrogenase, indomethacin, blocks the neuroprotective and anti-gliotic effects of both dihydroprogesterone and tetrahydroprogesterone, suggesting that both metabolites are necessary for the neuroprotective actions of progesterone (Ciriza et al., 2006). Dihydroprogesterone and tetrahydroprogesterone may exert complementary effects that contribute to neuroprotection. Dihydroprogesterone, which is neuroprotective at low concentrations (Ciriza et al., 2004a), may act on progestin receptors (Melcangi et al., 1999; Rupprecht et al., 1993) and may affect progesterone-receptor-mediated transcription of neuroprotective genes (Djebaili et al., 2005; Nilsen and Brinton, 2002b; Yao et al., 2005). Tetrahydroprogesterone, which is neuroprotective at high concentrations (Ciriza et al., 2004a), is an allosteric agonist of $GABA_A$ receptors (Lambert et al., 2003; Majewska, 1992; Puia et al., 1990); this interaction may contribute to the neuroprotective effects of progesterone (Frye and Scalise, 2000; Melcangi et al., 2001). The enzyme 3α-hydroxysteroid dehydrogenase may regulate the optimal levels of both metabolites in the brain.

The role of progesterone metabolism in the neuroprotective and anti-gliotic effects of the hormone is highly relevant for hormone therapy in humans using synthetic progestins. For instance, in contrast to the neuroprotective effects of progesterone, the synthetic progestin medroxyprogesterone acetate (MPA, Provera) used in hormonal therapy in postmenopausal women, in clinical studies such as the Women's Health Initiative of the NIH (Maki, 2005), and as a widely used female contraceptive (Hapgood et al., 2004), is unable to prevent gliosis and neuronal loss in the hilus of animals injected with kainic acid (Ciriza et al., 2006). Furthermore, while progesterone and estradiol protect hippocampal neurons in culture against glutamate toxicity, MPA is not neuroprotective; it reduces the protective effects of estradiol and blocks estrogen-induced over-expression of the antiapoptotic molecule Bcl-2 (Nilsen and Brinton, 2002a). In addition, both estradiol and progesterone exert a potentiation of glutamate-mediated rises in intracellular calcium in neurons, while MPA blocks the effect of estradiol (Nilsen and Brinton, 2002b). Furthermore, MPA decreases the neuroprotective effect of oral conjugated estrogens in the subcortical brain regions after experimental stroke in rats (Littleton-Kearney et al., 2005). Among other possible causes for the different treatments outcomes with progesterone and MPA are their different effects on the levels of active progesterone metabolites, since the administration of progesterone significantly increases plasma and hippocampal dihydroprogesterone and tetrahydroprogesterone levels, while MPA does not (Ciriza et al., 2006). The finding that both dihydroprogesterone and tetrahydroprogesterone are necessary for the neuroprotective effect of progesterone may in part explain why MPA, which cannot be converted into dihydroprogesterone or tetrahydroprogesterone, has no neuroprotective effects. In addition, MPA inhibits the enzyme 3α-hydroxysteroid dehydrogenase, involved in the reversible conversion between dihydroprogesterone and tetrahydroprogesterone; therefore, it may affect the local actions of dihydroprogesterone and tetrahydroprogesterone in the brain (Belelli and Herd, 2003). Other differences in the mechanisms of action of progesterone and MPA, including the action of MPA on androgen receptors (Bentel et al., 1999) and glucocorticoid receptors (Wiegratz and Kuhl, 2004), may also contribute to their different effects on neuronal survival.

Estradiol and Estrogens

The effects of estradiol on neuronal plasticity after a brain injury are well documented. Since the pioneering work of Matsumoto and Arai (1979), it has been shown that estradiol may promote synaptic sprouting in response to injury. These authors tested the effect of estradiol in the arcuate nucleus after deafferentation, a treatment that results in a loss of axodendritic synapses. Treatment with estradiol benzoate for three weeks (beginning on the day of surgery) effectively restored the axodendritic synaptic population of the deafferented arcuate nucleus in adult ovariectomized rats (Matsumoto and Arai, 1979, 1981). Further studies showed that the arcuate nucleus of aged female rats still retains plasticity to react to deafferentation under the influence of estrogen (Matsumoto et al., 1985). Other studies have shown that estrogen enhances synaptic sprouting in the hippocampus of ovariectomized female rats after entorhinal cortex lesions (Morse et al., 1986, 1992), and that estrogen accelerates the regeneration rates of axotomized facial motoneurons (Islamov et al., 2002; Tanzer and Jones, 1997). Estradiol may influence synaptic sprouting by regulating the expression or activity of a variety of molecules that participate in the process of axonal growth and axonal target recognition, including cytoskeletal components, adhesion and guidance molecules, and soluble factors, such as growth factors and neurotrophins. Estradiol induces the expression of the microtubule-associated protein tau in axons (Diaz et al., 1992; Ferreira and Caceres, 1991; Lorenzo et al., 1992), and regulates tau phosphorylation in the brain (Alvarez-de-la-Rosa et al., 2005; Cardona-Gomez et al., 2004; Goodenough et al., 2005); this may result in the stabilization of microtubules and the promotion of axonal growth. Another molecule that may be involved in estrogen-induced axonal regeneration is GAP43, a presynaptic protein implicated in the growth and regeneration of axons (Oestreicher et al., 1997). The expression of GAP43 is modulated by estrogen in the mediobasal hypothalamus of adult rats (Lustig et al., 1991), in the preoptic area of developing, adult, and aged rats (Shughrue and Dorsa, 1993; Singer et al., 1996a), and in the medial septum and vertical limb of the diagonal band of Broca in aged rats (Ferrini et al., 2002).

Apolipoprotein E (ApoE) may also participate in the effect of estrogen on synaptic sprouting. ApoE is involved in lipid and cholesterol metabolism, and in the mobilization and reutilization of lipid in the repair, growth, and maintenance of myelin and axonal membranes (both during development and after injury). Furthermore, the epsilon 4 allele of ApoE has a direct impact on the cholinergic function in Alzheimer's disease (Poirier, 1994), and is a risk factor for the development of age-related chronic neurological diseases (Struble et al., 2007). The synthesis of ApoE is dramatically increased after an injury of peripheral nerves (Ignatius et al., 1986; LeBlanc and Poduslo, 1990), and in the central nervous system (Poirier, 1994). Although nerve regeneration may occur in ApoE-deficient mice (de Chaves et al., 1997; Popko et al., 1993), these animals show increased central neuronal damage after a cerebral ischemia and other forms of cerebral injury (Chen Y et al., 1997; Horsburgh et al., 1999; Sheng et al., 1999), suggesting that ApoE is a factor involved in brain repair. Stone and associates (1997, 1998) have shown that estrogen enhances ApoE expression by astroglia and microglia, and that it induces synaptic sprouting in response to an entorhinal cortex lesion in wild-type mice, not ApoE-knockout mice. Furthermore, synaptic sprouting is increased by estrogen in the same regions where sprouting is dependent on ApoE (Teter et al., 1999). ApoE has been also shown to be involved in the effects of estradiol on axonal growth in vitro (Nathan et al., 2004). There is also evidence that ApoE is involved in the neuroprotective actions of estradiol against a cerebral ischemia (Horsburgh et al., 2002). Different ApoE alleles affect the neuroprotective and neuroplastic actions of estradiol. For instance, the antiinflammatory effects of the hormone are reduced in microglia from mice with the ApoE4 genotype compared to microglia from ApoE3 mice (Brown et al., 2008). In addition, estradiol enhances long-term synaptic potentiation in the dentate gyrus of mice expressing the human ApoE allele, but does not affect long-term synaptic potentiation mice expressing human ApoE3 (Yun et al., 2007). In agreement with these experimental findings, different ApoE alleles seem to determine the neuroprotective outcome of estrogen therapy in humans (Burkhardt et al., 2004; Struble et al., 2007; Wang et al., 2006; Yaffe et al., 2000).

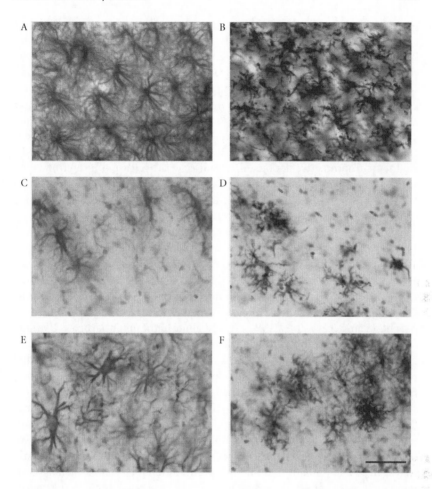

Figure 9.1. Hormonal regulation of reactive gliosis after brain injury. Immuno-reactivity for vimentin, a marker of reactive astrocytes (panels A, C, E) and for major histocompatibility complex-II (MHC-II), a marker of reactive microglia (panels B, D, F) in the CA1 stratum radiatum of the hippocampus at a distance of approximately 100–200 μm from the lateral border of a stab wound. The panels illustrate representative examples from orchidectomized rats after the administration of vehicle (A, B), testosterone (C, D), or estradiol (E, F) on days 0, 1 and 2 after injury. Both testosterone and estradiol reduce reactive gliosis. All figures are at the same magnification. Scale bar, 50 μm. (Courtesy of Dr. George Barreto. Based on Barreto et al., 2007.)

Another important action of estradiol on the remodeling of neural tissue under pathological conditions is the regulation of the plastic modifications of glial cells (Fig. 9.1). The effect of estradiol on astroglia differs depending on whether it is acting under physiological or pathological conditions. Thus, estradiol increases glial fibrillary acidic protein (GFAP) expression and promotes the extension of GFAP immunoreactive processes under physiological conditions, while the hormone decreases GFAP and vimentin expression in gliotic injured tissue (Ciriza et al., 2004b; Garcia-Estrada et al., 1999; Hoyk et al., 2004). For instance, estradiol decreases astrocyte proliferation and glial scar formation after a stab wound injury in the cerebral cortex and hippocampus (Barreto et al., 2007; Garcia-Estrada et al., 1993, 1999), decreases reactive astrogliosis in the hippocampus after kainic acid administration (Ciriza et al., 2004b), and decreases proliferation and increases cell death in primary cortical astrocytic cultures (Zhang et al., 2002). In addition, astrocytes may mediate the neuroprotective actions of estradiol by the release of growth factors, such as transforming growth factor β1 (TGF-β1), in response to the steroid (Dhandapani et al., 2005; Sortino et al., 2004). Furthermore, as mentioned earlier, estradiol increases the expression of ApoE in astrocytes; this may contribute to the reorganization of brain tissue after an injury (Stone et al., 1997, 1998). Estradiol also increases the expression of heat shock proteins in astrocytes (Mydlarski et al., 1995), an effect that has been observed in striatal astrocytes after global ischemia in gerbils (Lu et al., 2002), and may be related to the protective effects of the hormone in animal models of brain ischemia. Estradiol increases glutamate uptake in astrocytes derived from Alzheimer's patients (Liang et al., 2002). This may contribute to the potential protective hormonal effect against this neurodegenerative disease, in which the extracellular glutamate concentration appears to be increased. On the other hand, estradiol regulation of the expression of aquaporin-4 by astrocytes may reduce brain edema, and may contribute to the neuroprotective effects of this steroid in a stroke (Tomas-Camardiel et al., 2005). Estradiol also reduces brain inflammation acting on astrocytes, decreasing the activation of nuclear factor-kappaB induced by amyloid Aβ(1–40) and lipopolysacharide in cultured astrocytes (Dodel et al., 1999). Since nuclear factor-kappaB is a potent immediate-early transcriptional regulator of numerous proinflammatory genes, the hormonal regulation of this molecule in astrocytes may play a crucial role in the neuroprotective effects of estrogens.

Estradiol also exerts its antiinflammatory actions in the brain, acting on microglia (Fig. 9.1). Several studies have analyzed the effect of estradiol on microglia, in search of a basis for the neuroprotective effects of this steroid (Mor et al., 1999; Vegeto et al., 2006). As already mentioned, estradiol enhances ApoE secretion by microglia in the brain (Stone et al., 1997) and inhibits apoptosis in microglia cultures by a receptor-mediated enhancement of BNIP2 protein production (Vegeto et al., 1999). Subsequent studies in microglia cultures have shown that estradiol inhibits the induction of inducible nitric oxide synthase and several other inflammatory mediators in response to lipopolysacharide and to proinflammatory cytokines (Baker et al., 2004; Bruce-Keller et al., 2000, 2001; Dimayuga et al., 2005; Drew and Chavis, 2000b; Vegeto et al., 2001, 2006). In addition, the hormone reduces the number of reactive microglia in different models of brain inflammation (Tapia-Gonzalez et al., 2008; Vegeto et al., 2003, 2006) and brain injury (Barreto et al., 2007) in vivo. Estradiol is also able to enhance the uptake of the β-amyloid peptide by microglia derived from the human cortex (Li R et al., 2000), an effect that may be relevant for the protective effect of this hormone against Alzheimer's disease. In APP23 mice (an animal model of Alzheimer's disease), estradiol reduces microglia activation around β-amyloid plaques (Vegeto et al., 2006). Furthermore, Yue and associates (2005) have recently examined the importance of brain estrogen on β-amyloid peptide deposition by crossing the estrogen-synthesizing enzyme aromatase gene knockout mice with APP23 transgenic mice to produce estrogen-deficient APP23 mice. Compared with APP23 transgenic control mice, estrogen-deficient APP23 mice exhibited greatly reduced brain estrogen, and early-onset and increased β-amyloid peptide deposition. Interestingly, microglia cultures prepared from the brains of these mice were impaired in β-amyloid peptide clearance/degradation.

Estradiol also regulates adult neurogenesis under pathological conditions; this action may contribute to the regeneration of injured neural circuits. For instance, the hormone restores cell proliferation in the dentate gyrus and the subventricular zone in diabetic rats (Saravia et al., 2004, 2006), and increases neurogenesis in the subventricular zone following an ischemic stroke (Suzuki et al., 2007b). The hormone also partially compensates for the impairment in hippocampal neurogenesis in aged rats (Perez-Martin et al., 2005). Since adult hippocampal neurogenesis is necessary for the behavioral actions of antidepressants (Santarelli et al., 2003), and since changes in the rate of neurogenesis are correlated with modifications in cognition and affection (Abrous et al., 2005; Dupret et al., 2007; Llorens-Martín et al., 2007; Sahay and Hen, 2007; Trejo et al., 2007), it is conceivable that the effects of estradiol on adult hippocampal neurogenesis (see Chapter 4) may be involved in the hormonal antidepressive and procognitive effects.

In addition to the effects of estradiol in the reorganization of neural tissue under pathological conditions, regulating axonal sprouting, gliosis, and neurogenesis, the hormone exerts protective effects on neurons, preventing neurodegeneration. Many studies have documented the neuroprotective actions of estradiol in vitro. Estradiol promotes the survival of hypothalamic neurons (Chowen et al., 1992; Dueñas et al., 1996), amygdala neurons (Arimatsu and Hatanaka, 1986), neocortical neurons (Brinton et al., 1997), hippocampal neurons (Sudo et al., 1997), and dorsal root ganglion neurons (Patrone et al., 1999) in culture. Furthermore, estradiol prevents neuronal loss in primary mesencephalic cultures exposed to glutamate, superoxide anions, or hydrogen peroxide (Sawada et al., 1998), and also hippocampal cultures exposed to NMDA (Weaver et al., 1997). It has also been reported that estradiol protects cortical neurons in culture from death induced by different stimuli, such as iron (Vedder et al., 1999), glutamate toxicity (Singer et al., 1996b; Zaulyanov et al., 1999), AMPA toxicity (Zaulyanov et al., 1999), the pro-oxidant hemoglobin (Regan and Guo, 1997), anoxia (Zaulyanov et al., 1999), cytochrome oxidase inhibitor sodium azide, kainite, or NMDA (Regan and Guo, 1997). Other studies have used neuronal cell lines to demonstrate the neuroprotective effects of estradiol. For instance, estradiol protects NT2 neurons, PC12 cells, and mouse neuroblastoma (Neuro-2a) cells from H_2O_2 or glutamate-induced cell death (Bonnefont et al., 1998; Singer et al., 1998), SK-N-SH human neuroblastoma cells from serum deprivation (Green et al., 1997), hippocampal HT-22 cells from lipid peroxidation (Vedder et al., 1999) and B103 cells (Mook-Jung et al., 1997), PC12 cells and Neuro-2a cells (Bonnefont et al., 1998) from neurotoxic effects of β-amyloid.

Estradiol has shown neuroprotective activity in several different experimental models of neurodegeneration in vivo. For instance, estradiol prevents neuronal loss in the hippocampus induced by the systemic administration of kainic acid, a widely used experimental model of neurodegeneration (Azcoitia et al., 1998, 2001; Picazo et al., 2003; Reibel et al., 2000; Veliskova et al., 2000). This finding is relevant for human pathology since excitotoxicity is a common cause of neuronal loss in many neurodegenerative diseases. Of critical importance with regard to the neuroprotective effects of estrogen is the effect of kainic acid on hilar neurons in intact female rats, which differs depending on the day of the estrus cycle on which the neurotoxin is injected. No significant neuronal loss is observed when a low dose of kainic acid (7 mg/Kg b.w.) is injected on the morning of estrus (one day after the peak of estrogen levels in plasma). In contrast, there is a significant loss of hilar neurons when the same dose of kainic acid is injected in the morning of proestrus (before the peak of estrogen levels in plasma), and when it is injected into ovariectomized rats (Azcoitia et al., 1999a). These findings suggest that the natural fluctuation of ovarian hormones during the estrus cycle influences the vulnerability of hilar neurons to excitotoxicity.

Of great relevance for human pathology are the studies showing that estradiol is neuroprotective in experimental models of Parkinson's disease. Several research teams have studied the effects of estradiol on the nigrostriatal system, showing that the hormone exerts a regulation of the nigrostriatal dopaminergic system in normal animals and in experimental models of Parkinson's disease. Ovariectomy, per se, reduces dopamine concentrations in the striatum; estradiol replacement prevents this reduction (Callier et al., 2000; Dluzen, 2000). Several toxins that induce a loss of dopaminergic neurons in the substantia nigra and the consequent decrease of dopamine in the striatum in rodents and monkeys have been widely used to imitate Parkinson's disease in humans. Estradiol therapy prevents the loss of substantia nigra dopaminergic neurons and the loss of dopaminergic innervation in the striatum in these animal models. For instance, estradiol reduces dyskinesia caused by the administration of MPTP in cynomolgus monkeys (Gomez-Mancilla and Bedard, 1992). Estradiol also prevents the reduction in dopamine caused by the injection of 6-hydroxydopamine in the striatum of mice (Dluzen, 1997). Estrogen also has neuroprotective properties against MPTP-induced neurotoxicity in the nigrostriatal dopaminergic system of castrated males, preventing reductions in corpus striatum dopamine concentrations (Dluzen et al., 1996a, b). In addition to preventing the degeneration of substantia nigra neurons, estradiol may in part protect the nigrostriatal system by the regulation of dopamine release, and via the inhibition of dopamine uptake by decreasing the affinity of the transporter for dopamine (Disshon and Dluzen, 1997; Disshon et al., 1998; Dluzen, 2000). As mentioned regarding the neurodegenerative effect of kainic acid in the hippocampus, the degeneration of nigrostriatal dopaminergic neurons in experimental models of Parkinson's disease also depends on the endogenous fluctuation of gonadal hormones during the estrus cycle (Datla et al., 2003).

Experimental forebrain ischemia is another highly relevant model for human pathology where neuroprotective effects of estradiol have been assessed. The protective effects of estrogen in this model were documented by several pioneering studies in rats (Dubal et al., 1998; Pelligrino et al., 1998; Rusa et al., 1999; Simpkins et al., 1997b; Wang et al., 1999; Zhang et al., 1998), mice (Culmsee et al., 1999), and gerbils (Chen J et al., 1998; Sudo et al., 1997). For instance, James W. Simpkins and his collaborators (Shi et al., 1998; Simpkins et al., 1997b) showed that a pretreatment with 17 β-estradiol reduces animal mortality, ischemic area, and expression of the β-amyloid precursor protein mRNA in ovariectomized rats after a middle cerebral artery occlusion. Interestingly, the isomer 17 α-estradiol was able to reduce mortality, and the ischemic area as well. Both systemic and intracerebral administration of 17 β-estradiol was protective in this model. Phyllis Wise and her group (Dubal et al., 1998) showed that systemic estradiol pretreatment significantly reduced overall infarct volume compared with oil injected controls. This group also analyzed the expression of estrogen receptors and the antiapoptotic molecule Bcl-2 after an ischemia, and provided important cues on the neuroprotective mechanisms of estrogen in this model. In gerbils, 17 β-estradiol infused into the lateral cerebral ventricle prevents learning disability and neuronal loss at early stages after a transient forebrain ischemia (Chen J et al., 1998; Sudo et al., 1997). These early studies also showed that the neuroprotective effect of estradiol in this model is not restricted to females. Thus, Thomas J. K. Toung and collaborators in the laboratory of Patricia D. Hurn reported that either acute or chronic administration of 17 β-estradiol reduced cortical and caudate infarct volume in the male rat brain after an experimental stroke, using two hours of reversible middle cerebral artery occlusion. Furthermore, castration did not alter the ischemic outcome, whereas estrogen replacement reduced infarct volume in castrated animals (Toung et al., 1998). Further studies have confirmed these initial findings (Gibson et al., 2006; McCullough and Hurn, 2003; Merchenthaler et al., 2003; Wise et al., 2001; Yang et al., 2005) and indicate that estradiol not only prevents neuronal death but also protects against alterations in functional synaptic plasticity induced by ischemia (Dai et al., 2007).

Clinical data on the protective actions of estrogens against Alzheimer's disease are controversial (Asthana et al., 2001; Fillit et al., 1986; Henderson et al., 2000; Mulnard et al., 2000; Paganini-Hill and Henderson, 1996; Shaywitz and Shaywitz, 2000; Wang et al., 2000). The results of estrogen therapy on cognitive function and Alzheimer's disease in postmenopausal women will be discussed further in Chapter 10. Experimental studies suggest that estradiol may exert therapeutic effects for some aspects of the pathology. The hormone enhances the function of basal forebrain cholinergic neurons (Bora et al., 2005; Granholm et al., 2003; Rabbani et al., 1997), and decreases the hyperphosphorylation of tau (Alvarez-de-la-Rosa et al., 2005; Cardona-Gomez et al., 2004), which is characteristic of Alzheimer's disease. Furthermore, estradiol protects neurons against amyloid-β peptide neurotoxicity (Bonnefont et al., 1998; Marin et al., 2003; Mook-Jung et al., 1997; Quintanilla et al., 2005), and may decrease the generation and secretion of β-amyloid peptides (Xu et al., 2006) and amyloid precursor protein accumulation in the striatum of an animal model of Alzheimer's disease (Granholm et al., 2003). However, it has been shown that the hormone is unable to decrease amyloid precursor protein levels and β-amyloid deposits in the hippocampus and cortex in animal models of Alzheimer's disease (Granholm et al., 2003; Green et al., 2005; Heikkinen et al., 2004).

The neuroprotective effects of estradiol may be, at least in part, exerted by the activation of classical nuclear estrogen receptors. There is evidence that estrogen receptors are involved in the regulation of neuronal survival in vitro. Estrogen enhancement of neuronal survival in primary hypothalamic cultures in the serum-free medium and in cortical cultures exposed to glutamate is blocked by the estrogen receptor selective modulator tamoxifen (Chowen et al., 1992; Singer et al., 1996b) and by the estrogen receptor antagonist ICI 182780 (Dueñas et al., 1996; Singer et al., 1999). In addition, antiestrogens abolish the neuroprotective action of estradiol in cultures of dorsal root ganglion neurons deprived of nerve growth factor (NGF) (Patrone et al., 1999) and the protective effect of the hormone in a murine cholinergic cell line (SN56) against amyloid-β–induced toxicity (Marin et al., 2003). Furthermore, estradiol enhances the survival of PC12 cells transfected with the full-length rat estrogen receptor α, but does not affect the survival of control cells transfected with vector DNA alone (Gollapudi and Oblinger, 1999a, b; Lustig, 1996). In addition, selective agonists for both estrogen receptor α and β protect hippocampal neurons in vitro against glutamate excitotoxicity, suggesting that both forms of estrogen receptors are involved in neuroprotective mechanisms (Zhao et al., 2004).

The dependence of the neuroprotective effects of estradiol on estrogen receptors has been demonstrated in vivo as well. For instance, the intracerebroventricular administration of the estrogen receptor antagonist ICI 182780 inhibits the neuroprotective effect of estradiol in hippocampal hilar neurons of ovariectomized rats exposed to systemic kainic acid (Azcoitia et al., 1999b). In addition, neuroprotective actions of estradiol against an ischemic brain injury are lost in estrogen receptor-α–deficient mice but are preserved in estrogen receptor-β knockout mice, indicating that estrogen receptor α is indispensable for the neuroprotective effects (Dubal et al., 2001, 2006). Estrogen receptor-α knockout mice also show an increased depletion in striatal dopamine after a neurotoxic lesion of substantia nigra neurons in an experimental model of

Parkinson's disease. However, the neuroprotective effect of estradiol against striatal dopamine terminal loss is prevented in both estrogen receptor-α and estrogen receptor-β knockout mice, indicating that both receptors are involved in the neuroprotective mechanism of the hormone in this model (Morissette et al., 2007), likely mediating different protective mechanisms (D'Astous et al., 2006; Morissette et al., 2008).

Some of the neuroprotective effects of estradiol may be independent of estrogen receptor activation. Christian Behl and his collaborators were among the first to convincingly document that estradiol has antioxidant properties, and suppresses the oxidative stress in neurons and neuronal cell lines induced by hydrogen peroxide, superoxide anions, and other pro-oxidants (Behl, 1999; Behl et al, 1995, 1997). Both 17 β- and 17 α-estradiol (and some estradiol derivatives) can prevent intracellular peroxide accumulation and degeneration of cultured neurons and clonal hippocampal cells. The antioxidant activity of estrogens is dependent on the presence of the hydroxyl group in the C3 position on the A ring of the steroid molecule, and is independent of an activation of estrogen receptors (Behl et al., 1995, 1997; Culmsee et al., 1999; Moosmann and Behl, 1999; Regan and Guo, 1997). In addition to antioxidant effects, estradiol may use other possible neuroprotective mechanisms that are independent of nuclear estrogen receptor activation. Estradiol may interact with estrogen binding sites in the plasma membrane (Ramirez and Zheng, 1996), and may have many different rapid effects on neuronal excitability and neuronal transmission, affecting rapid cytoplasmic signaling in neurons and glial cells (Bicknell, 1998; Brann et al., 2007; Kelly et al., 2005; Lee and McEwen, 2001; Moss and Gu, 1999). These actions may be mediated through putative nonnuclear estrogen receptors located in the cytoplasmic and membrane compartments of neurons and glial cells. Estradiol may also exert neuroprotection through nonspecific receptors, such as neurotransmitter ion channels (Weaver et al., 1997). The actions of estradiol via the membrane, cytoplasmic, and nuclear receptors are undoubtedly, in many cases, inextricably linked because the gene products generated by the estradiol-dependent activation of nuclear receptors and transcription can be post-transcriptionally modified by cell signals activated by membrane estrogen receptors. Transcription itself can be augmented or reduced by coactivators and corepressors previously modified through membrane-associated estrogen receptor actions. Estradiol not only drives the transcription of genes whose promoters bind nuclear estrogen receptors, but also of genes that are transactivated by other transcription factors modified after membrane estradiol signaling. The extranuclear functions of estradiol may be mediated in part by receptors identical to the classical nuclear estrogen receptors, but in some way modified in order to prevent, at least temporarily, their translocation to the nucleus. While the predominant localization of classical estrogen receptors is in the cell nucleus, ultrastructural analyses have demonstrated that estrogen receptor α immunoreactivity is also present in dendritic spines, axons, synapses, and glial cell processes, in a position that could favor nonnuclear signaling (Woolley, 2007). Membrane-associated estrogen receptors may be part of macromolecular entities aggregated in specific plasma membrane domains, the caveolae, where they can hypothetically interact with G proteins, receptor tyrosine kinases, nonreceptor kinases, and other signaling partners (Marin et al., 2008; Toran-Allerand, 2004). Estrogen receptors can directly contact G proteins or transactivate other G-protein–coupled receptors, leading to the stimulation of ion channels and phospholipase C (Hewitt et al., 2005; Kelly et al., 2002; Revankar et al., 2005). Estrogenic induction of phospholipase C activation initiates a cascade of signals through increases in intracellular Ca^{+2} and activation of protein kinase C and protein kinase A, leading to the modulation of other ion channels and cAMP response element-binding protein-dependent transcription. Of particular relevance are glutamate-mediated increases in intracellular Ca^{+2} concentration that are potentiated by estradiol (Beyer et al., 2003), because this has been proposed to modulate cognitive function. The risk of calcium overload in neurons exposed to estrogenic compounds that could occur under an excitotoxic condition is attenuated through enhancing mitochondrial sequestration of Ca^{+2}. The estradiol-elicited intracellular rise in calcium may result in a rapid stimulation of PI3K signaling cascade (Beyer et al., 2003).

Neuroprotective effects of estradiol and estrogenic compounds may involve, at least in part, a modulation of the expression of molecules implicated in the control of cell death. Estradiol has been shown to increase the expression of the antiapoptotic molecule Bcl-2 in NT2 neurons (Singer et al., 1998), in hippocampal neurons in vitro (Nilsen and Brinton, 2003a; Wu et al., 2005; Zhao et al., 2004), in adult hypothalamic neurons in vivo (Cardona-Gomez et al., 2001; Garcia-Segura et al., 1998), and in the cerebral cortex after a brain ischemia (Dubal et al., 1999). In addition to preventing neuronal death, Bcl-2 may also promote axonal growth and regeneration (Chen DF et al., 1997; Holm and Isacson, 1999). Therefore, by the induction of Bcl-2, estradiol may promote neuronal survival after injury by both Bcl-2–induced inhibition of cell death and Bcl-2–induced facilitation of regeneration of neuronal connectivity. Furthermore, Bcl-2 attenuates the generation of reactive oxygen species (Bogdanov et al., 1999); therefore, estradiol may reduce oxidative stress in neural tissue by the induction of Bcl-2 expression. Estradiol also increases the expression of the antiapoptotic molecule Bcl-xl in PC12 cells (Gollapudi and Oblinger, 1999a, b; Koski et al., 2004), developing dorsal root ganglion cells (Patrone et al., 1999) and cultured hippocampal neurons (Pike, 1999). In addition, the mRNA for the Bcl-2 interacting protein BNIP2 is decreased by estrogen treatment in human neuroblastoma SK-ER3 cells (Belcredito et al., 2001; Garnier et al., 1997) and monoblastoid cells (Vegeto et al., 1999). Since BNIP-2 is a negative regulator of Bcl-2, estrogen may promote Bcl-2 expression by this mechanism. In addition, estradiol may directly affect transcription of the Bcl-2 gene, since several putative estrogen-responsive sites are present in the Bcl-2 promoter (Teixeira et al., 1995).

Some studies have observed that estradiol induces changes in the expression of the members of the Bcl-2 family in conditions in which the hormone prevents neuronal death, suggesting that hormonal regulation of these proteins is associated with the neuroprotective effects of estradiol. For instance, estradiol enhances the survival of PC12 cells transfected with the full-length rat estrogen receptor α, and this effect is associated with an increased expression of Bcl-XL and a reduced expression of BAD (Gollapudi and Oblinger, 1999b). An increased expression of Bcl-2 is also observed when the hormone protects NT2 neurons from H_2O_2 or glutamate-induced cell death (Singer et al., 1998). The reduction by estradiol of apoptosis induced by β-amyloid in primary neuronal cultures is accompanied by a significant increase in the expression of the antiapoptotic protein Bcl-XL, the up-regulation of Bcl-w, and the down-regulation of Bim (Pike, 1999; Yao et al., 2007). Furthermore, estradiol increases the survival of cultured dorsal root ganglion neurons deprived of NGF; this effect is associated with an increased expression of Bcl-X without affecting the expression of BAX (Patrone et al., 1999). Dubal and colleagues (1999) have found that estradiol prevents the down-regulation of Bcl-2 expression in the rat cerebral cortex induced by ischemia, and this is accompanied by decreased tissue damage. In addition, the selective estrogen receptor-α agonist 4,4',4"-(4-propyl-[1H]-pyrazole-1,3,5-triyl)tris-phenol (PPT) prevents the decrease in the ratio between the striatal Bcl-2 and BAD levels, and the decrease in striatal dopamine in experimental Parkinson's disease in mice (D'Astous et al., 2006).

Another target of estradiol that regulates cell death is the prostate apoptosis response-4 (Par-4), the product of a gene up-regulated in prostate cancer cells undergoing apoptosis. Par-4 expression is induced in neurons after exposure to trophic factor deprivation and apoptotic insults (Chan et al., 1999; Duan et al., 1999a, b; Guo et al., 1998) and is up-regulated in vulnerable neurons in Alzheimer's disease brains (Guo et al., 1998). Par-4 antisense treatment suppresses mitochondrial dysfunction and caspase activation in synaptosomes, and prevents cell death of cultured hippocampal neurons following exposure to excitotoxic and apoptotic insults (Duan et al., 1999a). Interestingly, both Par-4 induction and cell death induced by trophic factor deprivation in cultured hippocampal neurons are largely prevented by pretreatment of the cultures with 17 β-estradiol (Chan et al., 1999). Since increases in Par-4 expression follow an increase of reactive oxygen species and precede mitochondrial membrane depolarization, caspase activation, and nuclear chromatin condensation/fragmentation, the down-regulation of Par-4 expression by estradiol may be one of the mechanisms involved in the antioxidant and neuroprotective effects of the hormone.

Interaction with growth factors and neurotrophins is another important component of the mechanisms participating in the plastic regenerative changes induced by estradiol after injury. Since the pioneering work of Toran-Allerand and colleagues (Toran-Allerand, 1996; Toran-Allerand et al., 1999), it has been well established that estradiol and neurotrophins interact in many areas of the nervous system. Estradiol regulates the expression of neurotrophins and their receptors, and neurotrophins regulate the expression of estrogen receptors in different neuronal populations. For instance, NGF significantly increases nuclear estrogen binding in cortical explants (Miranda et al., 1996). In turn, estradiol regulates the expression of NGF receptors p75 and TrkA in dorsal root ganglion neurons from adult rats (Sohrabji et al., 1994a) and in PC12 cells (Sohrabji et al., 1994b). The hormone regulates the expression of mRNA for NGF in the hippocampus and frontal cortex (Simpkins et al., 1997a), decreases the expression of NGF in the hippocampus and TrkA in the medial septum and nucleus basalis magnocellularis (Gibbs et al., 1994), and increases the expression of TrkA in the basal forebrain of adult female rats (McMillan et al., 1996). Neurons that produce BDNF in the forebrain express estrogen receptors (Miranda et al., 1993); estradiol regulates BDNF expression in many brain regions of adult ovariectomized rats (Sohrabji and Lewis, 2006) and promotes BDNF retrograde transport in the forebrain (Jezierski and Sohrabji, 2003). Several of the neuroprotective, antiinflammatory, and affective effects of estradiol may be mediated by the regulation of BDNF brain levels (Murphy et al., 1998a; Scharfman and MacLusky, 2005; Sohrabji and Lewis, 2006) and by the interaction of estradiol with neurotrophin receptors (Carrer et al., 2005; Nordell et al., 2005). The interaction of neurotrophins and estrogen receptors may occur in the same neuron, since estrogen receptors and neurotrophin receptors are coexpressed in some cells. In 1992, Toran-Allerand and colleagues reported that estrogen receptors colocalize with p75, the low-affinity NGF receptor, in cholinergic neurons of the basal forebrain. Further studies have shown a widespread colocalization of estrogen and neurotrophin receptors within estrogen and neurotrophin targets, including neurons of the cerebral cortex, sensory ganglia, and PC12 cells (Miranda et al., 1994; Sohrabji et al., 1994a, b; Toran-Allerand, 1996; Toran-Allerand et al., 1999). These findings indicate that estrogens and growth factors may act in concert on the same neuron to regulate the expression of specific genes that may influence neuronal survival, axonal regeneration, and dendritic and glial reorganization after injury.

The interaction of estradiol and growth factors in neuroprotection may involve glia. Sortino and colleagues (2004) showed that conditioned medium from astrocytes pre-exposed to estradiol increases the viability of cortical neurons treated with β-amyloid protein. This effect seems to be mediated by the release of TGF-β1 from astrocytes in response to estradiol. Dhandapani and colleagues (2005) similarly showed that estradiol and the selective estrogen receptor modulator tamoxifen protect cortical neurons from apoptosis induced by camptothecin in co-cultures of neurons and glial cells, but not in purified cortical neuronal cultures. The neuroprotective effect seems to be mediated by the glial release of TGF-β. Estradiol and tamoxifen induce the release of TGF-β1 and TGF-β2 from cortical astrocytes; TGF-β immunoneutralization in the co-cultures prevents the neuroprotective effect. TGF-β released by astrocytes may also mediate estrogenic neuroprotection of noncortical neurons. For instance, TGF-β released by hypothalamic astrocytes treated with estradiol protects GT1–7 neurons from serum deprivation (Mahesh et al., 2006). The release of other growth factors by astrocytes in response to estradiol may also be involved in the neuroprotective effect of the hormone. For instance, the release of glial cell line-derived neurotrophic factor (GDNF) by astrocytes treated with estradiol protects spinal cord motoneurons from excitotoxic cell death in a co-culture system in which pure motoneurons are treated with AMPA and then transferred to a culture of astrocytes pretreated with estradiol (Platania et al., 2005). Brain injury also induces the synthesis of IGF-I and estradiol by reactive astrocytes (Garcia-Estrada et al., 1992; Garcia-Segura et al., 1999b; Hwang et al., 2004) and up-regulates estrogen receptors, IGF-I receptors, and IGF-binding proteins in reactive glia (Beilharz et al., 1998; Blurton-Jones and Tuszynski, 2001; Chung et al., 2003; Garcia-Ovejero et al., 2002). Therefore, estradiol and IGF-I released by reactive glia may act directly on these cells or on neighboring neurons, regulating reactive gliosis, neuronal survival, and the reorganization of neural tissue after injury. Indeed, IGF-I and estradiol interact to regulate the plastic response of the brain after injury and during neurodegenerative conditions. This has been assessed in ovariectomized rats in vivo, using systemic administration of kainic acid to induce excitotoxic degeneration of hippocampal hilar neurons (Azcoitia et al., 1999b). Both the systemic administration of estradiol and the intracerebroventricular infusion of IGF-I prevent hilar neuronal loss induced by kainic acid. The neuroprotective effect of estradiol is blocked by the intracerebroventricular infusion of the peptide JB1, an IGF-I receptor antagonist, while the neuroprotective effect of IGF-I is blocked by the intracerebroventricular infusion of the estrogen receptor antagonist ICI 182780. Similar results have been obtained in ovariectomized rats after the unilateral infusion of 6-hydroxdopamine into the medial forebrain bundle to lesion the nigrostriatal dopaminergic pathway (Quesada and Micevych, 2004), a model of Parkinson's disease. Pretreatment with estrogen or IGF-I significantly prevents the loss of substantia nigra compacta neurons, the decrease in dopaminergic innervation of the striatum, and the related motor disturbances. Blockage of the IGF-I receptor by intracerebroventricular JB1 attenuates the neuroprotective effects of both estrogen and IGF-I. Furthermore, the neuroprotective action of estradiol against MPTP toxicity in the nigrostriatal system of male mice is associated with the regulation of IGF-I receptor signaling (D'Astous et al., 2006). These findings suggest that the neuroprotective actions of estradiol and IGF-I after a brain injury depend on the coactivation of both estrogen receptors and IGF-I receptor in neural cells.

Activation of the PI3K/Akt signaling pathway may be involved in the interaction of the neuroprotective effects of IGF-I and estradiol. PI3K and Akt mediate neuroprotection by estrogen in different experimental models (Honda et al., 2000; Marin et al., 2005; Wang R et al., 2006; Yu et al., 2004; Zhang et al., 2001). Via the activation of Akt, estradiol may also activate the MAPK pathway (Mannella and Brinton, 2006), which is also involved in the neuroprotective effects of the hormone (Guerra et al., 2004; Kuroki et al., 2001; Marin et al., 2005). In addition, Akt regulates several transcription factors that may be involved in the control of neuronal survival, such as cAMP response element-binding proteins, nuclear factor-kappaB and several members of the forkhead family. In addition, the activation of Akt results in the phosphorylation of the Bcl-2 family member BAD; this may suppress BAD-induced cell death. Furthermore, Akt activation enhances Bcl-2 promoter activity; IGF-I and estrogen both induce Bcl-2 expression in neurons. Interestingly, IGF-I receptor activation is necessary for the induction of Bcl-2 by estradiol in the adult brain (Cardona-Gomez et al., 2002a). The activation of Akt by estradiol also has implications for the regulation of neuronal function and survival via the modulation of GSK3β activity (Cardona-Gomez et al., 2004; Goodenough et al., 2005; Quintanilla et al., 2005). Physiological phosphorylation of microtubule-associated proteins by GSK3β may be involved in the regulation of microtubule dynamics, neuritic growth, synaptogenesis, and synaptic plasticity. However, under pathological conditions, GSK3β may be responsible for the hyperphosphorylation of tau in Alzheimer's disease, and its inhibition is associated with the activation of survival pathways in neurons. Interestingly, estradiol regulates the activity of GSK3β and decreases the phosphorylation of tau in the hippocampus (Cardona-Gomez et al., 2004). Immunoprecipitation studies suggest that in this brain region GSK3β forms a macromolecular complex with tau, β-catenin, and the p85 subunit of the PI3K and another complex with estrogen receptor α and β-catenin. Estradiol increases the amount of phosphorylated GSK3β associated with the first complex and reduces the amount of β-catenin associated with the second complex. By the modulation of these macromolecular interactions between cytoskeletal and signaling proteins, estradiol may regulate microtubule dynamics, synaptic plasticity, and neuronal survival (Cardona-Gomez et al., 2004; Garcia-Segura et al., 2006; Mendez et al., 2005, 2006).

Testosterone

Testosterone has been shown to regulate regeneration of nerve cells after an injury in both the peripheral and central nervous system. The hormone accelerates regeneration and functional recovery in rodent peripheral nerve injury models (Huppenbauer et al., 2005; Jones et al., 2001; Tanzer and Jones, 2004), and also promotes motor axon regeneration in axotomized motoneurons (Jones, 1994; Perez and Kelley, 1996; Tetzlaff et al., 2006; Yu, 1982). In addition, removal of circulating androgens by castration decreases mRNA levels of the myelin proteins P0 and PMP22 in the sciatic nerve of adult male rats. Treatment with dihydrotestosterone, a metabolite of testosterone with a high affinity for androgen receptors, restores the levels of P0, while 5 α-androstane-3 α, 17 β-diol, a metabolite of dihydrotestosterone, restores the levels of both P0 and PMP22 (Magnaghi et al., 1999, 2004). Testosterone metabolites are also able to reduce functional and morphological impairments in the rat sciatic nerve induced by diabetes (Roglio et al., 2007).

Although some studies have reported increased neurodegeneration after testosterone administration in experimental models of cerebral hypoxia and ischemia (Hawk et al., 1998; Nishino et al., 1998), in general, testosterone exerts no effects or promotes the survival of specific neuronal populations in the central nervous system after different forms of neural injury (Jones, 1994; Perez and Kelley, 1996; Rasika et al., 1999; Tetzlaff et al., 2006; Yu, 1982). Testosterone prevents the hyperphosphorylation of the microtubule-associated protein tau (Papasozomenos, 1997), which is abnormally hyperphosphorylated in Alzheimer's disease, reduces neuronal secretion of β-amyloid peptides associated with Alzheimer's disease (Gouras et al., 2000), attenuates β-amyloid toxicity (Pike, 2001), protects granule and hilar neurons of the dentate gyrus from adrenalectomy (Frye and McCormick, 2000) and excitotoxicity (Azcoitia et al., 2001), respectively, and decreases apolipoprotein E4-induced cognitive deficits (Raber et al., 2002). Part of the neuroprotective properties of testosterone may be a result of the activation of androgen receptors (Ahlbom et al., 2001; Hammond et al., 2001; Jones et al., 2001). Testosterone may also exert neuroprotection by its metabolism into estradiol (Azcoitia et al., 2001; see below).

The control of gliosis may be one of the mechanisms involved in the neuroprotective effects of testosterone (Fig. 9.1). During brain development, testosterone and its metabolite estradiol affect the differentiation of GFAP immunoreactive astrocytes and generate sex differences in astroglia (Chowen et al., 1995; Conejo et al., 2005; Garcia-Segura et al., 1988c; Mong et al., 1999; see Chapter 6). In the adult brain, testosterone regulates the expression of GFAP in the hippocampus (Day et al., 1990, 1993) and reduces the increase of GFAP associated with aging in the cerebellum (Day et al., 1998). In addition, testosterone reduces GFAP immunoreactivity in the border of a stab wound in the cerebral cortex and hippocampus (Barreto et al., 2007; Garcia-Estrada et al., 1993, 1999), decreases GFAP immunostaining and astrocyte hypertrophy around the infarct area after a middle cerebral artery occlusion (Pan et al., 2005), and attenuates the astroglial reaction in the red nucleus after a rubrospinal tract transection (Storer and Jones, 2003). Testosterone has also been shown to reduce reactive microglia in the border of a stab wound in the cerebral cortex and hippocampus (Barreto et al., 2007). Effects of testosterone on gliosis may be a contributing factor to neural regeneration. This is suggested by the studies of Kathryn J. Jones and her collaborators on the effects of testosterone on the regulation of the central astrocytic response to peripheral nerve injury. In adult male hamsters, testosterone propionate administration reduces the increase of GFAP mRNA in the facial nucleus after a facial nerve axotomy (Coers et al., 2002; Jones et al., 1997b, 1999), attenuates glial-mediated synaptic stripping of axotomized motoneurons (Jones et al., 1997a, 1999), and increases facial nerve regeneration (Kujawa et al., 1991). These results suggest that the regulation of astrogliosis may contribute to the regenerative mechanisms of testosterone on facial motoneurons. Part of the effects of testosterone on gliosis may be mediated by its metabolism into dihydrotestosterone and estradiol within the brain (Barreto et al., 2007).

As we have seen in Chapter 4, aromatase is involved in the regulatory effects of androgens, via conversion into estrogens, on brain plasticity under physiological conditions. In addition, local estrogen formation by aromatase in the nervous system may influence the reorganization of brain tissue after injury. Different forms of neurotoxic and mechanical lesions in the brains of rats and mice increase aromatase activity and induce de novo expression of the enzyme in reactive glia (Garcia-Segura et al., 1999a, b, 2003). Aromatase expression is also induced in glial cells after an experimental stroke (Carswell et al., 2005). The morphology and ultrastructure of aromatase-immunoreactive glial cells, together with the coexpression of the astroglial marker GFAP, indicate that most, if not all, aromatase-expressing glial cells are astrocytes. The induction of aromatase expression in astrocytes after a brain injury is accompanied by a significant increase in aromatase enzymatic activity. Aromatase-expressing astrocytes are observed in both sexes and in all injured brain areas, including the cortex, corpus callosum, striatum, hippocampus, thalamus, and hypothalamus. This indicates that astrocytes from most rodent brain areas have the potential for expressing aromatase, and therefore the potential to produce estradiol in response to injury. Furthermore, Richard Scott Peterson, Barney A. Schlinger, Colin J. Saldanha, and their collaborators (Peterson et al., 2001, 2004; Saldanha et al., 2005) have shown that aromatase mRNA and protein are rapidly and locally up-regulated in glial cells following neural injury in the zebra finch brain. This finding suggests that injury-dependent up-regulation of aromatase may be a conserved characteristic of the vertebrate brain, and an important component of the initial response of neural tissue to injury.

The increased expression of aromatase in injured brain areas suggests that this enzyme may be involved in the reorganization of the nervous tissue by increasing local estradiol levels. Estradiol formed by astrocytes may be released as a trophic factor for damaged neurons, and may be involved in the compensatory restructuring of injured brain tissue. Thus, estradiol released by astroglia may potentially affect synaptic function, selective regeneration of neuronal processes and local cerebral blood flow, contributing to the facilitation of neuronal recovery and reduction of neuronal death. To determine the influence of aromatase on the response of brain tissue to injury, we injected a low dose of a neurotoxin, domoic acid, to aromatase knockout (ArKO) male mice and their wild-type male littermates. At the low dose selected in this study, domoic acid does not induce neurodegeneration in the hippocampus of normal mice. The number of neurons was then assessed in the hilus of the dentate gyrus using unbiased morphometric techniques. The number of hilar neurons was not significantly different between ArKO mice and their wild-type littermates, indicating that aromatase deficiency does not affect per se the development and survival of hilar neurons, at least in young adult animals. However, the number of hilar neurons in ArKO mice injected with domoic acid was significantly decreased compared to control ArKO mice, to wild-type controls and to wild-type mice injected with domoic acid (Azcoitia et al., 2001). This finding indicates that aromatase deficiency increases the vulnerability of hilar neurons to neurotoxic degeneration.

We obtained further proof of the neuroprotective role of aromatase in intact male rats that were implanted with an osmotic minipump containing the aromatase inhibitor fadrozole. Kainic acid, another well characterized neurotoxin for hilar neurons in the rat, was administered at a low dose that does not affect hilar neurons in intact male rats, but results in significant neuronal loss in the hilus of castrated rats. As expected, the number of hilar neurons was not affected by kainic acid in control animals that were not treated with fadrozole. Furthermore, fadrozole alone did not affect the number of hilar neurons, indicating that fadrozole is not neurotoxic by itself. However, animals that were treated with both fadrozole and kainic acid had a significant decrease in the number of hilar neurons compared to animals treated with vehicle, to animals treated with kainic acid alone, and to animals treated with fadrozole alone (Azcoitia et al., 2001). The loss of hilar neurons was accompanied by an increase in the number of neurons stained with Fluoro-Jade, a marker of dying cells. These findings further support the results obtained with the ArKO mice, and confirm that aromatase is neuroprotective against excitotoxicity.

To determine whether the formation of estradiol is involved in the neuroprotective effect of aromatase, male rats were treated with fadrozole, kainic acid, and estradiol. Estradiol treatment prevented the neurodegenerative effect of kainic acid in animals treated with fadrozole. The number of hilar neurons in animals treated with fadrozole, kainic acid, and estradiol was not significantly different from control animals, and was significantly higher than in animals treated with fadrozole and kainic acid (Azcoitia et al., 2001). This finding, showing that the neurodegenerative effect of aromatase deficiency is counterbalanced by the aromatase product estradiol, strongly suggests that the neuroprotective properties of aromatase lies in its ability to catalyze the formation of estradiol rather than reducing testosterone levels. Similar results have been obtained in ArKO mice after a reversible middle cerebral artery occlusion. Brain damage in this model is greater in female homozygous ArKO mice compared with wild-type female littermates; estradiol treatment prevents the increased susceptibility of ArKO mice to brain damage (McCullough et al., 2003).

Another experimental model in which the neuroprotective effects of aromatase have been detected is cerebellar ataxia in a rat produced by the degeneration of the inferior olivary nucleus after treatment with 3-acetylpirydine (3AP), an antimetabolite of nicotinamide. Olivary neurons have a very high metabolic rate and are, therefore, very sensitive to 3AP toxicity. The destruction of the inferior olive results in a loss of climbing fiber input to the cerebellar Purkinje neurons (Baetens et al., 1982); this deafferentiation leads to ataxia (Fernandez et al., 1999). Inferior olivary neurons express aromatase (Lavaque et al., 2006a; Sierra et al., 2003a) and estrogen receptors (Shughrue et al., 1997), and their activity is affected by estradiol (Smith, 1998). In addition, estradiol is neuroprotective for inferior olivary neurons (Sierra et al., 2003a). We observed that the inhibition of aromatase with fadrozole enhanced the injury produced by 3AP in the inferior olive of intact male rats. Fadrozole treatment decreased the number of neurons that survived from 3AP and increased the number of Fluoro-Jade stained dying cells (Sierra et al., 2003a), indicating that aromatase is neuroprotective for inferior olivary neurons. The neuronal loss induced by the aromatase inhibitor fadrozole in the inferior olivary nucleus of male rats treated with the neurotoxic 3AP was prevented by the administration of estradiol (Sierra et al., 2003a). This indicates that, as concluded in the hippocampus studies, the toxic effect of fadrozole is due to the inhibition of aromatase and not to another unknown effect of the drug. Therefore, estradiol formation also mediates the neuroprotective effect of aromatase in the inferior olivary nucleus. The action of estradiol and aromatase in this nucleus may be important for the maintenance of motor function that is under the control of the olivo–cerebellar system. Indeed, postmenopausal women receiving estrogen have a decreased risk of falling and better postural balance than nonestrogen users (Naessen et al., 1997; Randell et al., 2001).

In addition to preventing neuronal death, aromatase activity may also regulate brain cell proliferation after injury. Traumatic brain injury in the zebra finch hippocampus induces high levels of cell proliferation. Peterson and collaborators have found that the rate of cell proliferation, assessed by BrdU labeling, is correlated with the amount of expression of aromatase in glial cells around the lesion site, and that cell proliferation is reduced by an ovariectomy and by aromatase inhibition (Peterson et al., 2007).

The studies mentioned above, on ArKO mice and on rats and zebra finches after systemic administration of the aromatase inhibitor fadrozole, indicate that aromatase is neuroprotective. However, these studies did not differentiate between brain aromatase and the peripheral enzyme. The role of extragonadal estradiol synthesis in neuroprotection is suggested by the fact that brain injury after a reversible middle cerebral artery occlusion is increased in ArKO female mice and in female wild-type mice chronically treated with fadrozole, compared to ovariectomized wild-type mice (McCullough et al., 2003). Furthermore, aromatase inhibition in ovariectomized rats also increases neurodegeneration in the hippocampus of animals treated with kainic acid (Veiga et al., 2005a). To test the role of local brain aromatase activity in neuroprotection, the aromatase inhibitor fadrozole was infused into the right lateral cerebral ventricle of a group of male rats (Azcoitia et al., 2001). Fadrozole was administered at a concentration within the range previously shown to inhibit aromatase in the rat brain. The number of hilar neurons in the hippocampal formation was assessed after an injection of a low dose of kainic acid that does not induce neurodegeneration in intact males. Indeed, the number of hilar neurons was not affected by this low dose of kainic acid in control animals. Furthermore, the infusion of fadrozole in the cerebral ventricle did not affect the number of hilar neurons in control animals. This is a further indication that aromatase activity is not indispensable for maintaining hilar neuron survival under normal circumstances. However, animals that were treated with both fadrozole and kainic acid showed a significant decrease in the number of hilar neurons, compared to animals treated with vehicle, animals treated with kainic acid alone, and animals treated with fadrozole alone. These findings indicate that brain aromatase activity exerts an endogenous mechanism of neuroprotection. Similar findings have been obtained in the zebra finch brain. The size of the penetrating mechanical brain injury induced by a needle is greater when fadrozole is injected in the injured hemisphere compared to the injection of vehicle. Furthermore, a greater number of apoptotic cell nuclei are detected around the fadrozole-associated lesion relative to vehicle, and estradiol replacement reduces the effect of fadrozole (Saldanha et al., 2005; Wynne and Saldanha, 2004).

In conclusion, the endogenous response of neural tissue to cope with neurodegenerative insults may include the induction of aromatase and the consecutive increase in the local production of estradiol. Locally formed estradiol may act on estrogen receptors, which are known to mediate neuroprotection by estradiol in several experimental models of neurodegeneration (Azcoitia et al., 1999b; Sawada et al., 2000; Veliskova et al., 2000; Wilson et al., 2000; Wise et al., 2001). In addition, aromatase may also promote neuroprotection by increasing local estradiol concentration to levels compatible with the antioxidant neuroprotective effects of the molecule (Behl and Holsboer, 1999). Since aromatase is expressed in the adult human brain, including the hippocampus and the cerebral cortex (Stoffel-Wagner, 2001; Stoffel-Wagner et al., 1999; Yague et al., 2006), this enzyme may represent a new molecular target for the therapy or prevention of neurodegenerative diseases, such as Parkinson's, Alzheimer's, and other aging-associated brain neurodegenerative disorders. In this regard, it is important to note that estradiol is decreased in the cerebrospinal fluid of older women (Murakami et al., 1999), likely reflecting a decrease in local cerebral levels of the hormone. Furthermore, estradiol is decreased both in plasma and the cerebrospinal fluid of women with Alzheimer's disease (Manly et al., 2000; Schonknecht et al., 2001), suggesting that aromatase activity or expression may be decreased in these patients.

The role of brain aromatase in neuroprotection calls for the development of new therapeutic strategies aimed at the up-regulation of the enzyme in the brain without affecting its expression in other tissues. Considering the possible health risks of hormonal therapy, the regulation of local brain estradiol synthesis may offer an interesting therapeutic alternative for neuroprotection. Since the expression of the human aromatase gene, CYP19, in the various tissues is regulated by the use of tissue-specific promoters that are regulated by different transcription factors and signaling pathways, it is possible to envisage the development of selective aromatase modulators specific for brain tissue (DonCarlos et al., 2007).

Neurosteroids

In addition to estradiol, the synthesis of other steroids is also increased in the central nervous system after injury; this may also represent an endogenous neuroprotective response. It is now well accepted that the central nervous system is a steroidogenic tissue that expresses enzymes involved in the synthesis and metabolism of steroids (Baulieu, 1997, 1998; Lavaque et al., 2006b; Mellon et al., 2001; Stoffel-Wagner, 2001, 2003). These include the cytochrome P450side-chain-cleavage (P450scc) enzyme, which catalyzes the conversion of cholesterol into pregnenolone, the precursor for glucocorticoids, mineralocorticoids, and sex steroids. The synthesis of pregnenolone is the first enzymatic step in steroidogenesis. However, there is a previous step that is rate-limiting and hormonally regulated: the transfer of cholesterol from the outer to the inner mitochondrial membrane, where P450scc is located. Proteins located in the mitochondrial membranes, such as the peripheral benzodiazepin receptor (renamed translocator protein 18kDa [TSPO]) (Lacor et al., 1999; Papadopoulos et al., 2006) and the steroidogenic acute regulatory protein (StAR) (Stocco, 2001) allow cholesterol to cross the hydrophilic intermembrane space (Hauet et al., 2005) to reach P450scc.

TSPO was initially described on peripheral tissues as a second binding site for diazepam, which binds with a higher affinity to $GABA_A$ receptors on the nervous system (Braestrup and Squires, 1977). Since then, many studies have demonstrated that TSPO is pharmacologically and structurally distinct from the central benzodiazepine/$GABA_A$ receptors. TSPO is an 18kDa peptide located predominantly in mitochondrial membranes (Anholt et al., 1986; Papadopoulos et al., 1994), and represents a critical component of the permeability transition pore, a multiprotein complex implicated in the regulation of apoptosis (Chelli et al., 2004; Galiegue et al., 2003; Kunduzova et al., 2004; Marselli et al., 2004; Veenman et al., 2004). In addition, TSPO has been related to the regulation of several physiological events, including the control of steroidogenesis (Brown and Papadopoulos, 2001; Casellas et al., 2002; Lacapere and Papadopoulos, 2003; Papadopoulos et al., 1997). TSPO is expressed in the nervous system, predominantly in glial cells (Casellas et al., 2002; Kuhlmann and Guilarte, 2000; Vowinckel et al., 1997; Wilms et al., 2003). In addition, different forms of neural injury and different neuropathological conditions result in the induction of the expression of TSPO in the regions of the nervous system involved in the neurodegenerative events (Lang, 2002). The induction of TSPO expression after injury in the central nervous system is restricted mainly to microglia and astrocytes (Casellas et al., 2002; Kuhlmann and Guilarte, 2000; Vowinckel et al., 1997; Wilms et al., 2003), although a study has shown induction of TSPO in dorsal root ganglion neurons following an injury to the sciatic nerve (Karchewski et al., 2004). The induction of TSPO expression after a neural injury suggests that this molecule may be involved in the response of the neural tissue to cope with the neurodegenerative process. Indeed, it has been reported that SSR180575, a pyridazinoindole derivative that possesses a high affinity for TSPO, increases the survival of facial nerve motoneurons after an axotomy, and promotes the regeneration of peripheral nerves (Ferzaz et al., 2002). Another TSPO ligand, the benzodiazepine 7-chloro-5-(4-chlorophenyl)-1,   3-dihydro-1-methyl-2H-1,4-benzodiazepin-2-one (Ro5–4864), prevents the loss of neurons induced by kainic acid in the rat hippocampal formation (Veiga et al., 2005b). TSPO ligands are also able to reduce the activation of astroglia and microglia after a brain injury (Veiga et al., 2005b, 2007). These neuroprotective effects of TSPO ligands may be mediated by an increased steroid synthesis, although other alternative or complementary mechanisms cannot be excluded.

TSPO is closely associated with StAR in mitochondrial membranes, and both proteins interact in the transfer of cholesterol across the outer mitochondrial membrane to the inner mitochondrial membrane (Hauet et al., 2005). StAR was first characterized in murine MA-10 Leydig tumor cells as a mitochondrial protein responsible for the acute induction of steroidogenesis (Clark et al., 1994). StAR is formed as a 37-kDa protein, which is rapidly transported into mitochondria where it is cleaved, generating a mature 30-kDa intramitochondrial StAR protein that is inactive (Bose et al., 2002). StAR has been extensively studied in classical steroidogenic tissues, such as the adrenal gland and the ovary (Stocco, 2001). In addition, several studies have shown the expression of StAR in the central nervous system (Furukawa et al., 1998; Inoue et al., 2002; Kim et al., 2002, 2003a, 2004; Kimoto et al., 2001; King et al., 2002; Lavaque et al., 2006a; MacKenzie et al., 2002; Sierra et al., 2003b; Wehrenberg et al., 2001). StAR appears to be widely distributed throughout the brain, although different levels of expression have been detected between different brain areas. Furthermore, StAR expression seems to be restricted to very specific neuronal and astroglial populations in each brain area (Sierra, 2004). High levels of StAR mRNA expression have been detected in the cerebral cortex, hippocampus, dentate gyrus, olfactory bulb, cerebellar granular layer, and cerebellar Purkinje cells of rodents (Furukawa et al., 1998; Kim et al., 2002, 2003a; King et al., 2002; Wehrenberg et al., 2001). StAR mRNA has also been detected in the human brain (Inoue et al., 2002; Kim et al., 2003b; King et al., 2002). Western blot and immunohistochemical analyses have confirmed that StAR protein is widely expressed throughout the adult central nervous system (Kimoto et al 2001; Sierra et al., 2003b). This may implicate that steroidogenesis is a generalized process in the central nervous system. In addition, StAR is colocalized in the same neural cells with cytochrome P450scc and other steroidogenic enzymes (Furukawa et al., 1998; Kimoto et al., 2001; King et al., 2002, 2004a; Wehrenberg et al., 2001), suggesting that individual neural cells may synthesize several steroids directly from cholesterol.

StAR immunoreactivity has been detected in several neuronal populations, in ependymocytes, and in some astroglial cells in the brain (King et al., 2002; Sierra et al., 2003b). The immunoreactive signal is located in the cytoplasm and has a punctate aspect compatible with mitochondrial localization. Strong StAR immunoreactivity is observed in the soma of large neurons, such as the motoneurons of the motor cranial nerves, large rombencephalic motoneurons, neurons of the deep cerebellar nuclei, Purkinje cells of the cerebellar cortex, and pyramidal neurons of the cerebral cortex. These large neurons are characterized by a high mitochondrial content. In general, there is good agreement between data from in situ mRNA localization and data from immunohistochemical studies. Brain regions where neuronal perikarya with high StAR expression have been detected include (i) areas involved in the transmission, processing, and integration of sensory information, such as the olfactory bulb, olfactory nuclei, somatosensory cerebral cortex, lateral geniculate nucleus, superior olive, superior colliculus, vestibular and cochlear nuclei, or the spinal trigeminal nucleus; (ii) areas involved in motor coordination and control, such as the motor cerebral cortex, the globus pallidus, some thalamic nuclei, the cerebellum, or several motor nuclei in the brainstem; (iii) areas involved in the control of brain activity and cognition, such as the locus coeruleus, the reticular formation, and the hippocampal formation (Sierra et al., 2003b). Therefore, StAR is expressed in brain areas with different functions. This broad distribution of StAR corresponds to what should be expected, considering the variety of brain functions affected by locally produced steroids (Baulieu, 1998; Compagnone and Mellon, 2000; Mellon et al., 2001; Stoffel-Wagner, 2003).

Although StAR is predominantly expressed by neurons in the central nervous system, astrocytes also express StAR, both in vivo and in vitro (King et al., 2002; Sierra et al., 2003b). Immunoreactivity for both StAR and the astroglial marker GFAP is observed in the gray matter of specific brain areas such as the molecular layer of the hippocampus and the superficial layers of the cerebral cortex. In the white matter, StAR expression is exclusively restricted to astrocytes. In some white matter areas in proximity to the pia mater, long StAR immunoreactive cell processes are observed perpendicular to the brain surface. These cell processes are immunoreactive for both GFAP and vimentin, and likely correspond to marginal glia. In other areas of white matter, including the hippocampal fimbria, the corpus callosum or the corticospinal tract, immunoreactivity for both GFAP and StAR is observed in the soma and processes of astrocytes (Sierra et al., 2003b). This suggests that a subpopulation of astroglial cells is able to synthesize steroids from cholesterol in vivo, in agreement with the ability of astrocytes to synthesize pregnenolone, progesterone, dehydroepiandrosterone, androstenedione, and testosterone in vitro (Zwain and Yen, 1999a, b), and with the localization of P450scc in brain white matter (Le Goascogne et al., 1987). The local production of steroids, such as progesterone, by astrocytes in the white matter may influence oligodendrocyte differentiation and myelination (Gago et al., 2001; Jung-Testas et al., 1996). Finally, it should be mentioned that StAR (Kim et al., 2003b) and steroidogenic enzymes (Papadopoulos et al., 1992; Yague et al., 2004; Zhang et al., 1995) are expressed in gliomas and may be potentially be involved in tumor progression.

Like TSPO, StAR expression is responsive to neurodegenerative insults: StAR mRNA and protein levels increase acutely and transiently in the brain after injury (Lavaque et al., 2006a; Sierra et al., 2003b). This raises the possibility that the up-regulation of the expression of TSPO and StAR and subsequent formation of neuroprotective steroids may be part of the mechanisms used by the nervous system to cope with neurodegeneration. In addition, the up-regulation of the expression of StAR and TSPO after injury is coordinated with the up-regulation of steroidogenic enzymes and steroid receptors (Blurton-Jones and Tuszynski, 2001; di Michele et al., 2000; Garcia-Ovejero et al., 2002, 2005; Labombarda et al., 2006b; Lavaque et al., 2006a). TSPO and StAR allow the formation of pregnenolone by nerve cells (Baulieu et al., 2001; Kimoto et al., 2001), which in turn may be converted into other steroids, since the nervous tissues express the necessary enzymatic machinery to synthesize a variety of steroids (Baulieu, 1997, 1998; London et al., 2006; Melcangi et al., 2008; Mellon et al., 2001; Stoffel-Wagner, 2003;). Pregnenolone, the first steroid synthesized from cholesterol by P450scc, is neuroprotective. For instance, pregnenolone reduces neuronal death in brain cell cultures (Bologa et al., 1987), and protects mouse hippocampal HT22 cells against glutamate and amyloid-β protein toxicity (Gursoy et al., 2001). In vivo, pregnenolone protects hippocampal neurons from kainic acid toxicity (Veiga et al., 2003). Furthermore, pregnenolone and its sulfate derivative enhance memory and cognitive function in different animal models (Darnaudery et al., 2002; Flood et al., 1992; Vallée et al., 1997a, 2001) and increase neurogenesis in the adult rat hippocampus (Mayo et al., 2001). Pregnenolone may exert its neuroprotective actions by several mechanisms, including the rapid modulation of $GABA_A$, NMDA, and sigma 1 receptors (Irwin et al., 1992; Majewska, 1992; Maurice et al., 2001; Wu et al., 1991). In addition, pregnenolone is able to bind to microtubule-associated protein 2 (MAP2) and stimulate microtubule assembly (Murakami et al., 2000; Plassart-Schiess and Baulieu, 2001), and therefore may exert effects on the neuronal cytoskeleton. The neuroprotective effects of pregnenolone may also be in part exerted by its metabolites. As it has been mentioned before in this chapter, progesterone, one of the metabolites of pregnenolone, also has neuroprotective properties. DHEA, which is an intermediate in the metabolic pathway from pregnenolone to estradiol, is also neuroprotective, as is testosterone, the direct precursor of estradiol. Therefore, the nervous system may react to injury-enhancing endogenous protection by increasing the synthesis of these neuroprotective steroids. Some of the neuroprotective steroids, such as pregnenolone, DHEA, and testosterone may exert neuroprotection, at least in part, after conversion to estradiol (Azcoitia et al., 2001; Veiga et al., 2003). For instance, the intracerebroventricular infusion of the aromatase inhibitor fadrozole in castrated male rats prevents the neuroprotective effects of pregnenolone, DHEA, and testosterone in the hippocampus against kainic acid (Azcoitia et al., 2001; Veiga et al., 2003). The aromatase inhibitor fadrozole also results in the blockage of the inhibitory action of DHEA on astrogliosis induced by deafferentation in the olfactory bulb (Hoyk et al., 2004). Therefore, estradiol formation by aromatase may mediate the neuroprotective and antigliotic effects of DHEA. This conclusion does not exclude alternative or complementary mechanisms for the neuroprotective effects of DHEA, including the formation of 7-hydroxylated metabolites (Jellinck et al., 2001).

Finally, an important question is whether the central nervous tissue is a source of substrates for brain aromatase. Glial cells in vitro may convert pregnenolone to DHEA and may then metabolize DHEA to testosterone (Zwain and Yen, 1999 a, b). In addition, studies by Suguru Kawato and his collaborators have demonstrated that estradiol is synthesized in the adult rat brain from cholesterol through pregnenolone, dehydroepiandrosterone, and testosterone (Hojo et al., 2004; Ishii et al., 2007). However, it is still unclear whether the brain of some species, including the human brain, expresses all the enzymes needed to transform cholesterol into estradiol.

CHAPTER SUMMARY

In previous chapters of this book I have analyzed how physiological modifications in brain plasticity affect the activity of endocrine glands, and how physiological changes in hormonal levels impacts brain plasticity in order to maintain a functional homeodynamic equilibrium in the organism. The cross talk between the brain and endocrine glands also shows adaptive changes under pathological conditions. Alterations in brain plasticity due to brain pathology provoke modifications in the levels of hormonal secretions. Some of these hormonal secretions may in turn have an impact in the damaged brain and affect the reorganization of the injured neural tissue. I have examined the extensive evidence indicating that numerous hormones affect brain reorganization after injury and neurodegeneration. Some hormones exert neuroprotective and regenerative actions, promoting a reparative remodeling of the damaged brain, spinal cord, and peripheral nerves. However, deficits in hormonal levels or in hormonal signaling due to endocrine diseases or other causes has a negative impact in the central nervous system, promoting impairments of glial plasticity, synaptic plasticity, and neurogenesis. The alteration in the physiological homeodynamic equilibrium between the brain and endocrine glands due to endocrine diseases may result in cognitive alterations, and may represent a risk factor for the onset of neurodegenerative diseases. Aging is another situation in which alterations in the homeodynamic equilibrium between endocrine glands and brain plasticity represent a risk for the onset of brain pathology. I will examine the interaction between hormones and brain remodeling during aging in the next chapter.

Chapter 10

Life Stages, Hormones, and Brain Remodeling: Aging

INTRODUCTION: CHANGES IN BRAIN PLASTICITY AND ENDOCRINE FUNCTION WITH AGING

In previous chapters I have reviewed many examples of brain plastic changes that are modulated by hormonal signals during the developmental and adult periods of life. These examples have been presented in support of the central hypothesis of this book, which is that hormones play an essential role in the modulation of the endogenous mutability of the central nervous system, regulating plasticity and metaplasticity in adaptation to the environmental, biological, and social context, as well as endogenous body needs. Although some forms of brain plasticity may be affected by aging, during this period of life the brain continues its process of continual reorganization and suffers a substantial remodeling. This remodeling may in part represent an adaptation to the extensive physiological modifications that occur in the organism with the aging process, but it also reflects that the endogenous programming of the brain for mutability is still active in older ages.

Hormones play an essential role in the adaptation to aging by providing information regarding body changes to the brain. Thus, the impact of hormones on brain plasticity is also highly relevant during this final stage of the individual life cycle. The mutual interactions of the endocrine and nervous systems, which allows for the regulation of body homeodynamics during juvenile and adult life, are also maintained in older individuals. As in previous life periods, these interactions involve the remodeling of neuronal structure and function in parallel with the endocrine modifications. Aging is a period of profound changes in the body; this is reflected in the profound changes that occur in the communication between the endocrine organs and the brain as well. As for other periods of intense reorganization during life (such as early development and puberty), aging represents a moment where the fragility of the homeodynamic system is maximal and where this system is therefore more exposed to disequilibrium and to the consecutive onset of pathological alterations. Therefore, one of the difficulties in analyzing hormonal influences on brain plasticity in older individuals is to distinguish those aspects of brain remodeling that corresponds to physiological adaptive modifications from those that reflect pathological alterations. However, it is important to keep in mind that not all aspects of brain remodeling during aging necessarily reflect a loss of function or pathology and that some aspects may represent physiological adaptations.

The causes that produce the extensive physiological modifications of body functions with aging are still a matter of debate. Indeed, the causes of aging are still a mystery, as well as the relation, if any, of aging and lifespan. We do not yet have complete and fully satisfactory answers to many basic questions related to the aging process. It is even difficult to define with precision what the process of aging consists of. However, we know that aging is a period of transformation and reorganization of the homeodynamic systems of the body, and is associated with a restructuring of the homeodynamic equilibrium between the brain, the hormones, and the immune system.

One landmark of the aging process is a decline in immune function (Grubeck-Loebenstein and Wick, 2002; Miller, 1996). The involution of the thymus with aging is the cause of alterations in cellular and humoral immunity (Gruver et al., 2007), which affects all tissues and organs, including the nervous system. The brain is also affected by changes in hormonal levels during aging. In turn, aging-associated brain remodeling may be involved in the alterations of the endocrine and immune systems. Likely, the immune, endocrine, and nervous systems closely interact with mutual influences during the aging process (Fig. 10.1). The brain via the autonomic nervous system and hypothalamic regulation of pituitary hormones (such as growth hormone) may affect thymic involution and T-cell-mediated immune responses in aged animals (Burgess et al., 1999; Fabris et al., 1995; Kelley et al., 1988; Savino et al., 1999). Immune responses and cytokines released by the thymus, in turn, may affect the endocrine glands and the brain. Aging is associated with increased levels of various cytokines in plasma (Ershler, 1993; Hager et al., 1994; Roubenoff et al., 1998; Wei et al., 1992), and there is substantial evidence that peripheral cytokines can cross the blood–brain barrier (Dunn, 1992; Gutierrez, 1993, 1994) and directly affect brain function or may

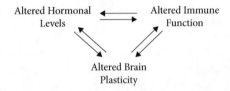

Figure 10.1. Aging is associated with alterations in brain plasticity, in hormonal levels, and in immune function. Alterations in hormonal levels may impact the immune system; alterations in immune function impact the activity of endocrine glands. Brain plasticity is affected by the modifications in hormonal levels and in endocrine function. In turn, aging-associated changes in brain plasticity affect the activity of endocrine glands and the immune system.

indirectly affect the brain via vagal afferents (Dantzer et al., 1998; Hansen et al., 1998). Acting on the brain, cytokines may induce reactive gliosis and central inflammatory responses, alter synaptic function and synaptic plasticity, affect behavior, impair cognition, alter sleep, and promote depression (Craig et al., 2002). In addition, the endocrine thymus produces hormones, such as thymulin, homeostatic thymus hormone, thymus factor, thymosin fraction 5, thymosin α-1, and thymosin β-4, which may affect the activity of the hypothalamus–pituitary axis acting on β-endorphin, adrenocorticotropic hormone (ACTH), glucocorticoids, luteinizing-hormone-releasing hormone, and luteinizing hormone secretion (Goya and Bolognani, 1999; Goya et al., 1999). Therefore, thymic involution with aging may also result in alterations in pituitary hormonal secretions.

Several hormones may affect immune responses with aging, including melatonin and thyroid hormones. In addition, it is well established that the hypothalamic–pituitary–adrenal axis, which shows activation with aging and is known to modulate brain plasticity (see Chapters 3 and 5), exerts a strong regulation of immune function (McEwen et al., 1997). Indeed, glucocorticoids have been used as immunosuppressive agents since the 1940s (Hench, 1952; Webster et al., 2002). Emotional stress, which may also be enhanced in elderly people showing impaired social cognition, affects immune function (Butcher and Lord, 2004; McEwen et al., 1997) and regulates brain plasticity (see Chapter 8). Therefore, brain remodeling, alteration of hormonal levels, and modifications of immune responses occur in parallel during aging, and are likely closely interrelated. Although our attention in this chapter focuses on the relations between hormonal changes and brain remodeling during aging, it is important to keep in mind that the reshaping of the neuroendocrine equilibrium with aging occurs in a context in which the immune system is also suffering a prominent reorganization, which may be actively involved in the endocrine and neural modifications.

Before analyzing the mutual influences of the endocrine and nervous system during aging, let us briefly summarize the main modifications that occur in the aged brain. Aging is a period of life accompanied by remarkable structural remodeling and volume changes of different brain regions. Studies with noninvasive brain imaging of living subjects have revealed that the human brain decreases in volume with aging. In particular, very interesting changes have been detected in the white matter, which shows a decline in volume in the later years of life. Myelin may represent one of the most vulnerable structures to aging (Bartzokis, 2004; Salat et al., 2005); myelin loss implies less functional neuronal connections, and may therefore have a strong impact on brain function and cognition. While the decrease in volume of the white matter with aging seems to be uniform, some regions of the gray matter are more affected by aging than others (Alexander et al., 2008; Esiri, 2007). For instance, the frontal and parietal regions of the cerebral cortex seem to be more affected than temporal and occipital cortical regions. Histological studies have also detected structural changes associated with aging in the brains of different species, such as a loss of neurons and myelinated fibers, increased numbers of astrocytes and microglia, reduced neurogenesis in the subventricular zone and the dentate gyrus of the hippocampus, reduced dendritic branching, reduced number of dendritic spines and synapses, and reduced size of perforated postsynaptic densities (Esiri, 2007; Finch, 2003; Geinisman et al., 1992; Hof and Morrison, 2004; Kempermann et al., 1998; Kuhn et al., 1996; Luo et al., 2006; Masliah et al., 2006; Nicholson et al., 2004; Scheibel, 1979; Scheibel et al., 1976; Seki and Arai, 1995). As just mentioned for the findings with noninvasive imaging techniques, histological studies in the brains of animals and humans have also detected that not all brain regions appear to be equally affected by aging, suggesting that some neuronal populations or brain regions are more vulnerable than others. This may be in part due to differences in vascularization or metabolic activity. However, there is a striking concordance between the brain regions that are more affected by aging and those in which hormones exert more profound regulatory actions on the plasticity of neural tissue.

The hippocampus, amygdala, and prefrontal cortex are highly sensitive to hormones, and also show strong structural remodeling with aging. For instance, synaptic loss and decreased dendritic branching has been detected in the prefrontal cortex, medial temporal lobe structures, and hippocampus of older humans and rodents (Bondareff and Geinisman, 1976; de Brabander et al., 1998; Geinisman et al., 1986; Grill and Riddle, 2002; Hof and Morrison, 2004; Markham and Juraska, 2002; Rosenzweig and Barnes, 2003; Scheibel, 1979; Scheibel et al., 1976; Uylings and de Brabander, 2002), and moderate neuronal loss has been detected in the prefrontal cortex of aging monkeys (Smith et al., 2004) and in the medial prefrontal cortex, visual cortex, and the hilus of the dentate gyrus of the hippocampus of aged rats (Azcoitia et al., 2005; Yates et al., 2008), although generalized neuronal loss with aging is an uncommon finding (Gazzaley et al., 1997; Keuker et al., 2003; Merrill et al., 2000, 2001; Pakkenberg and Gundersen, 1997; Peters et al., 1994; Rapp and Gallagher, 1996; Rasmussen et al., 1996; West et al., 1994). Most likely, nonpathological changes in brain function during aging are predominantly related to decreased myelination, selective and regional-specific dendritic remodeling, regional modifications in the number of synaptic inputs, and regional modifications of synaptic function and plasticity, and are not the consequence of a massive neuronal or synaptic loss. For instance, aging is associated with a decrease in the number of dendritic spines in the apical dendrites of layer V cortical pyramidal neurons of the rat visual cortex. However, in older individuals, this decrease is not homogeneous along the whole length of the apical dendritic shaft, being more pronounced in the segments of the dendrite crossing layers II/III and IV than in dendritic segments crossing deep layers (Ruiz-Marcos et al., 1992). This likely reflects a selective reorganization of neuronal circuits with aging rather than an unspecific alteration in all synaptic contacts on dendritic spines. The selective reorganization of neuronal connectivity is associated with selective functional modifications in neuronal excitability, calcium homeodynamics, and functional synaptic plasticity (Barnes, 2003; Chapman, 2005; Foster and Norris, 1997; Landfield, 1988; Rosenzweig and Barnes, 2003). For instance, synaptic long-term potentiation is impaired in the brain of aged rats, although with regional specificity (Barnes, 2003; Burke and Barnes, 2006; Lynch et al., 2006; Rosenzweig and Barnes, 2003; Toescu et al., 2004).

Cognitive processes that rely on the medial temporal lobe and prefrontal cortex, such as learning, memory, and executive function, show considerable aging-related impairments (Burke and Barnes, 2006). Spatial memory is one of the modalities more affected in elder people, and this may reflect an increased vulnerability of the hippocampus. Altered synaptic function and plasticity in the hippocampus with aging may impair the process of encoding new information (Wilson et al., 2006). Decreased neurogenesis may also contribute to impaired hippocampal function with aging (Darnaudery et al., 2006; Drapeau et al., 2003). Working memory, which is dependent on the prefrontal cortex and declarative memory (which is dependent on the hippocampus and other medial temporal lobe regions) are also affected in elderly persons. Older people may also be affected by depression; mainly those with chronic illnesses and cognitive impairment (Alexopoulos, 2005). Sensation and motor control are also affected in older ages. All these functional losses may be associated with alterations in brain plasticity with aging (Mahncke et al., 2006).

What are the causes of these modifications? As mentioned at the beginning of this chapter, some causes may represent physiological adaptations; others may reflect pathological alterations. It is not an easy task to distinguish what is physiological and what is not. Is the decrease in some cognitive modalities adaptive or pathological? We tend to think that aging modifications in brain reflect a generalized decline in its function. However, it cannot be excluded that the selective loss of a specific cognitive function, the selective decrease in the branching of some dendritic trees, or the selective modifications of functional synaptic plasticity in specific brain regions may reflect adaptations. As I have already mentioned, not all cognitive functions (and not all brain regions) are equally affected by aging. Remodeling in some brain regions may thus represent, at least in part, a process of adaptation to the new physiological conditions. What, then, are the causes of pathological alterations with aging? Although the probability of developing a neurodegenerative disorder (such as Alzheimer's or Parkinson's diseases) increases in elderly people, age per se is not the cause of brain pathological alterations. If we compare different elderly people of the same age, we will find a great variability in the degrees of cognitive, neurological, or affective alterations. Some people will have a completely normal brain function; and in others we will find neurodegenerative disorders. For instance, cognitive decline in elderly people ranges from normal cognitive aging, through mild cognitive impairment, to the dementias. Thus, there is an obvious individual variability in terms of brain deterioration with aging (for instance, see Perls, 2004; Wilson R.S. et al., 2002).

Several factors impact the variability of normal cognitive aging. According to the Scottish Mental Surveys of 1932 and 1947, the most important determining factor for cognitive aging is childhood intelligence (Deary et al., 2004). In addition, a variety of medical, psychological, social, and lifestyle factors interacting with genetic contributions also influence normal cognitive aging. Early events during fetal life (Whalley et al., 2006) may also impact late cognitive decline (see Chapter 6). The development of neurodegenerative alterations also depends on different interactions between life events and environmental and genetic factors. A restricted caloric diet, exercise, and exposure to a rich environment are among the environmental factors that may promote healthy brain aging. Some genes appear to be associated with healthy brain aging, and other genes increase the risk of neurodegeneration (Mattson and Magnus, 2006).

The function of endocrine organs is also affected by aging. In consequence, the levels of several hormones change in plasma with aging: some of them decrease, others increase, and others do not change. It should be noted that the change in the levels of hormones with aging and the nature of the changes are not identical in all species. For instance, menopause in women, caused by the loss of ovarian secretions, is associated with a dramatic decrease of estradiol levels in plasma. In contrast, reproductive aging in rats, caused by hypothalamic failure to properly regulate ovarian secretions, is often associated with high estradiol levels in plasma. Dehydroepiandrosterone (DHEA) levels decrease with aging in humans, a change that does not occur in rodents where DHEA levels are undetectable in plasma. In humans, growth hormone, ghrelin, insulin-like growth factor-I (IGF-I), DHEA, sex hormones, and thyroid-stimulating hormone are among the hormones that decrease with aging. In contrast, other hormones, like parathyroid hormone and prolactin, follicle-stimulating hormone, and luteinizing hormone increase in elderly people (Chahal and Drake, 2007). Aging-associated changes in hormonal levels may involve differences in secretion, metabolism, or both. For instance, both thyroid hormone secretion and metabolism decrease with aging, and serum thyroxine (T4) concentrations are not affected. However, as a result of the decreased metabolism of T4 into triiodothyronine (T3), the levels of T3 decrease with aging (Mariotti et al., 1995). Additionally, hormonal changes with aging are not necessarily linear. Good examples of this are the hormonal changes during menopause in women (Djahanbakhch et al., 2007; Johnson, 1998; Sherman et al., 1976). Compared to younger women, estradiol and inhibin B levels are lower, follicle stimulating hormone concentrations are higher, and luteinizing hormone levels are unchanged during the follicular phase in women of advanced reproductive age with ovulatory cycles. Then, after menopause, estrogen concentrations fall and follicle stimulating hormone and luteinizing hormone levels rise above premenopausal concentrations. Follicle stimulating hormone and luteinizing hormone levels also show a tendency to increase with aging in men.

In addition to changes in hormonal levels with aging, there are also altera-tions in circadian hormonal secretion rhythm. This is the case for testosterone in men in which circadian rhythm of plasma levels, higher in the morning than in the evening, is generally lost with aging (Bremner et al., 1983). The amplitude of the nocturnal pulses of thyroid stimulating hormone secretion is also lower in elderly subjects (Greenspan et al., 1991); there are also altera-tions in circadian rhythms of plasma cortisol in elderly people (Sherman et al., 1985; Van et al., 1996).

It is also important to consider that hormonal signaling and the cross talk between the brain and the endocrine glands in older ages may be altered with-out major changes in basal hormonal levels. One example is insulin resistance in the aged brain (Cole and Frautschy, 2007; García-San Frutos et al., 2007), which results in alterations in the regulation of brain plasticity and may cause cerebral atrophy and may have deleterious consequences for cognitive func-tion in elderly people (Reagan, 2007; see also Chapter 9). Another example is brain resistance to leptin (Fernandez-Galaz et al., 2001; Muzumdar et al., 2006; Scarpace et al., 2001), which may also potentially impact the plasticity of the aging brain (see Chapter 5). This is also the case with hormones regulated by the hypothalamo–pituitary–adrenal axis. Although there are no apparent changes in the levels of adrenal corticosteroids with aging (Waltman et al., 1991), the response to stress may be accentuated in elderly people (Bergendahl et al., 2000; Seeman and Robbins, 1994). Alterations in their capacity to pro-cess incoming information and to adequately adapt their responses to the changing environmental and social conditions are among the causes and consequences of their difficulties in coping with stressors (Fig. 10.2). Thus, decreases in the volume of the hippocampus in elderly people may reduce their capacity to process information and adapt to the social and environmen-tal context (Lupien et al., 2007).

Information processing in elderly people is further impaired by the fact that sensory organs provide unreliable information to the brain as sensory deficits progress with aging. In addition, the responses of elderly people to sensory inputs are also altered due to their decreased muscular strength, as well as impairments in motor coordination and postural balance (Stern and Carstensen, 2000). Other factors, such as alterations in circadian rhythms, may also contribute to the impaired response to stress in older ages. Moreover, social isolation is common in elderly individuals and may also contribute to their difficulties to cope with social stress. The psychological consequences of their nonadaptive responses to the changing environmental and social con-text further increase their nonadaptive responses to stressors—a vicious loop that may finally cause or facilitate the onset of depression and other affective and cognitive pathologies (Fig. 10.2).

Changes in hormonal levels and/or in hormonal responsiveness with aging are associated in time with the progression of neurodegenerative disorders, increased depressive symptoms, and other psychological disturbances. This suggests that the alteration of the cross talk between the endocrine glands and

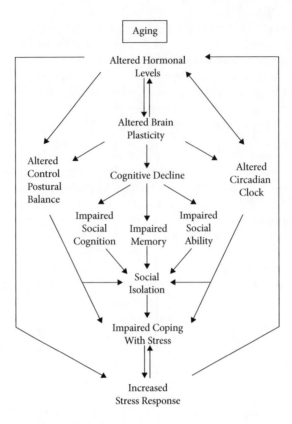

Figure 10.2. Modifications in brain plasticity and ability to process sensory information in older people may cause impairments in their cognitive skills, affecting social cognition, memory, and their ability to interact with other individuals. Alterations in physical strength and postural balance, together with alterations in the circadian clock, further contribute to social isolation, which causes an impaired ability to cope with stress and an increased stress response. This generates a vicious circle that results in further instability of the system: the increased stress response results in hormonal changes that will further affect brain plasticity, physical strength, motor control, circadian rhythms, and cognition.

the brain may be a risk factor for the development of neurodegenerative diseases or affective disorders of different etiologies in elderly people. Thus, the modification in hormone levels or hormonal signaling with aging may have a negative impact on the regulation of brain plasticity, and may in some way contribute to brain alterations with aging. However, the fact that two events occur at the same time is not proof of a causal relationship. Hormones may change and brain may suffer alterations in its plasticity and function by different causes; one event does not necessarily have to influence the other. I will analyze this question in detail in this chapter, and will argue in favor of the importance of the cross talk between the brain and endocrine organs in the regulation of physiological and pathological brain remodeling with aging.

Let me start with some basic questions on hormonal changes with aging. Are these hormonal alterations linked directly with the aging process? Do they reflect a physiological or a pathological alteration? If the alteration is pathological, does it promote aging-associated disorders or, on the contrary, represent a compensatory mechanism to cope with other aging-associated alterations? And finally, are the aging-associated hormonal changes good, bad, or irrelevant for brain function? It is easier to address by experimentation some of these questions than others; none have a direct short answer. In the next sections will focus on the trio of subjects that are involved: the hormones, the brain, and the aging process. I will discuss whether the decrease in plasma levels of several hormones that occur with aging represents a positive adaptation to the new physiological conditions of the aged individual or, on the contrary, represents a genuine deficit, negatively impacting brain function. The paradox that exists—the signaling of some hormones (growth hormone, IGF-I) is neuroprotective, yet at the same time it reduces longevity—will be discussed. How hormonal deprivation with aging affects the brain will also be covered, as well as a review of the studies dealing with the effects of hormonal therapies (gonadal hormones, DHEA, growth hormone, melatonin, and so forth) on the plasticity and function of the aging brain, including the human brain.

BIOLOGICAL SIGNIFICANCE OF ENDOCRINE FUNCTION CHANGES WITH AGING

As has been noted many times in this book, the regulation of hormone synthesis and metabolism is an essential mechanism to maintain body homeodynamics. Therefore, hormonal plasma levels fluctuate to maintain proper physiological function. Growth, reproduction, metabolism, temperature control, ionic concentration and water balance, and behavior: all body functions are tamely and timely regulated by changes in hormonal levels. Thus, plasma hormone levels increase and decrease according to physiological demands. Changes in the rate of hormonal synthesis and in the rate of hormonal metabolism participate in this physiological adaptation. However, hormonal levels in plasma may also change as a consequence of a pathological disequilibrium. This change may be the direct consequence of the pathology. In this case, hormone levels may change because its metabolism or synthesis is directly altered by pathology. Pathological alterations in the synthesis or metabolism of hormones are common in humans, and is the cause of many clinical syndromes. Many people suffer from an alteration in their pancreatic islets characterized by a massive or complete loss of β cells, the cells that produce insulin. This cellular loss leads to a decrease in insulin levels. In this case, pathology—the loss of β cells—is the direct cause of a change in hormonal production. As a secondary consequence, the homeodynamic function of insulin for the regulation of glucose metabolism is defective, and a new pathology emerges: diabetes mellitus. In other cases, however, a change in hormonal levels in plasma may represent a compensatory reaction to a pathological status. Hormonal secretion is then altered to cope with the pathological situation in an attempt to reach a new homeodynamic equilibrium. For instance, serum levels of insulin are increased in patients with insulin resistance. This is probably caused by both an increase of insulin secretion and a decrease in insulin degradation. By this compensatory mechanism, some people may maintain adequate glucose levels even if insulin signaling is defective.

Hormonal changes in plasma may thus correspond to at least three different situations, reflecting: i) a homeodynamic adaptation to changing physiological conditions; ii) a homeodynamic compensatory response to pathology; or iii) the direct consequence of a pathological alteration that, in turn, may result in a secondary pathology as a consequence of the hormonal misbalance. In which one of these categories should the changes in hormonal levels associated with aging be classified? This is not a semantic or purely academic question. In my view, it is important to understand the biological meaning of the hormonal changes associated with aging. If they were the consequence of a pathological situation, then it would be advisable to try to counteract the effects of the hormonal alteration. For instance, hormonal therapy would be adequate as a treatment to compensate for a decreased hormonal production with aging in this case. However, if the decrease of such a hormone with aging is a physiological homeodynamic adaptation or a compensatory response to pathology, then hormonal therapy could do more harm than good. Therefore, we should try to understand the causes and the biological significance of the hormonal changes with aging.

BRAIN MUTABILITY REGULATES AGING-ASSOCIATED CHANGES IN ENDOCRINE FUNCTION

The relation of hormones, the brain, and aging has two complementary faces: on one side, hormonal changes associated with the aging of endocrine glands may affect the brain; on the other side, brain remodeling associated with aging of the nervous tissue may alter hormonal production. Since the brain is the most important center for endocrine control, brain aging may have a strong impact on hormonal levels. Brain plasticity with aging may result in a reorganization of the circuits involved in sensing hormones and controlling hormone release. Indeed, there is evidence indicating that the hypothalamic circuits regulating hormonal production suffer marked alterations with aging. During aging, there is a decrease in the ordered rhythmic pattern of hormone release that likely reflects a modification of neuronal circuits regulating pituitary secretions (Smith et al., 2005; Wise, 1987, 1999; Wise et al., 1999). Indeed, aging is associated with a dramatic reorganization of the serotonergic and noradrenergic hypothalamic systems, as well as the tuberoinfundibular dopaminergic system (Hung et al., 2003; Reymond, 1990; Rossi et al., 1992;

Weiland et al., 1989). There is also a decrease in the expression of receptors for hormones, neuropeptides, and neurotransmitters (Brann and Mahesh, 2005; Gore, 2001; Sadow and Rubin, 1992), reorganization of neural membranes (Garcia-Segura et al., 1991a), and alterations in glial plasticity (Cashion et al., 2003) in brain regions regulating hormonal secretions.

All these changes affect the secretion of several hormones, such as luteinizing hormone and growth hormone. The pulse amplitude of these hormones is affected because of the hypothalamic alterations of the secretions of gonado-tropin-releasing hormone and growth-hormone-releasing hormone (GHRH), respectively. In turn, aging-associated modifications in growth hormone result in a reduced production of IGF-I in the liver, and alterations in gonado-tropins affect the release of sex steroid hormones. Thus, it is likely that the reorganization of specific neuronal circuits may initiate the hormonal changes associated with aging. If this were the case, the hormonal changes would be a consequence of brain aging. Reproductive aging in rodents is an example of how the aging of the brain may affect hormonal secretion. Contrary to women, in which menopause is mainly the consequence of a failure of the ovaries to respond to gonadotropins, reproductive aging in rodents is believed to be caused by the hypothalamic failure to regulate gonadotropin secretion, and thus, ovarian function. Areas of the hypothalamus of rodents that regu-late gonadotropin secretion show structural and functional changes in aged females (Brann and Mahesh, 2005; Garcia-Segura et al., 1991a; Gore, 2001; Hung et al., 2003; Sadow and Rubin, 1992). The hypothalamus is then unable to support cyclic ovarian function regulation and the animal enters the period of reproductive aging. Consequently, ovarian hormones do not show the cyclic changes observed in young females. Therefore, in this case, brain remodeling is the cause of the hormonal changes. Hypothalamic reorganization may also be the cause of changes in the control of gonadotropins that are involved in the irregularity of menstrual cycles in the perimenopausal period in women (Wise, 1999; Wise et al., 1999).

HORMONES REGULATE AGING-ASSOCIATED CHANGES IN BRAIN MUTABILITY

From the above, we may then assume that some hormonal changes associated with aging are initiated by specific plastic alterations in the brain circuits that regulate endocrine secretions. The question then becomes: what triggers these modifications in brain plasticity? Are we dealing with an endogenous mecha-nism of brain aging or a metaplastic adaptation of neuronal networks to previ-ous hormonal changes? We could imagine a scenario in which subtle hormonal changes initiate a modification in brain plasticity. Then, the reorganized neuronal circuits will result in a modification in the regulation of endocrine secretions. Subsequently, the distorted hormone levels in turn will produce new modifications in brain plasticity that will result in an amplification of the hormonal changes. This may reflect a situation where the equilibrium is broken in a temporal point of maximal instability. The temporal point in which equilibrium is broken may be reached by the cumulative sum of small changes in hormonal levels and brain plastic modifications, and may represent an example of brain metaplasticity. For instance, Frederick Naftolin and James R. Brawer proposed that the hypothalamic failure to maintain ovarian cycles in rodents is the result of accumulative estrogen input to the hypothalamic arcuate nucleus, which is involved in the cycling regulation of gonadotropin secretion (Brawer et al., 1980; Naftolin and Brawer, 1978). According to this hypothesis (re-elaborated with the concept of metaplasticity), accumulative regulatory actions of estradiol on synaptic and glial plasticity in the arcuate nucleus during each estrus cycle (see Chapter 8) would gradually alter future synaptic and glial plastic responses to ovarian hormones in this brain region (Horvath et al., 1997b; Hung et al., 2003; Leedom et al., 1994) and will finally result in the impaired function of specific neuronal circuits that regulate gonadotropin secretion, such as those in which β-endorphin neurons are involved (Desjardins et al., 1995). Thus, regulation of metaplasticity in the arcuate nucleus by estradiol will result in an altered regulation of ovarian secretions, which finally will lead to reproductive aging.

The complexity of the cross talk between hormones and brain plasticity in the aging process is also well illustrated by the effects of stress on brain aging. Substantial evidence supports the existence of a link between stress, hypothalamo–pituitary–adrenal axis dysfunction, memory disorders, and aging (McEwen, 2002; Sapolsky et al., 1986). Here, it is important to consider the different effects that stress hormones have on the brain, depending on whether we are facing acute stress or chronic, unpredictable stress. Acute stress is essential for proper physiological function; overcoming acute stress is a source of psychological enjoyment. We all need acute stress, and actively search for it. Chronic or repetitive, unpredictable stress is something very different. Chronic, unpredictable stress is a source of despair and depression; nobody likes to suffer from it. Overcoming acute stress has a positive impact on the brain, and is essential for memory formation. We remember much better those past situations that were impregnated with positive or negative emotions than those that were emotionally indifferent. Basal levels of glucocorticoids associated with acute stress are important for memory formation. In contrast, repetitive glucocorticoid action, during repeated or chronic stress, has a negative impact on the brain, resulting in memory and cognitive alterations.

Two important concepts, already introduced in this book, may help us understanding the different effects of acute and repetitive stress, and the rupture of homeodynamic equilibrium in aging: allostasis and allostatic load (McEwen, 2002; see also Chapter 3). Allostasis is the adaptation exerted by the neuroendocrine system, autonomic nervous system, and the immune system to the challenges of daily life. These systems maintain stability through change—their action is initiated when needed, and is shut off when no longer needed. These changes, such as the acute stress response, are adaptive in the short run. However, the action of the regulatory systems may be damaging if it is not shut off in due time. The regulatory signals may then cause alterations in the target tissues that may lead to pathological damage. This is the situation termed *allostatic load*. Thus, the acute actions of glucocorticoids may represent an allostatic response, maintaining proper function of the brain. However, if the action of glucocorticoids is not efficiently terminated, if we are unable to overcome stress, our brain and its capacity to program adaptive control of endocrine glands and behavior will be affected. Then, the new endocrine adjustments will further affect the brain, initiating a cascade of alterations that will produce brain damage and permanent hormonal imbalance in the end.

This is the basis of the so-called "glucocorticoid cascade hypothesis" of aging, a theory postulating that changes in specific brain areas, as a result of allostatic load, initiate the process of aging (Sapolsky, 1992). According to this hypothesis, one of the key brain regions involved in this process is the hippocampus, which is involved in episodic, declarative, spatial, and contextual memory, and is also an important integration center for the regulation of autonomic, neuroendocrine, and immune responses. Interestingly, the hippocampus is one of the brain regions more vulnerable to damage caused by repetitive stress. Neuronal death in the hippocampus after chronic glucocorticoid exposure may occur in some species and under certain conditions (Sapolsky, 1992; Sapolsky et al., 1985). However, hippocampal cell loss after chronic glucocorticoid exposure is not a generalized finding in all species (Conrad, 2006; Fuchs et al., 2001; Leverenz et al., 1999; Vollmann-Honsdorf et al., 1997) and does not occur in humans (Bao et al., 2008; Swaab et al., 2005). This may be due to the fact that the primate hippocampus expresses lower levels of glucocorticoid receptors than the hippocampus of rodents (Sanchez et al., 2000), which show neuronal death after chronic glucocorticoid exposure (Sapolsky, 1992; Sapolsky et al., 1985).

Although neuronal loss is not involved in all species, structural plastic changes in the hippocampus is likely a generalized response to the allostatic load caused by glucocorticoids. Chronic stress produces remodeling of dendrites and dendritic spines in the hippocampal neurons, decreases hippocampal neurogenesis, induces gliosis, and finally may promote the impairment of hippocampal function (Fuchs et al., 2001; McEwen, 2002; Mirescu and Gould, 2006; Sapolsky et al., 1985; see also Chapter 3). As a consequence, memory, cognition, autonomic control, endocrine secretions, and the immune system will be altered. Not only can unpredictable repetitive stress in adulthood increase hippocampal damage, repetitive stress during the prenatal period may even result in alterations in hippocampal synaptic plasticity and neurogenesis at older ages (see Chapter 6). Prenatal stress in rats induces an increased anxiety-like behavior and permanent dysfunction of the hypothalamo–pituitary–adrenal axis system in adult life. Aged rats that were stressed during prenatal life show spatial hippocampal-dependent learning impairments (Darnaudery et al., 2006; Vallée et al., 1999) compared to normal older animals.

Stress hormones affect other brain regions, such as the cerebral cortex and the amygdala (see Chapter 3). Repeated stress causes dendritic remodeling in the amygdala, increasing the dendritic length and spine synapse formation. In contrast, dendritic length in neurons from the medial prefrontal cortex is decreased by chronic stress (McEwen, 1999, 2005). It is remarkable that the brain regions more vulnerable to chronic stress, such as the hippocampus, the amygdala, and the prefrontal cortex, are also those regions that are more affected by aging. The effect of stress hormones on brain aging may also be envisaged as an example of metaplasticity. According to this view, developmental plastic changes induced by stress hormones during fetal and early postnatal life, and its regulatory actions on brain plasticity during puberty and adult life, will predetermine future plastic brain responses during aging. Metaplastic brain modifications induced by stress hormones throughout life may explain the long-term effects that their actions have on affection, behavior, and cognition in older ages.

A PARADOX: UNEXPECTED RELATIONSHIP BETWEEN BRAIN AGING, HORMONES, AND LONGEVITY

How stress hormones may affect brain aging has been previously discussed; an analysis of the effects that other hormonal changes during aging have on brain function is in order. As seen from Chapter 9, animal studies have shown that several hormones may protect neurons from different neurodegenerative stimuli. These include growth hormone, IGF-I, DHEA, and sex hormones. All these hormones have been shown to regulate plasticity and exert neuroprotective actions in the aging brain. Therefore, it is possible that the decrease in the levels of these hormones in elderly people may result in altered brain plasticity and decreased protection against the environmental and genetic factors that promote neurodegeneration. Some hormones, such as estradiol and IGF-I, antagonize the damaging effects of adrenal steroids. IGF-I attenuates spatial learning deficits in aged rats and promotes neurogenesis in the hippocampus. Chronic IGF-I infusion in the brain restores the spatial learning abilities of aged rats that were stressed during prenatal life. IGF-I also upregulates neurogenesis in the hippocampus of these animals, and reduces their hypothalamo–pituitary–adrenal axis dysfunction (Darnaudery et al., 2006). Interestingly, IGF-I increases estradiol levels in the plasma of aged rats that were submitted to prenatal stress. Estradiol, in turn, is known to increase neurogenesis in the hippocampus of old rats (Perez-Martin et al., 2005) and prevents hippocampal damage induced by excitotoxic injuries (Azcoitia et al., 1998). In addition, the signaling of estradiol and IGF-I interacts to promote neuroprotection (Azcoitia et al., 1999b; Garcia-Segura et al., 2006; Quesada and Micevych, 2004) and to regulate hippocampal neurogenesis (Perez-Martin et al., 2003). Therefore, different hormones affected by the aging process may act in cooperation or antagonistically. In consequence, decreased levels of protective hormones (such as IGF-I) with aging may increase the risk of neural damage induced by the allostatic load of stress hormones.

Thus, we may conclude that the decrease in plasma levels of some hormones in older individuals may have a negative impact on healthy brain aging. We may then be tempted to interpret the alterations in the levels of some hormones with aging as a pathological alteration that in turn may result in a secondary pathology, as a consequence of the hormonal misbalance. However, the situation is not so simple. First, the decrease in some neuroprotective hormones with aging may hardly be defined as pathological. For instance, the levels of the neuroprotective hormones estradiol and progesterone drop with menopause, which is not a pathological situation. Furthermore, we have reasons to suspect that the decrease in some hormones with aging may represent a positive adaptation to increase lifespan. The pioneering work of Cynthia Kenyon and coworkers (Kenyon et al., 1993) showed that mutations in single genes related to the IGF/insulin signaling pathways could considerably enhance lifespan in the nematode *Caenorhabditis elegans*. We know today that in *C. elegans*, insulin/IGF-I-like molecules through the activity of the DAF-2/insulin/ IGF-I-like receptor, and the DAF-16/FKHRL1/FOXO transcription factor may regulate lifespan. Targeted genetic manipulation of homologous genes in Drosophila has confirmed the involvement of this signaling pathway in the regulation of longevity (Tatar et al., 2001). Similar genes in vertebrates may have the same function (Bluher et al., 2003; Holzenberger et al., 2003; Kenyon, 2005; Tatar et al., 2003). For instance, growth hormone/IGF-I deficiency in dwarf mice is associated with an increase in longevity. Let us for a moment examine what dwarf mice may tell us about the relationship of hormones and longevity.

In 1929, George Snell described a recessive autosomal mutation in mice that results in a strong decrease in postnatal growth and adult body size (Snell, 1929). We know today that the cause for this dwarfism is a loss-of-function mutation of pituitary factor 1 (Pit-1), a homeobox transcription factor involved in the differentiation of the somatotrophs, the lactotrophs, and the thyrotrophs (Li et al., 1990). Therefore, Snell dwarf mice have a defect in the development of the anterior pituitary and a deficit in growth hormone, thyroid-stimulating hormone, and prolactin. As a consequence of the deficit in growth hormone, Snell dwarf mice have a reduced postnatal growth and undetectable peripheral levels of IGF-I. These animals are hypothyroid due to the lack of thyroid-stimulating hormone; females are sterile, due to luteal function failure as a consequence of the deficit in prolactin (Bartke and Brown-Borg, 2004). Ames dwarf mice were discovered by Schaible and Gowen (1961) at Iowa State University in Ames, Iowa. These animals have a mutation in a gene (Prop-1) that is expressed before Pit-1, which is necessary for the development of Pit-1-expressing cells that will differentiate into somatotrophs, lactotrophs, and thyrotrophs. Ames dwarf mice have similar deficits in growth hormone, prolactin, and thyroid-stimulating hormone that Snell mice have (Bartke and Brown-Borg, 2004). Another type of dwarfism in mice was obtained by the targeted disruption of the growth hormone receptor/growth-hormone-binding protein (GHR/GHBP) gene (Zhou et al., 1997). These mice have the same deficit than people who have Laron syndrome: they lack growth hormone receptors and consequently are growth hormone resistant. In consequence, IGF-I levels in plasma are dramatically decreased in these mice (Bartke and Brown-Borg, 2004).

Snell mice, Ames mice, and Laron mice have something else in common, in addition to hormonal deficits and being dwarfs: they live longer than normal mice. Both the average and maximal life span are increased in these mice (Bartke and Brown-Borg, 2004). As mentioned before, mutations of genes that codify for proteins analogous to those involved in mammalian IGF-I signaling increase longevity in *C. elegans* and the fruit fly, *Drosophila melanogaster*. In Snell, Ames, and Laron mice, IGF-I is undetectable in plasma; therefore, reduced IGF-I signaling may contribute to the increased longevity of these animals. Indeed, longevity is also increased in heterozygous IGF-I receptor knockout mice (homozygous IGF-I receptor knockout mice are not viable), even if these mice are not dwarf. Snell, Ames, and Laron mice have also reduced plasma insulin and glucose levels; this may also be a contributing factor for the increase in longevity. Reduced thyroid hormones may also be involved in the increased life span. Changes in metabolism, oxidative stress, decreased incidence of cancer, or other causes may account for the increased longevity of these mice. However, independent of what the cause or the causes of the increased longevity is, it seems that the reduced levels of certain hormones may have a positive impact on this parameter. Thus, it is tempting to speculate that the decrease in the levels of some hormones with aging may possibly be a positive adaptation.

Of course, longevity is only one aspect of the picture. An increased life span does not necessary imply a reduction in brain aging. Since IGF-I and IGF-I signaling are neuroprotective, and decreased IGF-I levels in plasma are associated with an increase in neurological alterations, it could be expected that Snell, Ames, and Laron mice, with undetectable IGF-I levels in plasma, would have increased brain deterioration. We would then have mice that live longer but that suffer more neurological alterations. The price of increased longevity would be an increase in brain deterioration. This prediction sounds reasonable, and yet it is completely wrong. Nature is not as simple as our predictions. What is surprising and unexpected is that Ames and Laron mice appear to have a delay in brain aging—an age-related decline in learning and memory is postponed in these animals. In addition, Ames dwarf mice exhibit an increase in hippocampal neurogenesis (Sun et al., 2005b). This is rather puzzling, since we know that IGF-I administration to normal animals increases hippocampal neurogenesis and prevents aging-associated cognitive decline, and that IGF-I is highly protective for the brain. Furthermore, reduced IGF-I levels in plasma are a common marker for several neurodegenerative diseases (Carro et al., 2002). Yet, these dwarf mice have undetectable levels of IGF-I in plasma and still show reduced brain aging. How would this be? Growth hormone is also neuroprotective, has positive effects on learning and memory, and prevents brain aging. Yet, Ames and Laron mice have undetectable levels of growth hormone in plasma, and in spite of this profound hormonal deficit, these animals exhibit apparently normal cognitive functions and maintain such into an advanced age. Can the positive effects of IGF-I and growth hormone administration for brain aging, combined with the lack of a negative impact of IGF-I and growth hormone deficiency in the brain of aged dwarf mice, be reconciled?

Andrzej Bartke and his colleagues have proposed a solution to this problem. They decided to assess growth hormone and IGF-I levels in the hippocampus of Ames dwarf mice. As we have seen in previous chapters (for instance, see Chapter 5), growth hormone and IGF-I are locally produced in the brain. Thus, in addition to being hormones, they are locally produced factors. Bartke and his colleagues found that growth hormone and IGF-I protein levels were increased in the hippocampus of Ames dwarf mice compared with normal mice. They also assessed the signaling of growth hormone and IGF-I and discovered that Ames dwarf mice had 70% higher levels of phosphorylated Akt in the hippocampus when compared to normal controls. A significant increase in the phosphorylation of cyclic AMP response element-binding protein (CREB) was also detected in the hippocampus of Ames dwarf mice (Sun et al., 2005a). Thus, Ames dwarf mice have an increased synthesis of growth hormone and IGF-I in the hippocampus, and an increased activation of growth hormone and IGF-I signaling in this brain area. In addition, the increased local production of growth hormone and IGF-I in the hippocampus of Ames dwarf mice is associated with an increased neurogenesis in the dentate gyrus and an increased activation of antiapoptotic signaling, which may contribute to maintaining hippocampal function (Sun et al., 2005b; Sun and Bartke, 2007). Therefore, Bartke and his colleagues have proposed that the increase in hippocampal growth hormone and IGF-I expression and subsequent activation of the phosphoinositide 3-kinase (PI3K)/Akt-CREB signal transduction cascade might contribute to the maintenance of cognitive function and neuronal structure in aged dwarf mice.

Thus, the brain may adapt its local synthesis of growth hormone and IGF-I as a compensatory mechanism for the deficit in the peripheral levels of these hormones. This may explain why Ames dwarf mice (and likely the other dwarf mice deficient in growth hormone and IGF-I) do not show brain deterioration in spite of the decreased plasma levels of growth hormone and IGF-I. These mice may have an increased longevity due to the decreased levels of growth hormone and IGF-I in plasma and the consequential changes in metabolism, oxidative stress, or growth of tumor cells. At the same time, the loss of growth hormone and IGF-I in plasma does not affect the brain of these animals, since this organ is able to increase its local production of these factors, which are so important for maintaining brain function. Of course, it is possible that Ames dwarf mice, which are permanently deprived of growth hormone and IGF-I throughout life, may develop compensatory mechanisms through the local production of these molecules in their brains that normal animals do not usually develop. Therefore, the deprivation of growth hormone and IGF-I with aging in normal animals may have a stronger negative impact on brain function. However, the data obtained by Bartke and his colleagues suggests that, at least during some specific circumstances, the brain may modulate the local synthesis of growth hormone and IGF-I in adaptation to plasma levels of these molecules. Could the brain do the same for other neuroprotective hormones? This brings us to another important consideration—do peripheral hormonal levels predict the brain levels of these molecules? I will analyze these questions further on in this chapter, but beforehand, we need to take a look at the outcomes of brain function with hormone therapies in elderly people.

HORMONE THERAPY AND HEALTHY BRAIN AGING

Revisiting the question regarding whether hormonal changes with aging are due to a homeodynamic adaptation to changing physiological or pathological conditions, or to a pathological alteration, we have seen in previous sections that hormonal alterations (such as those associated with repetitive stress) may promote alterations in brain plasticity and function during aging. However, the decrease of some hormones with aging may, at least in part, reflect a physiological adaptation to minimize aging-associated pathological alterations in metabolism, tumor growth, and oxidative stress. Thus, changes in the levels of some hormones with aging may reflect an allostatic response aimed at compensating for other imbalances associated with aging. Therefore, at least in theory, the administration of these hormones might be inadequate as a therapeutic approach of taking care of aging-associated symptoms. However, once again, the situation is not so simple. In fact, the decline of levels of certain hormones during aging might negatively impact some tissues, like bones or the brain. Actually, the same hormones that may potentially promote tumor growth, such as growth hormone, IGF-I, or estradiol, are also protective growth factors for normal cells. Thus, hormones that may promote tumor growth in aged animals may also promote neuronal survival and bone calcification. For instance, decreased levels of estradiol and IGF-I in plasma after menopause may be a protective physiological adaptation to minimize the risk of mammary tumors. However, at the same time, the decreased levels of these hormones in plasma are a risk factor for osteoporosis, and likely for neurodegenerative diseases as well. Therefore, hormonal therapies may be justified in treating or preventing the collateral effects of hormonal changes with aging. The question, and it is not an easy one, is to determine the appropriate age for treatment, the hormonal composition, dose, pattern of administration, and length of treatment that would result in positive effects. Unfortunately, we know very little regarding the effects of hormonal treatments for brain function in humans.

While basic studies on animals strongly suggest that several hormones are neuroprotective (see Chapter 9), the situation is not so clear when analyzing information collected from human studies. The effect of different hormonal therapies on brain function has been assessed in aged men and women with uncertain results. Below is a brief examination of the available information related to growth hormone, IGF-I, melatonin, DHEA, testosterone, and ovarian hormones.

Growth hormone deficiency in humans is associated with sleep disturbances, memory loss, feeling of diminished well-being, and other cognitive impairments. Several studies have reported a positive effect of growth hormone therapy in the cognitive performances of growth-hormone-deficient patients. In animal models, growth hormone has been shown to protect the brain and spinal cord from different forms of neurodegenerative stimuli, and promote neuronal survival after hypoxic-ischemic injury (see Chapter 9). Growth hormone deficiency in rats is associated with cognitive deficits, such as impaired spatial learning; short-term synaptic plasticity and growth hormone therapy attenuates these deficits (Ramsey et al., 2004). In addition, growth hormone has been shown to be effective in decreasing neurodegenerative changes in the hippocampus of aged rats (Azcoitia et al., 2005). A potential alternative to hormonal therapy with growth hormone is ghrelin, the endogenous ligand for the growth hormone secretagogue receptor. Ghrelin has potent growth-hormone-releasing activity, and ghrelin receptor agonists may represent a potential treatment for brain-aging alterations (Delgado-Rubin de Celix et al., 2006; Smith et al., 2007).

Neuroprotective effects of growth hormone may be mediated by direct actions on growth hormone receptors in the brain or by its effect in the liver, increasing the production of IGF-I, a potent neuroprotective hormone (see Chapter 9). Furthermore, it has been reported that growth hormone administration to old rats increases IGF-I expression in the brain (Frago et al., 2002; Lopez-Fernandez et al., 1996). The decrease of IGF-I levels with aging correlates with cognitive decline, and IGF-I levels are lower in several neurodegenerative diseases. In addition, the administration of IGF-I to aged rats exerts protective effects in the brain (Lichtenwalner et al., 2001; Lynch et al., 2001). However, we do not have enough data on the IGF-I effects in the brain of elderly people.

Melatonin is another neuroprotective hormone that may have an affect on brain mutability with aging (Srinivasan et al., 2005). Some studies have reported a decreased production of melatonin with aging, which is also associated with a significant reduction in the quality and continuity of sleep. Diminished nocturnal melatonin secretion has been detected in patients with Alzheimer's disease. Some of these patients also show severe disturbances in their sleep/wake rhythm. Clinical trials involving elderly insomniacs and Alzheimer's patients suffering from sleep disturbances suggest that treatment with melatonin may be effective in improving sleep. Interestingly, treatment with melatonin appears to be more effective in those individuals with low endogenous levels of melatonin, pointing to the possible influence of endogenous hormone levels in the outcome of hormonal therapies, an interesting question that will be analyzed further in this chapter.

Plasma levels of DHEA show a strong decline in humans with aging (Ferrari et al., 2001; Lamberts et al., 1997). DHEA has memory-enhancing effects in aging rodents, and counteracts the negative actions of glucocorticoids on memory (Vallée et al., 2001). DHEA therapy has considerable effects on mood, well-being, and sexuality in patients with adrenal insufficiency; some studies suggest that this steroid may improve cognition, promote a sense of well-being, and reduce depressive symptoms in normal elderly men and women (Morales et al., 1994), although other studies do not support this conclusion (Allolio and Arlt, 2002; Baulieu et al., 2000; Huppert et al., 2000; van Niekerk et al., 2001). There are also conflicting results regarding the relationship of DHEA-sulfate levels in human plasma and cognition (Vallée et al., 2001).

Testosterone declines in plasma with aging in both men and women. Testosterone deprivation has been associated with poor memory in men; some studies have suggested that testosterone loss may be a risk factor for cognitive decline and possibly dementia. Thus, men with low levels of free circulating testosterone appear to be at higher risk of developing Alzheimer's disease than men with higher serum levels of this hormone (Moffat et al., 2004). Higher testosterone levels are associated with better cognitive performance in elderly men (Muller et al., 2005); some studies have shown that testosterone supplementation enhances working memory and spatial cognition in elderly men (Janowsky, 2006). However, levels of testosterone that are too high may be unable to improve verbal and spatial memory (Cherrier et al., 2007). Although testosterone therapy may have positive effects on cognition, it is unclear whether it is an effective treatment for depressive symptoms in elderly men (Carnahan and Perry, 2004; Shamlian and Cole, 2006).

Many more studies have analyzed the effects on the brain of therapies with female hormones. Therapies with estrogen and progestin (HT) or estrogen-only therapies (ET) are currently used (and have been for many years) for the treatment of symptoms of menopause. Many postmenopausal women have received HT or ET, we therefore have much more information on the effects on the aged human brain of female sex hormones than for other hormones. Both progesterone and estradiol have been shown to be neuroprotective in animal studies, and for preventing cognitive and neuronal loss in several experimental animal models of neurodegeneration (see Chapter 9). ET in humans is associated with an increase in the hippocampus volume (Lord et al., 2008), and most studies suggest that ET increases memory and cognitive function in healthy women (Henderson, 2000; Yaffe et al., 1998). For example, in the Baltimore Longitudinal Study of Aging, nondemented postmenopausal women receiving HT performed better on tests of verbal and visual memory compared with never-treated women in samples in which both groups of women were comparable with respect to educational attainment, general medical health, and performance on a test of verbal knowledge (Resnick and

Maki, 2001). In addition, short-term ET has been shown to improve prefrontal cortex-dependent cognitive functions in postmenopausal women (Krug et al., 2006).

HT may also be an effective treatment of depression for perimenopausal women (Birkhauser, 2002), and may reduce the negative symptoms of schizophrenia in postmenopausal women (Stevens, 2002). Some studies have suggested that estrogen may reduce the motor disability associated with Parkinson's disease (Cyr et al., 2002; Dluzen and Horstink, 2003; Saunders-Pullman et al., 1999; Tsang et al., 2000). There is also evidence from observational studies suggesting that moderate exposure to exogenous estrogen may decrease the risk of stroke in postmenopausal women (Paganini-Hill, 1995, 2001). Furthermore, some studies suggest that ET may prevent or delay the onset of Alzheimer's disease (Paganini-Hill and Henderson, 1996); some randomized trials using estradiol also suggest that the hormone may improve cognition for women with Alzheimer's disease (Asthana et al., 2001). However, evidence of a protective effect of estrogens in the human brain is not without controversy. Some studies indicate that ET or HT have no effect on Parkinson disease (Saunders-Pullman, 2003). Other studies indicate that estradiol does not reduce mortality or the recurrence of stroke in postmenopausal women with cerebrovascular disease (Viscoli et al., 2001). In addition, some randomized trials do not support the argument for protective effects of estrogens for Alzheimer's disease (Henderson et al., 2000; Mulnard et al., 2000; Wang et al., 2000). Some studies even suggest that HT may have a negative impact on cognition in postmenopausal women with Alzheimer's disease (Shaywitz and Shaywitz, 2000). Furthermore, the Women's Health Initiative (WHI) randomized trial, where participants received one daily tablet of 0.625 mg of conjugated equine estrogens plus 2.5 mg of medroxyprogesterone acetate, or a matching placebo, suggests an increased risk of dementia and stroke as a result of long-lasting hormonal treatment several years after menopause (Shumaker et al., 2003; Wassertheil-Smoller et al., 2003; Yaffe, 2003). Therefore, there is an apparent discrepancy between the potent neuroprotective effect of sex steroids in animal models and the high variability of results in human studies; the question as to the source of these discrepancies naturally arises.

One potential source for the discrepancies in the literature is that there is a considerable variation in the exact hormonal composition and pattern of administration of HT in humans. Usually, a mixture of different natural or synthetic estrogens and natural progestins is administered. Differences in formulation, dose, route of administration, length of treatment, and sample size have been proposed as explanations for the disparity of results between different studies. For instance, different progestins may have very different effects on the brain. Medroxyprogesterone acetate, used in the WHI study, may have several undesirable effects. In animals, the neuroprotective effects of progesterone are blocked by the inhibition of its metabolism into dihydroprogesterone and tetrahydroprogesterone, and both progesterone metabolites seem necessary to exert neuroprotection (Ciriza et al., 2006). In contrast, medroxyprogesterone acetate cannot be metabolized into dihydroprogesterone and tetrahydroprogesterone, is not neuroprotective in animals (Ciriza et al., 2006), and may even block neuroprotection by estradiol (Nilsen and Brinton, 2002a, b; Nilsen et al., 2006). It cannot be excluded therefore that natural progesterone, being able to be transformed into the neuroprotective metabolites dihydroprogesterone and tetrahydroprogesterone by neural tissue may have better cognitive effects in the human brain than medroxyprogesterone acetate (see also Chapter 9). However, the estrogens-alone portion of the WHI study has not provided support for the expected beneficial effects of estrogens in the brain. However, the WHI did not use estradiol but equine estrogens. This may be the source of the discrepancy (Sherwin and Henry, 2008).

Two other parameters that may be highly relevant in explaining the different results is the age of the women receiving the treatment, or the previous duration of hormonal deprivation. The focus of the WHI study on women who were already many years beyond the onset of menopause is a serious limitation, since there are reasons to think that perimenopause may be a critical period for the highest efficacy of hormonal therapy on the prevention of brain disorders. Indeed, most studies that have analyzed the outcome of HT or ET treatments during the perimenopausal period have found positive cognitive effects (Henderson et al., 2005; Maki, 2006a, b). It is conceivable that during this critical period the brain may be adapting to the changing hormonal conditions. Another important consideration is the influence of an extended period of gonadal hormone deprivation on the neuroprotective effects of estrogen. The laboratory of Phyllis Wise has reported that estradiol loses neuroprotective and antiinflammatory actions against brain ischemia in mice after a long period of hypoestrogenicity. Estradiol exerts neuroprotective and antiinflammatory actions when administered immediately after an ovariectomy, but not when administered 10 weeks after an ovariectomy (Suzuki et al., 2007a). These results are important when explaining the discrepancy between the findings of basic research and those of the WHI study in which the majority of women were treated with hormone therapy after an extended period of hormonal deprivation. Therefore, the length of hormonal deprivation may affect brain responsiveness to ovarian hormones. In addition, age is another important factor to consider. It should be noted that the WHI data are relevant for long-term hormonal therapy started in women aged 65 and over; it could be that the brain may also lose responsiveness to hormones with age. This question will be analyzed further in the next section.

DOES AGING AFFECT BRAIN RESPONSIVENESS TO HORMONES?

Most studies in animal models have used young adult rodents submitted to different forms of brain injury to assess the neuroprotective effects of hormones (see Chapter 9). Very little is known about the effects of hormone therapies in the brains of older animals. The aged brain shows a reduced sensitivity to several hormones (Smith et al., 2005). For instance, the brains of old rats are less sensitive to leptin. The infusion of this hormone is more effective in reducing food consumption in young rats than in old rats. In addition, leptin induces an increase in oxygen consumption in young rats but not in old rats. The different effects of leptin in young and aged animals may be related to the fact that the hormone reduces neuropeptide Y levels in the hypothalamus of young animals but not in old animals. The aging brain is also less sensitive to ghrelin. The administration of ghrelin increases growth hormone levels in plasma. However, this response to ghrelin is reduced in elderly people due to age-dependent changes in hypothalamic responsiveness to the hormone. The limited evidence available suggests that, at least in rodents, sex steroids may still exert some neuroprotection in the aged brain. Sex steroids, and their precursors pregnenolone and DHEA, decrease age-related memory deficits in rodents (Vallée et al., 2001). Progesterone exerts neuroprotective effects against traumatic brain injury in aged rats (Cutler et al., 2007), and motoneurons of aged male rats retain synaptic plasticity in response to androgens (Matsumoto, 2001). Furthermore, it has been shown that estradiol decreases gliosis in the brain of aged mice (Lei et al., 2003; Saravia et al., 2007) and protects the brain of middle-aged rats (9–12 months) from a middle cerebral artery occlusion (Dubal and Wise, 2001). Estradiol also has similar effects on long-term synaptic potentiation and long-term synaptic depression in the hippocampus of adult (3–5-month-old) and aged (18–24-month-old) male rats, although the effect on long-term synaptic potentiation is smaller in aged rats (Foy et al., 2008). Furthermore, estradiol is still protective in aged rats against the effects of behavioral stress on synaptic plasticity (Foy et al., 2008). However, other studies suggest that some forms of plasticity in response to estrogen are abolished in the brain of old rats (Adams et al., 2001). Estradiol is also able to promote hippocampal neurogenesis in middle-aged mice (Saravia et al., 2007) and old rats (Perez-Martin et al., 2005), although it is not able to restore the rate of hippocampal neurogenesis to the level observed in young animals (Perez-Martin et al., 2005).

As mentioned at the beginning of this chapter, myelin loss may be one of the most important contributors to brain dysfunction with aging (Bartzokis, 2004; Salat et al., 2005). Therefore, it is important to search for potential treatments to promote remyelination in the aged brain. In this regard, it is highly relevant that progesterone may exert a modest but significant reversal of the age-associated decline in brain remyelination in middle-aged rats (Ibanez et al., 2004). Peripheral myelin is also responsive to progesterone in aged rats, although aging affects the responsiveness of peripheral nerves to the hormone. The aging process induces important biochemical and morphological changes in peripheral nerves; the prevalence of peripheral neuropathy in humans rises from about 2.4% to 8% with aging. Aging is associated with a decrease in the synthesis of myelin proteins, such as P0 and PMP22. In parallel, large myelinated fibers undergo atrophy, while myelin sheaths increase in thickness and show various irregularities, like myelin ballooning, splitting, infolding, reduplication, and remyelination. A reduction in the number and density of myelinated fibers has been reported with aging in peripheral nerves of several animal species; this effect is particularly evident in myelinated fibers of small caliber. Indeed, more than 60% of the myelinated fibers with a diameter under 5 μm are lost in aged animals. Moreover, alterations in the size and shape of myelinated fibers also occur with aging.

Roberto C. Melcangi and his collaborators at the University of Milan have detected that treatments with progesterone and dihydroprogesterone are able to increase the levels of the myelin protein P0 in the sciatic nerve of aged male rats, while tetrahydroprogesterone significantly increases the protein levels of PMP22 (Melcangi et al., 2003, 2005). Moreover, the treatments with progesterone or its metabolites have clear effects on the number and shape of myelinated fibers, as well as on the frequency of myelin abnormalities. One of the most striking effects of the steroids is on the number of myelinated fibers of a small caliber (<5 μm), which is significantly increased by progesterone and its metabolites in the nerves of old rats. This is accompanied by a decrease of similar magnitude in the number of unmyelinated axons, and in particular, to large (>3 μm) unmyelinated axons. Moreover, the morphometric analysis suggests that the increase in the number of myelinated fibers reflects an increased remyelination of small fibers in aged sciatic nerves. Another significant effect of the treatments of old rats with progesterone, dihydroprogesterone, and tetrahydroprogesterone is the reduction in the frequency of axons with myelin abnormalities. These steroids significantly reduce the frequency of axons with myelin infoldings (one of the structural alterations that increases in aged nerves), and reduce the proportion of fibers with irregular shapes. Therefore, progesterone therapy may contribute to the preservation of the functional and structural integrity of peripheral nerves with aging (Azcoitia et al., 2003; Melcangi et al., 2003, 2005). However, Roberto C. Melcangi and his collaborators have also detected a decreased capacity of the aged peripheral nerves to metabolize progesterone into dihydroprogesterone and tetrahydroprogesterone. Interestingly, the peripheral nerves of aged rats, although responsive to progesterone, are less sensitive to the neuroprotective effects of progesterone than the nerves of young rats. Therefore, aging may affect the responsiveness of peripheral nervous system to progesterone, due to the reduced capacity of the aged nerves to metabolize progesterone into the neuroprotective metabolites dihydroprogesterone and tetrahydroprogesterone (Melcangi et al., 2000b). A similar situation may occur in the central nervous system. It is clear that more studies are needed to determine to what extent sex steroid metabolism is altered in the brain of old animals.

In addition, neuroprotective effects of sex steroids that depend on the activation of their nuclear receptors may be impaired in the aged nervous system, because aging may affect the expression of steroid receptors and steroid receptor coactivators (Jezierski and Sohrabji, 2001; Matsumoto and Prins, 2002). Therefore, sex steroid receptor signaling may be very different in young and older brains; consequently, the effects of sex steroids in the brain of young animals may not be predictive of the effects of the same molecules in aged brains.

In addition to changes in steroid receptor expression and signaling, there is at least one other good reason to explain why neuroprotective effects of sex steroids may be reduced in the aged brain: aging may also deplete other substances that may be necessary for the effects of sex steroids. These may include growth factors, neuromodulators, neurotransmitters, and their receptors. For instance, Forger and her colleagues (Xu et al., 2001) have shown that the induction of motoneuron cell survival by testosterone in the spinal nucleus of the bulbocavernosus muscle (SNB) of rats is prevented by an acute blockade of the neurotrophin receptors TrkB and TrkC, as well as the blockade of the ciliary neurotrophic factor receptor-α. These findings indicate that endogenously produced trophic factors are necessary for the effect that testosterone has on neuronal survival. Another growth factor involved in the actions of sex steroids is IGF-I. Evidence has accumulated to support the idea that the actions of estrogen and IGF-I in the brain are interdependent. As seen in Chapters 5, 6, and 9, the interdependence between estrogen and IGF-I, or between estrogen receptors and IGF-I receptors, has been documented for neuronal differentiation, synaptic plasticity, adult neurogenesis, and neuroprotection (Cardona-Gomez et al., 2001; Garcia-Segura et al., 2007; Mendez et al., 2005, 2006). Plasma levels of IGF-I decrease with aging, and IGF-I treatment to old rats ameliorate several age-related deficits in the brain (Lichtenwalner et al., 2001; Lynch et al., 2001). Since brain IGF-I and IGF-I receptor levels are affected by aging (Sonntag et al., 1999), the effect of estrogen receptor activation may be very different in young and old brains because aging decreases the availability of this key synergist.

DOES THE BRAIN HAVE MECHANISMS TO COUNTERBALANCE HORMONAL CHANGES WITH AGING?

As seen in previous chapters, several hormones that affect brain plasticity and function are also produced by nerve cells as autocrine or paracrine factors. These molecules therefore have the duality of being hormones and locally produced neural factors. As hormones, they are involved in endocrine signaling. As local molecules, they may act as neuromodulators or growth factors acting by paracrine or autocrine mechanisms. Very little is known regarding how local synthesis of these factors is regulated in the brain. We have noted how Ames dwarf mice are able to increase the local synthesis of growth hormone and IGF-I in the brain to counterbalance the peripheral deficiency of these molecules. It may be assumed that, under physiological conditions, the brain may also adapt the local synthesis of these molecules and their receptors, at least in part. Indeed, we know that local synthesis of IGF-I in most brain regions is elevated during development, and declines dramatically in adulthood. In contrast, IGF-I plasma levels are high during adulthood. Thus, low levels of IGF-I synthesis in the brain are associated with high plasma levels of IGF-I in adults. This suggests that the actions of peripheral IGF-I predominate in the adult brain, while local actions of IGF-I predominate in the developing brain. Do high peripheral IGF-I levels present in the plasma in adults down-regulate local IGF-I synthesis in the brain? The studies of Andrzej Bartke and his colleagues on Ames dwarf mice suggest that peripheral IGF-I levels in some way may regulate the synthesis of IGF-I in the brain. Thus, it is conceivable that physiological changes affecting IGF-I plasma levels may be accompanied by physiological modifications in the synthesis of IGF-I by nerve cells. However, we do not have enough data yet to answer this question, and we do not know if the brain is regulating IGF-I synthesis to counteract the decline of IGF-I levels in plasma with aging.

A similar situation occurs for other hormones, such as sex steroids. As analyzed in Chapter 4, the capability to synthesize steroids is not only a peculiarity of the classical steroidogenic tissues (such as the gonads and adrenal gland), but may also be ascribed to the nervous system. Cholesterol is transformed into pregnenolone by the cholesterol side-chain cleavage enzyme (P450scc) in nerve cells, and pregnenolone is metabolized into progesterone by the enzyme 3β-hydroxysteroid dehydrogenase. Progesterone may then be transformed into its reduced metabolites dihydroprogesterone and tetrahydroprogesterone via the enzymatic complex formed by the 5α-reductase and 3α-hydroxysteroid dehydrogenase. Dihydroprogesterone and tetrahydroprogesterone mediate several effects of progesterone in the brain, acting via different mechanisms. Dihydroprogesterone acts on progesterone receptors, while tetrahydroprogesterone regulates the activity of ion channels associated with neurotransmitter receptors, such as the $GABA_A$ and NMDA receptors. By these actions on neurotransmitter receptors, tetrahydroprogesterone has anxiolytic and antidepressive effects. It is conceivable that physiological changes in progesterone levels in plasma during the ovarian cycle, during pregnancy, and after delivery may affect progesterone and tetrahydroprogesterone levels in the brain. This influence of peripheral progesterone in the brain may be related to the changes in mood that some women experience during the menstrual cycle or with postpartum depression, when the brain is suddenly deprived of progesterone as a consequence of the drop in the levels of this hormone after delivery. Progesterone in plasma is very high during pregnancy; therefore, the brain has an abundant peripheral supply of progesterone to produce tetrahydroprogesterone. However, progesterone decreases abruptly after delivery and the brain looses this abundant peripheral supply for the synthesis of the endogenous anxiolytic tetrahydroprogesterone. The brain likely has to adapt its local synthesis of progesterone and tetrahydroprogesterone to compensate for the changing peripheral input of these molecules. We know from animal studies that the levels of progesterone, dihydroprogesterone, and tetrahydroprogesterone in the brain do not necessarily match the changing levels of these molecules in plasma. This suggests that the brain regulates progesterone synthesis and metabolism in order to maintain the adequate local levels, independent of the changing peripheral abundance of progesterone. It is also conceivable that individual differences in the adaptation of local synthesis of progesterone and tetrahydroprogesterone may result in individual differences in the ability of the brain to compensate for the changing hormonal input. We may assume that not all female brains would be able to counterbalance the changes in peripheral hormones with the same accuracy. Indeed, it is evident that not all women experience the same depressive symptoms in the post-partum period, and not all experience the same mood changes during the menstrual cycle. However, I want to emphasize that it would be a flagrant, unjustified contribution to reductionism to ascribe all the individual differences in mood during the menstrual cycle or after parturition to individual differences in the synthesis and metabolism of progesterone. It is obvious that many other causes may affect the psychological situation of women in these circumstances. What I would like to suggest is that individual differences in brain progesterone synthesis and metabolism may represent a risk factor, or a contributing factor, for the different individual responses to hormonal changes that, no doubt, are influenced by many other biological, psychological, and social circumstances.

The decrease of progesterone levels in plasma after menopause may also affect progesterone and tetrahydroprogesterone levels in the brain, and influence the appearance of depressive symptoms and affective disorders in post-menopausal women. Once again, not all postmenopausal women experience the same symptoms after menopause; this suggests that the brain is able to counterbalance the hormonal changes after menopause. It may be hypothesized that the compensation for hormonal loss by local synthesis or other mechanisms may differ among individuals. Hormonal therapy may then possibly have a negative impact for those individuals in which the brain has adapted to hormonal loss. The same argument may be raised for other neuroprotective hormones that decrease in plasma with aging, such as IGF-I. The brain may have endogenous mechanisms to counterbalance this deficit; local synthesis of these neuroprotective molecules may be one of them. However, the brain of some individuals may be unable to adequately counterbalance the hormonal alterations with aging, and this may contribute to impairment in brain function and the development of brain disorders. In these particular cases, hormonal therapy may be an option to consider as a compensatory treatment.

For therapies with ovarian hormones, the perimenopause may represent a critical period when the brain may be adapting local steroid synthesis to the new situation created by the loss of ovarian function. Steroid receptor machinery and steroid synthesis in the brain is likely not yet severely affected by the new situation. In contrast, several years after menopause, the brain of many women may have counterbalanced the hormonal deficit, either by adapting its local steroid synthesis or by other unknown mechanisms. For instance, we know that steroid hormone receptors may be activated by growth factors (estrogen receptors) or dopamine (progesterone receptors) (Blaustein, 2004). It is conceivable that these factors may activate steroid receptors in the aged brain, compensating for the absence of steroids. It is therefore plausible that hormonal therapy and estrogen therapy may have a negative impact on these brains that are now in a different homeodynamic condition, having adapted to functioning with low levels of circulating ovarian hormones.

Unfortunately, we know very little regarding the levels of hormones in the human brain, and very little about levels of hormones in the brain of aging animals. We do know, however, that plasma levels of hormones in experimental animals do not necessarily reflect the brain hormonal levels. There are a few reports regarding the levels of hormones on cerebrospinal fluid in elderly individuals. Some studies have found a decrease with age in estradiol and an increase in cortisol levels in the cerebrospinal fluid of women with age, especially after menopause (Murakami et al., 1999). Increased cortisol levels have also been detected in the cerebrospinal fluid of elderly men; some studies also suggest a decrease in DHEA levels (Guazzo et al., 1996). Still, we ignore the degree to which cerebrospinal fluid levels of these hormones adequately reflect their levels in brain tissue; in general, our information regarding possible changes and individual differences in brain hormonal levels with aging is clearly unsatisfactory.

OPPORTUNITIES FOR THERAPEUTIC INTERVENTION: HORMONE THERAPIES AND BEYOND

We are still a long way from being able to design rational protocols for hormonal therapies to protect the brain from the effects of aging. More studies into understanding the mechanisms of the action of hormones in the aging brain are necessary. More information is needed on the interaction of hormones with other neuronal survival factors that are affected by the aging process. Moreover, it is not clear yet whether hormones may be protective from some types of damage but deleterious in the case of other types of brain insult. Alternative strategies to hormonal therapies that may be clinically more effective can be experimentally tested. Gene therapy directed toward increasing the levels of peptide hormones in specific brain areas may be experimentally tested as a therapeutic approach to reduce brain deficits associated with aging. Experimental gene therapy in rats, by the stereotaxic administration of an adenoviral vector expressing IGF-I, has given positive results in preventing the loss of hypothalamic tuberoinfundibular dopaminergic neurons with aging (Herenu et al., 2006, 2007).

It may also be useful to exploit the endogenous capacity of the brain to synthesize (as local paracrine or autocrine factors) some of the hormones affected by aging, such as growth hormone, ghrelin, IGF-I, and sex steroids. For instance, one approach to increase growth hormone and IGF-I levels in aged people is the administration of GHRH (growth-hormone-releasing hormone) analogs, or the use of molecules that increase the production of GHRH in the hypothalamus. For instance, L-dopa increases GHRH release in old rats, resulting in a pulsatile growth hormone profile typical to that observed in young rats (Smith et al., 2005). IGF-I local synthesis in the brain may be enhanced by the administration of growth hormone. The use of new synthetic agonists for the growth hormone secretagogue receptor may represent an option to increase growth hormone and IGF-I levels in elderly people.

For steroids, possible targets for therapeutic approaches are the proteins that participate in the transport of cholesterol from the cytoplasm to the inner mitochondrial membrane. Cholesterol is converted into pregnenolone in the mitochondria, then pregnenolone is converted into DHEA or progesterone in the endoplasmic reticulum. The transport of cholesterol to the inner mito-chondrial membrane is the rate-limiting step for steroid synthesis, and is highly regulated. Two proteins located in the mitochondrial membrane, the steroidogenic acute regulatory protein (StAR) (Stocco, 2001) and the periph-eral-type benzodiazepine receptor, recently renamed as 18kDa translocator protein (TSPO) (Lacor et al., 1999; Papadopoulos et al., 2006) are involved in this transport (see Chapter 4), and may represent good candidates for pharma-cological treatments to increase steroid synthesis in the aging brain. In agree-ment with this hypothesis, it has been shown that the TSPO ligand Ro5–4864 exerts neuroprotective effects in the brain of young animals (Chapter 9) and a beneficial effect on morphological parameters of the sciatic nerve of aged male rats (Leonelli et al., 2005). The treatment with this TSPO ligand significantly increased the total number of myelinated fibers and decreased the percentage of fibers with myelin decompaction. In contrast to the neuroprotective effects exerted by Ro5–4864, the TSPO ligand PK11195, which binds to a different site in the TSPO structure, did not significantly affect any of the parameters analyzed (Leonelli et al., 2005). In addition to increasing local synthesis of neuroprotective steroids, other functions of TSPO may also be important to maintain sciatic nerve integrity. These include the regulation of oxidative pro-cesses, since TSPO may modulate mitochondrial sensitivity to reactive oxygen species. Reactive oxygen species have been implicated in several neurodegen-erative events; these become generally worse during the aging process. For instance, it is well known that the rate and degree of recovery after peripheral nerve lesions decline with age, and it has been proposed that reactive oxy-gen species contribute to this delayed recovery. Consequently, Ro5–4864 may in part protect peripheral nerves by reducing sensitivity to reactive oxygen-species-induced damage. Given these promising results, TSPO ligands and other molecules that may enhance steroidogenesis in the nervous system should be systematically tested in aged animals. Compounds that regulate StAR activity may also be explored and developed.

Other proteins of potential therapeutic interest are the enzymes respon-sible for sex steroid formation and metabolism, such as 5α-reductase and aromatase. More information is needed on the levels of expression of these enzymes in the aged human brain, since a potential mechanism to locally increase sex steroid levels in the brain is to change the expression or activity of these enzymes specifically in the nervous system. For instance, the aromatase gene is under the control of different tissue-specific promoters (Honda et al., 1999; Yague et al., 2006), and it is conceivable that it will be possible to develop specific selective aromatase modulators that will enhance the expression of this enzyme in the brain but not in other tissues. In addition, gene therapy can be envisaged to increase the production of steroidogenic enzymes in specific brain regions. Finally, other potential candidates for pharmacological targeting are the hormone receptors. Selective modulators for androgen and estrogen receptors are under development. Several studies have shown that some synthetic selective estrogen receptor modulators (SERMs), such as tamoxifen, raloxifene, or bazedoxifene, and some natural SERMs, such as genistein, are neuroprotective in vitro and in vivo (Azcoitia et al., 2006; Callier et al., 2001; Ciriza et al., 2004b; Dhandapani and Brann, 2002; Grandbois et al., 2000; Kimelberg et al., 2003; Kokiko et al., 2006; Mehta et al., 2003; Mickley and Dluzen, 2004; Rossberg et al., 2000; Tapia-Gonzalez et al., 2008; Zhao et al., 2005, 2006). SERMs interact with estrogen receptors, and have tissue-specific effects distinct from those of estradiol, acting as estrogen receptor agonists in some tissues and as antagonists in others. Therefore, some SERMs may have estrogenic actions in some brain regions but an absence of estrogenic actions, or even anti-estrogenic effects, in other brain regions or peripheral tissues. However, before the therapeutic use of these drugs as neuroprotectants is considered, it is essential to learn much more about the expression and regulation of sex steroid receptors and their cofactors in the aging brain, and also the impact of aging on the convergence of sex steroid receptor signaling with other signaling pathways. In addition, SERMs may also exert protection by antioxidant actions (Zhang Y et al., 2007). Antioxidant nongenomic effects of estradiol and other estrogenic compounds are the basis for the development of estrogen derivatives with neuroprotective potency (Prokai and Simpkins, 2007). Among these, a group of interesting molecules are the so-called non-feminizing estrogens, such as 17α-estradiol, and the estratriene derivatives, which share the neuroprotective effects of 17β-estradiol but do not activate estrogen receptors in the reproductive tract (Dykens et al., 2003; Simpkins et al., 2004, 2005).

In conclusion, potential alternatives to the treatment with neuroprotective hormonal factors might be either the treatment with molecules able to induce their local synthesis in the brain, or with molecules able to interact with their receptors and signaling cascades, or a combination of both. However, before considering broad clinical applications, it is still necessary for more basic research to clarify the mechanisms of action and potential risks of some of these treatments. More important, those aspects of brain remodeling with aging that represent a positive adaptive response still need to be delineated from those that reflect a pathological alteration, to better define the adequate goals of therapeutic interventions.

HORMONES AND BRAIN AGING: SUMMARY

I have analyzed in this chapter the interaction of hormones and brain plasticity during aging. There is an additional component that is important for understanding the brain and endocrine changes with aging: the immune system.

The immune, endocrine, and nervous systems suffer a remarkable adjustment with aging. The reorganization of the immune, endocrine, and nervous interactions may engage in a substantial reorganization of hypothalamic circuits controlling hormonal secretions, and are also accompanied by modifications of plastic responses in other brain regions (such as the hippocampus, amygdala, and the frontal cortex) involved in cognition and emotions. It is conceivable that the important changes observed in brain white matter with aging may be related with general alterations of immune and endocrine functions. Plastic reorganization in brain gray matter with aging appears to have regional specificity, and may in part involve specific neural remodeling as an adaptation to endocrine alterations. In this regard, it is noticeable that brain areas involved with emotions and cognition are among those more affected by aging, and also among those where hormones exert a stronger regulation of structural and functional plasticity. Our hypothesis is that hormones exert selective regulation on some forms of neural plasticity in certain brain regions during aging. Furthermore, neuroplastic effects of hormones during previous periods of life predetermine the outcome of hormonal regulation of brain plasticity during aging. Therefore, hormones exert plastic and metaplastic effects on the brain to adapt brain function to the new physiological conditions in older ages.

Although increasing age is a risk factor for the development of neurodegenerative and affective disorders, age per se is not the cause of brain disorders, and not all plastic changes in the aged brain reflect pathological alterations. Genetic factors, environmental influences, and general health status may affect brain function, resulting in a considerable degree of individual variation in the grade of cognitive and affective alterations in elderly people. The endocrine system is also reorganized with age, and the instability associated with the physiological remodeling of brain neuronal and glial networks in adaptation to these endocrine changes may also represent a risk factor for the onset of brain pathological alterations. In turn, brain remodeling with aging may cause further endocrine alterations. Therefore, although hormonal regulation of brain plasticity during aging may in part represent an allostatic adaptation to maintain stable body function, in some cases it may result in a nonadaptive modification caused by the impossibility to reach an adequate homeodynamic equilibrium. These nonadaptive modifications may eventually cause pathological alterations that, for the brain, may be manifested as cognitive decline, depressive symptoms, or psychological disturbances.

As highlighted earlier in this chapter, an important factor that should be taken in consideration is the capacity of the aging brain to functionally adapt to the hormonal changes. Previous chapters have shown that many hormones affect brain function, and regulate morphological and functional synaptic plasticity and neurogenesis in adult animals. In some aspects, these hormones act as trophic neuroplastic factors that maintain a proper brain activity. Thus, the decline in the levels of some of these hormones with aging, such as DHEA, estradiol, progesterone, growth hormone, and IGF-I, may represent a challenge for brain tissue, and may result in alterations in the regulation of brain plasticity and a decreased protection of neurons and glial cells against environmental and genetic factors that promote neurodegeneration. Apparently, one of the mechanisms that the brain uses to cope with the hormonal changes is to regulate the local synthesis of the same molecules, although we still do not know to what extent local synthesis in the aged brain is able to compensate for the modifications in peripheral hormone levels.

Hormone therapies for elderly people may in part help the brain to adapt to the endocrine changes associated with aging. In general, however, there is limited information regarding the risks and benefits associated with some of these therapies in humans. There is also limited and fragmentary information about whether the responsiveness of the human brain to hormones is or is not affected by aging. Therefore, we do not have enough information yet to design rational protocols for hormonal therapies to protect the aging brain. Some alternatives to hormonal therapies for the aging brain are currently being experimentally tested, including gene therapies or the use of pharmacological agents that activate hormone receptors or regulate hormone synthesis and metabolism.

Concluding Summary

As mentioned in the preface, the main aims of this book were to show that brain plasticity plays an essential role in the regulation of hormonal levels and that hormones orchestrate the multiple endogenous plastic events of the brain for the generation of adequate physiological and behavioral responses in adaptation to and prediction of changing life conditions. I hope to have been able to cover these aims by depicting in detail the continuous cross-talk between the endocrine glands and the nervous system to modulate brain plasticity and hormonal levels along lifespan.

Looking back now to the previous pages I feel that the book also illustrates how our view of the brain, which was still considered a static structure in the middle of the twentieth century, has dramatically changed in a few decades. In parallel, our view on the role of hormones in the modulation of brain function has also experienced a drastic modification during this time. The book also shows that numerous hormones have a much broader range of actions on the brain than originally conceived.

At the end of my quest, and after reviewing an extensive amount of literature, I would like to propose several principles that may help to elaborate a unitary view on how hormones act on brain plasticity:

a. *Hormones are regulators of brain plasticity.* In my view, one of the most important principles is that hormones act as regulators and not as causative agents of a specific form of brain plasticity. Brain plasticity may be elicited in vitro in absence of hormones, and we have seen in the book numerous examples indicating that the same hormone, depending on the context, may have different effects on the same mechanism of plasticity.

b. *One single hormone regulates different forms of brain plasticity.* Another principle is that the neuroplastic response to a given hormone integrates multiple mechanisms of action. Thus, a given hormone may regulate different mechanisms of plasticity, including cellular plasticity, cellular replacement, and functional synaptic plasticity.

c. *Divergent actions on brain plasticity.* Hormones exert divergent actions and the same hormone may regulate plasticity in different brain regions. In some cases, the hormone may enhance a specific form of brain plasticity in a given brain region and have the opposite effect in another brain region.

    d. *Convergent actions on brain plasticity.* Conversely, we have also seen that the action of multiple hormones converge and interact to regulate the same form of plasticity in a given brain region.

    e. *Coordinated hormonal actions over space and time.* Hormones regulate metaplasticity. Multiple coordinated hormonal actions on plasticity in different brain regions are integrated to generate the final functional response. In addition, all hormonal actions on brain plasticity in different brain regions and all the neuroplastic events regulating hormonal release are integrated over time, under the form of metaplasticity, to produce the adequate behavioral and physiological homeodynamic responses within the context of different life stages and different life conditions.

BIBLIOGRAPHY

Åberg MA, Aberg ND, Hedbacker H, Oscarsson J, Eriksson PS. (2000) Peripheral infusion of IGF-I selectively induces neurogenesis in the adult rat hippocampus. *J Neurosci* 20:2896–2903.

Åberg ND, Brywe KG, Isgaard J. (2006) Aspects of growth hormone and insulin-like growth factor-I related to neuroprotection, regeneration, and functional plasticity in the adult brain. *Scientific WorldJournal* 6:53–80.

Åberg ND, Johansson UE, Aberg MA, Hellstrom NA, Lind J, Bull C, Isgaard J, Anderson MF, Oscarsson J, Eriksson PS. (2007) Peripheral infusion of insulin-like growth factor-I increases the number of newborn oligodendrocytes in the cerebral cortex of adult hypophysectomized rats. *Endocrinology* 148:3765–3772.

Abizaid A, Mezei G, Sotonyi P, Horvath TL. (2004) Sex differences in adult suprachiasmatic nucleus neurons emerging late prenatally in rats. *Eur J Neurosci* 19:2488–2496.

Abizaid A, Liu ZW, Andrews ZB, Shanabrough M, Borok E, Elsworth JD, Roth RH, Sleeman MW, Picciotto MR, Tschop MH, Gao XB, Horvath TL. (2006) Ghrelin modulates the activity and synaptic input organization of midbrain dopamine neurons while promoting appetite. *J Clin Invest* 116:3229–3239.

Abraham WC, Bear MF. (1996) Metaplasticity: The plasticity of synaptic plasticity. *Trends Neurosci* 19:126–130.

Abraham WC, Tate WP. (1997) Metaplasticity: A new vista across the field of synaptic plasticity. *Prog Neurobiol* 52:303–323.

Abrous DN, Koehl M, Le Moal M. (2005) Adult neurogenesis: From precursors to network and physiology. *Physiol Rev* 85:523–569.

Absil P, Pinxten R, Balthazart J, Eens M. (2003) Effects of testosterone on Reelin expression in the brain of male European starlings. *Cell Tissue Res* 312:81–93.

Acerini CL, Tasker RC. (2007) Traumatic brain injury induced hypothalamic–pituitary dysfunction: A paediatric perspective. *Pituitary* 10:373–380.

Acerini CL, Tasker RC, Bellone S, Bona G, Thompson CJ, Savage MO. (2006) Hypopituitarism in childhood and adolescence following traumatic brain injury: The case for prospective endocrine investigation *Eur J Endocrinol* 155:663–669.

Adamec RE, Blundell J, Burton P. (2006) Relationship of the predatory attack experience to neural plasticity, pCREB expression and neuroendocrine response. *Neurosci Biobehav Rev* 30:356–375.

Adams MM, Shah RA, Janssen WG, Morrison JH. (2001) Different modes of hippocampal plasticity in response to estrogen in young and aged female rats. *Proc Natl Acad Sci USA* 98:8071–8076.

Adams VL, Goodman RL, Salm AK, Coolen LM, Karsch FJ, Lehman MN. (2006) Morphological plasticity in the neural circuitry responsible for seasonal breeding in the ewe. *Endocrinology* 147:4843–4851.

Adkins-Regan E, Mansukhani V, Seiwert C, Thompson R. (1994) Sexual differentiation of brain and behavior in the zebra finch: Critical periods for effects of early estrogen treatment. *J Neurobiol* 25:865–877.

Agate RJ, Grisham W, Wade J, Mann S, Wingfield J, Schanen C, Palotie A, Arnold AP. (2003) Neural, not gonadal, origin of brain sex differences in a gynandromorphic finch. *Proc Natl Acad Sci USA* 100:4873–4878.

Agrati P, Garnier M, Patrone C, Pollio G, Santagati S, Vegeto E, Maggi A. (1997) SK-ER3 neuroblastoma cells as a model for the study of estrogen influence on neural cells. *Brain Res Bull* 44:519–523.

Aguado F, Rodrigo J, Cacicedo L, Mellstrom B. (1993) Distribution of insulin-like growth factor-I receptor mRNA in rat brain. Regulation in the hypothalamo-neurohypophysial system. *J Mol Endocrinol* 11:231–239.

Ahima RS, Prabakaran D, Flier JS. (1998) Postnatal leptin surge and regulation of circadian rhythm of leptin by feeding. Implications for energy homeostasis and neuroendocrine function. *J Clin Invest* 101:1020–1027.

Ahima RS, Bjorbaek C, Osei S, Flier JS. (1999) Regulation of neuronal and glial proteins by leptin: Implications for brain development. *Endocrinology* 140:2755–2762.

Ahlbom E, Prins GS, Ceccatelli S. (2001) Testosterone protects cerebellar granule cells from oxidative stress-induced cell death through a receptor mediated mechanism. *Brain Res* 892:255–262.

Ahlgren SC, Wallace H, Bishop J, Neophytou C, Raff MC. (1997) Effects of thyroid hormone on embryonic oligodendrocyte precursor cell development in vivo and in vitro. *Mol Cell Neurosci* 9:420–432.

Ahmed T, Frey JU, Korz V. (2006) Long-term effects of brief acute stress on cellular signaling and hippocampal LTP. *J Neurosci* 26:3951–3958.

Aimaretti G, Ambrosio MR, Di Somma C, Fusco A, Cannavo S, Gasperi M, Scaroni C, De Marinis L, Benvenga S, degli Uberti EC, Lombardi G, Mantero F, Martino E, Giordano G, Ghigo E. (2004) Traumatic brain injury and subarachnoid haemorrhage are conditions at high risk for hypopituitarism: Screening study at 3 months after the brain injury. *Clin Endocrinol* 61:320–326.

Aizenman Y, de Vellis J. (1987) Synergistic action of thyroid hormone, insulin and hydrocortisone on astrocyte differentiation. *Brain Res* 414:301–308.

Ajo R, Cacicedo L, Navarro C, Sanchez-Franco F. (2003) Growth hormone action on proliferation and differentiation of cerebral cortical cells from fetal rat. *Endocrinology* 144:1086–1097.

Akbari E, Naghdi N, Motamedi F. (2006) Functional inactivation of orexin 1 receptors in CA1 region impairs acquisition, consolidation and retrieval in Morris water maze task. *Behav Brain Res* 173:47–52.

Albrecht D. (2007) Angiotensin-(1-7)-induced plasticity changes in the lateral amygdala are mediated by COX-2 and NO. *Learn Mem* 14:177–184.

Aldskogius H, Liu L, Svensson M. (1999) Glial responses to synaptic damage and plasticity. *J Neurosci Res* 58:33–41.

Aleisa AM, Alzoubi KH, Gerges NZ, Alkadhi KA. (2006) Chronic psychosocial stress-induced impairment of hippocampal LTP: Possible role of BDNF. *Neurobiol Dis* 22:453–462.

Alejandre-Gomez M, Garcia-Segura LM, Gonzalez-Burgos I. (2007) Administration of an inhibitor of estrogen biosynthesis facilitates working memory acquisition in male rats. *Neurosci Res* 58:272–277.

Alexander GE, Chen K, Aschenbrenner M, Merkley TL, Santerre-Lemmon LE, Shamy JL, Skaggs WE, Buonocore MH, Rapp PR, Barnes CA. (2008) Age-related regional network of magnetic resonance imaging gray matter in the rhesus macaque. *J Neurosci* 28:2710-2718.

Alexopoulos GS. (2005) Depression in the elderly. *Lancet* 365:1961-1970.

Alfarez DN, Wiegert O, Joëls M, Krugers HJ. (2002) Corticosterone and stress reduce synaptic potentiation in mouse hippocampal slices with mild stimulation. *Neuroscience* 115:1119-1126.

Alfarez DN, Karst H, Velzing EH, Joëls M, Krugers HJ. (2008) Opposite effects of glucocorticoid receptor activation on hippocampal CA1 dendritic complexity in chronically stressed and handled animals. *Hippocampus* 18:20-28.

Alkayed NJ, Harukuni I, Kimes AS, London ED, Traystman RJ, Hurn PD. (1998) Gender-linked brain injury in experimental stroke. *Stroke* 29:159-165.

Allolio B, Arlt W. (2002) DHEA treatment: Myth or reality? *Trends Endocrinol Metab* 13:288-294.

Almazan G, Honegger P, Matthieu JM. (1985) Triiodothyronine stimulation of oligodendroglial differentiation and myelination. A developmental study. *Dev Neurosci* 7:45-54.

Alonso G. (2000) Prolonged corticosterone treatment of adult rats inhibits the proliferation of oligodendrocyte progenitors present throughout white and gray matter regions of the brain. *Glia* 31:219-231.

Alonso R, Griebel G, Pavone G, Stemmelin J, Le Fur G, Soubrié P. (2004) Blockade of CRF(1) or V(1b) receptors reverses stress-induced suppression of neurogenesis in a mouse model of depression. *Mol Psychiatry* 9:278-286.

Alonso SJ, Arevalo R, Afonso D, Rodriguez M. (1991) Effects of maternal stress during pregnancy on forced swimming test behavior of the offspring. *Physiol Behav* 50:511-517.

Alvarez E, Martinez MD, Roncero I, Chowen JA, Garcia-Cuartero B, Gispert JD, Sanz C, Vazquez P, Maldonado A, de Caceres J, Desco M, Pozo MA, Blazquez E. (2005) The expression of GLP-1 receptor mRNA and protein allows the effect of GLP-1 on glucose metabolism in the human hypothalamus and brainstem. J Neurochem 92:798-806.

Alvarez VA, Sabatini BL. (2007) Anatomical and physiological plasticity of dendritic spines. *Annu Rev Neurosci* 30:79-97.

Alvarez-Buylla A, Kirn JR. (1997) Birth, migration, incorporation, and death of vocal control neurons in adult songbirds. *J Neurobiol* 33:585-601.

Alvarez-Buylla A, Kirn JR, Nottebohm F. (1990) Birth of projection neurons in adult avian brain may be related to perceptual or motor learning. *Science* 249:1444-1446.

Alvarez-de-la-Rosa M, Silva I, Nilsen J, Perez MM, Garcia-Segura LM, Avila J, Naftolin F. (2005) Estradiol prevents neural tau hyperphosphorylation characteristic of Alzheimer's disease. *Ann N Y Acad Sci* 1052:210-224.

Alzoubi KH, Bedawi AS, Aleisa AM, Alkadhi KA. (2004) Hypothyroidism impairs long-term potentiation in sympathetic ganglia: lectrophysiologic and molecular studies. *J Neurosci Res* 78:393-402.

Alzoubi KH, Gerges NZ, Alkadhi KA. (2005) Levothyroxin restores hypothyroidism-induced impairment of LTP of hippocampal CA1: Electrophysiological and molecular studies. *Exp Neurol* 195:330-341.

Ambrogini P, Cuppini R, Ferri P, Mancini C, Ciaroni S, Voci A, Gerdoni E, Gallo G. (2005) Thyroid hormones affect neurogenesis in the dentate gyrus of adult rat. *Neuroendocrinology* 81:244–253.

Anderson CH. (1982) Changes in dendritic spine density in the preoptic area of the female rat at puberty. *Brain Res Bull* 8:261–265.

Anderson SA, Classey JD, Conde F, Lund JS, Lewis DA. (1995) Synchronous development of pyramidal neuron dendritic spines and parvalbumin-immunoreactive chandelier neuron axon terminals in layer III of monkey prefrontal cortex. *Neuroscience* 67:7–22.

Andersson IK, Edwall D, Norstedt G, Rozell B, Skottner A, Hansson HA. (1988) Differing expression of insulin-like growth factor I in the developing and in the adult rat cerebellum. *Acta Physiol Scand* 132:167–173.

Ando H, Zhou J, Macova M, Imboden H, Saavedra JM. (2004) Angiotensin II AT1 receptor blockade reverses pathological hypertrophy and inflammation in brain microvessels of spontaneously hypertensive rats. *Stroke* 35:1726–1731.

Anholt RR, Pedersen PL, De Souza EB, Snyder SH. (1986) The peripheral-type benzodiazepine receptor. Localization to the mitochondrial outer membrane. *J Biol Chem* 261:576–583.

Aoki H, Kimoto K, Hori N, Toyoda M. (2005) Cell proliferation in the dentate gyrus of rat hippocampus is inhibited by soft diet feeding. *Gerontology* 51:369–374.

Aragno M, Mastrocola R, Brignardello E, Catalano M, Robino G, Manti R, Parola M, Danni O, Boccuzzi G. (2000) Dehydroepiandrosterone modulates nuclear factor-kappaB activation in hippocampus of diabetic rats. *Diabetes* 49:1924–1931.

Arai O, Taniguchi I, Saito N. (1989) Correlation between the size of song control nuclei and plumage color change in orange bishop birds. *Neurosci Lett* 98:144–148.

Arai Y, Matsumoto A. (1978) Synapse formation of the hypothalamic arcuate nucleus during post-natal development in the female rat and its modification by neonatal estrogen treatment. *Psychoneuroendocrinology* 3:31–45.

Araque A, Parpura V, Sanzgiri RP, Haydon PG. (1999) Tripartite synapses: Glia, the unacknowledged partner. *Trends Neurosci* 22:208–215.

Araque A, Carmignoto G, Haydon PG. (2001) Dynamic signaling between astrocytes and neurons. *Annu Rev Physiol* 63:795–813.

Arendt T, Stieler J, Strijkstra AM, Hut RA, Rudiger J, Van der Zee EA, Harkany T, Holzer M, Hartig W. (2003) Reversible paired helical filament-like phosphorylation of tau is an adaptive process associated with neuronal plasticity in hibernating animals. *J Neurosci* 23:6972–6981.

Arimatsu Y, Hatanaka H. (1986) Estrogen treatment enhances survival of cultured fetal rat amygdala neurons in a defined medium. *Dev Brain Res* 26:151–159.

Armstrong DL, Garcia EA, Ma T, Quinones B, Wayner MJ. (1996) Angiotensin II blockade of long-term potentiation at the perforant path-granule cell synapse in vitro. *Peptides* 17:689–693.

Arnold AP. (2004) Sex chromosomes and brain gender. *Nat Rev Neurosci* 5:701–708.

Arnold AP, Breedlove SM. (1985) Organizational and activational effects of sex steroids on brain and behavior: A reanalysis. *Horm Behav* 19:469–498.

Arnold AP, Gorski RA. (1984) Gonadal steroid induction of structural sex differences in the central nervous system. *Annu Rev Neurosci* 7:413–442.

Arnold AP, Bottjer SW, Brenowitz EA, Nordeen EJ, Nordeen KW. (1986) Sexual dimorphisms in the neural vocal control system in song birds: Ontogeny and phylogeny. *Brain Behav Evol* 28:22–31.

Artola A, Brocher S, Singer W. (1990) Different voltage-dependent thresholds for inducing long-term depression and long-term potentiation in slices of rat visual cortex. *Nature* 347:69–72.

Artola A, Singer W. (1993) Long-term depression of excitatory synaptic transmission and its relationship to long-term potentiation. *Trends Neurosci* 16:480–487.

Artola A, Hensch T, Singer W. (1996) Calcium-induced long-term depression in the visual cortex of the rat in vitro. *J Neurophysiol* 76:984–994.

Artola A, Kamal A, Ramakers GM, Biessels GJ, Gispen WH. (2005) Diabetes mellitus concomitantly facilitates the induction of long-term depression and inhibits that of long-term potentiation in hippocampus. *Eur J Neurosci* 22:169–178.

Artola A, von Frijtag JC, Fermont PC, Gispen WH, Schrama LH, Kamal A, Spruijt BM. (2006) Long-lasting modulation of the induction of LTD and LTP in rat hippocampal CA1 by behavioural stress and environmental enrichment. *Eur J Neurosci* 23:261–272.

Arwert LI, Veltman DJ, Deijen JB, van Dam PS, Drent ML. (2006) Effects of growth hormone substitution therapy on cognitive functioning in growth hormone deficient patients: A functional MRI study. *Neuroendocrinology* 83:12–19.

Asbury ET, Fritts ME, Horton JE, Isaac WL. (1998) Progesterone facilitates the acquisition of avoidance learning and protects against subcortical neuronal death following prefrontal cortex ablation in the rat. *Behav Brain Res* 97:99–106.

Aste N, Cozzi B, Stankov B, Panzica G. (2001) Sexual differences and effect of photoperiod on melatonin receptor in avian brain. *Microsc Res Tech* 55:37–47.

Asthana S, Baker LD, Craft S, Stanczyk FZ, Veith RC, Raskind MA, Plymate SR. (2001) High-dose estradiol improves cognition for women with AD: Results of a randomized study. *Neurology* 57:605–612.

Auger AP. (2001) Ligand-independent activation of progestin receptors: Relevance for female sexual behaviour. *Reproduction* 122:847–855.

Auso E, Lavado-Autric R, Cuevas E, Del Rey FE, Morreale De Escobar G, Berbel P. (2004) A moderate and transient deficiency of maternal thyroid function at the beginning of fetal neocorticogenesis alters neuronal migration. *Endocrinology* 145:4037–4047.

Austin MP, Hadzi-Pavlovic D, Leader L, Saint K, Parker G. (2005) Maternal trait anxiety, depression and life event stress in pregnancy: Relationships with infant temperament. *Early Hum Dev* 81:183–190.

Avital A, Segal M, Richter-Levin G. (2006) Contrasting roles of corticosteroid receptors in hippocampal plasticity. *J Neurosci* 26:9130–9134.

Ayhan S, Markal N, Siemionow K, Araneo B, Siemionow M. (2003) Effect of subepineurial dehydroepiandrosterone treatment on healing of transected nerves repaired with the epineurial sleeve technique. *Microsurgery* 23:49–55.

Azcoitia I, Sierra A, Garcia-Segura LM. (1998) Estradiol prevents kainic acid-induced neuronal loss in the rat dentate gyrus. *NeuroReport* 9:3075–3079.

Azcoitia I, Fernandez-Galaz MC, Sierra A, Garcia-Segura LM. (1999a) Gonadal hormones affect neural vulnerability to excitoxin-induced degeneration. *J Neurocytol* 28:699–710.

Azcoitia I, Sierra A, Garcia-Segura LM. (1999b) Neuroprotective effects of estradiol in the adult rat hippocampus: Interaction with insulin-like growth factor-I signaling. *J Neurosci Res* 58:815–822.

Azcoitia I, Sierra A, Veiga S, Honda S, Harada N, Garcia-Segura LM. (2001) Brain aromatase is neuroprotective. *J Neurobiol* 47:318–329.

Azcoitia I, DonCarlos LL, Garcia-Segura LM. (2002) Estrogen and brain
vulnerability. *Neurotox Res* 4:235–245.

Azcoitia I, Leonelli E, Magnaghi V, Veiga S, Garcia-Segura LM, Melcangi RC. (2003)
Progesterone and its derivatives dihydroprogesterone and tetrahydroprogesterone
reduce myelin fiber morphological abnormalities and myelin fiber loss in the
sciatic nerve of aged rats. *Neurobiol Aging* 24:853–860.

Azcoitia I, Perez-Martin M, Salazar V, Castillo C, Ariznavarreta C, Garcia-Segura
LM, Tresguerres JA. (2005) Growth hormone prevents neuronal loss in the aged
rat hippocampus. *Neurobiol Aging* 26:697–703.

Azcoitia I, Moreno A, Carrero P, Palacios S, Garcia-Segura LM. (2006)
Neuroprotective effects of soy phytoestrogens in the rat brain. *Gynecol Endocrinol*
22:63–69.

Baas D, Bourbeau D, Sarlieve LL, Ittel ME, Dussault JH, Puymirat J. (1997)
Oligodendrocyte maturation and progenitor cell proliferation are independently
regulated by thyroid hormone. *Glia* 19:324–332.

Baetens D, Garcia-Segura LM, Perrelet A. (1982) Effects of climbing fiber destruction
on large dendrite spines of Purkinje cells. *Exp Brain Res* 48:256–262.

Baimoukhametova DV, Hewitt SA, Sank CA, Bains JS. (2004) Dopamine modulates
use-dependent plasticity of inhibitory synapses. *J Neurosci* 24:5162–5171.

Baker AE, Brautigam VM, Watters JJ. (2004) Estrogen modulates microglial
inflammatory mediator production via interactions with estrogen receptor beta.
Endocrinology 145:5021–5032.

Bakker J, Baum MJ. (2000) Neuroendocrine regulation of GnRH release in induced
ovulators. *Front Neuroendocrinol* 21:220–262.

Balazs R, Brooksbank BW, Davison AN, Eayrs JT, Wilson DA. (1969) The effect of
neonatal thyroidectomy on myelination in the rat brain. *Brain Res* 15:219–232.

Ball GF, MacDougall-Shackleton SA. (2001) Sex differences in songbirds 25 years
later: What have we learned and where do we go? *Microsc Res Tech* 54:327–334.

Ball GF, Auger C, Bernard DJ, Charlier TC, Sartor JJ, Riters LV, Balthazart J. (2004)
Seasonal plasticity in the song control system: Steroid metabolism, brain sites and
mechanism of hormone action. *Ann NY Acad Sci* 1016:586–610.

Balthazart J, Ball GF. (2006) Is brain estradiol a hormone or a neurotransmitter?
Trends Neurosci 29: 241–249.

Balthazart J, Baillien M, Ball GF. (2006a) Rapid control of brain aromatase activity
by glutamatergic inputs. *Endocrinology* 147:359–366.

Balthazart J, Cornil CA, Taziaux M, Charlier TD, Baillien M, Ball GF. (2006b)
Rapid changes in production and behavioral action of estrogens. *Neuroscience*
138:783–791.

Banasr M, Hery M, Brezun JM, Daszuta A. (2001) Serotonin mediates oestrogen
stimulation of cell proliferation in the adult dentate gyrus. *Eur J Neurosci*
14:1417–1424.

Bancroft J. (2005) The endocrinology of sexual arousal. *J Endocrinol* 186:411–427.

Banks JA, Freeman ME. (1980) Inhibition of the daily LH release mechanism by
progesterone acting at the hypothalamus. *Biol Reprod* 22:217–227.

Bao AM, Meynen G, Swaab DF. (2008) The stress system in depression and
neurodegeneration: Focus on the human hypothalamus. *Brain Res Rev*
57:531–553.

Barakat-Walter I. (1999) Role of thyroid hormones and their receptors in peripheral
nerve regeneration. *J Neurobiol* 40:541–559.

Barakat-Walter I, Kraftsik R, Schenker M, Kuntzer T. (2007) Thyroid hormone in biodegradable nerve guides stimulates sciatic nerve regeneration: A potential therapeutic approach for human peripheral nerve injuries. *J Neurotrauma* 24:567–577.

Barbazanges M, Piazza PV, Le Moal M, Maccari S. (1996) Maternal glucocorticoid secretion mediates long-term effects of prenatal stress. *J Neurosci* 16:7783–7790.

Barger SW, Chavis JA, Drew PD. (2000) Dehydroepiandrosterone inhibits microglial nitric oxide production in a stimulus-specific manner. *J Neurosci Res* 62:503–509.

Barker DJ. (2004) The developmental origins of chronic adult disease. *Acta Paediatr Suppl* 93:26–33.

Barker DJ, Osmond C. (1986) Infant mortality, childhood nutrition, and ischaemic heart disease in England and Wales. *Lancet* 1(8489):1077–1081.

Barnea A, Nottebohm F. (1994) Seasonal recruitment of hippocampal neurons in adult free-ranging black-capped chickadees. *Proc Natl Acad Sci USA* 91:11217–11221.

Barnes CA. (2003) Long-term potentiation and the ageing brain. *Philos Trans R Soc Lond B Biol Sci* 358:765–772.

Barnes CA, McNaughton BL, Goddard GV, Douglas RM, Adamec R. (1977) Circadian rhythm of synaptic excitability in rat and monkey central nervous system. *Science* 197:91–92.

Barnes CA, Jung MW, McNaughton BL, Korol DL, Andreasson K, Worley PF. (1994) LTP saturation and spatial learning disruption: Effects of task variables and saturation levels. *J Neurosci* 14:5793–5806.

Baroncini M, Allet C, Leroy D, Beauvillain JC, Francke JP, Prevot V. (2007) Morphological evidence for direct interaction between gonadotrophin-releasing hormone neurones and astroglial cells in the human hypothalamus. *J Neuroendocrinol* 19:691–702.

Barraclough CA, Camp P, Weiland N, Akabori A. (1986) Stimulatory versus inhibitory effects of progesterone on estrogen-induced phasic LH and prolactin secretion correlated with estrogen nuclear and progestin cytosol receptor concentration in brain and pituitary gland. *Neuroendocrinology* 42:6–14.

Barres BA, Lazar MA, Raff MC. (1994) A novel role for thyroid hormone, glucocorticoids and retinoic acid in timing oligodendrocyte development. *Development* 120:1097–1108.

Barreto G, Veiga S, Azcoitia I, Garcia-Segura LM, Garcia-Ovejero D. (2007) Testosterone decreases reactive astroglia and reactive microglia after brain injury in male rats: Role of its metabolites oestradiol and dihydrotestosterone. *Eur J Neurosci* 25:3039–3046.

Bartke A, Brown-Borg H. (2004) Life extension in the dwarf mouse. *Curr Top Dev Biol* 63:189–225.

Bartz JA, Hollander E. (2006) The neuroscience of affiliation: Forging links between basic and clinical research on neuropeptides and social behavior. *Horm Behav* 50:518–528.

Bartzokis G. (2004) Related age-related myelin breakdown: A developmental model of cognitive decline and Alzheimer's disease. *Neurobiol Aging* 25:5–18.

Bastianetto S, Ramassamy C, Poirier J, Quirion R. (1999) Dehydroepiandrosterone (DHEA) protects hippocampal cells from oxidative stress-induced damage. *Mol Brain Res* 66:35–41.

Bateman JM, McNeill H. (2006) Insulin/IGF signaling in neurogenesis. *Cell Mol Life Sci* 63:1701–1705.

Baulieu EE. (1997) Neurosteroids: Of the nervous system, by the nervous system, for the nervous system. *Rec Prog Hormone Res* 52:1–32.

Baulieu EE. (1998) Neurosteroids: A novel function of the brain. *Psychoneuroendocrinology* 23:963–987.

Baulieu EE, Schumacher M. (2000) Progesterone as a neuroactive neurosteroid, with special reference to the effect of progesterone on myelination. *Steroids* 65:605–612.

Baulieu EE, Thomas G, Legrain S, Lahlou N, Roger M, Debuire B, Faucounau V, Girard L, Hervy MP, Latour F, Leaud MC, Mokrane A, Pitti-Ferrandi H, Trivalle C, de Lacharriere O, Nouveau S, Rakoto-Arison B, Souberbielle JC, Raison J, Le Bouc Y, Raynaud A, Girerd X, Forette F. (2000) Dehydroepiandrosterone (DHEA), DHEA sulfate, and aging: Contribution of the DHEAge Study to a sociobiomedical issue. *Proc Natl Acad Sci USA* 97:4279–4284.

Baulieu EE, Robel P, Schumacher M. (2001) Neurosteroids: Beginning of the story. *Int Rev Neurobiol* 46:1–32.

Bauman WA. (1990) Seasonal changes in pancreatic insulin and glucagon in the little brown bat (Myotis lucifugus). *Pancreas* 5:342–346.

Bayatti N, Zschocke J, Behl C. (2003) Brain region-specific neuroprotective action and signaling of corticotropin-releasing hormone in primary neurons. *Endocrinology* 144:4051–4060.

Bayatti N, Behl C. (2005) The neuroprotective actions of corticotropin releasing hormone. *Ageing Res Rev* 4:258–270.

Baydas G, Nedzvetskii VS, Tuzcu M, Yasar A, Kirichenko SV. (2003) Increase of glial fibrillary acidic protein and S-100B in hippocampus and cortex of diabetic rats: Effects of vitamin E. *Eur J Pharmacol* 462:67–71.

Beauchet O. (2006) Testosterone and cognitive function: Current clinical evidence of a relationship. *Eur J Endocrinol* 155:773–781.

Becquet D, Girardet C, Guillaumond F, François-Bellan AM, Bosler O. (2008) Ultrastructural plasticity in the rat suprachiasmatic nucleus. Possible involvement in clock entrainment. *Glia* 56:294–305.

Behl C. (1999) Alzheimer's disease and oxidative stress: Implications for novel therapeutic approaches. *Prog Neurobiol* 57:301–323.

Behl C, Widmann M, Trapp T, Holsboer F. (1995) 17-beta estradiol protects neurons from oxidative stress-induced cell death in vitro. *Biochem Biophys Res Commun* 216:473–482.

Behl C, Skutella T, Lezoualch F, Post A, Widmann M, Newton CJ, Holsboer F. (1997) Neuroprotection against oxidative stress by estrogens: Structure–activity relationship. *Mol Pharmacol* 51:535–541.

Behl C, Holsboer F. (1999) The female sex hormone oestrogen as a neuroprotectant. *Trends Pharmacol Sci* 20:441–444.

Behringer RR, Lewin TM, Quaife CJ, Palmiter RD, Brinster RL, D'Ercole AJ. (1990) Expression of insulin-like growth factor I stimulates normal somatic growth in growth hormone-deficient transgenic mice. *Endocrinology* 127:1033–1040.

Beilharz EJ, Russo VC, Butler G, Baker NL, Connor B, Sirimanne ES, Dragunow M, Werther GA, Gluckman PD, Williams CE, Scheepens A. (1998) Coordinated and cellular specific induction of the components of the IGF/IGFBP axis in the rat brain following hypoxic-ischemic injury. *Mol Brain Res* 59:119–134.

Belanger A, Lavoie N, Trudeau F, Massicotte G, Gagnon S. (2004) Preserved LTP and water maze learning in hyperglycaemic-hyperinsulinemic ZDF rats. *Physiol Behav* 83:483–494.

Belcredito S, Vegeto E, Brusadelli A, Ghisletti S, Mussi P, Ciana P, Maggi A. (2001) Estrogen neuroprotection: The involvement of the Bcl-2 binding protein BNIP2. *Brain Res Rev* 37:335–342.

Belelli D, Herd MB. (2003) The contraceptive agent Provera enhances GABA(A) receptor-mediated inhibitory neurotransmission in the rat hippocampus: Evidence for endogenous neurosteroids? *J Neurosci* 23:10013–10020.

Belelli D, Lambert JJ. (2005) Neurosteroids: Endogenous regulators of the GABA(A) receptor. *Nat Rev Neurosci* 6:565–575.

Bender CM, Sereika SM, Brufsky AM, Ryan CM, Vogel VG, Rastogi P, Cohen SM, Casillo FE, Berga SL. (2007) Memory impairments with adjuvant anastrozole versus tamoxifen in women with early-stage breast cancer. *Menopause* 14:995–998.

Bennur S, Shankaranarayana Rao BS, Pawlak R, Strickland S, McEwen BS, Chattarji S. (2007) Stress-induced spine loss in the medial amygdala is mediated by tissue-plasminogen activator. *Neuroscience* 144:8–16.

Bentel JM, Birrell SN, Pickering MA, Holds DJ, Horsfall DJ, Tilley WD. (1999) Androgen receptor agonist activity of the synthetic progestin, medroxyprogesterone acetate, in human breast cancer cells. *Mol Cell Endocrinol* 154:11–20.

Bentley GE. (2001) Unraveling the enigma: The role of melatonin in seasonal processes in birds. *Microsc Res Tech* 53:63–71.

Bentley GE, Van't Hof TJ, Ball GF. (1999) Seasonal neuroplasticity in the songbird telencephalon: A role for melatonin. *Proc Natl Acad Sci USA* 96:4674–4679.

Benvenga S. (2005) Brain injury and hypopituitarism: The historical background. *Pituitary* 8:193–195.

Berbel P, Guadaño-Ferraz A, Angulo A, Ramón Cerezo J. (1994) Role of thyroid hormones in the maturation of interhemispheric connections in rats. *Behav Brain Res* 64:9–14.

Berbel P, Ausó E, Garcia-Velasco JV, Molina ML, Camacho M. (2001) Role of thyroid hormones in the maturation and organisation of rat barrel cortex. *Neuroscience* 107:383–394.

Berbel P, Obregón MJ, Bernal J, Escobar del Rey F, Morreale de Escobar G. (2007) Iodine supplementation during pregnancy: A public health challenge. *Trends Endocrinol Metab* 18:338–343.

Bereiter DA, Jeanrenaud B. (1979) Altered neuroanatomical organization in the central nervous system of the genetically obese (ob/ob) mouse. *Brain Res* 165:249–260.

Bergan JF, Ro P, Ro D, Knudsen EI. (2005) Hunting increases adaptive auditory map plasticity in adult barn owls. *J Neurosci* 25:9816–9820.

Bergendahl M, Iranmanesh A, Mulligan T, Veldhuis JD. (2000) Impact of age on cortisol secretory dynamics basally and as driven by nutrient-withdrawal stress. *J Clin Endocrinol Metab* 85:2203–2214.

Bergeron R, de Montigny C, Debonnel G. (1996) Potentiation of neuronal NMDA response induced by dehydroepiandrosterone and its suppression by progesterone: Effects mediated via σ receptors. *J Neurosci* 16:1193–1202.

Bernard C. (1878–1879) Leçons sur les Phénomènes de la Vie Communs aux Animaux et aux Végétaux. 2 Vols. Baillière. Paris.

Bernard DJ, Ball GF. (1997) Photoperiodic condition modulates the effects of testosterone on song control nuclei volumes in male European starlings. *Gen Comp Endocrinol* 105:276–283.

Bernard DJ, Wilson FE, Ball GF. (1997) Testis-dependent and -independent effects of photoperiod on volumes of song control nuclei in American tree sparrows (Spizella arborea). *Brain Res* 760:163–169.

Bernaudin M, Marti HH, Roussel S, Divoux D, Nouvelot A, MacKenzie ET, Petit E. (1999) A potential role for erythropoietin in focal permanent cerebral ischemia in mice. *J Cereb Blood Flow Metab* 19:643–651.

Bernaudin M, Bellail A, Marti HH, Yvon A, Vivien D, Duchatelle I, Mackenzie ET, Petit E. (2000) Neurons and astrocytes express EPO mRNA: Oxygen-sensing mechanisms that involve the redox-state of the brain. *Glia* 30:271–278.

Berton O, McClung CA, Dileone RJ, Krishnan V, Renthal W, Russo SJ, Graham D, Tsankova NM, Bolanos CA, Rios M, Monteggia LM, Self DW, Nestler EJ. (2006) Essential role of BDNF in the mesolimbic dopamine pathway in social defeat stress. *Science* 311:864–868.

Bessis A, Bechade C, Bernard D, Roumier A. (2007) Microglial control of neuronal death and synaptic properties. *Glia* 55:233–238.

Beyer C, Pawlak J, Brito V, Karolczak M, Ivanova T, Kuppers E. (2003) Regulation of gene expression in the developing midbrain by estrogen: Implication of classical and nonclassical steroid signaling. *Ann N Y Acad Sci* 1007:17–28.

Bi R, Foy MR, Vouimba RM, Thompson RF, Baudry M. (2001) Cyclic changes in estradiol regulate synaptic plasticity through the MAP kinase pathway. *Proc Natl Acad Sci USA* 98:13391–13395.

Bialek M, Zaremba P, Borowicz KK, Czuczwar SJ. (2004) Neuroprotective role of testosterone in the nervous system. *Pol J Pharmacol* 56:509–518.

Bicknell RJ. (1998) Sex-steroid actions on neurotransmission. *Curr Opin Neurol* 11:667–671.

Bielsky IF, Young LJ. (2004) Oxytocin, vasopressin, and social recognition in mammals. *Peptides* 25:1565–1574.

Biessels GJ, Kamal A, Ramakers GM, Urban IJ, Spruijt BM, Erkelens DW, Gispen WH. (1996) Place learning and hippocampal synaptic plasticity in streptozotocin-induced diabetic rats. *Diabetes* 45:1259–1266.

Biessels GJ, Kamal A, Urban IJ, Spruijt BM, Erkelens DW, Gispen WH. (1998) Water maze learning and hippocampal synaptic plasticity in streptozotocin-diabetic rats: Effects of insulin treatment. *Brain Res* 800:125–135.

Billon N, Jolicoeur C, Tokumoto Y, Vennstrom B, Raff M. (2002) Normal timing of oligodendrocyte development depends on thyroid hormone receptor α1 (TRα1). *EMBO J* 21:6452–6460.

Birkhauser M. (2002) Depression, menopause and estrogens: Is there a correlation? *Maturitas* 41(Suppl 1):3–8.

Blair HT, Schafe GE, Bauer EP, Rodrigues SM, Ledoux JE. (2001) Synaptic plasticity in the lateral amygdala: A cellular hypothesis of fear conditioning. *Learn Mem* 8:229–242.

Blakemore SJ. (2008) The social brain in adolescence. *Nat Rev Neurosci* 9:267–277.

Blaustein JD. (2004) Minireview: Neuronal steroid hormone receptors: They're not just for hormones anymore. *Endocrinology* 145:1075–1081.

Bleier R, Byne W, Siggelkow I. (1982) Cytoarchitectonic sexual dimorphisms of the medial preoptic and anterior hypothalamic areas in guinea pig, rat, hamster, and mouse. *J Comp Neurol* 212:118–130.

Bliss TV, Gardner-Medwin AR. (1973) Long-lasting potentiation of synaptic transmission in the dentate area of the unanaestetized rabbit following stimulation of the perforant path. *J Physiol* 232:357–374.

Bliss TV, Lømo T. (1973) Long-lasting potentiation of synaptic transmission in the dentate area of the anaesthetized rabbit following stimulation of the perforant path. *J Physiol* 232:331–356.

Bloch B, Ling N, Benoit R, Wehrenberg WB, Guillemin R. (1984) Specific depletion of immunoreactive growth hormone-releasing factor by monosodium glutamate in rat median eminence. *Nature* 307:272–273.

Blüher M, Kahn BB, Kahn CR. (2003) Extended longevity in mice lacking the insulin receptor in adipose tissue. Science 299:572–574.

Blüher S, Mantzoros CS. (2007) Leptin in reproduction. *Curr Opin Endocrinol Diabetes Obes* 14:458–464.

Blurton-Jones M, Tuszynski MH. (2001) Reactive astrocytes express estrogen receptors in the injured primate brain. *J Comp Neurol* 433:115–123.

Blutstein T, Devidze N, Choleris E, Jasnow AM, Pfaff DW, Mong JA. (2006) Oestradiol up-regulates glutamine synthetase mRNA and protein expression in the hypothalamus and hippocampus: Implications for a role of hormonally responsive glia in amino acid neurotransmission. *J Neuroendocrinol* 18:692–702.

Bobak JB, Salm AK. (1996) Plasticity of astrocytes of the ventral glial limitans subjacent to the supraoptic nucleus. *J Comp Neurol* 376:188–197.

Bogdanov MB, Ferrante RJ, Mueller G, Ramos LE, Martinou JC, Beal MF. (1999) Oxidative stress is attenuated in mice overexpressing BCL-2. *Neurosci Lett* 262:33–36.

von Bohlen und Halbach O, Albrecht D. (1998) Angiotensin II inhibits long-term potentiation within the lateral nucleus of the amygdala through AT1 receptors. *Peptides* 19:1031–1036.

Bologa L, Sharma J, Roberts E. (1987) Dehydroepiandrosterone and its sulfated derivative reduce neuronal death and enhance astrocytic differentiation in brain cell cultures. *J Neurosci Res* 17:225–234.

Bondanelli M, Ambrosio MR, Zatelli MC, De Marinis L, degli Uberti EC. (2005) Hypopituitarism after traumatic brain injury. *Eur J Endocrinol* 152:679–691.

Bondanelli M, Ambrosio MR, Cavazzini L, Bertocchi A, Zatelli MC, Carli A, Valle D, Basaglia N, Uberti EC. (2007) Anterior pituitary function may predict functional and cognitive outcome in patients with traumatic brain injury undergoing rehabilitation. *J Neurotrauma* 24:1687–1698.

Bondareff W, Geinisman Y. (1976) Loss of synapses in the dentate gyrus of the senescent rat. *Am J Anat* 145:129–136.

Bondy CA, Cheng CM. (2004) Signaling by insulin-like growth factor 1 in brain. *Eur J Pharmacol* 490:25–31.

Bonfanti L. (2006) PSA-NCAM in mammalian structural plasticity and neurogenesis. *Prog Neurobiol* 80:129–164.

Bonfanti L, Olive S, Poulain DA, Theodosis DT. (1992) Mapping of the distribution of polysialylated neural cell adhesion molecule throughout the central nervous system of the adult rat: An immunohistochemical study. *Neuroscience* 49:419–436.

Bonnefont AB, Munoz FJ, Inestrosa NC. (1998) Estrogen protects neuronal cells from the cytotoxicity induced by acetylcholinesterase-amyloid complexes. *FEBS Lett* 441:220–224.

Boonstra R, Hubbs AH, Lacey EA, McColl CJ. (2001) Seasonal changes in glucocorticoid and testosterone concentrations in free-living arctic ground squirrels from the boreal forest of the Yukon. *Can J Zool* 79:49–58.

Bora SH, Liu Z, Kecojevic A, Merchenthaler I, Koliatsos VE. (2005) Direct, complex effects of estrogens on basal forebrain cholinergic neurons. *Exp Neurol* 194:506–522.

Borlongan CV, Yamamoto M, Takei N, Kumazaki M, Ungsuparkorn C, Hida H, Sanberg PR, Nishino H. (2000) Glial cell survival is enhanced during melatonin-induced neuroprotection against cerebral ischemia. *FASEB J* 14:1307–1317.

Bose HS, Lingappa VR, Miller WL. (2002) Rapid regulation of steroidogenesis by mitochondrial protein import. *Nature* 417:87–91.

Boseret G, Carere C, Ball GF, Balthazart J. (2006) Social context affects testosterone-induced singing and the volume of song control nuclei in male canaries (Serinus canaria). *J Neurobiol* 66:1044–1060.

Boswell T, Woods SC, Kenagy GJ. (1994) Seasonal changes mass, insulin, and glucocorticoids of free-living golden-ground squirrels. *Gen Comp Endocrinol* 96:339–346.

Brabham T, Phelka A, Zimmer C, Nash A, Lopez JF, Vazquez DM. (2000) Effects of prenatal dexamethasone on spatial learning and response to stress is influenced by maternal factors. *Am J Physiol Regul Integr Comp Physiol* 279:R1899–R1909.

Braestrup C, Squires RF. (1977) Specific benzodiazepine receptors in rat brain characterized by high-affinity (3H)diazepam binding. *Proc Natl Acad Sci USA* 74:3805–3809.

Brailoiu E, Dun SL, Brailoiu GC, Mizuo K, Sklar LA, Oprea TI, Prossnitz ER, Dun NJ. (2007) Distribution and characterization of estrogen receptor G protein-coupled receptor 30 in the rat central nervous system. *J Endocrinol* 193:311–321.

Brain SD, Grant AD. (2004) Vascular actions of calcitonin gene-related peptide and adrenomedullin. *Physiol Rev* 84:903–934.

Brann DW, Mahesh VB. (2005) The aging reproductive neuroendocrine axis. *Steroids* 70:273–283.

Brann DW, Dhandapani K, Wakade C, Mahesh VB, Khan MM. (2007) Neurotrophic and neuroprotective actions of estrogen: Basic mechanisms and clinical implications. *Steroids* 72:381–405.

Brannvall K, Bogdanovic N, Korhonen L, Lindholm D. (2005) 19-Nortestosterone influences neural stem cell proliferation and neurogenesis in the rat brain. *Eur J Neurosci* 21:871–878.

Brawer JR, Naftolin F, Martin J, Sonnenschein C. (1978) Effects of a single injection of estradiol valerate on the hypothalamic arcuate nucleus and on reproductive function in the female rat. *Endocrinology* 103:501–512.

Brawer JR, Schipper H, Naftolin F. (1980) Ovary-dependent degeneration in the hypothalamic arcuate nucleus. Endocrinology 107:274–279.

Breedlove SM, Arnold AP. (1980) Hormone accumulation in a sexually dimorphic motor nucleus of the rat spinal cord. *Science* 210:564–566.

Breedlove SM, Arnold AP. (1981) Sexually dimorphic motor nucleus in the rat lumbar spinal cord: Response to adult hormone manipulation, absence in androgen-insensitive rats. *Brain Res* 225:297–307.

Breedlove SM, Arnold AP. (1983) Hormonal control of a developing neuromuscular system. I. Sensitive periods for the androgen-induced masculinization of the rat spinal nucleus of the bulbocavernosus. *J Neurosci* 3:424–432.

Bremner JD, Randall P, Vermetten E, Staib L, Bronen RA, Mazure C, Capelli S, McCarthy G, Innis RB, Charney DS. (1997) Magnetic resonance imaging-based measurement of hippocampal volume in posttraumatic stress disorder related to childhood physical and sexual abuse—a preliminary report. *Biol Psychiatry* 41:23–32.

Bremner WJ, Vitiello MV, Prinz PN. (1983) Loss of circadian rhythmicity in blood testosterone levels with aging in normal men. *J Clin Endocrinol Metab* 56:1278–1281.

Brenowitz EA, Nalls B, Wingfield JC, Kroodsma DE. (1991) Seasonal changes in avian song nuclei without seasonal changes in song repertoire. *J Neurosci* 11:1367–1374.

Brenowitz EA, Baptista LF, Lent K, Wingfield JC. (1998) Seasonal plasticity of the song control system in wild Nuttall's white-crowned sparrows. *J Neurobiol* 34:69–82.

Brezun JM, Daszuta A. (1999) Serotonin depletion in the adult rat produces differential changes in highly polysialylated form of neural cell adhesion molecule and tenascin-C immunoreactivity. *J Neurosci Res* 55:54–70.

Brines ML, Ghezzi P, Keenan S, Agnello D, de Lanerolle NC, Cerami C, Itri LM, Cerami A. (2000) Erythropoietin crosses the blood-brain barrier to protect against experimental brain injury. *Proc Natl Acad Sci USA* 97:10526–10531.

Brinton RD, Tran J, Proffitt P, Montoya, M. (1997) 17 beta-Estradiol enhances the outgrowth and survival of neocortical neurons in culture. *Neurochem Res* 22:1339–1351.

Brinton RE, Gruener R. (1987) Vasopressin promotes neurite growth in cultured embryonic neurons. *Synapse* 1:329–334.

Brixey SN, Gallagher BJ, McFalls JA, Parmelee LF. (1993) Gestational and neonatal factors in the etiology of schizophrenia. *J Clin Psychol* 49:447–456.

Brown CM, Choi E, Xu Q, Vitek MP, Colton CA. (2008) The APOE4 genotype alters the response of microglia and macrophages to 17beta-estradiol. *Neurobiol Aging* 29:1783–1794.

Brown DD, Cai L. (2007) Amphibian metamorphosis. *Dev Biol* 306:20–33.

Brown RC, PapadopoulosV. (2001) Role of the peripheral-type benzodiazepine receptor in adrenal and brain steroidogenesis. *Int Rev Neurobiol* 46:117–143.

Brown SD, Bottjer SW. (1993) Testosterone-induced changes in adult canary brain are reversible. *J Neurobiol* 24:627–640.

Bruce-Keller AJ. (1999) Microglial-neuronal interactions in synaptic damage and recovery. *J Neurosci Res* 58:191–201.

Bruce-Keller AJ, Keeling JL, Keller JN, Huang FF, Camondola S, Mattson MP. (2000) Anti-inflammatory effects of estrogen on microglial activation. *Endocrinology* 141:3646–3656.

Bruce-Keller AJ, Barger SW, Moss NI, Pham JT, Keller JN, Nath A. (2001) Pro-inflammatory and pro-oxidant properties of the HIV protein Tat in a microglial cell line: Attenuation by 17 beta-estradiol. *J Neurochem* 78:1315–1324.

Brummelte S, Pawluski JL, Galea LA. (2006) High post-partum levels of corticosterone given to dams influence postnatal hippocampal cell proliferation and behavior of offspring: A model of post-partum stress and possible depression. *Horm Behav* 50:370–382.

Brun VH, Ytterbø K, Morris RGM, Moser MB, Moser EI. (2001) Retrograde amnesia for spatial memory induced by NMDA receptor-mediated long-term potentiation. *J Neurosci* 21:356–362.

Bruns J, Hauser WA. (2003) The epidemiology of traumatic brain injury: A review. *Epilepsia* 44(Suppl 10):2–10.

Brunson KL, Eghbal-Ahmadi M, Bender R, Chen Y, Baram TZ. (2001) Long-term, progressive hippocampal cell loss and dysfunction induced by early-life administration of corticotropin-releasing hormone reproduce the effects of early-life stress. *Proc Natl Acad Sci USA* 98:8856–8861.

Brunson KL, Kramár E, Lin B, Chen Y, Colgin LL, Yanagihara TK, Lynch G, Baram TZ. (2005) Mechanisms of late-onset cognitive decline after early-life stress. *J Neurosci* 25:9328–9338.

Brunton PJ, Russell JA. (2008) The expectant brain: Adapting for motherhood. *Nat Rev Neurosci* 9:11–25.

Brussaard AB, Kits KS, Baker RE, Willems WP, Leyting-Vermeulen JW, Voorn P, Smit AB, Bicknell RJ, Herbison AE. (1997) Plasticity in fast synaptic inhibition of adult oxytocin neurons caused by switch in GABA(A) receptor subunit expression. *Neuron* 19:1103–1114.

Brywe KG, Leverin AL, Gustavsson M, Mallard C, Granata R, Destefanis S, Volante M, Hagberg H, Ghigo E, Isgaard J. (2005a) Growth hormone-releasing peptide hexarelin reduces neonatal brain injury and alters Akt/glycogen synthase kinase-3beta phosphorylation. *Endocrinology* 146:4665–4672.

Brywe KG, Mallard C, Gustavsson M, Hedtjärn M, Leverin A.L, Wang X, Blomgren K, Isgaard J, Hagberg H. (2005b) IGF-1 neuroprotection in the immature brain after hypoxia-ischemia, involvement of Akt and GSK3b. *Eur J Neurosci* 21:1489–1502.

Buck CL, Barnes BM. (2000) Effects of ambient temperature on metabolic rate, respiratory quotient, and torpor in an arctic hibernator. *Am J Physiol* 279:R255–R262.

Buijs RM, Pévet P, Masson-Pévet M, Pool CW, deVries GJ, Canguilhem B, Vivien-Roels B. (1986) Seasonal variation in vasopressin innervation in the brain of the European hamster (Cricetus cricetus). *Brain Res* 371:193–196.

Burd GD. (1991) Development of the olfactory nerve in the African clawed frog, Xenopus laevis: I. Normal development. *J Comp Neurol* 304:123–134.

Burd GD. (1992) Development of the olfactory nerve in the clawed frog, Xenopus laevis: II. Effects of hypothyroidism. *J Comp Neurol* 315:255–263.

Burd GD, Nottebohm F. (1985) Ultrastructural characterization of synaptic terminals formed on newly generated neurons in a song control nucleus of the adult canary forebrain. *J Comp Neurol* 240:143–152.

Burgess W, Liu Q, Zhou J, Tang Q, Ozawa A, VanHoy R, Arkins S, Dantzer R, Kelley KW. (1999) The immune-endocrine loop during aging: Role of growth hormone and insulin-like growth factor-I. *Neuroimmunomodulation* 6:56–68.

Burke SN, Barnes CA. (2006) Neural plasticity in the ageing brain. *Nat Rev Neurosci* 7:30–40.

Burkhardt MS, Foster JK, Laws SM, Baker LD, Craft S, Gandy SE, Stuckey BG, Clarnette R, Nolan D, Hewson-Bower B, Martins RN. (2004) Oestrogen replacement therapy may improve memory functioning in the absence of APOE epsilon4. *J Alzheimer's Dis* 6:221–228.

Burmeister SS, Kailasanath V, Fernald RD. (2007) Social dominance regulates androgen and estrogen receptor gene expression. *Horm Behav* 51:164–170.

Busiguina S, Fernandez AM, Barrios V, Clark R, Tolbert DL, Berciano J, Torres-Alemán I. (2000) Neurodegeneration is associated to changes in serum insulin-like growth factors. *Neurobiol Dis* 7:657–665.

Butcher SK, Lord JM. (2004) Stress responses and innate immunity: Aging as a contributory factor. *Aging Cell* 3:151–160.

Buwalda B, Kole MH, Veenema AH, Huininga M, de Boer SF, Korte SM, Koolhaas JM. (2005) Long-term effects of social stress on brain and behavior: A focus on hippocampal functioning. *Neurosci Biobehav Rev* 29:83–97.

Cagnoli CM, Atabay C, Kharlamova E, Manev H. (1995) Melatonin protects neurons from singlet oxygen-induced apoptosis. *J Pineal Res* 18:222–226.

Cai D, McCarron RM, Yu EZ, Li Y, Hallenbeck J. (2004) Akt phosphorylation and kinase activity are down-regulated during hibernation in the 13-lined ground squirrel. *Brain Res* 1014:14–21.

Cai L, Brown DD. (2004) Expression of type II iodothyronine deiodinase marks the time that a tissue responds to thyroid hormone-induced metamorphosis in Xenopus laevis. *Dev Biol* 266:87–95.

Calapai G, Marciano MC, Corica F, Allegra A, Parisi A, Frisina N, Caputi AP, Buemi M. (2000) Erythropoietin protects against brain ischemic injury by inhibition of nitric oxide formation. *Eur J Pharmacol* 401:349–356.

Caldwell HK, Lee HJ, Macbeth AH, Young WS. (2008) Vasopressin: Behavioral roles of an "original" neuropeptide. *Prog Neurobiol* 84:1–24.

Calizo LH, Flanagan-Cato LM. (2000) Estrogen selectively regulates spine density within the dendritic arbor of rat ventromedial hypothalamic neurons. *J Neurosci* 20:1589–1596.

Calizo LH, Flanagan-Cato LM. (2002) Estrogen-induced dendritic spine elimination on female rat ventromedial hypothalamic neurons that project to the periaqueductal gray. *J Comp Neurol* 447:234–248.

Callier S, Morisette M, Grandbois M, Di Paolo T. (2000) Stereospecific prevention by 17β-estradiol of MPTP-induced dopamine depletion in mice. *Synapse* 37:245–251.

Callier S, Morissette M, Grandbois M, Pelaprat D, Di Paolo T. (2001) Neuroprotective properties of 17beta-estradiol, progesterone, and raloxifene in MPTP C57Bl/6 mice. *Synapse* 41:131–138.

Calzà L, Fernandez M, Giuliani A, D'Intino G, Pirondi S, Sivilia S, Paradisi M, Desordi N, Giardino L. (2005) Thyroid hormone and remyelination in adult central nervous system: A lesson from an inflammatory-demyelinating disease. *Brain Res Rev* 48:339–346.

Camarero G, Leon Y, Gorospe I, De Pablo F, Alsina B, Giraldez F, Varela-Nieto I. (2003) Insulin-like growth factor 1 is required for survival of transit-amplifying neuroblasts and differentiation of otic neurons. *Dev Biol* 262:242–253.

Cambiasso MJ, Colombo JA, Carrer HF. (2000) Differential effect of oestradiol and astroglia-conditioned media on the growth of hypothalamic neurons from male and female rat brains. *Eur J Neurosci* 12:2291–2298.

Cameron HA, Dayer AG. (2008) New interneurons in the adult neocortex: Small, sparse, but significant? *Biol Psychiatry* 63:650–655.

Campagne C, Bouret SG, Beauvillain JC, Prevot V. (2006) Expression of Semaphorin3A and Neuropilin-1 in the adult median eminence. *Front Neuroendocrinol* 27:74 (Abstract).

Campbell S, MacQueen G. (2006) An update on regional brain volume differences associated with mood disorders. *Curr Opin Psychiatry* 19:25–33.

Cannon WB. (1929) Organization for physiological homeostasis. *Physiol Rev* 9:399–343.

Cardona-Gomez GP, Chowen JA, Garcia-Segura LM. (2000a) Estradiol and progesterone regulate the expression of insulin-like growth factor-I receptor and insulin-like growth factor binding protein-2 in the hypothalamus of adult female rats. *J Neurobiol* 43:269–281.

Cardona-Gomez GP, DonCarlos L, Garcia-Segura LM. (2000b) Insulin-like growth factor I receptors and estrogen receptors colocalize in female rat brain. *Neuroscience* 99: 751–760.

Cardona-Gomez GP, Trejo JL, Fernandez AM, Garcia-Segura LM. (2000c) Estrogen receptors and insulin-like growth factor-I receptors mediate estrogen-dependent synaptic plasticity. *NeuroReport* 11:1735–1738.

Cardona-Gomez GP, Mendez P, DonCarlos LL, Azcoitia I, Garcia-Segura LM. (2001) Interactions of estrogens and insulin-like growth factor-I in the brain: Implications for neuroprotection. *Brain Res Rev* 37:320–334.

Cardona-Gomez GP, Mendez P, DonCarlos LL, Azcoitia I, Garcia-Segura LM. (2002a) Interactions of estrogen and insulin-like growth factor-I in the brain: Molecular mechanisms and functional implications. *J Steroid Biochem Mol Biol* 83:211–217.

Cardona-Gomez GP, Mendez P, Garcia-Segura LM. (2002b) Synergistic interaction of estradiol and insulin-like growth factor-I in the activation of PI3K/Akt signaling in the adult rat hypothalamus. *Mol Brain Res* 107:80–88.

Cardona-Gomez GP, Perez M, Avila J, Garcia-Segura LM, Wandosell F. (2004) Estradiol inhibits GSK3 and regulates interaction of estrogen receptors, GSK3, and beta-catenin in the hippocampus. *Mol Cell Neurosci* 25:363–373.

Cardona-Gomez GP, Arango-Davila C, Gallego-Gomez JC, Barrera-Ocampo A, Pimienta H, Garcia-Segura LM. (2006) Estrogen dissociates Tau and alpha-amino-3-hydroxy-5-methylisoxazole-4-propionic acid receptor subunit in postischemic hippocampus. *NeuroReport* 17:1337–1341.

Cardounel A, Regelson W, Kalimi M. (1999) Dehydroepiandrosterone protects hippocampal neurons against neurotoxin-induced cell death: Mechanism of action. *Proc Soc Exp Biol Med* 222:145–149.

Carnahan RM, Perry PJ. (2004) Depression in aging men: The role of testosterone. *Drugs Aging* 21:361–376.

Carrer HF, Aoki A. (1982). Ultrastructural changes in the hypothalamic ventromedial nucleus of ovariectomized rats after estrogen treatment. *Brain Res* 240:221–233.

Carrer HF, Cambiasso MJ. (2002) Sexual differentiation of the brain: Genes, estrogen, and neurotrophic factors. *Cell Mol Neurobiol* 22:479–500.

Carrer HF, Cambiasso MJ, Gorosito S. (2005) Effects of estrogen on neuronal growth and differentiation. *J Steroid Biochem Mol Biol* 93:319–323.

Carro E, Nunez A, Busiguina S, Torres-Alemán I. (2000) Circulating insulin-like growth factor I mediates effects of exercise on the brain. *J Neurosci* 20:2926–2933.

Carro E, Trejo JL, Busiguina S, Torres-Alemán I. (2001) Circulating insulin-like growth factor I mediates the protective effects of physical exercise against brain insults of different etiology and anatomy. *J Neurosci* 21:5678–5684.

Carro E, Trejo JL, Gomez-Isla T, LeRoith D, Torres-Alemán I. (2002) Serum insulin-like growth factor I regulates brain amyloid-beta levels. *Nat Med* 8:1390–1397.

Carro E, Trejo JL, Nunez A, Torres-Alemán I. (2003) Brain repair and neuroprotection by serum insulin-like growth factor I. *Mol Neurobiol* 27:153–162.

Carro E, Torres-Alemán I. (2004) The role of insulin and insulin-like growth factor I in the molecular and cellular mechanisms underlying the pathology of Alzheimer's disease. *Eur J Pharmacol* 490:127–133.

Carro E, Trejo JL, Spuch C, Bohl D, Heard JM, Torres-Alemán I. (2006) Blockade of the insulin-like growth factor I receptor in the choroid plexus originates Alzheimer's-like neuropathology in rodents: New cues into the human disease? *Neurobiol Aging* 27:1618–1631.

Carswell HV, Dominiczak AF, Garcia-Segura LM, Harada N, Hutchison JB, Macrae IM. (2005) Brain aromatase expression after experimental stroke: Topography and time course. *J Steroid Biochem Mol Biol* 96:89–91.

Casellas P, Galiegue S, Basile AS. (2002) Peripheral benzodiazepine receptors and mitochondrial function. *Neurochem Int* 40:475–486.

Cashion AB, Smith MJ, Wise PM. (2003) The morphometry of astrocytes in the rostral preoptic area exhibits a diurnal rhythm on proestrus: Relationship to the luteinizing hormone surge and effects of age. *Endocrinology* 144:274–280.

Castellano JM, Navarro VM, Fernandez-Fernandez R, Nogueiras R, Tovar S, Roa J, Vazquez MJ, Vigo E, Casanueva FF, Aguilar E, Pinilla L, Dieguez C, Tena-Sempere M. (2005) Changes in hypothalamic KiSS-1 system and restoration of pubertal activation of the reproductive axis by kisspeptin in undernutrition. *Endocrinology* 146:3917–3925.

Castro-Alamancos MA, Torres-Alemán I. (1993) Long-term depression of glutamate-induced gamma-aminobutyric acid release in cerebellum by insulin-like growth factor I. *Proc Natl Acad Sci USA* 90:7386–7390.

Castro-Alamancos MA, Torres-Alemán I. (1994) Learning of the conditioned eye-blink response is impaired by an antisense insulin-like growth factor I oligonucleotide. *Proc Natl Acad Sci USA* 91:10203–10207.

Castro-Alamancos MA, Arevalo MA, Torres-Alemán I. (1996) Involvement of protein kinase C and nitric oxide in the modulation by insulin-like growth factor-I of glutamate-induced GABA release in the cerebellum. *Neuroscience* 70:843–847.

Catania MA, Marciano MC, Parisi A, Sturiale A, Buemi M, Grasso G, Squadrito F, Caputi AP, Calapai G. (2002) Erythropoietin prevents cognition impairment induced by transient brain ischemia in gerbils. *Eur J Pharmacol* 437:147–150.

Celik M, Gokmen N, Erbayraktar S, Akhisaroglu M, Konakc S, Ulukus C, Genc S, Genc K, Sagiroglu E, Cerami A, Brines M. (2002) Erythropoietin prevents motor neuron apoptosis and neurologic disability in experimental spinal cord ischemic injury. *Proc Natl Acad Sci USA* 99:2258–2263.

Celotti F, Melcangi RC, Martini L. (1992) The 5 alpha-reductase in the brain: Molecular aspects and relation to brain function. *Front Neuroendocrinol* 13:163–215.

Cerqueira JJ, Pêgo JM, Taipa R, Bessa JM, Almeida OF, Sousa N. (2005) Morphological correlates of corticosteroid-induced changes in prefrontal cortex-dependent behaviors. *J Neurosci* 25:7792–7800.

Cerqueira JJ, Mailliet F, Almeida OF, Jay TM, Sousa N. (2007) The prefrontal cortex as a key target of the maladaptive response to stress. *J Neurosci* 27:2781–2787.

Cervantes M, Gonzalez-Vidal MD, Ruelas R, Escobar A, Morali G. (2002) Neuroprotective effects of progesterone on damage elicited by acute global cerebral ischemia in neurons of the caudate nucleus. *Arch Med Res* 33:6–14.

Cesa R, Strata P. (2005) Axonal and synaptic remodeling in the mature cerebellar cortex. *Prog Brain Res* 148:45–56.

Chabot C, Massicotte G, Milot M, Trudeau F, Gagné J. (1997) Impaired modulation of AMPA receptors by calcium-dependent processes in streptozotocin-induced diabetic rats. *Brain Res* 768:249–256.

Chahal HS, Drake WM. (2007) The endocrine system and ageing. *J Pathol* 211:173–180.

Champagne DL, Bagot RC, van Hasselt F, Ramakers G, Meaney MJ, de Kloet ER, Joëls M, Krugers H. (2008) Maternal care and hippocampal plasticity: Evidence for experience-dependent structural plasticity, altered synaptic functioning, and differential responsiveness to glucocorticoids and stress. *J Neurosci* 28:6037–6045.

Champagne FA, Meaney MJ. (2006) Stress during gestation alters postpartum maternal care and the development of the offspring in a rodent model. *Biol Psychiatry* 59:1227–1235.

Chan SL, Tammariello SP, Estus S, Mattson MP. (1999) Prostate apoptosis response-4 mediates trophic factor withdrawal-induced apoptosis of hippocampal neurons: Actions prior to mitochondrial dysfunction and caspase activation. *J Neurochem* 73:502–512.

Chang DC, Reppert SM. (2001) The circadian clocks of mice and men. *Neuron* 29:555–558.

Chapman DB, Theodosis DT, Montagnese C, Poulain DA, Morris JF. (1986) Osmotic stimulation causes structural plasticity of neuron-glia relationships of the oxytocin but not vasopressin secreting neurons in the hypothalamic supraoptic nucleus. *Neuroscience* 17:679–686.

Chapman PF. (2005) Cognitive aging: Recapturing the excitation of youth? *Curr Biol* 15:R31–R33.

Chaudhury D, Wang LM, Colwell CS. (2005) Circadian regulation of hippocampal long-term potentiation. *J Biol Rhythms* 20:225–236.

Chaouloff F, Hémar A, Manzoni O. (2008) Local facilitation of hippocampal metabotropic glutamate receptor-dependent long-term depression by corticosterone and dexamethasone. *Psychoneuroendocrinology* 33:686–691.

Chavez-Delgado ME, Gomez-Pinedo U, Feria-Velasco A, Huerta-Viera M, Castaneda SC, Toral FA, Párducz A, Anda SL, Mora-Galindo J, Garcia-Estrada J. (2005) Ultrastructural analysis of guided nerve regeneration using progesterone- and pregnenolone-loaded chitosan prostheses. *J Biomed Mater Res B Appl Biomater* 74:589–600.

Chelli B, Lena A, Vanacore R, Pozzo ED, Costa B, Rossi L, Salvetti A, Scatena F, Ceruti S, Abbracchio MP, Gremigni V, Martini C. (2004) Peripheral benzodiazepine receptor ligands: Mitochondrial transmembrane potential depolarization and apoptosis induction in rat C6 glioma cells. *Biochem Pharmacol* 68:125–134.

Chen C, Díaz Brinton RD, Shors TJ, Thompson RF. (1993) Vasopressin induction of long-lasting potentiation of synaptic transmission in the dentate gyrus. *Hippocampus* 3:193–203.

Chen C, Leonard JP. (1996) Protein tyrosine kinase-mediated potentiation of currents from cloned NMDA receptors. *J Neurochem* 67:194–200.

Chen DF, Schneider GE, Martinou JC, Tonegawa S. (1997) Bcl-2 promotes regeneration of severed axons in mammalian CNS. *Nature* 385:434–439.

Chen J Adachi N, Liu K, Arai T. (1998) The effects of 17beta-estradiol on ischemia-induced neuronal damage in the gerbil hippocampus. *Neuroscience* 87:817–822.

Chen J, Chopp M, Li Y. (1999) Neuroprotective effects of progesterone after transient middle cerebral artery occlusion in rat. *J Neurol Sci* 171:24–30.

Chen L, Lund PK, Burgess SB, Rudisch BE, McIlwain DL. (1998) Growth hormone, insulin-like growth factor I, and motoneuron size. *J Neurobiol* 32:202–212.

Chen Q, Patel R, Sales A, Oji G, Kim J, Monreal AW, Brinton RD. (2000) Vasopressin-induced neurotrophism in cultured neurons of the cerebral cortex: Dependency on calcium signaling and protein kinase C activity. *Neuroscience* 101:19–26.

Chen WP, Witkins JW, Silverman AJ. (1990) Sexual dimorphism in the synaptic input to gonadotrophin releasing hormone neurones. *Endocrinology* 126:695–702.

Chen Y, Lomnitski L, Michaelson DM, Shohami E. (1997) Motor and cognitive deficits in apolipoprotein E-deficient mice after closed head injury. *Neuroscience* 80:1255–1262.

Cherrier MM. (2005) Androgens and cognitive function. *J Endocrinol Invest* 28:65–75.

Cherrier MM, Matsumoto AM, Amory JK, Ahmed S, Bremner W, Peskind ER, Raskind MA, Johnson M, Craft S. (2005) The role of aromatization in testosterone supplementation effects on cognition in older men. *Neurology* 64:290–296.

Cherrier MM, Matsumoto AM, Amory JK, Johnson M, Craft S, Peskind ER, Raskind MA. (2007) Characterization of verbal and spatial memory changes from moderate to supraphysiological increases in serum testosterone in healthy older men. *Psychoneuroendocrinology* 32:72–79.

Cherry JA, Basham ME, Weaver CE, Krohmer RW, Baum MJ. (1990) Ontogeny of the sexually dimorphic male nucleus in the preoptic/anterior hypothalamus of ferrets and its manipulation by gonadal steroids. *J Neurobiol* 21:844–857.

Cherry JA, Tobet SA, DeVoogd TJ, Baum MJ. (1992) Effects of sex and androgen treatment on dendritic dimensions of neurons in the sexually dimorphic preoptic/anterior hypothalamic area of male and female ferrets. *J Comp Neurol* 323:577–585.

Chesik D, Wilczak N, De Keyser J. (2007) The insulin-like growth factor system in multiple sclerosis. *Int Rev Neurobiol* 79:203–226.

Chiba S, Suzuki M, Yamanouchi K, Nishihara M. (2007) Involvement of granulin in estrogen-induced neurogenesis in the adult rat hippocampus. *J Reprod Dev* 53:297–307.

Chong ZZ, Kang JQ, Maiese K. (2002) Hematopoietic factor erythropoietin fosters neuroprotection through novel signal transduction cascades. *J Cereb Blood Flow Metab* 22:503–514.

Chong ZZ, Kang JQ, Maiese K. (2003) Erythropoietin fosters both intrinsic and extrinsic neuronal protection through modulation of microglia, Akt1, Bad, and caspase-mediated pathways. *Br J Pharmacol* 138:1107–1118.

Chowen JA, Torres-Alemán I, Garcia-Segura LM. (1992) Trophic effects of estradiol on fetal rat hypothalamic neurons. *Neuroendocrinology* 56:895–901.

Chowen JA, Argente J, Gonzalez-Parra S, Garcia-Segura LM. (1993) Differential effects of the neonatal and adult sex steroid environments on the organization and activation of hypothalamic growth hormone-releasing hormone and somatostatin neurons. *Endocrinology* 136:2792–2802.

Chowen JA, Busiguina S, Garcia-Segura LM. (1995) Sexual dimorphism and sex steroid modulation of glial fibrillary acidic protein messenger RNA and immunoreactivity levels in the rat hypothalamus. *Neuroscience* 69:519–532.

Chowen JA, Rodriguez de Fonseca F, Alvarez E, Navarro M, Garcia-Segura LM, Blazquez E. (1999) Increased glucagon-like peptide-1 receptor expression in glia after mechanical lesion of the rat brain. *Neuropeptides* 33:212–215.

Christiansen, K. (2001) Behavioural effects of androgen in men and women. *J Endocrinol* 170:39–48.

Christie BR, Cameron HA. (2006) Neurogenesis in the adult hippocampus. *Hippocampus* 16:199–207.

Christie JM, Wenthold RJ, Monaghan DT. (1999) Insulin causes a transient tyrosine phosphorylation of NR2A and NR2B NMDA receptor subunits in rat hippocampus. *J Neurochem* 72:1523–1528.

Christophe J. (1998) Is there appetite after GLP-1 and PACAP? *Ann NY Acad Sci* 865:323–335.

Christou H, Serdy S, Mantzoros CS. (2002) Leptin in relation to growth and developmental processes in the fetus. *Semin Reprod Med* 20:123–130.

Chugani HT, Behen ME, Muzik O, Juhasz C, Nagy F, Chugani DC. (2001) Local brain functional activity following early deprivation: A study of postinstitutionalized Romanian orphans. *Neuroimage* 14:1290–1301.

Chung SK, Pfaff DW, Cohen RS. (1988) Estrogen-induced alterations in synaptic morphology in the midbrain central gray. *Exp Brain Res* 69:522–530.

Chung SY, Han SH. (2003) Melatonin attenuates kainic acid-induced hippocampal neurodegeneration and oxidative stress through microglial inhibition. *J Pineal Res* 34:95–102.

Chung WC, De Vries GJ, Swaab DF. (2002) Sexual differentiation of the bed nucleus of the stria terminalis in humans may extend into adulthood. *J Neurosci* 22:1027–1033.

Chung YH, Joo KM, Shin CM, Lee YJ, Shin DH, Lee KH, Cha CI. (2003) Immunohistochemical study on the distribution of insulin-like growth factor I (IGF-I) receptor in the central nervous system of SOD1(G93A) mutant transgenic mice. *Brain Res* 994:253–259.

Ciana P, Raviscioni M, Mussi P, Vegeto E, Que I, Parker MG, Lowik C, Maggi A. (2002) In vivo imaging of transcriptionally active estrogen receptors. *Nature Med* 9:82–86.

Ciofi P, Lapirot OC, Tramu G. (2007) An androgen-dependent sexual dimorphism visible at puberty in the rat hypothalamus. *Neuroscience* 146:630–642.

Ciriza I, Azcoitia I, Garcia-Segura LM. (2004a) Reduced progesterone metabolites protect rat hippocampal neurones from kainic acid excitotoxicity in vivo. *J Neuroendocrinol* 16:58–63.

Ciriza I, Carrero P, Azcoitia I, Lundeen SG, Garcia-Segura LM. (2004b) Selective estrogen receptor modulators protect hippocampal neurons from kainic acid excitotoxicity: Differences with the effect of estradiol. *J Neurobiol* 61:209–221.

Ciriza I, Carrero P, Frye CA, Garcia-Segura LM. (2006) Reduced metabolites mediate neuroprotective effects of progesterone in the adult rat hippocampus.

The synthetic progestin medroxyprogesterone acetate (Provera) is not neuroprotective. *J Neurobiol* 66:916–928.

Clark BJ, Wells J, King SR, Stocco DM. (1994) The purification, cloning, and expression of a novel luteinizing hormone-induced mitochondrial protein in MA-10 mouse Leydig tumor cells. Characterization of the steroidogenic acute regulatory protein (StAR). *J Biol Chem* 269:28314–28322.

Clarke AS, Schneider ML. (1993) Prenatal stress has long-term effects on behavioral responses to stress in juvenile rhesus monkeys. *Dev Psychobiol* 26:293–304.

Clarke AS, Wittwer DJ, Abbott DH, Schneider ML. (1994) Long-term effects of prenatal stress on HPA axis activity in juvenile rhesus monkeys. *Dev Psychobiol* 27:257–269.

Clasadonte J, Poulain P, Beauvillain JC, Prevot V. (2008) Activation of neuronal nitric oxide release inhibits spontaneous firing in adult gonadotropin-releasing hormone neurones: A possible local synchronizing signal. *Endocrinology* 149:587–596.

Clower RP, Nixdorf BE, DeVoogd TJ. (1989) Synaptic plasticity in the hypoglossal nucleus of female canaries: Structural correlates of season, hemisphere, and testosterone treatment. *Behav Neural Biol* 52:63–77.

Coe CL, Kramer M, Czeh B, Gould E, Reeves AJ, Kirschbaum C, Fuchs E. (2003) Prenatal stress diminishes neurogenesis in the dentate gyrus of juvenile rhesus monkeys. *Biol Psychiatry* 54:1025–1034.

Coers S, Tanzer L, Jones KJ. (2002) Testosterone treatment attenuates the effects of facial nerve transection on glial fibrillary acidic protein (GFAP) levels in the hamster facial motor nucleus. *Metab Brain Dis* 17:55–63.

Cohen RS, Pfaff DW. (1981) Ultrastructure of neurons in the ventromedial nucleus or the hypothalamus in ovariectomized rats with or without estrogen treatment. *Cell Tissue Res* 217:451–470.

Cole GM, Frautschy SA. (2007) The role of insulin and neurotrophic factor signaling in brain aging and Alzheimer's Disease. *Exp Gerontol* 42:10–21.

Collins DR, Davies SN. (1997) Melatonin blocks the induction of long-term potentiation in an N-methyl-D-aspartate independent manner. *Brain Res* 767:162–165.

Compagnone NA, Mellon SH. (2000) Neurosteroids: Biosynthesis and function of these novel neuromodulators. *Front Neuroendocrinol* 21:1–56.

Conejo NM, Gonzalez-Pardo H, Cimadevilla JM, Arguelles JA, Diaz F, Vallejo-Seco G, Arias JL. (2005) Influence of gonadal steroids on the glial fibrillary acidic protein-immunoreactive astrocyte population in young rat hippocampus. *J Neurosci Res* 79:488–494.

Connolly PB, Resko JA. (1994) Prenatal testosterone differentiates brain regions controlling gonadotropin release in guinea pigs. *Biol Reprod* 51:125–130.

Conrad CD. (2006) What is the functional significance of chronic stress-induced CA3 dendritic retraction within the hippocampus? *Behav Cogn Neurosci Rev* 5:41–60.

Conrad CD, Magariños AM, LeDoux JE, McEwen BS. (1999) Repeated restraint stress facilitates fear conditioning independently of causing hippocampal CA3 dendritic atrophy. *Behav Neurosci* 113:902–913.

Conrad CD, McLaughlin KJ, Harman JS, Foltz C, Wieczorek L, Lightner E, Wright RL. (2007) Chronic glucocorticoids increase hippocampal vulnerability to neurotoxicity under conditions that produce CA3 dendritic retraction but fail to impair spatial recognition memory. *J Neurosci* 27:8278–8285.

Cook SC, Wellman CL. (2004) Chronic stress alters dendritic morphology in rat medial prefrontal cortex. *J Neurobiol* 60:236–248.

Cooke BM. (2006) Steroid-dependent plasticity in the medial amygdale. *Neuroscience* 138:997–1005.

Cooke BM, Hegstrom CD, Villeneuve LS, Breedlove SM. (1998) Sexual differentiation of the vertebrate brain: Principles and mechanisms. *Front Neuroendocrinol* 19:323–362.

Cooke BM, Tabibnia G, Breedlove SM. (1999) A brain sexual dimorphism controlled by adult circulating androgens. *Proc Natl Acad Sci USA* 96:7538–7540.

Cooke BM, Hegstrom CD, Breedlove SM. (2002a) Photoperiod-dependent response to androgen in the medial amygdala of the Siberian hamster, Phodopus sungorus. *J Biol Rhythms* 17:147–154.

Cooke BM, Hegstrom CD, Keen A, Breedlove SM. (2002b) Photoperiod and social cues influence the medial amygdala but not the bed nucleus of the stria terminalis in the Siberian hamster. *Neurosci Lett* 312:9–12.

Cooke BM, Breedlove SM, Jordan CJ. (2003) Both estrogen receptors and androgen receptors contribute to testosterone-induced changes in the morphology of the medial amygdala and sexual arousal in male rats. *Horm Behav* 43:336–346.

Cooke BM, Stokas MR, Woolley CS. (2007) Morphological sex differences and laterality in the prepubertal medial amygdala. *J Comp Neurol* 501:904–915.

Cordero MI, Rodriguez JJ, Davies HA, Peddie CJ, Sandi C, Stewart MG. (2005) Chronic restraint stress down-regulates amygdaloid expression of polysialylated neural cell adhesion molecule. *Neuroscience* 133:903–910.

Cordoba Montoya DA, Carrer HF. (1997) Estrogen facilitates induction of long term potentiation in the hippocampus of awake rats. *Brain Res* 778:430–438.

Cornil CA, Ball GF, Balthazart J. (2006) Functional significance of the rapid regulation of brain estrogen action: Where do the estrogens come from? *Brain Res* 1126: 2–26.

Coss RG, Globus A. (1979) Social experience affects the development of dendritic spines and branches on tectal interneurons in the jewel fish. *Dev Psychobiol* 12:347–358.

Cotman CW, Berchtold NC. (2002) Exercise: A behavioral intervention to enhance brain health and plasticity. *Trends Neurosci* 25:295–301.

Cotter DR, Pariante CM, Everall IP. (2001) Glial cell abnormalities in major psychiatric disorders: The evidence and implications. *Brain Res Bull* 55:585–595.

Cottrell EC, Campbell RE, Han SK, Herbison AE. (2006) Postnatal remodeling of dendritic structure and spine density in gonadotropin-releasing hormone neurones. *Endocrinology* 147:3652–3661.

Cowley MA, Smith RG, Diano S, Tschop M, Pronchuk N, Grove KL, Strasburger CJ, Bidlingmaier M, Esterman M, Heiman ML, Garcia-Segura LM, Nillni EA, Mendez P, Low MJ, Sotonyi P, Friedman JM, Liu H, Pinto S, Colmers WF, Cone RD, Horvath TL. (2003) The distribution and mechanism of action of ghrelin in the CNS demonstrates a novel hypothalamic circuit regulating energy homeostasis. *Neuron* 37:649–661.

Craig MC, Daly EM, O'Gorman R, Rymer J, Lythgoe D, Ng G, Simmons A, Maki PM, Murphy DG. (2007) Effects of acute ovarian hormone suppression on the human brain: An in vivo 1H MRS study. *Psychoneuroendocrinology* 32:1128–1132.

Crawley JN, Chen T, Puri A, Washburn R, Sullivan TL, Hill JM, Young NB, Nadler JJ, Moy SS, Young LJ, Caldwell HK, Young WS. (2007) Social approach behaviors in oxytocin knockout mice: Comparison of two independent lines tested in different laboratory environments. *Neuropeptides* 41:145–163.

Crews D, Robker R, Mendonca M. (1993) Seasonal fluctuations in brain nuclei in the red-sided garter snake and their hormonal control. *J Neurosci* 13:5356–5364.

Crispino M, Stone DJ, Wei M, Anderson CP, Tocco G, Finch CE, Baudry M. (1999) Variations of synaptotagmin I, synaptotagmin IV, and synaptophysin mRNA levels in rat hippocampus during the estrous cycle. *Exp Neurol* 159:574–583.

Csakvari E, Hoyk Z, Gyenes A, Garcia-Ovejero D, Garcia-Segura LM, Párducz A. (2007) Fluctuation of synapse density in the arcuate nucleus during the estrous cycle. *Neuroscience* 144:1288–1292.

Csakvari E, Kurunczi A, Hoyk Z, Gyenes A, Naftolin F, Párducz A. (2008) Estradiol-induced synaptic remodeling of tyrosine hydroxylase immunopositive neurons in the rat arcuate nucleus. *Endocrinology* 149:4137–4141.

Cuevas E, Auso E, Telefont M, Morreale de Escobar G, Sotelo C, Berbel P. (2005) Transient maternal hypothyroxinemia at onset of corticogenesis alters tangential migration of medial ganglionic eminence-derived neurons. *Eur J Neurosci* 22:541–551.

Cui M, Yang Y, Yang J, Zhang J, Han H, Ma W, Li H, Mao R, Xu L, Hao W, Cao J. (2006) Enriched environment experience overcomes the memory deficits and depressive-like behavior induced by early life stress. *Neurosci Lett* 404:208–212.

Culmsee C, Vedder H, Ravati A, Junker V, Otto D, Ahlemeyer B, Krieg JC, Krieglstein J. (1999) Neuroprotection by estrogens in a mouse model of focal cerebral ischemia and in cultured neurons: Evidence for a receptor-independent antioxidative mechanism. *J Cereb Blood Flow Metab* 19:1263–1269.

Curras-Collazo MC, Dao J. (1999) Osmotic activation of the hypothalamo–neurohypophysial system reversibly downregulates the NMDA receptor subunit, NR2B, in the supraoptic nucleus of the hypothalamus. *Mol Brain Res* 70:187–196.

Cutler SM, Cekic M, Miller DM, Wali B, Vanlandingham JW, Stein DG. (2007) Progesterone improves acute recovery after traumatic brain injury in the aged rat. *J Neurotrauma* 24:1475–1486.

Cyr M, Calon F, Morissette M, Di Paolo T. (2002) Estrogenic modulation of brain activity: Implications for schizophrenia and Parkinson's disease. *J Psychiatry Neurosci* 27:12–27.

Cyran E. (1918) Hypophysenschadigung durch Schadelbasisfraktur. *Dtsch Med Wschr* 44:1261–1270.

Daan S, Barnes BM, Strijkstra AM. (1991) Warming up for sleep? Ground squirrels sleep during arousals from hibernation. *Neurosci Lett* 128:265–268.

Daftary SS, Gore AC. (2003) Developmental changes in hypothalamic insulin-like growth factor-1: Relationship to gonadotropin-releasing hormone neurones. *Endocrinology* 144:2034–2045.

Daftary SS, Gore AC. (2004) The hypothalamic insulin-like growth factor-1 receptor and its relationship to gonadotropin-releasing hormones neurones during postnatal development. *J Neuroendocrinol* 16:160–169.

Daftary SS, Gore AC. (2005) IGF-1 in the brain as a regulator of reproductive neuroendocrine function. *Exp Biol Med* (Maywood) 230:292–306.

Dai X, Chen L, Sokabe M. (2007) Neurosteroid estradiol rescues ischemia-induced deficit in the long-term potentiation of rat hippocampal CA1 neurons. *Neuropharmacology* 52:1124–1138.

Dalla C, Antoniou K, Papadopoulou-Daifoti Z, Balthazart J, Bakker J.(2004) Oestrogen-deficient female aromatase knockout (ArKO) mice exhibit depressive-like symptomatology. *Eur J Neurosci* 20:217–228.

Dalla C, Antoniou K, Papadopoulou-Daifoti Z, Balthazart J, Bakker J. (2005) Male aromatase-knockout mice exhibit normal levels of activity, anxiety and "depressive-like" symptomatology. *Behav Brain Res* 163:186–193.

Damasio A. (2003) Looking for Spinoza. Joy, sorrow, and the feeling brain. Harcourt: New York.

d'Anglemont de Tassigny X, Campagne C, Dehouck B, Leroy D, Holstein GR, Beauvillain JC, Buee-Scherrer V, Prevot V. (2007) Coupling of neuronal nitric oxide synthase to NMDA receptors via postsynaptic density-95 depends on estrogen and contributes to the central control of adult female reproduction. *J Neurosci* 27:6103–6114.

Dantzer R, Bluthe RM, Gheusi G, Cremona S, Laye S, Parnet P, Kelley KW. (1998) Molecular basis of sickness behavior. *Ann N Y Acad Sci* 856:132–138.

Darnaudéry M, Pallares M, Piazza P, Le Moal M, Mayo W. (2002) The neurosteroid pregnenolone sulfate infused into the medial septum nucleus increases hippocampal acetylcholine and spatial memory in rats. *Brain Res* 951:237–242.

Darnaudéry M, Perez-Martin M, Belizaire G, Maccari S, Garcia-Segura LM. (2006) Insulin-like growth factor 1 reduces age-related disorders induced by prenatal stress in female rats. *Neurobiol Aging* 27:119–127.

Darnaudéry M, Perez-Martin M, Del Favero F, Gomez-Roldan C, Garcia-Segura LM, Maccari S. (2007) Early motherhood in rats is associated with a modification of hippocampal function. *Psychoneuroendocrinology* 32:803–812.

Darrow JM, Tamarkin L, Duncan MJ, Goldman BD. (1986) Pineal melatonin rhythms in female Turkish hamsters: Effects of photoperiod and hibernation. *Biol Reprod* 35:74–83.

D'Astous M, Mendez P, Morissette M, Garcia-Segura LM, Di Paolo T. (2006) Implication of the phosphatidylinositol-3 kinase/protein kinase B signaling pathway in the neuroprotective effect of estradiol in the striatum of 1-methyl-4-phenyl-1,2,3,6-tetrahydropyridine mice. *Mol Pharmacol* 69:1492–1498.

Datla KP, Murray HE, Pillai AV, Gillies GE, Dexter DT. (2003) Differences in dopaminergic neuroprotective effects of estrogen during estrous cycle. *NeuroReport* 14:47–50.

Davis EC, Shryne JE, Gorski RA. (1995) A revised critical period for the sexual differentiation of the sexually dimorphic nucleus in the preoptic area in the rat. *Neuroendocrinology* 62:579–585.

Davis EC, Shryne JE, Gorski RA. (1996) Structural sexual dimorphisms in the anteroventral periventricular nucleus of the rat hypothalamus are sensitive to gonadal steroids perinatally, but develop peripubertally. *Neuroendocrinology* 63:142–148.

Dawley EM, Crowder J. (1995) Sexual and seasonal differences in the vomeronasal epithelium of the red-backed salamander (Plethodon cinereus). *J Comp Neurol* 359:382–390.

Day JR, Laping NJ, McNeill TH, Schreiber SS, Pasinetti G, Finch CE. (1990) Castration enhances expression of glial fibrillary acidic protein and sulfated glycoprotein-2 in the intact and lesion-altered hippocampus of the adult male rat. *Mol Endocrinol* 4:1995–2002.

Day JR, Laping NJ, Lampert-Etchells M, Brown SA, O'Callaghan JP, McNeill TH, Finch CE. (1993) Gonadal steroids regulate the expression of glial fibrillary acidic protein in the adult male rat hippocampus. *Neuroscience* 55:435–443.

Day JR, Frank AT, O'Callaghan JP, Jones BC, Anderson JE. (1998) The effect of age and testosterone on the expression of glial fibrillary acidic protein in the rat cerebellum. *Exp Neurol* 151:343–346.

Deary IJ, Whiteman MC, Starr JM, Whalley LJ, Fox HC. (2004) The impact of childhood intelligence on later life: Following up the Scottish Mental Surveys of 1932 and 1947. *J Pers Soc Psychol* 86:130–147.

De Bellis MD, Keshavan MS, Beers SR, Hall J, Frustaci K, Masalehdan A, Noll J, Boring AM. (2001) Sex differences in brain maturation during childhood and adolescence. *Cereb Cortex* 11:552–557.

De Bellis MD, Keshavan MS, Shifflett H, Lyengar S, Beers SR, Hall J, Moritz G. (2002) Brain structures in pediatric maltreatment-related posttraumatic stress disorder: A sociodemographically matched study. *Biol Psychiatry* 52:1066–1078.

de Brabander JM, Kramers RJ, Uylings HB. (1998) Layer-specific dendritic regression of pyramidal cells with ageing in the human prefrontal cortex. *Eur J Neurosci* 10:1261–1269.

de Chaves EI, Rusinol AE, Vance DE, Campenot RB, Vance JE. (1997) Role of lipoproteins in the delivery of lipids to axons during axonal regeneration. *J Biol Chem* 272:30766–30773.

Decker RS. (1976) Influence of thyroid hormones on neuronal death and differentiation in larval Rana pipiens. *Dev Biol* 49:101–118.

DeFelipe J. (2006) Brain plasticity and mental processes: Cajal again. *Nat Rev Neurosci* 7:811–817.

DeFelipe J, Jones EG. (1988) *Cajal on the cerebral cortex. An annotated translation of the complete writings.* Oxford University Press, New York.

Deisseroth K, Bito H, Schulman H, Tsien RW. (1995) Synaptic plasticity: A molecular mechanism for metaplasticity. *Curr Biol* 5:1334–1338.

de Kloet ER, Joëls M, Holsboer F. (2005) Stress and the brain: From adaptation to disease. *Nat Rev Neurosci* 6:463–475.

de Lecea L, Kilduff TS, Peyron C, Gao X, Foye PE, Danielson PE, Fukuhara C, Battenberg EL, Gautvik VT, Bartlett FS 2nd, Frankel WN, van den Pol AN, Bloom FE, Gautvik KM, Sutcliffe JG. (1998) The hypocretins: Hypothalamus-specific peptides with neuroexcitatory activity. *Proc Natl Acad Sci USA* 95:322–327.

Delgado-Rubin de Celix A, Chowen JA, Argente J, Frago LM. (2006) Growth hormone releasing peptide-6 acts as a survival factor in glutamate-induced excitotoxicity. *J Neurochem* 99:839–849.

De Nicola AF, Gonzalez SL, Labombarda F, Deniselle MC, Garay L, Guennoun R, Schumacher M. (2006) Progesterone treatment of spinal cord injury: Effects on receptors, neurotrophins, and myelination. *J Mol Neurosci* 28:3–15.

Denny JB, Polan-Curtain J, Wayner MJ, Armstrong DL. (1991) Angiotensin II blocks hippocampal long-term potentiation. *Brain Res* 567:321–324.

de Pablo F, Banner LR, Patterson PH. (2000) IGF-I expression is decreased in LIF-deficient mice after peripheral nerve injury. *NeuroReport* 11:1365–1368.

De Paola V, Arber S, Caroni P. (2003) AMPA receptors regulate dynamic equilibrium of presynaptic terminals in mature hippocampal networks. *Nat Neurosci* 6:491–500.

Désarnaud F, Do Thi AN, Brown AM, Lemke G, Baulieu EE, Schumacher M. (1998) Progesterone stimulates the activity of the promoters of peripheral myelin protein-22 and protein zero genes in Schwann cells. *J Neurochem* 71:1765–1768.

Désarnaud F, Bidichandani S, Patel PI, Baulieu EE, Schumacher M. (2000) Glucocorticosteroids stimulate the activity of the promoters of peripheral myelin protein-22 and protein zero genes in Schwann cells. *Brain Res* 865:12–16.

De Seranno S, Estrella C, Loyens A, Cornea A, Ojeda SR, Beauvillain JC, Prevot V. (2004) Vascular endothelial cells promote acute plasticity in ependymoglial cells of the neuroendocrine brain. *J Neurosci* 24:10353–10363.

De Seranno S, d'Anglemont de Tassigny X, Estrella C, Loyens A, Cornea A, Leroy D, Ojeda S, Beauvillain JC, Prevot V. (2005) Estrogen modulates endothelial cell-induced ependymoglial cell plasticity in cultured cells of the neuroendocrine brain. *Soc Neurosci Abst* 860.4.

Desjardins GC, Beaudet A, Meaney MJ, Brawer JR. (1995) Estrogen-induced hypothalamic beta-endorphin neuron loss: A possible model of hypothalamic aging. *Exp Gerontol* 30:253–267.

De Souza EB. (1987) Corticotropin-releasing factor receptors in the rat central nervous system: Characterization and regional distribution. *J Neurosci* 7:88–100.

Desouza LA, Ladiwala U, Daniel SM, Agashe S, Vaidya RA, Vaidya VA. (2005) Thyroid hormone regulates hippocampal neurogenesis in the adult rat brain. *Mol Cell Neurosci* 29:414–426.

DeVito WJ, Okulicz WC, Stone S, Avakian C. (1992) Prolactin-stimulated mitogenesis of cultured astrocytes. *Endocrinology* 130:2549–2556.

DeVoogd T, Nottebohm F. (1981) Gonadal hormones induce dendritic growth in the adult avian brain. *Science* 214:202–204.

DeVoogd TJ, Nixdorf B, Nottebohm F. (1985) Synaptogenesis and changes in synaptic morphology related to acquisition of a new behavior. *Brain Res* 329:304–308.

DeVries GJ, Best W, Sluiter AA. (1983) The influence of androgens on the development of a sex difference in the vasopressinergic innervation of the rat lateral septum. *Dev Brain Res* 8:377–380.

DeVries GJ, Bujis RM, Sluiter AA. (1984) Gonadal hormone actions on the morphology of the vasopressinergic innervation of the adult rat brain. *Brain Res* 298:141–145.

Dhandapani KM, Brann DW. (2002) Protective effects of estrogen and selective estrogen receptor modulators in the brain. *Biol Reprod* 67:1379–1385.

Dhandapani KM, Wade FM, Mahesh VB, Brann DW. (2005) Astrocyte-derived transforming growth factor-β mediates the neuroprotective effects of 17β-estradiol: Involvement of nonclassical genomic signaling pathways. *Endocrinology* 146:2749–2759.

Di S, Tasker JG. (2004) Dehydration-induced synaptic plasticity in magnocellular neurons of the hypothalamic supraoptic nucleus. *Endocrinology* 145:5141–5149.

Diamond DM, Bennett MC, Fleshner M, Rose GM. (1992) Inverted-U relationship between the level of peripheral corticosterone and the magnitude of hippocampal primed burst potentiation. *Hippocampus* 2:421–430.

Diamond MC, Krech D, Rosenzweig MR. (1964) The effects of an enriched environment on the histology of the rat cerebral cortex. *J Comp Neurol* 123:111–120.

Diamond MC, Law F, Rhodes H, Lindner B, Rosenzweig MR, Krech D, Bennett EL. (1966) Increases in cortical depth and glia numbers in rats subjected to enriched environment. *J Comp Neurol* 128:117–126.

Diano S, Farr SA, Benoit SC, McNay EC, da Silva I, Horvath B, Gaskin FS, Nonaka N, Jaeger LB, Banks WA, Morley JE, Pinto S, Sherwin RS, Xu L, Yamada KA, Sleeman MW, Tschop MH, Horvath TL. (2006) Ghrelin controls hippocampal spine synapse density and memory performance. *Nat Neurosci* 9:381–388.

Diaz H, Lorenzo A, Carrer HF, Caceres A. (1992) Time lapse study of neurite growth in hypothalamic dissociated neurons in culture: Sex differences and estrogen effects. *J Neurosci Res* 33:266–281.

Dicou E, Attoub S, Gressens P. (2001) Neuroprotective effects of leptin in vivo and in vitro. *NeuroReport* 12:3947–3951.

Dierssen M, Benavides-Piccione R, Martinez-Cue C, Estivill X, Florez J, Elston GN, DeFelipe J. (2003) Alterations of neocortical pyramidal cell phenotype in the Ts65Dn mouse model of Down syndrome: Effects of environmental enrichment. *Cereb Cortex* 13:758–764.

Digicaylioglu M, Bichet S, Marti HH, Wenger RH, Rivas LA, Bauer C, Gassmann M. (1995) Localization of specific erythropoietin binding sites in defined areas of the mouse brain. *Proc Natl Acad Sci USA* 92:3717–3720.

Digicaylioglu M, Lipton SA. (2001) Erythropoietin-mediated neuroprotection involves cross-talk between Jak2 and NF-kappaB signalling cascades. *Nature* 412:641–647.

Digicaylioglu M, Garden G, Timberlake S, Fletcher L, Lipton SA. (2004) Acute neuroprotective synergy of erythropoietin and insulin-like growth factor I. *Proc Natl Acad Sci USA* 101:9855–9860.

Di Luca M, Ruts L, Gardoni F, Cattabeni F, Biessels GJ, Gispen WH. (1999) NMDA receptor subunits are modified transcriptionally and post-translationally in the brain of streptozotocin-diabetic rats. *Diabetologia* 42:693–701.

DiLuigi L, Guidetti L, Baldari C, Gallotta MC, Sgro P, Perroni F, Romanelli F, Lenzi A. (2006) Cortisol, dehydroepiandrosterone sulphate and dehydroepiandrosterone sulphate/cortisol ratio responses to physical stress in males are influenced by pubertal development. *J Endocrinol Invest* 29:796–804.

Di Mario U, Morano S, Valle E, Pozzessere G. (1995) Electrophysiological alterations of the central nervous system in diabetes mellitus. *Diabetes Metab Rev* 11:259–277.

Dimayuga FO, Reed JL, Carnero GA, Wang C, Dimayuga ER, Dimayuga VM, Perger A, Wilson ME, Keller JN, Bruce-Keller AJ. (2005) Estrogen and brain inflammation: Effects on microglial expression of MHC, costimulatory molecules and cytokines. *J Immunol* 161:123–136.

di Michele F, Lekieffre D, Pasini A, Bernardi G, Benavides J, Romeo E. (2000) Increased neurosteroids synthesis after brain and spinal cord injury in rats. *Neurosci Lett* 284:65–68.

Dimopoulou I, Kouyialis AT, Tzanella M, Armaganidis A, Thalassinos N, Sakas DE, Tsagarakis S. (2004) High incidence of neuroendocrine dysfunction in long-term survivors of aneurysmal subarachnoid hemorrhage. *Stroke* 35:2884–2889.

Ding Q, Vaynman S, Akhavan M, Ying Z, Gomez-Pinilla F. (2006) Insulin-like growth factor I interfaces with brain-derived neurotrophic factor-mediated synaptic plasticity to modulate aspects of exercise-induced cognitive function. *Neuroscience* 140:823–833.

D'Intino G, Perretta G, Taglioni A, Calistri M, Falzone C, Baroni M, Giardino L, Calzà L. (2006) Endogenous stem and precursor cells for demyelinating diseases: An alternative for transplantation? *Neurol Res* 28:513–517.

Disshon KA, Dluzen DE. (1997) Estrogen as a neuromodulator of MPTP-induced neurotoxicity: Effects upon striatal dopamine release. *Brain Res* 764:9–16.

Disshon KA, Boja JW, Dluzen DE. (1998) Inhibition of striatal dopamine transporter activity by 17 β-estradiol. *Eur J Pharmacol* 345:207–211.

Djahanbakhch O, Ezzati M, Zosmer A. (2007) Reproductive ageing in women. *J Pathol* 211:219–231.

Djebaili M, Hoffman SW, Stein DG. (2004) Allopregnanolone and progesterone decrease cell death and cognitive deficits after a contusion of the rat pre-frontal cortex. *Neuroscience* 123:349–359.

Djebaili M, Guo Q, Pettus EH, Hoffman SW, Stein DG. (2005) The neurosteroids progesterone and allopregnanolone reduce cell death, gliosis, and functional deficits after traumatic brain injury in rats. *J Neurotrauma* 22:106–118.

Dluzen DE, McDermott JL, Liu B. (1996a) Estrogen as a neuroprotectant against MPTP-induced neurotoxicity in C57/B1 mice. *Neurotoxicol Teratol* 18:603–606.

Dluzen DE, McDermott JL, Liu B. (1996b) Estrogen alters MPTP-induced neurotoxicity in female mice: Effects on striatal dopamine concentrations and release. *J Neurochem* 66:658–666.

Dluzen DE. (1997) Estrogen decreases corpus striatal neurotoxicity in response to 6-hydroxydopamine. *Brain Res* 767:340–344.

Dluzen DE. (2000) Neuroprotective effects of estrogen upon the nigrostriatal dopaminergic system. *J Neurocytol* 29:387–399.

Dluzen DE, Horstink M. (2003) Estrogen as neuroprotectant of nigrostriatal dopaminergic system: Laboratory and clinical studies. *Endocrine* 21:67–75.

Dodel RC, Du Y, Bales KR, Gao F, Paul SM. (1999) Sodium salicylate and 17beta-estradiol attenuate nuclear transcription factor NF-kappaB translocation in cultured rat astroglial cultures following exposure to amyloid A beta(1-40) and lipopolysaccharides. *J Neurochem* 73:1453–1460.

Dodson RE, Shryne JE, Gorski RA. (1988) Hormonal modification of the number of total and late-arising neurons in the central part of the medial preoptic nucleus of the rat. *J Comp Neurol* 275:623–629.

Dominguez R, Jalali C, de Lacalle S. (2004) Morphological effects of estrogen on cholinergic neurons in vitro involves activation of extracellular signal-regulated kinases. *J Neurosci* 24:982–990.

Dominguez-Salazar E, Portillo W, Baum MJ, Bakker J, Paredes RG. (2002) Effect of prenatal androgen receptor antagonist or aromatase inhibitor on sexual behavior, partner preference and neuronal Fos responses to estrous female odors in the rat accessory olfactory system. *Physiol Behav* 75:337–346.

Donahue SW, Galley SA, Vaughan MR, Patterson-Buckendahl P, Demers LM, Vance JL, McGee ME. (2006) Parathyroid hormone may maintain bone formation in hibernating black bears (Ursus americanus) to prevent disuse osteoporosis. *J Exp Biol* 209:1630–1638.

DonCarlos LL, Greene GL, Morrell JI. (1989) Estrogen plus progesterone increases progestin receptor immunoreactivity in the brain of ovariectomized guinea pigs. *Neuroendocrinology* 50:613–623.

DonCarlos LL, Monroy E, Morrell JI. (1991) Distribution of estrogen receptor-immunoreactive cells in the forebrain of the female guinea pig. *J Comp Neurol* 305:591–612.

DonCarlos LL, Garcia-Ovejero D, Sarkey S, Garcia-Segura LM, Azcoitia I. (2003) Androgen receptor immunoreactivity in forebrain axons and dendrites in the rat. *Endocrinology* 144:3632–3638.

DonCarlos LL, Sarkey S, Lorenz B, Azcoitia I, Garcia-Ovejero D, Huppenbauer C, Garcia-Segura LM. (2006) Novel cellular phenotypes and subcellular sites for androgen action in the forebrain. *Neuroscience* 138:801–807.

DonCarlos LL, Azcoitia I, Garcia-Segura LM. (2007) In search of neuroprotective therapies based on the mechanisms of estrogens. *Expert Rev Endocrinol Metabol* 2: 387–397.

Donohue HS, Gabbott PL, Davies HA, Rodriguez JJ, Cordero MI, Sandi C, Medvedev NI, Popov VI, Colyer FM, Peddie CJ, Stewart MG. (2006) Chronic restraint stress induces changes in synapse morphology in stratum lacunosum-moleculare CA1 rat hippocampus: A stereological and three-dimensional ultrastructural study. *Neuroscience* 140:597–606.

Drapeau E, Mayo W, Aurousseau C, Le Moal M, Piazza PV, Abrous DN. (2003) Spatial memory performances of aged rats in the water maze predict levels of hippocampal neurogenesis. *Proc Natl Acad Sci USA* 100:14385–14390.

Drew KL, Buck CL, Barnes BM, Christian SL, Rasley BT, Harris MB. (2007) Central nervous system regulation of mammalian hibernation: Implications for metabolic suppression and ischemia tolerance. *J Neurochem* 102:1713–1726.

Drew PD, Chavis JA. (2000a) Inhibition of microglial cell activation by cortisol. *Brain Res Bull* 52:391–396.

Drew PD, Chavis JA. (2000b) Female sex steroids: Effects upon microglial cell activation. *J Neuroimmunol* 111:77–85.

Duan W, Rangnekar VM, Mattson MP. (1999a) Prostate apoptosis response-4 production in synaptic compartments following apoptotic and excitotoxic insults: Evidence for a pivotal role in mitochondrial dysfunction and neuronal degeneration. *J Neurochem* 72:2312–2322.

Duan W, Zhang Z, Gash DM, Mattson MP. (1999b) Participation of prostate apoptosis response-4 in degeneration of dopaminergic neurons in models of Parkinson's disease. *Ann Neurol* 46:587–597.

Dubal DB, Kashon ML, Pettigrew LC, Ren JM, Finklestein SP, Rau SW, Wise PM. (1998) Estradiol protects against ischemic injury. *J Cereb Blood Flow Metab* 18:1253–1258.

Dubal DB, Shughrue PJ, Wilson ME, Merchenthaler I, Wise PM. (1999) Estradiol modulates bcl-2 in cerebral ischemia: A potential role for estrogen receptors. *J Neurosci* 19:6385–6393.

Dubal DB, Wise PM. (2001) Neuroprotective effects of estradiol in middle-aged female rats. *Endocrinology* 142:43–48.

Dubal DB, Zhu B, Yu B, Rau SW, Shughrue PJ, Merchenthaler I, Kindy MS, Wise PM. (2001) Estrogen receptor-α, not -β, is a critical link in estradiol-mediated protection against brain injury. *Proc Natl Acad Sci USA* 98:1952–1957.

Dubal DB, Rau SW, Shughrue PJ, Zhu H, Yu J, Cashion AB, Suzuki S, Gerhold LM, Bottner MB, Dubal SB, Merchanthaler I, Kindy MS, Wise PM. (2006) Differential modulation of estrogen receptors (ERs) in ischemic brain injury: A role for ERalpha in estradiol-mediated protection against delayed cell death. *Endocrinology* 147:3076–3084.

Dubrovsky B, Tatarinov A, Gijsbers K, Harris J, Tsiodras A. (2003) Effects of arginine-vasopressin (AVP) on long-term potentiation in intact anesthetized rats. *Brain Res Bull* 59:467–472.

Dueñas M, Luquín S, Chowen JA, Torres-Alemán I, Naftolin F, Garcia-Segura LM. (1994) Gonadal hormone regulation of insulin-like growth factor-I-like immunoreactivity in hypothalamic astroglia of developing and adult rats. *Neuroendocrinology* 59:528–538.

Dueñas M, Torres-Alemán I, Naftolin F, Garcia-Segura LM. (1996) Interaction of insulin-like growth factor-1 and estradiol signaling pathways on hypothalamic neuronal differentiation. *Neuroscience* 74:531–539.

Dugovic C, Maccari S, Weibel L, Turek FW, Van Reeth O. (1999) High corticosterone levels in prenatally stressed rats predict persistent paradoxical sleep alterations. *J Neurosci* 19:8656–8664.

Dumesic DA, Abbott DH, Eisner JR, Goy RW. (1997) Prenatal exposure of female rhesus monkeys to testosterone propionate increases serum luteinizing hormone levels in adulthood. *Fertil Steril* 67:155–163.

Dungan HM, Clifton DK, Steiner RA. (2006) Minireview: Kisspeptin neurons as central processors in the regulation of gonadotropin-releasing hormone secretion. *Endocrinology* 147:1154–1158.

Dunlap KD, Castellano JF, Prendaj E. (2006) Social interaction and cortisol treatment increase cell addition and radial glia fiber density in the diencephalic periventricular zone of adult electric fish, Apteronotus leptorhynchus. *Horm Behav* 50:10–17.

Dunn AJ. (1992) Endotoxin-induced activation of cerebral catecholamine and serotonin metabolism: Comparison with interleukin-1. *J Pharmacol Exp Ther* 261:964–969.

Dupret D, Fabre A, Dobrossy MD, Panatier A, Rodriguez JJ, Lamarque S, Lemaire V, Oliet SH, Piazza PV, Abrous DN. (2007) Spatial learning depends on both the addition and removal of new hippocampal neurons. *PLoS Biol* 5:e214.

Dupret D, Revest JM, Koehl M, Ichas F, De Giorgi F, Costet P, Abrous DN, Piazza PV. (2008) Spatial relational memory requires hippocampal adult neurogenesis. *PLoS ONE* 3:e1959.

Durakoglugil M, Irving AJ, Harvey J. (2005) Leptin induces a novel form of NMDA receptor-dependent long-term depression. *J Neurochem* 95:396–405.

During MJ, Cao L, Zuzga DS, Francis JS, Fitzsimons HL, Jiao X, Bland RJ, Klugmann M, Banks WA, Drucker DJ, Haile CN. (2003) Glucagon-like peptide-1 receptor is involved in learning and neuroprotection. *Nat Med* 9:1173–1179.

Dykens JA, Simpkins JW, Wang J, Gordon K. (2003) Polycyclic phenols, estrogens and neuroprotection: A proposed mitochondrial mechanism. *Exp Gerontol* 38:101–107.

Dziedzic B, Prevot V, Lomniczi A, Jung H, Cornea A, Ojeda SR. (2003) Neuron-to-glia signaling mediated by excitatory amino acid receptors regulates ErbB receptor function in astroglial cells of the neuroendocrine brain. *J Neurosci* 23:915–926.

Eadie BD, Redila VA, Christie BR. (2005) Voluntary exercise alters the cytoarchitecture of the adult dentate gyrus by increasing cellular proliferation, dendritic complexity, and spine density. *J Comp Neurol* 486:39–47.

Eayrs JT, Taylor SH. (1951) The effect of thyroid deficiency induced by methylthiouracil on the maturation of the central nervous system. *J Anat* 85:350–358.

Eckenhoff MF, Rakic P. (1988) Nature and fate of proliferative cells in the hippocampal dentate gyrus during the life span of the rhesus monkey. *J Neurosci* 8:2729–2747.

Edinger KL, Frye CA. (2005) Testosterone's anti-anxiety and analgesic effects may be due in part to actions of its 5alpha-reduced metabolites in the hippocampus. *Psychoneuroendocrinology* 30:418–430.

Ehrenreich H, Hinze-Selch D, Stawicki S, Aust C, Knolle-Veentjer S, Wilms S, Heinz G, Erdag S, Jahn H, Degner D, Ritzen M, Mohr A, Wagner M, Schneider U, Bohn M, Huber M, Czernik A, Pollmacher T, Maier W, Siren AL, Klosterkotter J, Falkai P, Ruther E, Aldenhoff JB, Krampe H. (2007) Improvement of cognitive functions in chronic schizophrenic patients by recombinant human erythropoietin. *Mol Psychiatry* 12:206–220.

Ellenbroek BA, Cools AR. (1998) The neurodevelopment hypothesis of schizophrenia: Clinical evidence and animal models. *Neurosci Res Com* 22:127–136.

Ellenbroek BA, van den Kroonenberg PT, Cools AR. (1998) The effects of an early stressful life event on sensorimotor gating in adult rats. *Schizophr Res* 30:251–260.

El Majdoubi M, Poulain DA, Theodosis DT. (1996) The glutamatergic innervation of oxytocin- and vasopressin-secreting neurons in the rat supraoptic nucleus and its contribution to lactation-induced synaptic plasticity. *Eur J Neurosci* 8:1377–1389.

El Majdoubi M, Poulain DA, Theodosis DT. (1997) Lactation-induced plasticity in the supraoptic nucleus augments axodendritic and axosomatic GABAergic and glutamatergic synapses: An ultrastructural analysis using the disector method. *Neuroscience* 80:1137–1147.

Elmquist JK, Bjorbaek C, Ahima RS, Flier JS, Saper CB. (1998) Distributions of leptin receptor mRNA isoforms in the rat brain. *J Comp Neurol* 395:535–547.

Elsaesser F, Parvizi N. (1979) Estrogen feedback in the pig: Sexual differentiation and the effect of prenatal testosterone treatment. *Biol Reprod* 20:1187–1193.

El-Sherif Y, Tesoriero J, Hogan MV, Wieraszko A. (2003) Melatonin regulates neuronal plasticity in the hippocampus. *J Neurosci Res* 72:454–460.

Engert F, Bonhoeffer T. (1999) Dendritic spine changes associated with hippocampal long-term synaptic plasticity. *Nature* 399:66–70.

Ershler WB. (1993) Interleukin-6: A cytokine for gerontologists. *J Am Geriatr Soc* 41:176–181.

Escamilla RF, Lisser H. (1942) Simmond's disease. A clinical study with review of the literature; differentiation from anorexia nervosa by statistical analysis of 595 cases, 101 of which were proved pathologically. *J Clin Endocrinol* 2:65–96.

Esiri MM. (2007) Ageing and the brain. *J Pathol* 211:181–187.

Espinar A, Garcia-Oliva A, Isorna EM, Quesada A, Prada FA, Guerrero JM. (2000) Neuroprotection by melatonin from glutamate-induced excitotoxicity during development of the cerebellum in the chick embryo. *J Pineal Res* 28:81–88.

Estrella C, De Seranno S, Caron E, d'Anglemont de Tassigny X, Mitchell V, Beauvillain JC, Prevot V. (2004) Matrix metalloproteinases are expressed in the median eminence of the hypothalamus and their activities vary during the rat estrous cycle. Prog 86th Ann Mtg Endocrine Soc, New Orleans, LO, P3–266.

Evrard HC. (2006) Estrogen synthesis in the spinal dorsal horn: A new central mechanism for the hormonal regulation of pain. *Am J Physiol Regul Integr Comp Physiol* 291:R291–R299.

Evrard HC, Balthazart J. (2004) Rapid regulation of pain by estrogens synthesized in spinal dorsal horn neurons. *J Neurosci* 24:7225–7229.

Fabre-Nys C, Venier G. (1991) Sexual differentiation of sexual behaviour and preovulatory LH surge in ewes. *Psychoneuroendocrinology* 16:383–396.

Fabricius K, Wörtwein G, Pakkenberg B. (2008) The impact of maternal separation on adult mouse behaviour and on the total neuron number in the mouse hippocampus. *Brain Struct Funct* 212:403–416.

Fabris N, Mocchegiani E, Provinciali M. (1995) Pituitary-thyroid axis and immune system: A reciprocal neuroendocrine-immune interaction. *Horm Res* 43:29–38.

Faherty CJ, Kerley D, Smeyne RJ. (2003) A Golgi-Cox morphological analysis of neuronal changes induced by environmental enrichment. *Dev Brain Res* 141:55–61.

Falleti MG, Maruff P, Burman P, Harris A. (2006) The effects of growth hormone (GH) deficiency and GH replacement on cognitive performance in adults: A meta-analysis of the current literature. *Psychoneuroendocrinology* 31:681–691.

Fargo KN, Sengelaub DR. (2004) Testosterone manipulation protects motoneurons from dendritic atrophy after contralateral motoneuron depletion. *J Comp Neurol* 469:96–106.

Farmer J, Zhao X, van Praag H, Wodtke K, Gage FH, Christie BR. (2004) Effects of voluntary exercise on synaptic plasticity and gene expression in the dentate gyrus of adult male Sprague-Dawley rats in vivo. *Neuroscience* 124:71–79.

Faulconbridge LF, Cummings DE, Kaplan JM, Grill HJ. (2003) Hyperphagic effects of brainstem ghrelin administration. *Diabetes* 52:2260–2265.

Feng Z, Chang Y, Cheng Y, Zhang BL, Qu ZW, Qin C, Zhang JT. (2004) Melatonin alleviates behavioral deficits associated with apoptosis and cholinergic system dysfunction in the APP 695 transgenic mouse model of Alzheimer's disease. *J Pineal Res* 37:129–136.

Ferezou I, Haiss F, Gentet LJ, Aronoff R, Weber B, Petersen CCH. (2007) Spatiotemporal dynamics of cortical sensorimotor integration in behaving mice. *Neuron* 56: 907–923.

Fernandez AM, de la Vega AG, Torres-Alemán I. (1998) Insulin-like growth factor I restores motor coordination in a rat model of cerebellar ataxia. *Proc Natl Acad Sci USA* 95:1253–1258.

Fernandez AM, Gonzalez de la Vega AG, Planas B, Torres-Alemán I. (1999) Neuroprotective actions of peripherally administered insulin-like growth factor I in the injured olivo-cerebellar pathway. *Eur J Neurosci* 11:2019–2030.

Fernandez AM, Carro EM, Lopez-Lopez C, Torres-Alemán I. (2005) Insulin-like growth factor I treatment for cerebellar ataxia: Addressing a common pathway in the pathological cascade? *Brain Res Rev* 50:134–141.

Fernandez M, Pirondi S, Manservigi M, Giardino L, Calzà L. (2004a) Thyroid hormone participates in the regulation of neural stem cells and oligodendrocyte precursor cells in the central nervous system of adult rat. *Eur J Neurosci* 20:2059–2070.

Fernandez M, Giuliani A, Pirondi S, D'Intino G, Giardino L, Aloe L, Levi-Montalcini R, Calzà L. (2004b) Thyroid hormone administration enhances remyelination in chronic demyelinating inflammatory disease. *Proc Natl Acad Sci USA* 101:16363–16368.

Fernandez-Galaz MC, Torres-Alemán I, Garcia-Segura LM. (1996) Endocrine-dependent accumulation of IGF-I by hypothalamic glia. *NeuroReport* 8:373–377.

Fernandez-Galaz MC, Morschl E, Chowen JA, Torres-Alemán I, Naftolin F, Garcia-Segura LM. (1997) Role of astroglia and insulin-like growth factor-I in gonadal hormone-dependent synaptic plasticity. *Brain Res Bull* 44:525–531.

Fernandez-Galaz MC, Naftolin F, Garcia-Segura LM. (1999a) Phasic synaptic remodeling of the arcuate nucleus during the estrous cycle depends on insulin-like growth factor-I receptor activation. *J Neurosci Res* 55:286–292.

Fernandez-Galaz MC, Martinez Munoz R, Villanua MA, Garcia-Segura LM. (1999b) Diurnal oscillation in glial fibrillary acidic protein in a perisuprachiasmatic area and its relationship to the luteinizing hormone surge in the female rat. *Neuroendocrinology* 70:368–376.

Fernandez-Galaz MC, Fernández-Agulló T, Campoy F, Arribas C, Gallardo N, Andrés A, Ros M, Carrascosa JM. (2001) Decreased leptin uptake in hypothalamic nuclei with ageing in Wistar rats. *J Endocrinol* 171:23–32.

Ferrari E, Casarotti D, Muzzoni B, Albertelli N, Cravello L, Fioravanti M, Solerte SB, Magri F. (2001) Age-related changes of the adrenal secretory pattern: Possible role in pathological brain aging. *Brain Res Rev* 37:294–300.

Ferreira A, Caceres A. (1991) Estrogen-enhanced neurite growth: Evidence for a selective induction of tau and stable microtubules. *J Neurosci* 11:392–400.

Ferrini M, Bisagno V, Piroli G, Grillo C, Deniselle MC, De Nicola AF. (2002) Effects of estrogens on choline-acetyltransferase immunoreactivity and GAP-43 mRNA in the forebrain of young and aging male rats. *Cell Mol Neurobiol* 22:289–301.

Ferris CF. (2000) Adolescent stress and neural plasticity in hamsters: A vasopressin-serotonin model of inappropriate aggressive behaviour. *Exp Physiol* 85:85S–90S.

Ferzaz B, Brault E, Bourliaud G, Robert JP, Poughon G, Claustre Y, Marguet F, Liere P, Schumacher M, Nowicki JP, Fournier J, Marabout B, Sevrin M, George P, Soubrie P, Benavides J, Scatton B. (2002) SSR180575 (7-chloro-N,N,5-trimethyl-4-oxo-3-phenyl-3,5-dihydro-4H-pyridazino[4,5-b]i ndole-1-acetamide), a peripheral benzodiazepine receptor ligand, promotes neuronal survival and repair. *J Pharmacol Exp Ther* 301:1067–1078.

Fester L, Ribeiro-Gouveia V, Prange-Kiel J, von Schassen C, Bottner M, Jarry H, Rune GM. (2006) Proliferation and apoptosis of hippocampal granule cells require local oestrogen synthesis. *J Neurochem* 97:1136–1144.

Fillit H, Weinreb H, Cholst I, Luine V, McEwen B, Amador R, Zabriskie J. (1986) Observations in a preliminary open trial of estradiol therapy for senile dementia-Alzheimer's type. *Psychoneuroendocrinology* 11:337–345.

Finch CE. (2003) Neurons, glia, and plasticity in normal brain aging. *Neurobiol Aging 24* (Suppl 1):S123–S127.

Fink G, Sumner B, Rosie R, Wilson H, McQueen J. (1999) Androgen actions on central serotonin neurotransmission: Relevance for mood, mental state and memory. *Behav Brain Res* 105:53–68.

Flanagan-Cato LM. (2000) Estrogen-induced remodeling of hypothalamic neural circuitry. *Front Neuroendocrinol* 21:309–329.

Flanagan-Cato LM, Calizo LH, Griffin GD, Lee BJ, Whisner SY. (2006) Sexual behaviour induces the expression of activity-regulated cytoskeletal protein and modifies neuronal morphology in the female rat ventromedial hypothalamus. *J Neuroendocrinol* 18:857–864.

Fleming AS, Cheung U, Myhal N, Kessler Z. (1989) Effects of maternal hormones on 'timidity' and attraction to pup-related odors in female rats. *Physiol Behav* 46:440–453.

Flood JF, Morley JE, Roberts E. (1992) Memory-enhancing effects in male mice of pregnenolone and steroids metabolically derived from it. *Proc Natl Acad Sci USA* 89:1567–1571.

Florant GL, Rivera ML, Lawrence AK, Tamarkin L. (1984) Plasma melatonin concentrations in hibernating marmots: Absence of a plasma melatonin rhythm. *Am J Physiol* 247:R1062–R1066.

Flores F, Naftolin F, Ryan KJ, White RJ. (1973) Estrogen formation by the isolated perfused rhesus monkey brain. *Science* 180:1074–1075.

Foecking EM, Szabo M, Schwartz NB, Levine JE. (2005) Neuroendocrine consequences of prenatal androgen exposure in the female rat: Absence of luteinizing hormone surges, suppression of progesterone receptor gene expression, and acceleration of the gonadotropin-releasing hormone pulse generator. *Biol Reprod* 72:1475–1483.

Follesa P, Concas A, Porcu P, Sanna E, Serra M, Mostallino MC, Purdy RH, Biggio G. (2001) Role of allopregnanolone in regulation of GABA(A) receptor plasticity during long-term exposure to and withdrawal from progesterone. *Brain Res Rev* 37:81–90.

Font de Mora J, Brown M. (2000) AIB1 is a conduit for kinase-mediated growth factor signaling to the estrogen receptor. *Mol Cell Biol* 20:5041–5047.

Fordyce DE, Wehner JM. (1993) Physical activity enhances spatial learning performance with an associated alteration in hippocampal protein kinase C activity in C57BL/6 and DBA/2 mice. *Brain Res* 619:111–119.

Forger NG, Breedlove SM. (1986) Sexual dimorphism in human and canine spinal cord: Role of early androgen. *Proc Natl Acad Sci USA* 83:7527–7531.

Foster TC, Norris CM. (1997) Age-associated changes in Ca^{2+}-dependent processes: Relation to hippocampal synaptic plasticity. *Hippocampus* 7:602–612.

Fowler CD, Freeman ME, Wang Z. (2003) Newly proliferated cells in the adult male amygdala are affected by gonadal steroid hormones. *J Neurobiol* 57:257–269.

Fowler PA. (1988) Seasonal endocrine cycles in the European hedgehog, Erinaceus europaeus. *J Reprod Fertil* 84:259–272.

Fowler PA, Racey PA. (1990) Effect of melatonin administration and long day-length on endocrine cycles in the hedgehog Erinaceus europaeus. *J Pineal Res* 8:193–204.

Fox MW, Anderson RE, Meyer FB. (1993) Neuroprotection by corticotropin releasing factor during hypoxia in rat brain. *Stroke* 24:1072–1076.

Foy MR, Stanton ME, Levine S, Thompson RF. (1987) Behavioral stress impairs long-term potentiation in rodent hippocampus. *Behav Neural Biol* 48:138–149.

Foy MR, Xu J, Xie X, Brinton RD, Thompson RF, Berger TW. (1999) 17beta-estradiol enhances NMDA receptor-mediated EPSPs and long-term potentiation. *J Neurophysiol* 81:925–929.

Foy MR, Baudry M, Foy JG, Thompson RF. (2008) 17beta-estradiol modifies stress-induced and age-related changes in hippocampal synaptic plasticity. *Behav Neurosci* 122:301–309.

Frago LM, Paneda C, Dickson SL, Hewson AK, Argente J, Chowen JA. (2002) Growth hormone (GH) and GH-releasing peptide-6 increase brain insulin-like growth factor-I expression and activate intracellular signaling pathways involved in neuroprotection. *Endocrinology* 143:4113–4122.

Frank C, Sagratella S. (2000) Neuroprotective effects of allopregnenolone on hippocampal irreversible neurotoxicity in vitro. *Prog Neuropsychopharmacol Biol Psychiatry* 24:1117–1126.

Frankfurt M, Gould E, Woolley CS, McEwen BS. (1990) Gonadal steroids modify dendritic spine density in ventromedial hypothalamic neurons: A Golgi study in the adult rat. *Neuroendocrinology* 51:530–535.

Frankfurt M, McEwen BS. (1991) Estrogen increases axodendritic synapses in the VMN of rats after ovariectomy. *NeuroReport* 2:380–382.

Frederich RC, Lollmann B, Hamann A, Napolitano-Rosen A, Kahn BB, Lowell BB, Flier JS. (1995) Expression of ob m-RNA and its encoded protein in rodents. Impact of nutrition and obesity. *J Clin Invest* 96:1658–1663.

Freeman DA, Lewis DA, Kauffman AS, Blum RM, Dark J. (2004) Reduced leptin concentrations are permissive for display of torpor in Siberian hamsters. *Am J Physiol Regul Integr Comp Physiol* 287:R97–R103.

Fride E, Dan Y, Feldon J, Halevy G, Weinstock M. (1985) Prenatal stress impairs maternal behavior in a conflict situation and reduces hippocampal benzodiazepine receptors. *Life Sci* 36:2103–2109.

Fride E, Dan Y, Feldon J, Halevy G, Weinstock M. (1986) Effects of prenatal stress on vulnerability to stress in prepubertal and adult rats. *Physiol Behav* 37:681–687.

Frostig RD. (2006) Functional organization and plasticity in the adult rat barrel cortex: Moving out-of-the-box. *Curr Opin Neurobiol* 16:445–450.

Frye CA. (1995) The neurosteroid 3 alpha, 5 apha-THP has antiseizure and possible neuroprotective effects in an animal model of epilepsy. *Brain Res* 696:113–120.

Frye CA, McCormick CM. (2000) Androgens are neuroprotective in the dentate gyrus of adrenalectomized female rats. *Stress* 3:185–194.

Frye CA, Scalise TJ. (2000) Anti-seizure effects of progesterone and 3alpha, 5alpha-THP in kainic acid and perforant pathway models of epilepsy. *Psychoneuroendocrinology* 25:407–420.

Fuchs E, Flügge G, Ohl F, Lucassen P, Vollmann-Honsdorf GK, Michaelis T. (2001) Psychosocial stress, glucocorticoids, and structural alterations in the tree shrew hippocampus. *Physiol Behav* 73:285–291.

Fukunaga K, Horikawa K, Shibata S, Takeuchi Y, Miyamoto E. (2002) $Ca^{2+}/$calmodulin-dependent protein kinase II-dependent long-term potentiation in the rat suprachiasmatic nucleus and its inhibition by melatonin. *J Neurosci Res* 70:799–807.

Fumagalli F, Molteni R, Racagni G, Riva MA. (2007) Stress during development: Impact on neuroplasticity and relevance to psychopathology. *Prog Neurobiol* 81:197–217.

Furukawa A, Miyatake A, Ohnishi T, Ichikawa Y. (1998) Steroidogenic acute regulatory protein (StAR) transcripts constitutively expressed in the adult rat central nervous system: Colocalization of StAR, cytochrome P-450SCC (CYP XIA1), and 3beta-hydroxysteroid dehydrogenase in the rat brain. *J Neurochem* 71:2231–2238.

Furuta M, Bridges RS. (2005) Gestation-induced cell proliferation in the rat brain. *Dev Brain Res* 156:61–66.

Fusani L, Gahr M. (2006) Hormonal influence on song structure and organization: The role of estrogen. *Neuroscience* 138:939–946.

Gagné J, Milot M, Gélinas S, Lahsaïni A, Trudeau F, Martinoli MG, Massicotte G. (1997) Binding properties of glutamate receptors in streptozotocin-induced diabetes in rats. *Diabetes* 46:841–846.

Gago N, Akwa Y, Sananes N, Guennoun R, Baulieu EE, El Etr M, Schumacher M. (2001). Progesterone and the oligodendroglial lineage: Stage-dependent biosynthesis and metabolism. *Glia* 36:295–308.

Gahr M, Garcia-Segura LM. (1996) Testosterone-dependent increase of gap-junctions in HVC neurons of adult female canaries. *Brain Res* 712:69–73.

Galbiati M, Martini L, Melcangi RC. (2002) Oestrogens, via transforming growth factor alpha, modulate basic fibroblast growth factor synthesis in hypothalamic astrocytes: In vitro observations. *J Neuroendocrinol* 14: 829–835.

Galea LA, McEwen BS. (1999) Sex and seasonal differences in the rate of cell proliferation in the dentate gyrus of adult wild meadow voles. *Neuroscience* 89:955–964.

Galea LA, Spritzer MD, Barker JM, Pawluski JL. (2006) Gonadal hormone modulation of hippocampal neurogenesis in the adult. *Hippocampus* 16:225–232.

Galiegue S, Tinel N, Casellas P. (2003) The peripheral benzodiazepine receptor: A promising therapeutic drug target. *Curr Med Chem* 10:1563–1572.

Gao Q, Mezei G, Nie Y, Rao Y, Choi CS, Bechmann I, Leranth C, Toran-Allerand D, Priest CA, Roberts JL, Gao XB, Mobbs C, Shulman GI, Diano S, Horvath TL. (2007) Anorectic estrogen mimics leptin's effect on the rewiring of melanocortin cells and Stat3 signaling in obese animals. *Nat Med* 13:89–94.

Garay L, Deniselle MC, Lima A, Roig P, De Nicola AF. (2007) Effects of progesterone in the spinal cord of a mouse model of multiple sclerosis. *J Steroid Biochem Mol Biol* 107:228–237.

Garay L, Gonzalez Deniselle MC, Gierman L, Meyer M, Lima A, Roig P, De Nicola AF. (2008) Steroid protection in the experimental autoimmune encephalomyelitis model of multiple sclerosis. *Neuroimmunomodulation* 15:76–83.

Garcia R. (2001) Stress, hippocampal plasticity, and spatial learning. *Synapse* 40:180–183.

Garcia R. (2002) Stress, metaplasticity, and antidepressants. *Curr Mol Med* 2:629–638.

Garcia-Estrada J, Garcia-Segura LM, Torres-Alemán I. (1992) Expression of insulin-like growth factor I by astrocytes in response to injury. *Brain Res* 592:343–347.

Garcia-Estrada J, Del Rio JA, Luquín S, Soriano E, Garcia-Segura LM. (1993) Gonadal hormones down-regulate reactive gliosis and astrocyte proliferation after a penetrating brain injury. *Brain Res* 628:271–278.

Garcia-Estrada J, Luquín S, Fernandez AM, Garcia-Segura LM. (1999) Dehydroepiandrosterone, pregenenolone and sex steroids down-regulate reactive astroglia in the male rat brain after a penetrating brain injury. *Int J Dev Neurosci* 17: 145–151.

Garcia-Galloway E, Arango C, Pons S, Torres-Alemán I. (2003) Glutamate excitotoxicity attenuates insulin-like growth factor-I prosurvival signaling. *Mol Cell Neurosci* 24:1027–1037.

Garcia-Lopez P, Garcia-Marin V, Freire M. (2007) The discovery of dendritic spines by Cajal in 1888 and its relevance in the present neuroscience. *Prog Neurobiol* 83:110–130.

Garcia-Marin V, Garcia-Lopez P, Freire M. (2007) Cajal's contributions to glia research. *Trends Neurosci* 30:479–487.

Garcia-Ovejero D, Veiga S, Garcia-Segura LM, DonCarlos LL. (2002) Glial expression of estrogen and androgen receptors after rat brain injury. *J Comp Neurol* 450:256–271.

Garcia-Ovejero D, Azcoitia I, DonCarlos LL, Melcangi RC, Garcia-Segura LM. (2005) Glia-neuron crosstalk in the neuroprotective mechanisms of sex steroid hormones. *Brain Res Rev* 48:273–286.

García-San Frutos M, Fernández-Agulló T, De Solís AJ, Andrés A, Arribas C, Carrascosa JM, Ros M. (2007) Impaired central insulin response in aged Wistar rats: Role of adiposity. *Endocrinology* 148:5238–4247.

Garcia-Segura LM. (2002) Cajal and glial cells. *Prog Brain Res* 136:255–260.

Garcia-Segura LM, Baetens D, Naftolin F. (1985) Sex differences and maturational changes in arcuate nucleus neuronal plasma membrane organization. *Dev Brain Res* 19:146–149.

Garcia-Segura LM, Baetens D, Naftolin F. (1986) Synaptic remodeling in arcuate nucleus after injection of estradiol valerate in adult female rats. *Brain Res* 366:131–136.

Garcia-Segura LM, Olmos G, Tranque P, Aguilera P, Naftolin F. (1987a) Nuclear pores in rat hypothalamic arcuate neurons: Sex differences and changes during the oestrus cycle. *J Neurocytol* 16:469–475.

Garcia-Segura LM, Olmos G, Tranque P, Naftolin F. (1987b) Rapid effects of gonadal steroids upon hypothalamic neuronal membrane ultrastructure. *J Steroid Biochem* 27:615–623.

Garcia-Segura LM, Hernandez P, Olmos G, Tranque PA, Naftolin F. (1988a) Neuronal membrane remodeling during the oestrus cycle: A freeze-fracture study in the arcuate nucleus of the rat hypothalamus. *J Neurocytol* 17:377–383.

Garcia-Segura LM, Perez J, Tranque PA, Olmos G, Naftolin F. (1988b) Sexual differentiation of the neuronal plasma membrane: Neonatal levels of sex steroids modulate the number of exo-endocytotic images in the developing rat arcuate neurons. *Neurosci Lett* 91:19–23.

Garcia-Segura LM, Suarez I, Segovia S, Tranque PA, Cales JM, Aguilera P, Olmos G, Guillamón A, Segovia S, Del Abril A. (1988c) The distribution of glial fibrillary acidic protein in the adult rat brain is influenced by the neonatal levels of sex steroids. *Brain Res* 456:357–363.

Garcia-Segura LM, Perez J, Tranque PA, Olmos G, Naftolin F. (1989a) Sex differences in plasma membrane concanavalin A binding in the rat arcuate neurons. *Brain Res Bull* 22:651–655.

Garcia-Segura LM, Torres-Alemán I, Naftolin F. (1989b) Astrocytic shape and glial fibrillary acidic protein immunoreactivity are modified by estradiol in primary rat hypothalamic cultures. *Dev Brain Res* 47:298–302.

Garcia-Segura LM, Olmos G, Robbins RJ, Hernandez P, Meyer JH, Naftolin F. (1989c) Estradiol induces rapid remodeling of plasma membranes in developing rat cerebrocortical neurons in culture. *Brain Res* 498:339–343.

Garcia-Segura LM, Perez J, Jones E, Naftolin F. (1991a) Loss of sexual dimorphism in rat arcuate nucleus neuronal membranes with reproductive aging. *Expl Neurol* 112:125–128.

Garcia-Segura LM, Perez J, Pons S, Rejas MT, Torres-Alemán I. (1991b) Localization of insulin-like growth factor I (IGF-I)-like immunoreactivity in the developing and adult rat brain. *Brain Res* 560:167–174.

Garcia-Segura LM, Diolez-Bojda F, Lenoir V, Naftolin F, Kerdelhué B. (1992) Estrogen-like effects of the mammary carcinogen 7, 12-dimethylbenz (alpha) antracene on hypothalamic neuronal membranes. *Brain Res Bull* 28:625–628.

Garcia-Segura LM, Luquín S, Martinez P, Casas MT, Suau P. (1993) Differential expression and gonadal hormone regulation of histone H1° in the developing and adult brain. *Dev Brain Res* 73:63–70.

Garcia-Segura LM, Chowen JA, Párducz A, Naftolin F. (1994a) Gonadal hormones as promoters of structural synaptic plasticity: Cellular mechanisms. *Prog Neurobiol* 44:279–307.

Garcia-Segura LM, Luquín S, Párducz A, Naftolin F. (1994b) Gonadal hormone regulation of glial fibrillary acidic protein immunoreactivity and glial ultrastructure in the rat neuroendocrine hypothalamus. *Glia* 10:59–69.

Garcia-Segura LM, Canas B, Párducz A, Rougon G, Theodosis D, Naftolin F, Torres-Alemán I. (1995a) Estradiol promotion of changes in the morphology of astroglia growing in culture depends on the expression of polysialic acid of neural membranes. *Glia* 13:209–216.

Garcia-Segura LM, Dueñas M, Busiguina S, Naftolin F, Chowen JA. (1995b) Gonadal hormone regulation of neuronal–glial interactions in the developing neuroendocrine hypothalamus. *J Steroid Biochem Mol Biol* 53:293–298.

Garcia-Segura LM, Chowen JA, Naftolin F. (1996) Endocrine glia: Roles of glial cells in the brain actions of steroid and thyroid hormones and in the regulation of hormone secretion. *Front Neuroendocrinol* 17:180–211.

Garcia-Segura LM, Rodriguez JR, Torres-Alemán I. (1997) Localization of the insulin-like growth factor I receptor in the cerebellum and hypothalamus of adult rats: An electron microscopic study. *J Neurocytol* 26:479–490.

Garcia-Segura LM, Cardona-Gomez P, Naftolin F, Chowen JA. (1998) Estradiol upregulates Bcl-2 expression in adult brain neurons. *NeuroReport* 9:593–597.

Garcia-Segura LM, Naftolin F, Hutchison JB, Azcoitia I, Chowen JA. (1999a) Role of astroglia in estrogen regulation of synaptic plasticity and brain repair. *J Neurobiol* 40:574–584.

Garcia-Segura LM, Wozniak A, Azcoitia I, Rodriguez JR, Hutchison RE, Hutchison JB. (1999b) Aromatase expression by astrocytes after brain injury: Implications for local estrogen formation in brain repair. *Neuroscience* 89:567–578.

Garcia-Segura LM, Cardona-Gomez GP, Chowen JA, Azcoitia I. (2000) Insulin-like growth factor-I receptors and estrogen receptors interact in the promotion of neuronal survival and neuroprotection. *J Neurocytol* 29:425–437.

Garcia-Segura LM, Azcoitia I, DonCarlos LL. (2001) Neuroprotection by estradiol. *Prog Neurobiol* 63:29–60.

Garcia-Segura LM, Veiga S, Sierra A, Melcangi RC, Azcoitia I. (2003) Aromatase: A neuroprotective enzyme. *Prog Neurobiol* 71:31–41.

Garcia-Segura LM, McCarthy MM. (2004) Minireview: Role of glia in neuroendocrine function. *Endocrinology* 145:1082–1086.

Garcia-Segura LM, Melcangi RC. (2006) Steroids and glial cell function. *Glia* 54:485–98.

Garcia-Segura LM, Sanz A, Mendez P. (2006) Cross-talk between IGF-I and estradiol in the brain: Focus on neuroprotection. *Neuroendocrinology* 84:275–279.

Garcia-Segura LM, Diz-Chaves Y, Perez-Martin M, Darnaudéry M. (2007) Estradiol, insulin-like growth factor-I and brain aging. *Psychoneuroendocrinology* 32 (Suppl 1):S57–S61.

Garcia-Segura LM, Lorenz B, DonCarlos LL. (2008) The role of glia in the hypothalamus: Implications for gonadal steroid feedback and reproductive neuroendocrine output. *Reproduction* 135:419–429.

Gardoni F, Kamal A, Bellone C, Biessels GJ, Ramakers GM, Cattabeni F, Gispen WH, Di Luca M. (2002) Effects of streptozotocin-diabetes on the hippocampal NMDA receptor complex in rats. *J Neurochem* 80:438–447.

Garnier M, Di Lorenzo D, Albertini A, Maggi A. (1997) Identification of estrogen-responsive genes in neuroblastoma SK-ER3 cells. *J Neurosci* 17:4591–4599.

Gasparini L, Xu H. (2003) Potential roles of insulin and IGF-1 in Alzheimer's disease. *Trends Neurosci* 26:404–406.

Gasparini L, Gouras GK, Wang R, Gross RS, Beal MF, Greengard P, Xu H. (2001) Stimulation of beta-amyloid precursor protein trafficking by insulin reduces intraneuronal beta-amyloid and requires mitogen-activated protein kinase signaling. *J Neurosci* 21:2561–2570.

Gasparini L, Netzer WJ, Greengard P, Xu H. (2002) Does insulin dysfunction play a role in Alzheimer's disease? *Trends Pharmacol Sci* 23:288–293.

Gatewood JD, Morgan MD, Eaton M, McNamara IM, Stevens LF, Macbeth AH, Meyer EA, Lomas LM, Kozub FJ, Lambert KG, Kinsley CH. (2005) Motherhood mitigates aging related decrements in learning and memory and positively affects brain aging in the rat. *Brain Res Bull* 66:91–98.

Gault VA, Hölscher C. (2008) GLP-1 agonists facilitate hippocampal LTP and reverse the impairment of LTP induced by beta-amyloid. *Eur J Pharmacol* 587:112–117.

Gazzaley AH, Thakker MM, Hof PR, Morrison JH. (1997) Preserved number of entorhinal cortex layer II neurons in aged macaque monkeys. *Neurobiol Aging* 18:549–553.

Geinisman Y, de Toledo-Morrell L, Morrell F. (1986) Loss of perforated synapses in the dentate gyrus: Morphological substrate of memory deficit in aged rats. *Proc Natl Acad Sci USA* 83:3027–3031.

Geinisman Y, de Toledo-Morrell L, Morrell F, Persina IS, Rossi M. (1992) Age-related loss of axospinous synapses formed by two afferent systems in the rat dentate gyrus as revealed by the unbiased stereological dissector technique. *Hippocampus* 2:437–444.

Geiser F. (2004) Metabolic rate and body temperature reduction during hibernation and daily torpor. *Annu Rev Physiol* 66:239–274.

Geiser F, Kenagy GJ. (1988) Torpor duration in relation to temperature and metabolisms in hibernating ground squirrels. *Physiol Zool* 61:442–449.

Genazzani AR, Pluchino N, Luisi S, Luisi M. (2007) Estrogen, cognition and female ageing. *Hum Reprod Update* 13:175–187.

Genc K, Genc S, Baskin H, Semin I. (2006) Erythropoietin decreases cytotoxicity and nitric oxide formation induced by inflammatory stimuli in rat oligodendrocytes. *Physiol Res* 55:33–38.

Gendron A, Kouassi E, Nuara S, Cossette C, D'Angelo G, Geadah D, du Souich P, Teitelbaum J. (2004) Transient middle cerebral artery occlusion influence on systemic oxygen homeostasis and erythropoiesis in Wistar rats. *Stroke* 35:1979–1984.

Gerges NZ, Stringer JL, Alkadhi KA. (2001) Combination of hypothyroidism and stress abolishes early LTP in the CA1 but not dentate gyrus of hippocampus of adult rats. *Brain Res* 922:250–260.

Ghoumari AM, Ibanez C, El-Etr M, Leclerc P, Eychenne B, O'Malley BW, Baulieu EE, Schumacher M. (2003) Progesterone and its metabolites increase myelin basic protein expression in organotypic slice cultures of rat cerebellum. *J Neurochem* 86:848–859.

Ghoumari AM, Baulieu EE, Schumacher M. (2005) Progesterone increases oligodendroglial cell proliferation in rat cerebellar slice cultures. *Neuroscience* 135:47–58.

Giachino C, Galbiati M, Fasolo A, Peretto P, Melcangi R. (2003) Neurogenesis in the subependymal layer of the adult rat: A role for neuroactive derivatives of progesterone. *Ann N Y Acad Sci* 1007:335–339.

Giachino C, Galbiati M, Fasolo A, Peretto P, Melcangi RC. (2004) Effects of progesterone derivatives, dihydroprogesterone and tetrahydroprogesterone, on the subependymal layer of the adult rat. *J Neurobiol* 58:493–502.

Gibbs RB, Wu D, Hersh LB, Pfaff DW. (1994) Effects of estrogen replacement on the relative levels of choline acetyltransferase, trkA, and nerve growth factor messenger RNAs in the basal forebrain and hippocampal formation of adult rats. *Exp Neurol* 129:70–80.

Gibson CL, Murphy SP. (2004) Progesterone enhances functional recovery after middle cerebral artery occlusion in male mice. *J Cereb Blood Flow Metab* 24:805–813.

Gibson CL, Gray LJ, Murphy SP, Bath PM. (2006) Estrogens and experimental ischemic stroke: A systematic review. *J Cereb Blood Flow Metab* 26:1103–1113.

Giedd JN. (2004) Structural magnetic resonance imaging of the adolescent brain. *Ann NY Acad Sci* 1021:77–85.

Giedd JN, Castellanos FX, Rajapakse JC, Vaituzis AC, Rapoport JL. (1997) Sexual dimorphism of the developing human brain. *Prog Neuropsychopharmacol Biol Psychiatry* 21:1185–1201.

Giedd JN, Blumenthal J, Jeffries NO, Castellanos FX, Liu H, Zijdenbos A, Paus T, Evans AC, Rapoport JL. (1999) Brain development during childhood and adolescence: A longitudinal MRI study. *Nat Neurosci* 2:861–863.

Gies U, Theodosis DT. (1994) Synaptic plasticity in the rat supraoptic nucleus during lactation involves GABA innervation and oxytocin neurons: A quantitative immunocytochemical analysis. *J Neurosci* 14:2861–2869.

Gispen WH, Biessels GJ. (2000) Cognition and synaptic plasticity in diabetes mellitus. *Trends Neurosci* 23:542–549.

Giusti P, Lipartiti M, Franceschini D, Schiavo N, Floreani M, Manev H. (1996) Neuroprotection by melatonin from kainate-induced excitotoxicity in rats. *FASEB J* 10:891–896.

Glass JD, Lee W, Shen H, Watanabe M. (1994) Expression of immunoreactive polysialylated neural cell adhesion molecule in the suprachiasmatic nucleus. *Neuroendocrinology* 60:87–95.

Glass JD, Chen L. (1999) Serotonergic modulation of astrocytic activity in the hamster suprachiasmatic nucleus. *Neuroscience* 94:1253–1259.

Gluck EF, Stephens N, Swoap SJ. (2006) Peripheral ghrelin deepens torpor bouts in mice through the arcuate nucleus neuropeptide Y signaling pathway. *Am J Physiol Regul Integr Comp Physiol* 291:R1303–1309.

Goel N, Bale TL. (2007) Identifying early behavioral and molecular markers of future stress sensitivity. *Endocrinology* 148:4585–4591.

Gogtay N, Giedd JN, Lusk L, Hayashi KM, Greenstein D, Vaituzis AC, Nugent TF, Herman DH, Clasen LS, Toga AW, Rapoport JL, Thompson PM. (2004) Dynamic mapping of human cortical development during childhood through early adulthood. *Proc Natl Acad Sci USA* 101:8174–8179.

Gold SM, Voskuhl RR. (2006) Testosterone replacement therapy for the treatment of neurological and neuropsychiatric disorders. *Curr Opin Investig Drugs* 7:625–630.

Goldman SA, Nottebohm F. (1983) Neuronal production, migration, and differentiation in a vocal control nucleus of the adult female canary brain. *Proc Natl Acad Sci USA* 80:2390–2394.

Goldstein LA, Kurz EM, Sengelaub DR. (1990) Androgen regulation of dendritic growth and retraction in the development of a sexually dimorphic spinal nucleus. *J Neurosci* 10:935–946.

Goldstein LA, Sengelaub DR. (1992) Timing and duration of dihydrotestosterone treatment affect the development of motoneuron number and morphology in a sexually dimorphic rat spinal nucleus. *J Comp Neurol* 326:147–157.

Gollapudi L, Oblinger MM. (1999a) Stable transfection of PC12 cells with estrogen receptor (ERα): Protective effects of estrogen on cell survival after serum deprivation. *J Neurosci Res* 56:99–108.

Gollapudi L, Oblinger MM. (1999b) Estrogen and NGF synergistically protect terminally differentiated, ERα-transfected PC12 cells from apoptosis. *J Neurosci Res* 56:471–481.

Gomez DM, Newman SW. (1991) Medial nucleus of the amygdale in the adult Syrian hamster a quantitative Golgi analysis of gonadal hormonal regulation of neuronal morphology. *Anat Rec* 231:498–509.

Gomez L, Carrascosa A, Teste D, Potau N, Rique S, Ruiz-Cuevas P, Almar J. (1999) Leptin values in placental cord blood of human newborns with normal intrauterine growth after 30–42 weeks of gestation. *Horm Res* 51:10–14.

Gomez-Mancilla B, Bedard PJ. (1992) Effect of estrogen and progesterone on L-dopa induced dyskinesia in MPTP-treated monkeys. *Neurosci Lett* 135:129–132.

Gomez-Pinilla F, Ying Z, Roy RR, Molteni R, Edgerton VR. (2002) Voluntary exercise induces a BDNF-mediated mechanism that promotes neuroplasticity. *J Neurophysiol* 88: 2187–2195.

Gompf HS, Allen CN. (2004) GABAergic synapses of the suprachiasmatic nucleus exhibit a diurnal rhythm of short-term synaptic plasticity. *Eur J Neurosci* 19:2791–2798.

Gonzalez SL, Labombarda F, Gonzalez Deniselle MC, Guennoun R, Schumacher M, De Nicola AF. (2004) Progesterone up-regulates neuronal brain-derived neurotrophic factor expression in the injured spinal cord. *Neuroscience* 125:605–614.

Gonzalez SL, Labombarda F, Deniselle MC, Mougel A, Guennoun R, Schumacher M, De Nicola AF. (2005) Progesterone neuroprotection in spinal cord trauma involves up-regulation of brain-derived neurotrophic factor in motoneurons. *J Steroid Biochem Mol Biol* 94:143–149.

González-Burgos I, Letechipía-Vallejo G, López-Loeza E, Moralí G, Cervantes M. (2007) Long-term study of dendritic spines from hippocampal CA1 pyramidal cells, after neuroprotective melatonin treatment following global cerebral ischemia in rats. *Neurosci Lett* 423:162–166.

Gonzalez Deniselle MC, Lopez-Costa JJ, Saavedra JP, Pietranera L, Gonzalez SL, Garay L, Guennoun R, Schumacher M, De Nicola AF. (2002) Progesterone neuroprotection in the Wobbler mouse, a genetic model of spinal cord motor neuron disease. *Neurobiol Dis* 11:457–468.

Gonzalez Deniselle MC, Garay L, Gonzalez S, Guennoun R, Schumacher M, De Nicola AF. (2005) Progesterone restores retrograde labeling of cervical motoneurons in Wobbler mouse motoneuron disease. *Exp Neurol* 195:518–523.

Gonzalez Deniselle MC, Garay L, Gonzalez S, Saravia F, Labombarda F, Guennoun R, Schumacher M, De Nicola AF. (2007) Progesterone modulates brain-derived neurotrophic factor and choline acetyltransferase in degenerating Wobbler motoneurons. *Exp Neurol* 203:406–414.

Good M, Day M, Muir JL. (1999) Cyclical changes in endogenous levels of oestrogen modulate the induction of LTD and LTP in the hippocampal CA1 region. *Eur J Neurosci* 11:4476–4480.

Goodenough S, Schleusner D, Pietrzik C, Skutella T, Behl C. (2005) Glycogen synthase kinase 3beta links neuroprotection by 17beta-estradiol to key Alzheimer's processes. *Neuroscience* 132:581–589.

Goodson JL, Bass AH. (2001) Social behavior functions and related anatomical characteristics of vasotocin/vasopressin systems in vertebrates. *Brain Res Rev* 35:246–265.

Gordon GR, Baimoukhametova DV, Hewitt SA, Rajapaksha WR, Fisher TE, Bains JS. (2005) Norepinephrine triggers release of glial ATP to increase postsynaptic efficacy. *Nat Neurosci* 8:1078–1086.

Gordon GR, Bains JS. (2006) Can homeostatic circuits learn and remember? *J Physiol* 576:341–347.

Gore AC. (2001) Gonadotropin-releasing hormone neurones, NMDA receptors, and their regulation by steroid hormones across the reproductive life cycle. *Brain Res Rev* 37:235–248.

Gorio A, Gokmen N, Erbayraktar S, Yilmaz O, Madaschi L, Cichetti C, Di Giulio AM, Vardar E, Cerami A, Brines M. (2002) Recombinant human erythropoietin counteracts secondary injury and markedly enhances neurological recovery from experimental spinal cord trauma. *Proc Natl Acad Sci USA* 99:9450–9455.

Gorski RA, Gordon JH, Shryne JE, Southam AM. (1978) Evidence for a morphological sex difference within the medial preoptic area of the rat brain. *Brain Res* 148:333–346.

Gorski RA, Harlan RE, Jacobson CO, Shryne JE, Southam AM. (1980) Evidence for the existence of a sexually dimorphic nucleus in the preoptic area of the rat. *J Comp Neurol* 198:529–539.

Gould E. (2007) How widespread is adult neurogenesis in mammals? *Nat Rev Neurosci* 8:481–488.

Gould E, Butcher LL. (1989) Developing cholinergic basal forebrain neurons are sensitive to thyroid hormone. *J Neurosci* 9:3347–3358.

Gould E, Woolley CS, Frankfurt M, McEwen BS. (1990a) Gonadal steroids regulate dendritic spine density in hippocampal pyramidal cells in adulthood. *J Neurosci* 10:1286–1291.

Gould E, Westlind-Danielsson A, Frankfurt M, McEwen BS. (1990b) Sex differences and thyroid hormone sensitivity of hippocampal pyramidal cells. *J Neurosci* 10:996–1003.

Gould E, Woolley CS, McEwen BS. (1991) The hippocampal formation: Morphological changes induced by thyroid, gonadal and adrenal hormones. *Psychoneuroendocrinology* 16:67–84.

Gould E, Cameron HA, Daniels DC, Woolley CS, McEwen BS. (1992) Adrenal hormones suppress cell division in the adult rat dentate gyrus. *J Neurosci* 12:3642–3650.

Gould E, McEwen BS, Tanapat P, Galea LA, Fuchs E. (1997) Neurogenesis in the dentate gyrus of the adult tree shrew is regulated by psychosocial stress and NMDA receptor activation. *J Neurosci* 17: 2492–2498.

Gould E, Tanapat P. (1999) Stress and hippocampal neurogenesis. *Biol Psychiatr* 46:1472–1479.

Gouras GK, Xu H, Gross RS, Greenfield JP, Hai B, Wang R, Greengard P. (2000) Testosterone reduces neuronal secretion of Alzheimer's beta-amyloid peptides. *Proc Natl Acad Sci USA* 97:1202–1205.

Goya RG, Bolognani F. (1999) Homeostasis, thymic hormones and aging. *Gerontology* 45:174–178.

Goya RG, Brown OA, Bolognani F. (1999) The thymus–pituitary axis and its changes during aging. *Neuroimmunomodulation* 6:137–142.

Graf W, Baker R. (1983) Adaptive changes of the vestibulo-ocular reflex in flatfish are achieved by reorganization of central nervous pathways. *Science* 221:777–779.

Graf W, Baker R. (1990) Neuronal adaptation accompanying metamorphosis in the flatfish. *J Neurobiol* 21:1136–1152.

Grandbois M, Morisette M, Callier S, Di Paolo T. (2000) Ovarian steroids and raloxifene prevent MPTP-induced dopamine depletion in mice. *NeuroReport* 11:343–346.

Granholm AC, Sanders L, Seo H, Lin L, Ford K, Isacson O. (2003) Estrogen alters amyloid precursor protein as well as dendritic and cholinergic markers in a mouse model of Down syndrome. *Hippocampus* 13:905–914.

Grant S, Keating MJ. (1986) Ocular migration and the metamorphic and postmetamorphic maturation of the retinotectal system in Xenopus laevis: An autoradiographic and morphometric study. *J Embryol Exp Morphol* 92:43–69.

Green PS, Bishop J, Simpkins JW. (1997) 17 alpha-estradiol exerts neuroprotective effects on SK-N-SH cells. *J Neurosci* 17:511–515.

Green PS, Bales K, Paul S, Bu G. (2005) Estrogen therapy fails to alter amyloid deposition in the PDAPP model of Alzheimer's disease. *Endocrinology* 146:2774–2781.

Greenough WT, Carter CS, Steerman C, DeVoogd TJ. (1977) Sex differences in dendritic patterns in hamster preoptic area. *Brain Res* 126:63–72.

Greenspan SL, Klibanski A, Rowe JW, Elahi D. (1991) Age-related alterations in pulsatile secretion of TSH: Role of dopaminergic regulation. *Am J Physiol* 260:E486–E491.

Greenwood AK, Fernald RD. (2004) Social regulation of the electrical properties of gonadotropin-releasing hormone neurons in a cichlid fish (*Astatotilapia burtoni*). *Biol Reprod* 71:909–918.

Greenwood AK, Wark AR, Fernald RD, Hofmann HA. (2008) Expression of arginine vasotocin in distinct preoptic regions is associated with dominant and subordinate behaviour in an African cichlid fish. *Proc Biol Sci* 275:2393–2402.

Greer ER, Diamond MC, Murphy GM. (1982) Increased branching of basal dendrites on pyramidal neurons in the occipital cortex of homozygous Brattleboro rats in standard and enriched environmental conditions: A Golgi study. *Exp Neurol* 76:254–262.

Gregg C, Shikar V, Larsen P, Mak G, Chojnacki A, Yong VW, Weiss S. (2007) White matter plasticity and enhanced remyelination in the maternal CNS. *J Neurosci* 27:1812–1823.

Gregory WA, Tweedle CD, Hatton GI. (1980) Ultrastructure of neurons in the paraventricular nucleus of normal, dehydrated and rehydrated rats. *Brain Res Bull* 5:301–306.

Grenier J, Tomkiewicz C, Trousson A, Rajkowski KM, Schumacher M, Massaad C. (2005) Identification by microarray analysis of aspartate aminotransferase and glutamine synthetase as glucocorticoid target genes in a mouse Schwann cell line. *J Steroid Biochem Mol Biol* 97:342–352.

Griffin WC, Skinner HD, Salm AK, Birkle DL. (2003) Mild prenatal stress in rats is associated with enhanced conditioned fear. *Physiol Behav* 79:209–215.

Grill JD, Riddle DR. (2002) Age-related and laminar-specific dendritic changes in the medial frontal cortex of the rat. *Brain Res* 937:8–21.

Grillo CA, Piroli GG, Wood GE, Reznikov LR, McEwen BS, Reagan LP. (2005) Immunocytochemical analysis of synaptic proteins provides new insights into diabetes-mediated plasticity in the rat hippocampus. *Neuroscience* 136:477–486.

Grimm G, Stockenhuber F, Schneeweiss B, Madl C, Zeitlhofer J, Schneider B. (1990) Improvement of brain function in hemodialysis patients treated with erythropoietin. *Kidney Int* 38:480–486.

Grossman KJ, Goss CW, Stein DG. (2004) Effects of progesterone on the inflammatory response to brain injury in the rat. *Brain Res* 1008:29–39.

Gruart A, Munoz MD, Delgado-Garcia JM. (2006) Involvement of the CA3-CA1 synapse in the acquisition of associative learning in behaving mice. *J Neurosci* 26:1077–1087.

Gruart A, Delgado-García JM. (2007) Activity-dependent changes of the hippocampal CA3-CA1 synapse during the acquisition of associative learning in conscious mice. *Genes Brain Behav* 6 (Suppl 1):24–31.

Grubb MS, Thompson ID. (2004) The influence of early experience on the development of sensory systems. *Curr Opin Neurobiol* 14:503–512.

Grubeck-Loebenstein B, Wick G. (2002) The aging of the immune system. *Adv Immunol* 80:243–284.

Gruver AL, Hudson LL, Sempowski GD. (2007) Immunosenescence of ageing. *J Pathol* 211:144–156.

Guan J, Williams C, Gunning M, Mallard C, Gluckman P. (1993) The effects of IGF-1 treatment after hypoxic-ischemic brain injury in adult rats. *J Cereb Blood Flow Metab* 13:609–616.

Guan J, Bennet L, Gluckman PD, Gunn AJ. (2003) Insulin-like growth factor-1 and post-ischemic brain injury. *Prog Neurobiol* 70:443–462.

Guazzo EP, Kirkpatrick PJ, Goodyer IM, Shiers HM, Herbert J. (1996) Cortisol, dehydroepiandrosterone (DHEA), and DHEA sulfate in the cerebrospinal fluid of man: Relation to blood levels and the effects of age. *J Clin Endocrinol Metab* 81:3951–3960.

Gubernick DJ, Sengelaub DR, Kurz EM. (1993) A neuroanatomical correlate of paternal behavior in the biparental California mouse (Peromyscus californicus). *Behav Neurosci* 107:194–201.

Gudemez E, Ozer K, Cunningham B, Siemionow K, Browne E, Siemionow M. (2002) Dehydroepiandrosterone as an enhancer of functional recovery following crush injury to rat sciatic nerve. *Microsurgery* 22:234–241.

Gudino-Cabrera G, Nieto-Sampedro M. (1999) Estrogen receptor immunoreactivity in Schwann-like brain macroglia. *J Neurobiol* 40:458–470.

Gué M, Bravard A, Meunier J, Veyrier R, Gaillet S, Recasens M, Maurice T. (2004) Sex differences in learning deficits induced by prenatal stress in juvenile rats. *Behav Brain Res* 150:149–157.

Guennoun R, Benmessahel Y, Delespierre B, Gouezou M, Rajkowski KM, Baulieu EE, Schumacher M. (2001) Progesterone stimulates Krox-20 gene expression in Schwann cells. *Mol Brain Res* 90:75–82.

Guennoun R, Meffre D, Labombarda F, Gonzalez SL, Deniselle MC, Stein DG, De Nicola AF, Schumacher M. (2008) The membrane-associated progesterone-binding protein 25-Dx: Expression, cellular localization and up-regulation after brain and spinal cord injuries. *Brain Res Rev* 57:493–505.

Guerra B, Diaz M, Alonso R, Marin R. (2004) Plasma membrane oestrogen receptor mediates neuroprotection against beta-amyloid toxicity through activation of Raf-1/MEK/ERK cascade in septal-derived cholinergic SN56 cells. *J Neurochem* 91:99–109.

Guerra-Araiza C, Villamar-Cruz O, Gonzalez-Arenas A, Chavira R, Camacho-Arroyo I. (2003) Changes in progesterone receptor isoforms content in the rat brain during the oestrous cycle and after oestradiol and progesterone treatments. *J Neuroendocrinol* 15:984–990.

Guerra-Araiza C, Amorim MA, Camacho-Arroyo I, Garcia-Segura LM. (2007) Effects of progesterone and its reduced metabolites, dihydroprogesterone and tetrahydroprogesterone, on the expression and phosphorylation of glycogen synthase kinase-3 and the microtubule-associated protein tau in the rat cerebellum. *Dev Neurobiol* 67:510–520.

Guillamón A, Segovia S, Del Abril A. (1988) Early effects of gonadal steroids on the neuron number in the medial posterior region and the lateral division of the bed nucleus of the stria terminalis in the rat. *Dev Brain Res* 44:281–290.

Guillamón A, Segovia S. (1997) Sex differences in the vomeronasal system. *Brain Res Bull* 44:377–382.

Güldner FH. (1982) Sexual dimorphisms of axo-spine synapses and postsynaptic density material in the suprachiasmatic nucleus of the rat. *Neurosci Lett* 28:145–150.

Güldner FH, Ingham CA. (1979) Plasticity in synaptic appositions of optic nerve afferents under different lighting conditions. *Neurosci Lett* 14:235–240.

Güldner FH, Bahar E, Young CA, Ingham CA. (1997) Structural plasticity of optic synapses in the rat suprachiasmatic nucleus: Adaptation to long-term influence of light and darkness. *Cell Tissue Res* 287:43–60.

Gulledge CC, Deviche P. (1997) Androgen control of vocal control region volumes in a wild migratory songbird (Junco hyemalis) is region and possibly age dependent. *J Neurobiol* 32:391–402

Guo Q, Fu W, Xie J, Luo H, Sells SF, Geddes JW, Bondada V, Rangnekar VM, Mattson MP. (1998) Par-4 is a mediator of neuronal degeneration associated with the pathogenesis of Alzheimer's disease. *Nat Med* 4:957–962.

Guo Q, Sayeed I, Baronne LM, Hoffman SW, Guennoun R, Stein DG. (2006) Progesterone administration modulates AQP4 expression and edema after traumatic brain injury in male rats. *Exp Neurol* 198:469–478.

Gurney ME. (1981) Hormonal control of cell form and number in the zebra finch song system. *J Neurosci* 1:658–673.

Gursoy E, Cardounel A, Kalimi M. (2001) Pregnenolone protects mouse hippocampal (HT-22) cells against glutamate and amyloid beta protein toxicity. *Neurochem Res* 26:15–21.

Gustafson K, Hagberg H, Bengtsson BA, Brantsing C, Isgaard J. (1999) Possible protective role of growth hormone in hypoxia-ischemia in neonatal rats. *Pediatr Res* 45:318–323.

Gutierrez EG, Banks WA, Kastin AJ. (1993) Murine tumor necrosis factor alpha is transported from blood to brain in the mouse. *J Neuroimmunol* 47:169–176.

Gutierrez EG, Banks WA, Kastin AJ. (1994) Blood-borne interleukin-1 receptor antagonist crosses the blood brain barrier. *J Neuroimmunol* 55:153–160.

Gutman DA, Nemeroff CB. (2003) Persistent central nervous system effects of an adverse early environment: Clinical and preclinical studies. *Physiol Behav* 79:471–478.

Gutteling BM, de Weerth C, Willemsen-Swinkels SHN, Huizink AC, Mulder EJH, Visser GHA, Buitelaar JK. (2005) The effects of prenatal stress on temperament and problem behavior of 27-month-old toddlers. *Eur Child Adolesc Psychiatry* 14:41–51.

Hager K, Machein U, Krieger S, Platt D, Seefried G, Bauer J. (1994) Interleukin-6 and selected plasma proteins in healthy persons of different ages. *Neurobiol Aging* 15:771–772.

Hajszan T, MacLusky NJ, Leranth C. (2004) Dehydroepiandrosterone increases hippocampal spine synapse density in ovariectomized female rats. *Endocrinology* 145:1042–1045.

Hajszan T, MacLusky NJ. (2006) Neurologic links between epilepsy and depression in women: Is hippocampal neuroplasticity the key? *Neurology* 66 (6 Suppl 3):S13–S22.

Håkansson M, de Lecea L, Sutcliffe JG, Yanagisawa M, Meister B. (1999) Leptin receptor- and STAT3-immunoreactivities in hypocretin/orexin neurones of the lateral hypothalamus. *J Neuroendocrinol* 11:653–663.

Hales CN, Barker DJ. (2001) The thrifty phenotype hypothesis. *Br Med Bull* 60:5–20.

Hammer RP, Jacobson CO. (1984) Sex differences in dendritic development of the sexually dimorphic nucleus of the preoptic area in the rat. *Int J Devl Neurosci* 2:277–285.

Hammock EA, Young LJ. (2006) Oxytocin, vasopressin and pair bonding: Implications for autism. *Philos Trans R Soc Lond B Biol Sci* 361:2187–2198.

Hammond J, Le Q, Goodyer C, Gelfand M, Trifiro M, LeBlanc A. (2001) Testosterone-mediated neuroprotection through the androgen receptor in human primary neurons. *J Neurochem* 77:1319–1326.

Han SK, Abraham IM, Herbison AE. (2002) Effect of GABA on GnRH neurons switches from depolarization to hyperpolarization at puberty in the female mouse. *Endocrinology* 143:1459–1466.

Han SK, Gottsch ML, Lee KJ, Popa SM, Smith JT, Jakawich SK, Clifton DK, Steiner RA, Herbison AE. (2005) Activation of gonadotropin-releasing hormone neurones by kisspeptin as a neuroendocrine switch for the onset of puberty. *J Neurosci* 25:11349–11356.

Handa RJ, Pak TR, Kudwa AE, Lund TD, Hinds L. (2008) An alternate pathway for androgen regulation of brain function: Activation of estrogen receptor beta by the metabolite of dihydrotestosterone, 5alpha-androstane-3beta,17beta-diol. *Horm Behav* 53:741–752.

Hansen MK, Taishi P, Chen Z, Krueger JM. (1998) Vagotomy blocks the induction of interleukin-1beta (IL-1beta) mRNA in the brain of rats in response to systemic IL-1beta. *J Neurosci* 18:2247–2253.

Hao J, Janssen WG, Tang Y, Roberts JA, McKay H, Lasley B, Allen PB, Greengard P, Rapp PR, Kordower JH, Hof PR, Morrison JH. (2003) Estrogen increases the number of spinophilin-immunoreactive spines in the hippocampus of young and aged female rhesus monkeys. *J Comp Neurol* 465:540–550.

Hapgood JP, Koubovec D, Louw A, Africander D. (2004) Not all progestins are the same: Implications for usage. *Trends Pharmacol Sci* 25:554–557.

Hardin-Pouzet H, Giraudon P, Belin MF, Didier-Bazes M. (1996) Glucocorticoid upregulation of glutamate dehydrogenase gene expression in vitro in astrocytes. *Mol Brain Res* 37:324–328.

Harley CW, Malsbury CW, Squires A, Brown RA. (2000) Testosterone decreases CA1 plasticity in vivo in gonadectomized male rats. *Hippocampus* 10:693–697.

Harris, GW. (1970) Hormonal differentiation of the developing central nervous system with respect to patterns of endocrine function. *Phil Trans Roy Soc Lond B* 259:165–176.

Harris KM, Teyler TJ. (1983) Age differences in a circadian influence on hippocampal LTP. *Brain Res* 261:69–73.

Harris KM, Fiala JC, Ostroff L. (2003) Structural changes at dendritic spine synapses during long-term potentiation. *Phil Trans Roy Soc Lond B* 358:745–748.

Hart SA, Snyder MA, Smejkalova T, Woolley CS. (2007) Estrogen mobilizes a subset of estrogen receptor-alpha-immunoreactive vesicles in inhibitory presynaptic boutons in hippocampal CA1. *J Neurosci* 27:2102–2111.

Harvey J. (2007) Leptin regulation of neuronal excitability and cognitive function. *Curr Opin Pharmacol* 7:643–647.

Harvey J, Solovyova N, Irving A. (2006) Leptin and its role in hippocampal synaptic plasticity. *Prog Lipid Res* 45:369–378.

Harvey S, Kakebeeke M, Murphy AE, Sanders EJ. (2003) Growth hormone in the nervous system: Autocrine or paracrine roles in retinal function? *Can J Physiol Pharmacol* 81:371–384.

Harvey S, Baudet ML, Sanders EJ. (2006) Growth hormone and cell survival in the neural retina: Caspase dependence and independence. *NeuroReport* 17:1715–1718.

Hatton GI. (1986) Plasticity in the hypothalamic magnocellular neurosecretory system. *Fed Proc* 45:2328–2333.

Hatton GI. (1988) Pituicytes, glia and control of terminal secretion. *J Exp Biol* 139:67–79.

Hatton GI. (1990) Emerging concepts of structure-function dynamics in adult brain: The hypothalamo-neurohypophysial system. *Prog Neurobiol* 34:437–504.

Hatton GI. (1997) Function-related plasticity in hypothalamus. *Annu Rev Neurosci* 20:375–397.

Hatton GI, Walters JK. (1973) Induced multiple nucleoli, nucleolar margination, and cell size changes in supraoptic neurons during dehydration and rehydration in the rat. *Brain Res* 59:137–154.

Hatton GI, Tweedle CD. (1982) Magnocellular neuropeptidergic neurons in hypothalamus: Increases in membrane apposition and number of specialized synapses from pregnancy to lactation. *Brain Res Bull* 8:197–204.

Hatton GI, Perlmutter LS, Salm AK, Tweedle CD. (1984) Dynamic neuronal-glial interactions in hypothalamus and pituitary: Implications for control of hormone synthesis and release. *Peptides* 5 (Suppl 1):121–138.

Hauet T, Yao ZX, Bose HS, Wall CT, Han Z, Li W, Hales DB, Miller WL, Culty M, Papadopoulos V. (2005) Peripheral-type benzodiazepine receptor-mediated action of steroidogenic acute regulatory protein on cholesterol entry into Leydig cell mitochondria. *Mol Endocrinol* 19:540–554.

Hauser KF, Toran-Allerand D. (1989) Androgen increases the number of cells in fetal mouse spinal cord cultures: Implications for motoneuron survival. *Brain Res* 458:157–164.

Hauser KF, Gona AG. (1984) Purkinje cell maturation in the frog cerebellum during thyroxine-induced metamorphosis. *Neuroscience* 11:139–155.

Havrankova J, Roth J, Brownstein M. (1978) Insulin receptors are widely distributed in the central nervous system of the rat. *Nature* 272:827–829.

Hawk T, Zhang YQ, Rajakumar G, Day AL, Simpkins JW. (1998) Testosterone increases and estradiol decreases middle cerebral artery occlusion lesion size in male rats. *Brain Res* 796:296–298.

Hawrylak N, Fleming JC, Salm AK. (1998) Dehydration and rehydration selectively and reversibly alter glial fibrillary acidic protein immunoreactivity in the rat supraoptic nucleus and subjacent glial limitans. *Glia* 22:260–271.

Hayashi A, Nagaoka M, Yamada K, Ichitani Y, Miake Y, Okado N. (1998) Maternal stress induces synaptic loss and developmental disabilities of offspring. *Int J Dev Neurosci* 16:209–216.

He J, Hoffman SW, Stein DG. (2004) Allopregnanolone, a progesterone metabolite, enhances behavioral recovery and decreases neuronal loss after traumatic brain injury. *Restor Neurol Neurosci* 22:19–31.

He J, Crews FT. (2007) Neurogenesis decreases during brain maturation from adolescence to adulthood. *Pharmacol Biochem Behav* 86:327–333.

Hebb DO. (1949). *The organization of behavior.* Wiley, New York.

Hebbard PC, King RR, Malsbury CW, Harley CW. (2003) Two organizational effects of pubertal testosterone in male rats: Transient social memory and a shift away from long-term potentiation following a tetanus in hippocampal CA1. *Exp Neurol* 182:470–475.

Heger S, Mastronardi C, Dissen GA, Lomniczi A, Cabrera R, Roth CL, Jung H, Galimi F, Sippell W, Ojeda SR. (2007) Enhanced at puberty 1 (EAP1) is a new transcriptional regulator of the female neuroendocrine reproductive axis. *J Clin Invest* 117:2145–2154.

Heikkinen T, Kalesnykas G, Rissanen A, Tapiola T, Iivonen S, Wang J, Chaudhuri J, Tanila H, Miettinen R, Puolivali J. (2004) Estrogen treatment improves spatial learning in APP + PS1 mice but does not affect beta amyloid accumulation and plaque formation. *Exp Neurol* 187:105–117.

Heim C, Plotsky PM, Nemeroff CB. (2004) Importance of studying the contributions of early adverse experience to neurobiological findings in depression. *Neuropsychopharmacology* 29:641–648.

Heinicke E. (1977) Influence of exogenous triiodothyronine on axonal regeneration and wound healing in the brain of the rat. *J Neurol Sci* 31:293–305.

Hellner K, Walther T, Schubert M, Albrecht D. (2005) Angiotensin-(1-7) enhances LTP in the hippocampus through the G-protein-coupled receptor Mas. *Mol Cell Neurosci* 29:427–435.

Helmeke C, Ovtscharoff W, Poeggel G, Braun K. (2008) Imbalance of immunohistochemically characterized interneuron populations in the adolescent and adult rodent medial prefrontal cortex after repeated exposure to neonatal separation stress. *Neuroscience* 152:18–28.

Hench PS. (1952) The reversibility of certain rheumatic and nonrheumatic conditions by the use of cortisone or of the pituitary adrenocorticotropic hormone. *Ann Internal Med* 36:1–25.

Henderson VW, Paganini-Hill A, Miller BL, Elble RJ, Reyes PF, Shoupe D, McCleary CA, Klein RA, Hake AM, Farlow MR. (2000) Estrogen for Alzheimer's disease in women: Randomized, double-blind, placebo-controlled trial. *Neurology* 54:295–301.

Henderson VW, Benke KS, Green RC, Cupples LA, Farrer LA and MIRAGE Study Group (2005) Postmenopausal hormone therapy and Alzheimer's disease risk: Interaction with age. *J Neurol Neurosurg Psychiatry* 76:103–105.

Henderson VW, Sherwin BB. (2007) Surgical versus natural menopause: Cognitive issues. *Menopause* 14:572–579.

Hennessey AC, Camak L, Gordon F, Edwards DA. (1990) Connections between the pontine central gray and the ventromedial hypothalamus are essential for lordosis in female rats. *Behav Neurosci* 104:477–488.

Henry C, Kabbaj M, Simon H, Le Moal M, Maccari S. (1994) Prenatal stress increases the hypothalamo–pituitary–adrenal axis response in young and adult rats. *J Neuroendocrinol* 6:341–345.

Herbison AE, Pape JR, Simonian SX, Skynner MJ, Sim JA. (2001) Molecular and cellular properties of GnRH neurons revealed through transgenics in the mouse. *Mol Cell Endocrinol* 185:185–194.

Herbosa CG, Dahl GE, Evans NP, Pelt J, Wood RI, Foster DL. (1996) Sexual differentiation of the surge mode of gonadotropin secretion: Prenatal androgens abolish the gonadotropin-releasing hormone surge in sheep. *J Neuroendocrinol* 8:627–633.

Herenu CB, Brown OA, Sosa YE, Morel GR, Reggiani PC, Bellini MJ, Goya RG. (2006) The neuroendocrine system as a model to evaluate experimental gene therapy. *Curr Gene Ther* 6:125–129.

Herenu CB, Cristina C, Rimoldi OJ, Becu-Villalobos D, Cambiaggi V, Portiansky EL, Goya RG. (2007) Restorative effect of insulin-like growth factor-I gene therapy in the hypothalamus of senile rats with dopaminergic dysfunction. *Gene Ther* 14:237–245.

Hernandez-Sanchez C, Mansilla A, de la Rosa EJ, de Pablo F. (2006) Proinsulin in development: New roles for an ancient prohormone. *Diabetologia* 49:1142–1150.

Hewitt SC, Deroo BJ, Korach KS. (2005) Signal transduction. A new mediator for an old hormone? *Science* 307, 1572–1573.

Hidalgo A, Barami K, Iversen K, Goldman SA. (1995) Estrogens and non-estrogenic ovarian influences combine to promote the recruitment and decrease the turnover of new neurons in the adult female canary brain. *J Neurobiol* 27:470–487.

Higa-Taniguchi KT, Silva FC, Silva HM, Michelini LC, Stern JE. (2007) Exercise training-induced remodeling of paraventricular nucleus (nor)adrenergic innervation in normotensive and hypertensive rats. *Am J Physiol Regul Integr Comp Physiol* 292:R1717–1727.

Hill KM, DeVoogd TJ. (1991) Altered daylength affects dendritic structure in a song-related brain region in red-winged blackbirds. *Behav Neural Biol* 56:240–250.

Hill RA, McInnes KJ, Gong EC, Jones ME, Simpson ER, Boon WC. (2007) Estrogen deficient male mice develop compulsive behavior. *Biol Psychiatry* 61:359–366.

Hines M. (2003) Sex steroids and human behavior: Prenatal androgen exposure and sex-typical play behavior in children. *Ann N Y Acad Sci* 1007:272–282.

Hof PR, Morrison JH. (2004) The aging brain morphomolecular senescence of cortical circuits. *Trends Neurosci* 27:607–613.

Hofer SB, Mrsic-Flogel TD, Bonhoeffer T, Hübener M. (2006) Lifelong learning: Ocular dominance plasticity in mouse visual cortex. *Curr Opin Neurobiol* 16:451–459.

Hoffman GE, Moore N, Fiskum G, Murphy AZ. (2003) Ovarian steroid modulation of seizure severity and hippocampal cell death after kainic acid treatment. *Exp Neurol* 182:124–134.

Hofmann HA, Fernald RD. (2000) Social status controls somatostatin neuron size and growth. *J Neurosci* 20:4740–4744.

Hofman MA, Swaab DF. (1992) Seasonal changes in the suprachiasmatic nucleus of man. *Neurosci Lett* 139:257–260.

Hojo Y, Hattori TA, Enami T, Furukawa A, Suzuki K, Ishii HT, Mukai H, Morrison JH, Janssen WG, Kominami S, Harada N, Kimoto T, Kawato S. (2004) Adult male rat hippocampus synthesizes estradiol from pregnenolone by cytochromes P45017alpha and P450 aromatase localized in neurons. *Proc Natl Acad Sci USA* 101:865–870.

Hojvat S, Emanuele N, Baker G, Connick E, Kirsteins L, Lawrence AM. (1982) Growth hormone (GH), thyroid-stimulating hormone (TSH), and luteinizing hormone (LH)-like peptides in the rodent brain: Non-parallel ontogenetic development with pituitary counterparts. *Brain Res* 256:427–434.

Holm K, Isacson O. (1999) Factors intrinsic to the neuron can induce and maintain its ability to promote axonal outgrowth: A role for Bcl-2? *Trends Neurosci* 22:269–273.

Holmes MM, Wide JK, Galea LA. (2002) Low levels of estradiol facilitate, whereas high levels of estradiol impair, working memory performance on the radial-arm maze. *Behav Neurosci* 116:928–934.

Holzenberger M, Dupont J, Ducos B, Leneuve P, Geloen A, Even PC, Cervera P, Le Bouc Y. (2003) IGF-1 receptor regulates lifespan and resistance to oxidative stress in mice. *Nature* 421:182–187.

Honda K, Sawada H, Kihara T, Urushitani M, Nakamizo T, Akaile A, Shimohama S. (2000) Phosphatidylinositol 3-kinase mediates neuroprotection by estrogen in cultured cortical neurons. *J Neurosci Res* 60:321–327.

Honda S, Harada N, Abe-Dohmae S, Takagi Y. (1999) Identification of cis-acting elements in the proximal promoter region for brain-specific exon 1 of the mouse aromatase gene. *Mol Brain Res* 66:122–132.

Hong M, Lee VMY. (1997) Insulin and insulin-like growth factor-1 regulate tau phosphorylation in cultured human neurons. *J Biol Chem* 272:19547–19553.

Horsburgh K, Kelly S, McCulloch J, Higgins GA, Roses AD, Nicoll JA. (1999) Increased neuronal damage in apolipoprotein E-deficient mice following global ischaemia. *NeuroReport* 10:837–841.

Horsburgh K, Macrae IM, Carswell H. (2002) Estrogen is neuroprotective via an apolipoprotein E-dependent mechanism in a mouse model of global ischemia. *J Cereb Blood Flow Metab* 22:1189–1195.

Hortnagl H, Hansen L, Kindel G, Schneider B, el Tener A, Hanin I. (1993) Sex differences and estrous cycle-variations in the AF64A-induced cholinergic deficit in the rat hippocampus. *Brain Res Bull* 31:129–134.

Horvath TL. (2005) The hardship of obesity: A soft-wired hypothalamus. *Nat Neurosci* 8:561–565.

Horvath TL. (2006) Synaptic plasticity in energy balance regulation. *Obesity* (Silver Spring) 14 (Suppl 5):228S–233S.

Horvath TL, Garcia-Segura LM, Naftolin F. (1997a) Control of gonadotropin feedback: The possible role of estrogen-induced hypothalamic synaptic plasticity. *Gynecol Endocrinol* 11:139–143.

Horvath TL, Garcia-Segura LM, Naftolin F. (1997b) Lack of gonadotropin-positive feedback in the male rat is associated with lack of estrogen-induced synaptic plasticity in the arcuate nucleus. *Neuroendocrinology* 65:136–140.

Horvath TL, Roa-Pena L, Jakab RL, Simpson ER, Naftolin F. (1997c) Aromatase in axonal processes of early postnatal hypothalamic and limbic areas including the cingulate cortex. *J Steroid Biochem Mol Biol* 61:349–357.

Horvath TL, Diano S, van den Pol AN. (1999a) Synaptic interaction between hypocretin (orexin) and neuropeptide Y cells in the rodent and primate hypothalamus: A novel circuit implicated in metabolic and endocrine regulations. *J Neurosci* 19:1072–1087.

Horvath TL, Peyron C, Diano S, Ivanov A, Aston-Jones G, Kilduff TS, van den Pol AN. (1999b) Hypocretin (orexin) activation and synaptic innervation of the locus coeruleus noradrenergic system. *J Comp Neurol* 415: 145–159.

Horvath TL, Diano S. (2004) The floating blueprint of hypothalamic feeding circuits. *Nat Rev Neurosci* 5:662–667.

Horvath TL, Gao XB. (2005) Input organization and plasticity of hypocretin neurons: Possible clues to obesity's association with insomnia. *Cell Metab* 1:279–286.

Hoshooley JS, Sherry DF. (2007) Greater hippocampal neuronal recruitment in food-storing than in non-food-storing birds. *Dev Neurobiol* 67:406–414.

Hoskins SG. (1990) Metamorphosis of the amphibian eye. *J Neurobiol* 21:970–989.

Howdeshell KL. (2002) A model of the development of the brain as a construct of the thyroid system. *Environ Health Perspect* 110 (Suppl 3):337–348.

Howes OD, McDonald C, Cannon M, Arseneault L, Boydell J, Murray RM. (2004) Pathways to schizophrenia: The impact of environmental factors. *Int J Neuropsychopharmacol* 7 (Suppl 1):S7–S13.

Hoyk Z, Párducz A, Theodosis DT. (2001) The highly sialylated isoform of the neural cell adhesion molecule is required for estradiol-induced morphological synaptic plasticity in the adult arcuate nucleus. *Eur J Neurosci* 13:649–656.

Hoyk Z, Párducz A, Garcia-Segura LM. (2004) Dehydroepiandrosterone regulates astroglia reaction to denervation of olfactory glomeruli. *Glia* 48:207–216.

Hoyk Z, Varga C, Párducz A. (2006) Estrogen-induced region specific decrease in the density of 5-bromo-2-deoxyuridine-labeled cells in the olfactory bulb of adult female rats. *Neuroscience* 141:1919–1924.

Hsieh J, Aimone JB, Kaspar BK, Kuwabara T, Nakashima K, Gage FH. (2004) IGF-1 instructs multipotent adult neural progenitor cells to become oligodendrocytes. *J Cell Biol* 164:111–122.

Hsu HK, Yang RC, Shih HC, Hsieh YL, Chen UY, Hsu C. (2001) Prenatal exposure of testosterone prevents SDN-POA neurons of postnatal male rats from apoptosis through NMDA receptor. *J Neurophysiol* 86:2374–2380.

Huang CC, You JL, Lee CC, Hsu KS. (2003) Insulin induces a novel form of postsynaptic mossy fiber long-term depression in the hippocampus. *Mol Cell Neurosci* 24:831–841.

Huang CC, Lee CC, Hsu KS. (2004) An investigation into signal transduction mechanisms involved in insulin-induced long-term depression in the CA1 region of the hippocampus. *J Neurochem* 89:217–231.

Huang H, Marsh-Armstrong AN, Brown DD. (1999) Metamorphosis is inhibited in transgenic Xenopus laevis tadpoles that overexpress type III deiodinase. *Proc Natl Acad Sci USA* 96:962–967.

Huang H, Cai L, Remo BF, Brown DD. (2001) Timing of metamorphosis and the onset of the negative feedback loop between the thyroid gland and the pituitary is controlled by type II iodothyronine deiodinase in Xenopus laevis. *Proc Natl Acad Sci USA* 98: 7348–7353.

Huang L, DeVries GJ, Bittman EL. (1998) Photoperiod regulates neuronal bromodeoxyuridine labeling in the brain of a seasonally breeding mammal. *J Neurobiol* 36:410–420.

Huang WL, Harper CG, Evans SF, Newnham JP, Dunlop SA. (2001) Repeated prenatal corticosteroid administration delays myelination of the corpus callosum in fetal sheep. *Int J Dev Neurosci* 19:415–425.

Hubel DH, Wiesel TN. (1965). Binocular interaction in striate cortex of kittens reared with artificial squint. *J Neurophysiol* 28:1041–1059.

Huhman KL. (2006) Social conflict models: Can they inform us about human psychopathology? *Horm Behav* 50:640–646.

Huizink AC, Robles de Medina PG, Mulder EJH, Visser GHA, Buitelaar JK. (2003) Stress during pregnancy is associated with developmental outcome in infancy. *J Child Psychol Psychiatry* 44:810–818.

Huizink AC, Mulder EJH, Buitelaar JK. (2004) Prenatal stress and risk for psychopathology: Specific effects or induction of general susceptibility? *Psychol Bull* 130:115–142.

Hung AJ, Stanbury MG, Shanabrough M, Horvath TL, Garcia-Segura LM, Naftolin F. (2003) Estrogen, synaptic plasticity and hypothalamic reproductive aging. *Exp Gerontol* 38:53–59.

Hunt RK, Jacobson M. (1970) Brain enhancement in tadpoles: Increased DNA concentration after somatotrophin or prolactin. *Science* 170:342–344.

Hunt RK, Jacobson M. (1971) Neurogenesis in frogs after early larval treatment with somatotropin or prolactin. *Dev Biol* 26:100–124.

Huot RL, Thrivikraman KV, Meaney MJ, Plotsky PM. (2001) Development of adult ethanol preference and anxiety as a consequence of neonatal maternal separation in Long Evans rats and reversal with antidepressant treatment. *Psychopharmacology* 158:366–373.

Huot RL, Plotsky PM, Lenox RH, McNamara RK. (2002) Neonatal maternal separation reduces hippocampal mossy fiber density in adult Long Evans rats. *Brain Res* 950:52–63.

Huppenbauer CB, Tanzer L, DonCarlos LL, Jones KJ. (2005) Gonadal steroid attenuation of developing hamster facial motoneuron loss by axotomy: Equal efficacy of testosterone, dihydrotestosterone, and 17-beta estradiol. *J Neurosci* 25:4004–4013.

Huppert FA, Van Niekerk JK, Herbert J. (2000) Dehydroepiandrosterone (DHEA) supplementation for cognition and well-being. *Cochrane Database Syst Rev* (2):CD000304.

Hurley LL, Wallace AM, Sartor JJ, Ball GF. (2008) Photoperiodic induced changes in reproductive state of border canaries (*Serinus canaria*) are associated with marked variation in hypothalamic gonadotropin-releasing hormone immunoreactivity and the volume of song control regions. *Gen Comp Endocrinol* 158:10–19.

Husson I, Mesples B, Bac P, Vamecq J, Evrard P, Gressens P. (2002) Melatoninergic neuroprotection of the murine periventricular white matter against neonatal excitotoxic challenge. *Ann Neurol* 51:82–92.

Hut RA, Van der Zee EA, Jansen K, Gerkema MP, Daan S. (2002) Gradual reappearance of post-hibernation circadian rhythmicity correlates with numbers of vasopressin-containing neurons in the suprachiasmatic nuclei of European ground squirrels. *J Comp Physiol B* 172:59–70.

Hutchison JB. (1991) Hormonal control of behaviour: Steroid action in the brain. *Curr Opin Neurobiol* 1:562–570.

Huttunen MO, Machon RA, Mednick SA. (1994) Prenatal factors in the pathogenesis of schizophrenia. *Br J Psychiatr Suppl* :15–19.

Hwang IK, Yoo KY, Park SK, An SJ, Lee YL, Choi SY, Kang JK, Kwon YG, Kang TC, Won MH. (2004) Expression and changes of endogenous insulin-like growth factor-1 in neurons and glia in the gerbil hippocampus and dentate gyrus after ischemic insult. *Neurochem Int* 45:149–156.

Ibanez C, Shields SA, El-Etr M, Baulieu EE, Schumacher M, Franklin RJ. (2004) Systemic progesterone administration results in a partial reversal of the age-associated decline in CNS remyelination following toxin-induced demyelination in male rats. *Neuropathol Appl Neurobiol* 30:80–89.

Ignatius MJ, Gebicke-Harter PJ, Skene JH, Schilling JW, Weisgraber KH, Mahley RW, Shooter EM. (1986) Expression of apolipoprotein E during nerve degeneration and regeneration. *Proc Natl Acad Sci USA* 83:1125–1129.

Iliadou A, Cnattingius S, Lichtenstein P. (2004) Low birth weight and type 2 diabetes: A study on 11,162 Swedish twins. *Int J Epidemiol* 33:948–953.

Inagaki T, Dutchak P, Zhao G, Ding X, Gautron L, Parameswara V, Li Y, Goetz R, Mohammadi M, Esser V, Elmquist JK, Gerard RD, Burgess SC, Hammer RE, Mangelsdorf DJ, Kliewer SA. (2007) Endocrine regulation of the fasting response by PPARalpha-mediated induction of fibroblast growth factor 21. *Cell Metab* 5:415–425.

Inoue T, Akahira J, Suzuki T, Darnel AD, Kaneko C, Takahashi K, Hatori M, Shirane R, Kumabe T, Kurokawa Y, Satomi S, Sasano H. (2002) Progesterone production and actions in the human central nervous system and neurogenic tumors. *J Clin Endocrinol Metab* 87:5325–5331.

Inui Y, Miwa S. (1985) Thyroid hormone induces metamorphosis of flounder larvae. *Gen Comp Endocrinol* 60:450–454.

Ipina SL, Ruiz-Marcos A. (1986) Dendritic structure alterations induced by hypothyroidism in pyramidal neurons of the rat visual cortex. *Brain Res* 394:61–67.

Ipina SL, Ruiz-Marcos A, Escobar del Rey F, Morreale de Escobar G. (1987) Pyramidal cortical cell morphology studied by multivariate analysis: Effects of neonatal thyroidectomy, ageing and thyroxine-substitution therapy. *Brain Res* 465:219–229.

Irwin RP, Maragakis NJ, Rogawski MA, Purdy RH, Farb DH, Paul SM. (1992) Pregnenolone sulphate augments NMDA receptor mediated increases in intracellular Ca^{2+} in cultured rat hippocampal neurons. *Neurosci Lett* 141:30–34.

Ishikawa A, Ishiguro S, Tamai M. (1996) Accumulation of γ-aminobutyric acid in diabetic rat retinal Müller cells evidenced by electron microscopy immunohistochemistry. *Curr Eye Res* 15:958–964.

Ishiwata H, Shiga T, Okado N. (2005) Selective serotonin reuptake inhibitor treatment of early postnatal mice reverses their prenatal stress-induced brain dysfunction. *Neuroscience* 133:893–901.

Isgor C, Sengelaub DR. (1998) Prenatal gonadal steroids affect adult spatial behavior, CA1 and CA3 pyramidal cell morphology in rats. *Horm Behav* 34:183–198.

Isgor C, Watson SJ. (2005) Estrogen receptor alpha and beta mRNA expressions by proliferating and differentiating cells in the adult rat dentate gyrus and subventricular zone. *Neuroscience* 134:847–856.

Ishii H, Tsurugizawa T, Ogiue-Ikeda M, Asashima M, Mukai H, Murakami G, Hojo Y, Kimoto T, Kawato S. (2007) Local production of sex hormones and their modulation of hippocampal synaptic plasticity. *Neuroscientist* 13:323–334.

Ishunina TA, van Beurden D, van der Meulen G, Unmehopa UA, Hol EM, Huitinga I, Swaab DF. (2005) Diminished aromatase immunoreactivity in the hypothalamus, but not in the basal forebrain nuclei in Alzheimer's disease. *Neurobiol Aging* 26:173–194.

Islamov RR, Hendricks WA, Jones RJ, Lyall GJ, Spanier NS, Murashov AK. (2002) 17Beta-estradiol stimulates regeneration of sciatic nerve in female mice. *Brain Res* 943:283–286.

Israel JM, Poulain DA, Oliet SH. (2008) Oxytocin-induced postinhibitory rebound firing facilitates bursting activity in oxytocin neurons. *J Neurosci* 28:385–394.

Ito M. (2002) The molecular organization of cerebellar long-term depression. *Nat Rev Neurosci* 3:896–902.

Ito S, Murakami S, Yamanouchi K, Arai Y. (1986) Prenatal androgen exposure, preoptic area and reproductive functions in the female rat. *Brain Dev* 8:463–468.

Itti E, Gaw Gonzalo IT, Pawlikowska-Haddal A, Boone KB, Mlikotic A, Itti L, Mishkin FS, Swerdloff RS. (2006) The structural brain correlates of cognitive deficits in adults with Klinefelter's syndrome. *J Clin Endocrinol Metab* 91:1423–1427.

Ivanova T, Mendez P, Garcia-Segura LM, Beyer C. (2002) Rapid stimulation of the PI3-kinase/Akt signalling pathway in developing midbrain neurons by oestrogen. *J Neuroendocrinol* 14:73–79.

Izumi Y, Yamada KA, Matsukawa M, Zorumski CF. (2003) Effects of insulin on long-term potentiation in hippocampal slices from diabetic rats. *Diabetologia* 46:1007–1012.

Jackson-Guilford J, Leander JD, Nisenbaum LK. (2000) The effect of streptozotocin-induced diabetes on cell proliferation in the rat dentate gyrus. *Neurosci Lett* 293:91–94.

Jacob S, Poeggeler B, Weishaupt JH, Siren AL, Hardeland R, Bahr M, Ehrenreich H. (2002) Melatonin as a candidate compound for neuroprotection in amyotrophic lateral sclerosis (ALS): High tolerability of daily oral melatonin administration in ALS patients. *J Pineal Res* 33:186–187.

Jacobs LF. (1996) The economy of winter: Phenotypic plasticity in behavior and brain structure. *Biol Bull* 191:92–100.

Jacobson CD, Csernus VJ, Shryne JE, Gorski RA. (1981) The influence of gonadectomy, androgen exposure, or a gonadal graft in the neonatal rat brain on the volume of the sexually dimorphic nucleus of the preoptic area. *J Neurosci* 1:1142–1146.

Jaeger LB, Farr SA, Banks WA, Morley JE. (2002) Effects of orexin-A on memory processing. *Peptides* 23:1683–1688.

Jakab RL, Horvath TL, Leranth C, Harada N, Naftolin F. (1993) Aromatase immunoreactivity in the rat brain gonadectomy-sensitive hypothalamic neurons and an unresponsive "limbic ring" of the lateral septum-bed nucleus-amygdala complex. *J Steroid Biochem Mol Biol* 44:481–498.

Janowsky JS. (2006) The role of androgens in cognition and brain aging in men. *Neuroscience* 138:1015–1020.

Jansen HT, Cutter C, Hardy S, Lehman MN, Goodman RL. (2003) Seasonal plasticity within the gonadotropin-releasing hormone (GnRH) system of the ewe: Changes in identified GnRH inputs and glial association. *Endocrinology* 144:3663–3676.

Jelkmann W. (1992) Erythropoietin: Structure, control of production, and function. *Physiol Rev* 72:449–489.

Jelkmann W. (2007) Erythropoietin after a century of research: Younger than ever. *Eur J Haematol* 78:183–205.

Jellinck PH, Lee SJ, McEwen BS. (2001) Metabolism of dehydroepiandrosterone by rat hippocampal cells in culture: Possible role of aromatization and 7-hydroxylation in neuroprotection. *J Steroid Biochem Mol Biol* 78:313–317.

Jenkins VA, Fallowfield LJ, Schilling V, Howell A. (2002) Does hormone therapy for the treatment of breast cancer have a detrimental effect on memory and cognition? *Breast Cancer Res Treat* 76 (Suppl 1): S137.

Jernigan TL, Trauner DA, Hesselink JR, Tallal PA. (1991) Maturation of human cerebrum observed in vivo during adolescence. *Brain* 114(Pt 5):2037–2049.

Jezierski MK, Sohrabji F. (2001) Neurotrophin expression in the reproductively senescent forebrain is refractory to estrogen stimulation. *Neurobiol Aging* 22:309–319.

Jezierski MK, Sohrabji F. (2003) Estrogen enhances retrograde transport of brain-derived neurotrophic factor in the rodent forebrain. *Endocrinology* 144:5022–5029.

Jiang J, McMurtry J, Niedzwiecki D, Goldman SA. (1998) Insulin-like growth factor-1 is a radial cell-associated neurotrophin that promotes neuronal recruitment from the adult songbird edpendyma/subependyma. *J Neurobiol* 36:1–15.

Joëls M, Krugers HJ. (2007) LTP after stress: Up or down? *Neural Plast* 2007:93202.

Johnson F, Bottjer SW. (1992) Growth and regression of thalamic efferents in the song-control system of male zebra finches. *J Comp Neurol* 326:442–450.

Johnson F, Bottjer SW. (1993) Hormone-induced changes in identified cell populations of the higher vocal center in male canaries. *J Neurobiol* 24:400–418.

Johnson F, Bottjer S. (1995) Differential estrogen accumulation among populations of projection neurons in the higher vocal center of male canaries. *J Neurobiol* 26:87–108.

Johnson SR. (1998) Menopause and hormone replacement therapy. *Med Clin North Am* 82:297–320.

Jones DM, Tucker BA, Rahimtula M, Mearow KM. (2003) The synergistic effects of NGF and IGF-1 on neurite growth in adult sensory neurons: Convergence on the PI 3-kinase signaling pathway. *J Neurochem* 86:1116–1128.

Jones KJ. (1994) Androgenic enhancement of motor neuron regeneration. *Ann N Y Acad Sci* 743:141–161.

Jones KJ, Durica TE, Jacob SK. (1997a) Gonadal steroid preservation of central synaptic input to hamster facial motoneurons following peripheral axotomy. *J Neurocytol* 26:257–266.

Jones KJ, Kinderman NB, Oblinger MM. (1997b) Alterations in glial fibrillary acidic protein (GFAP) mRNA levels in the hamster facial motor nucleus: Effects of axotomy and testosterone. *Neurochem Res* 22:1359–1366.

Jones KJ, Coers S, Storer PD, Tanzer L, Kinderman NB. (1999) Androgenic regulation of the central glia response following nerve damage. *J Neurobiol* 40:560–573.

Jones KJ, Brown TJ, Damaser M. (2001) Neuroprotective effects of gonadal steroids on regenerating peripheral motoneurons. *Brain Res Rev* 37:372–382.

Jones SA, Jolson DM, Cuta KK, Mariash CN, Anderson GW. (2003) Triiodothyronine is a survival factor for developing oligodendrocytes. *Mol Cell Endocrinol* 199:49–60.

Jordan CL, Letinsky MS, Arnold AP. (1989) The role of gonadal hormones in neuromuscular synapse elimination in rats. I. Androgen delays the loss of multiple innervation in the levator ani muscle. *J Neurosci* 9:229–238.

Jourdain P, Bergersen LH, Bhaukaurally K, Bezzi P, Santello M, Domercq M, Matute C, Tonello F, Gundersen V, Volterra A. (2007) Glutamate exocytosis from astrocytes controls synaptic strength. *Nat Neurosci* 10:331–339.

Jung-Testas I, Schumacher M, Robel P, Baulieu EE. (1996) The neurosteroid progesterone increases the expression of myelin proteins (MBP and CNPase) in rat oligodendrocytes in primary culture. *Cell Mol Neurobiol* 16:439–443.

Junk AK, Mammis A, Savitz SI, Singh M, Roth S, Malhotra S, Rosenbaum PS, Cerami A, Brines M, Rosenbaum DM. (2002) Erythropoietin administration protects retinal neurons from acute ischemia-reperfusion injury. *Proc Natl Acad Sci USA* 99:10659–10664.

Juraska JM. (1991) Sex differences in "cognitive" regions of the rat brain. *Psychoneuroendocrinology* 16:105–119.

Juraska JM, Fitch JM, Henderson C, Rivers N. (1985) Sex differences in the dendritic branching of dentate granule cells following differential experience. *Brain Res* 333:73–80.

Juraska JM, Kopcik JR, Washburne DL, Perry DL. (1988) Neonatal castration of male rats affects the dendritic response to differential environments in granule neurons of the hippocampal dentate gyrus. *Psychobiology* 16:406–410.

Kaas JH, Florence SL. (2001) Reorganization of sensory and motor systems in adult mammals after injury. In: (Kaas, JH, ed), *The mutable brain. Dynamics and plastic features of the developing and mature brain.* Harwood Academic Publishers, Amsterdam, pp. 165–242.

Kaasik A, Kalda A, Jaako K, Zharkovsky A. (2001) Dehydroepiandrosterone sulphate prevents oxygen-glucose deprivation-induced injury in cerebellar granule cell culture. *Neuroscience* 102:427–432.

Kabelik D, Weiss SL, Moore MC. (2006) Steroid hormone mediation of limbic brain plasticity and aggression in free-living tree lizards, Urosaurus ornatus. *Horm Behav* 49:587–597.

Kamal A, Biessels GJ, Urban IJ, Gispen WH. (1999) Hippocampal synaptic plasticity in streptozotocin-diabetic rats: Impairment of long-term potentiation and facilitation of long-term depression. *Neuroscience* 90:737–745.

Kamal A, Biessels GJ, Ramakers GM, Gispen WH. (2005) The effect of short duration streptozotocin-induced diabetes mellitus on the late phase and threshold of long-term potentiation induction in the rat. *Brain Res* 1053:126–130.

Kamat A, Hinshelwood MM, Murry BA, Mendelson CR. (2002) Mechanisms in tissue-specific regulation of estrogen biosynthesis in humans. *Trends Endocrinol Metab* 13:122–128.

Kandel ER, Tauc L. (1965) Heterosynaptic facilitation in neurons of the abdominal ganglion of Aplysia depilans. *J Physiol* 181:1–27.

Karchewski LA, Bloechlinger S, Woolf CJ. (2004) Axonal injury-dependent induction of the peripheral benzodiazepine receptor in small-diameter adult rat primary sensory neurons. *Eur J Neurosci* 20:671–683.

Karishma KK, Herbert J. (2002) Dehydroepiandrosterone (DHEA) stimulates neurogenesis in the hippocampus of the rat, promotes survival of newly formed neurons and prevents corticosterone-induced suppression. *Eur J Neurosci* 16:445–453.

Karmarkar UR, Dan Y. (2006) Experience-dependent plasticity in adult visual cortex. *Neuron* 52:577–585.

Kash TL, Winder DG. (2006) Neuropeptide Y and corticotropin-releasing factor bi-directionally modulate inhibitory synaptic transmission in the bed nucleus of the stria terminalis. *Neuropharmacology* 51:1013–1022.

Kauffman AS, Clifton DK, Steiner RA. (2007) Emerging ideas about kisspeptin-GPR54 signaling in the neuroendocrine regulation of reproduction. *Trends Neurosci* 30:504–511.

Kaur G, Heera PK, Srivastava LK. (2002) Neuroendocrine plasticity in GnRH release during rat estrous cycle: Correlation with molecular markers of synaptic remodeling. *Brain Res* 954:21–31.

Kavushansky A, Richter-Levin G. (2006) Effects of stress and corticosterone on activity and plasticity in the amygdala. *J Neurosci Res* 84:1580–1587.

Kavushansky A, Vouimba RM, Cohen H, Richter-Levin G. (2006) Activity and plasticity in the CA1, the dentate gyrus, and the amygdala following controllable vs. uncontrollable water stress. *Hippocampus* 16:35–42.

Kawakami M, Sekiguchi M, Sato K, Kozaki S, Takahashi M. (2001) Erythropoietin receptor-mediated inhibition of exocytotic glutamate release confers neuroprotection during chemical ischemia. *J Biol Chem* 276:39469–39475.

Kehoe P, Bronzino JD. (1999) Neonatal stress alters LTP in freely moving male and female adult rats. *Hippocampus* 9:651–658.

Kelley DB. (1986) Neuroeffector for vocalization in Xenopus laevis: Hormonal regulation of sexual dimorphism. *J Neurobiol* 17:231–248.

Kelley DB, Dennison J. (1990) The vocal motor neurons of Xenopus laevis: Development of sex differences in axon number. *J Neurobiol* 21:869–882.

Kelley KW, Davila DR, Brief S, Simon J, Arkins S. (1988) A pituitary-thymus connection during aging. *Ann N Y Acad Sci* 521:88–98.

Kelly DF, Gonzalo IT, Cohan P, Berman N, Swerdloff R, Wang C. (2000) Hypopituitarism following traumatic brain injury and aneurysmal subarachnoid hemorrhage: A preliminary report. *Journal of Neurosurgery* 93:743–752.

Kelly MJ, Ronnekleiv OK, Ibrahim N, Lagrange AH, Wagner EJ. (2002) Estrogen modulation of K(+) channel activity in hypothalamic neurons involved in the control of the reproductive axis. *Steroids* 67:447–456.

Kelly MJ, Qiu J, Ronnekleiv OK. (2005) Estrogen signaling in the hypothalamus. *Vitam Horm* 71:123–145.

Kempermann G, Kuhn HG, Gage FH. (1998) Experience-induced neurogenesis in the senescent dentate gyrus. *J Neurosci* 18:3206–3212.

Kempermann G, van Praag H, Gage FH. (2000) Activity-dependent regulation of neuronal plasticity and self repair. *Prog Brain Res* 127:35–48.

Kennaway DJ, Rowe SA. (1995) Melatonin binding sites and their role in seasonal reproduction. *J Reprod Fertil* 49 (Suppl):423–435.

Kenyon C. (2005) The plasticity of aging: Insights from long-lived mutants. *Cell* 120:449–460.

Kenyon C, Chang J, Gensch E, Rudner A, Tabtiang R. (1993) A C. elegans mutant that lives twice as long as wild type. *Nature* 366:461–464.

Kester MH, Martinez de Mena R, Obregon MJ, Marinkovic D, Howatson A, Visser TJ, Hume R, Morreale de Escobar G. (2004) Iodothyronine levels in the human developing brain: Major regulatory roles of iodothyronine deiodinases in different areas. *J Clin Endocrinol Metab* 89:3117–3128.

Keuker JI, Luiten PG, Fuchs E. (2003) Preservation of hippocampal neuron numbers in aged rhesus monkeys. *Neurobiol Aging* 24:157–165.

Keverne EB, Curley JP. (2004) Vasopressin, oxytocin and social behaviour. *Curr Opin Neurobiol* 14:777–783.

Keyser-Marcus L, Stafisso-Sandoz G, Gerecke K, Jasnow AM, Nightingale L, Lambert KG, Gatewood J, Kinsley CH. (2001) Alteration of medial preoptic area neurons following pregnancy and pregnancy-like steroidal treatment in the rat. *Brain Res Bull* 55:737–745.

Kihslinger RL, Nevitt GA. (2006) Early rearing environment impacts cerebellar growth in juvenile salmon. *J Exp Biol* 209:504–509.

Kihslinger RL, Lema SC, Nevitt GA. (2006) Environmental rearing conditions produce forebrain differences in wild Chinook salmon Oncorhynchus tshawytscha. *Comp Biochem Physiol A Mol Integr Physiol* 145:145–151.

Kikuyama S, Miyakawa M, Arai Y. (1979) Influence of thyroid hormone on the development of peoptic-hypothalamic monoaminergic neurons in tadpoles of Bufo bufo japonicus. *Cell Tissue Res* 198:27–33.

Kilic E, Kilic Ü, Soliz J, Bassetti CL, Gassmann M, Hermann DM. (2005) Brain-derived erythropoietin protects from focal cerebral ischemia by dual activation of ERK-1/-2 and Akt pathways. *FASEB J* 19:2026–2028.

Kilic Ü, Kilic E,, Soliz J, Bassetti CI, Gassmann M, Hermann DM. (2005) Erythropoietin protects from axotomy-induced degeneration of retinal ganglion cells by activating ERK-1/-2. *FASEB J* 19:249–251.

Kim HJ, Park CH, Roh GS, Kang SS, Cho GJ, Choi WS. (2002) Changes of steroidogenic acute regulatory protein mRNA expression in postnatal rat development. *Dev Brain Res* 139:247–254.

Kim HJ, Ha M, Park CH, Park SJ, Youn SM, Kang SS, Cho GJ, Choi WS. (2003a) StAR and steroidogenic enzyme transcriptional regulation in the rat brain: Effects of acute alcohol administration. *Mol Brain Res* 115:39–49.

Kim HJ, Kim JE, Ha M, Kang SS, Kim JT, Park LS, Paek SH, Jung HW, Kim DG, Cho GJ, Choi WS. (2003b) Steroidogenic acute regulatory protein expression in the normal human brain and intracranial tumors. *Brain Res* 978:245–249.

Kim HJ, Kang SS, Cho GJ, Choi WS. (2004) Steroidogenic acute regulatory protein: Its presence and function in brain neurosteroidogenesis. *Arch Histol Cytol* 67:383–392.

Kim JJ, Foy MR, Thompson RF. (1996) Behavioral stress modifies hippocampal plasticity through N-methyl-D-aspartate receptor activation. *Proc Natl Acad Sci USA* 93:4750–4753.

Kim JJ, Yoon KS. (1998) Stress: Metaplastic effects in the hippocampus. *Trends Neurosci* 21:505–509.

Kim JJ, Song EY, Kosten TA. (2006) Stress effects in the hippocampus: Synaptic plasticity and memory. *Stress* 9:1–11.

Kim JS, Kim HY, Kim JH, Shin HK, Lee SH, Lee YS, Son H. (2002) Enhancement of rat hippocampal long-term potentiation by 17 beta-estradiol involves mitogen-activated protein kinase-dependent and -independent components. *Neurosci Lett* 332:65–69.

Kim SJ, Foster DL, Wood RI. (1999) Prenatal testosterone masculinizes synaptic input to gonadotropin-releasing hormone neurones in sheep. *Biol Reprod* 61:599–605.

Kimelberg HK, Jin Y, Charniga C, Feustel PJ. (2003) Neuroprotective activity of tamoxifen in permanent focal ischemia. *J Neurosurg* 99:138–142.

Kimonides VG, Khatibi NH, Svendsen CN, Sofroniew MV, Herbert J. (1998) Dehydroepiandrosterone (DHEA) and DHEA-sulfate (DHEAS) protect hippocampal neurons against excitatory amino acid-induced neurotoxicity. *Proc Natl Acad Sci USA* 95:1852–1857.

Kimonides VG, Spillantini MG, Sofroniew MV, Fawcett JW, Herbert J. (1999) Dehydroepiandrosterone antagonizes the neurotoxic effects of corticosterone and translocation of stress-activated protein kinase 3 in hippocampal primary cultures. *Neuroscience* 89:429–436.

Kimoto T, Tsurugizawa T, Ohta Y, Makino J, Tamura H, Hojo Y, Takata N, Kawato S. (2001) Neurosteroid synthesis by cytochrome p450-containing systems localized in the rat brain hippocampal neurons: N-methyl-D-aspartate and calcium-dependent synthesis. *Endocrinology* 142:3578–3589.

King CE, Rodger J, Bartlett C, Esmaili T, Dunlop SA, Beazley LD. (2007) Erythropoietin is both neuroprotective and neuroregenerative following optic nerve transection. *Exp Neurol* 205:48–55.

King JC, Williams TH, Gerall AA. (1974) Transformations of hypothalamic arcuate neurons. I. Changes associated with stages of the estrous cycle. *Cell Tissue Res* 153:497–515.

King JC, Letourneau RL. (1994) Luteinizing hormone-releasing hormone terminals in the median eminence of rats undergo dramatic changes after gonadectomy, as revealed by electron microscopic image analysis. *Endocrinology* 134: 1340–1351.

King JC, Rubin BS. (1994) Dynamic changes in LHRH neurovascular terminals with various endocrine conditions in adults. *Horm Behav* 28:349–356.

King SR, Manna PR, Ishii T, Syapin PJ, Ginsberg SD, Wilson K, Walsh LP, Parker KL, Stocco DM, Smith RG, Lamb DJ. (2002) An essential component in steroid synthesis, the steroidogenic acute regulatory protein, is expressed in discrete regions of the brain. *J Neurosci* 22:10613–10620.

King SR, Ginsberg SD, Ishii T, Smith RG, Parke KL, Lamb DJ. (2004a) The steroidogenic acute regulatory protein is expressed in steroidogenic cells of the day-old brain. *Endocrinology* 145:4775–4780.

King SR, Matassa AA, White EK, Walsh LP, Jo Y, Rao RM, Stocco DM, Reyland ME. (2004b) Oxysterols regulate expression of the steroidogenic acute regulatory protein. *J Mol Endocrinol* 32:507–517.

Kinsley CH, Madonia L, Gifford GW, Tureski K, Griffin GR, Lowry C, Williams J, Collins J, McLearie H, Lambert KG. (1999) Motherhood improves learning and memory. *Nature* 402:137–138.

Kinsley CH, Trainer R, Stafisso-Sandoz G, Quadros P, Marcus LK, Hearon C, Meyer EA, Hester N, Morgan M, Kozub FJ, Lambert KG. (2006) Motherhood and the hormones of pregnancy modify concentrations of hippocampal neuronal dendritic spines. *Horm Behav* 49:131–142.

Kipper-Galperin M, Galilly R, Danenberg HD, Brenner T. (1999) Dehydroepiandrosterone selectively inhibits production of tumor necrosis factor alpha and interleukin-6 in astrocytes. *Int J Dev Neurosci* 17:765–775.

Kirn JR, Alvarez-Buylla A, Nottebohm F. (1991) Production and survival of projection neurons in a forebrain vocal center of adult male canaries. *J Neurosci* 11:1756–1762.

Kirn JR, Nottebohm F. (1993) Direct evidence for loss and replacement of projection neurons in adult canary brain. *J Neurosci* 13:1654–1663.

Kirn J, O'Loughlin B, Kasparian S, Nottebohm F. (1994) Cell death and neuronal recruitment in the high vocal center of adult male canaries are temporally related to changes in song. *Proc Natl Acad Sci USA* 91:7844–7848.

Kis Z, Horvath S, Hoyk Z, Toldi J, Párducz A. (1999) Estrogen effects on arcuate neurons in rat. An in situ electrophysiological study. *NeuroReport* 10:3649–3652.

Klein DC, Moore RY, Reppert SM (eds). (1991) *Suprachiasmatic nucleus. The mind's clock.* Oxford University Press, New York.

Klotz DM, Hewitt SC, Ciana P, Raviscioni M, Lindzey JK, Foley J, Maggi A, DiAugustine RP, Korach KS (2002) Requirement of estrogen receptor-alpha in insulin-like growth factor-1 (IGF-1)-induced uterine responses and in vivo evidence for IGF-1/estrogen receptor cross-talk. *J Biol Chem* 277:8531–8537.

Kobayashi H, Wada M, Uemura H. (1972) The hypothalamic median eminence as a neuroendocrine organ. *Med J Osaka Univ* 23:43–55.

Koehl M, Barbazanges A, Le Moal M, Maccari S. (1997) Prenatal stress induces a phase advance of circadian corticosterone rhythm in adult rats which is prevented by postnatal stress. *Brain Res* 759:317–320.

Koehl M, Daurnaudery M, Dulluc J, Van Reeth O, Le Moal M, Maccari S. (1999) Prenatal stress alters circadian activity of hypothalamo–pituitary–adrenal axis and hippocampal corticosteroid receptors in adult rats of both gender. *J Neurobiology* 40:302–315.

Koenig HL, Schumacher M, Ferzaz B, Do Thi AN, Ressouches A, Guennoun R, Jung-Testas I, Robel P, Akwa Y, Baulieu EE. (1995) Progesterone synthesis and myelin formation by Schwann cells. *Science* 268:1500–1503.

Koenig JI, Elmer GI, Shepard PD, Lee PR, Mayo C, Joy B, Hercher E, Brady DL. (2005) Prenatal exposure to a repeated variable stress paradigm elicits behavioral and neuroendocrinological changes in the adult offspring: Potential relevance to schizophrenia. *Behav Brain Res* 156:251–261.

Koh KB, Lee BK. (1998) Reduced lymphocyte proliferation and interleukin-2 production in anxiety disorders. *Psychosom Med* 60:479–483.

Kohama SG, Goss JR, McNeill TH, Finch CE. (1995) Glial fibrillary acidic protein mRNA increases at proestrus in the arcuate nucleus of mice. *Neurosci Lett* 183:164–166.

Kojima M, Hosoda H, Date Y, Nakazato M, Matsuo H, Kangawa K. (1999) Ghrelin is a growth-hormone-releasing acylated peptide from stomach. *Nature* 402:656–660.

Kokay IC, Bull PM, Davis RL, Ludwig M, Grattan DR. (2006) Expression of the long form of the prolactin receptor in magnocellular oxytocin neurons is associated with specific prolactin regulation of oxytocin neurons. *Am J Physiol Regul Integr Comp Physiol* 290:R1216–R1225.

Kokiko ON, Murashov AK, Hoane MR. (2006) Administration of raloxifene reduces sensorimotor and working memory deficits following traumatic brain injury. *Behav Brain Res* 170:233–240.

Kokoeva MV, Yin H, Flier JS. (2005) Neurogenesis in the hypothalamus of adult mice: Potential role in energy balance. *Science* 310:679–683.

Kole MHP, Costoli T, Koolhaas JM, Fuchs E. (2004) Bi-directional shift in the Cornu Ammonis 3 pyramidal dendritic organization following brief stress. *Neuroscience* 125:337–347.

Kollros JJ, Bovbjerg AM. (1997) Growth and death of rohon-Beard cells in Rana pipiens and Ceratophrys ornata. *J Morphol* 232:67–78.

Kondo N, Kondo J. (1992) Identification of novel blood proteins specific for mammalian hibernation. *J Biol Chem* 267:473–478.

Kondo N, Sekijima T, Kondo J, Takamatsu N, Tohya K, Ohtsu T. (2006) Circannual control of hibernation by HP complex in the brain. *Cell* 125:161–172.

Konishi M, Akutagawa E. (1985) Neuronal growth, atrophy and death in a sexually dimorphic song nucleus in the zebra finch brain. *Nature* 315:145–147.

Konishi M, Akutagawa E. (1987) Hormonal control of cell death in a sexually dimorphic song nucleus in the zebra finch. *Ciba Found Symp* 126:173–185.

Konishi M, Akutagawa E. (1988) A critical period for estrogen action on neurons of the song control system in the zebra finch. *Proc Natl Acad Sci USA* 85:7006–7007.

Konishi Y, Chui DH, Hirose H, Kunishita T, Tabira T. (1993) Trophic effect of erythropoietin and other hematopoietic factors on central cholinergic neurons in vitro and in vivo. *Brain Res* 609:29–35.

Koo JW, Park CH, Choi SH, Kim NJ, Kim HS, Choe JC, Suh YH. (2003) The postnatal environment can counteract prenatal effects on cognitive ability, cell proliferation, and synaptic protein expression. *FASEB J* 17:1556–1558.

Koski CL, Hila S, Hoffman GE. (2004) Regulation of cytokine-induced neuron death by ovarian hormones: Involvement of antiapoptotic protein expression and c-JUN N-terminal kinase-mediated proapoptotic signaling. *Endocrinology* 145:95–103.

Kossut M. (1998) Experience-dependent changes in function and anatomy of adult barrel cortex. *Exp Brain Res* 123:110–116.

Kosten TA, Lee HJ, Kim JJ. (2006) Early life stress impairs fear conditioning in adult male and female rats. *Brain Res* 1087:142–150.

Kow LM, Pfaff DW. (1998) Mapping of neural and signal transduction pathways for lordosis in the search for estrogen actions on the central nervous system. *Behav Brain Res* 92:169–180.

Kozlowski GP, Coates PW. (1985) Ependymoneuronal specializations between LHRH fibers and cells of the cerebroventricular system. *Cell Tissue Res* 242:301–311.

Kramár EA, Armstrong DL, Ikeda S, Wayner MJ, Harding JW, Wright JW. (2001) The effects of angiotensin IV analogs on long-term potentiation within the CA1 region of the hippocampus in vitro. *Brain Res* 897:114–121.

Kramer AF, Hahn S, Cohen NJ, Banich MT, McAuley E, Harrison CR, Chason J, Vakil E, Bardell L, Boileau RA, Colcombe A. (1999) Ageing, fitness and neurocognitive function. *Nature* 400:418–419.

Kramer AF, Erickson KI, Colcombe SJ. (2006) Exercise, cognition, and the aging brain. *J Appl Physiol* 101:1237–1242.

Krantz SB. (1991) Erythropoietin. *Blood* 77:419–434.

Kravitz HM, Janssen I, Lotrich FE, Kado DM, Bromberger JT. (2006) Sex steroid hormone gene polymorphisms and depressive symptoms in women at midlife. *Am J Med* 119 (Suppl 1):S87–S93.

Kreitschmann-Andermahr I. (2005) Subarachnoid hemorrhage as a cause of hypopituitarism. *Pituitary* 8:219–225.

Kretz O, Fester L, Wehrenberg U, Zhou L, Brauckmann S, Zhao S, Prange-Kiel J, Naumann T, Jarry H, Frotscher M, Rune GM. (2004) Hippocampal synapses depend on hippocampal estrogen synthesis. *J Neurosci* 24:5913–5921.

Kriegsfeld LJ, Silver R. (2006) The regulation of neuroendocrine function: Timing is everything. *Horm Behav* 49:557–574.

Krilowicz BL, Glotzbach SF, Heller HC. (1988) Neuronal activity during sleep and complete bouts of hibernation. *Am J Physiol* 255:R1008–R1019.

Krizsan-Agbas D, Smith PG. (2002) Estrogen modulates myometrium-induced sympathetic neurite formation through actions on target and ganglion. *Neuroscience* 114:339–347.

Krug R, Born J, Rasch B. (2006) A 3-day estrogen treatment improves prefrontal cortex-dependent cognitive function in postmenopausal women. *Psychoneuroendocrinology* 31:965–975.

Krugers HJ, Alfarez DN, Karst H, Parashkouhi K, van Gemert N, Joëls M. (2005) Corticosterone shifts different forms of synaptic potentiation in opposite directions. *Hippocampus* 15:697–703.

Kuhlmann AC, Guilarte TR. (2000) Cellular and subcellular localization of peripheral benzodiazepine receptors after trimethyltin neurotoxicity. *J Neurochem* 74:1694–1704.

Kuhn ER, De Groef B, Van der Geyten S, Darras VM. (2005) Corticotropin-releasing hormone-mediated metamorphosis in the neotenic axolotl Ambystoma mexicanum: Synergistic involvement of thyroxine and corticoids on brain type II deiodinase. *Gen Comp Endocrinol* 143:75–81.

Kuhn HG, Dickinson-Anson H, Gage FH. (1996) Neurogenesis in the dentate gyrus of the adult rat: Age-related decrease of neuronal progenitor proliferation. *J Neurosci* 16:2027–2033.

Kuipers SD, Trentani A, Den Boer JA, Ter Horst GJ. (2003) Molecular correlates of impaired prefrontal plasticity in response to chronic stress. *J Neurochem* 85:1312–1323.

Kujawa KA, Emeric E, Jones KJ. (1991) Testosterone differentially regulates the regenerative properties of injured hamster facial motoneurons. *J Neurosci* 11:3898–3906.

Kullmann DM, Lamsa KP. (2007) Long-term synaptic plasticity in hippocampal interneurons. *Nat Rev Neurosci* 8:687–699.

Kumon Y, Kim SC, Tompkins P, Stevens A, Sakaki S, Loftus CM. (2000) Neuroprotective effect of postischemic administration of progesterone in spontaneously hypertensive rats with focal cerebral ischemia. *J Neurosurg* 92:848–852.

Kunduzova OR, Escourrou G, De La Farge F, Salvayre R, Seguelas MH, Leducq N, Bono F, Herbert JM, Parini A. (2004) Involvement of peripheral benzodiazepine receptor in the oxidative stress, death-signaling pathways, and renal injury induced by ischemia-reperfusion. *J Am Soc Nephrol* 15:2152–2160.

Kuroki Y, Fukushima K, Kanda Y, Mizuno K, Watanabe Y. (2001) Neuroprotection by estrogen via extracellular signal-regulated kinase against quinolinic acid-induced cell death in the rat hippocampus. *Eur J Neurosci* 13:472–476.

Kurz EM, Sengelaub DR, Arnold AP. (1986) Androgens regulate the dendritic length of mammalian motoneurons in adulthood. *Science* 232:395–298.

Kurz EM, Brewer RG, Sengelaub DR. (1991) Hormonally mediated plasticity of motoneuron morphology in the adult rat spinal cord: A cholera toxin-HRP study. *J Neurobiol* 22:976–988.

Labombarda F, Guennoun R, Gonzalez S, Roig P, Lima A, Schumacher M, De Nicola AF. (2000) Immunocytochemical evidence for a progesterone receptor in neurons and glial cells of the rat spinal cord. *Neurosci Lett* 288:29–32.

Labombarda F, Gonzalez SL, Gonzalez DM, Guennoun R, Schumacher M, De Nicola AF. (2002) Cellular basis for progesterone neuroprotection in the injured spinal cord. *J Neurotrauma* 19:343–355.

Labombarda F, Gonzalez SL, Deniselle MC, Vinson GP, Schumacher M, De Nicola AF, Guennoun R. (2003) Effects of injury and progesterone treatment on progesterone receptor and progesterone binding protein 25-Dx expression in the rat spinal cord. *J Neurochem* 87:902–913.

Labombarda F, Gonzalez S, Gonzalez Deniselle MC, Garay L, Guennoun R, Schumacher M, De Nicola AF. (2006a) Progesterone increases the expression of myelin basic protein and the number of cells showing NG2 immunostaining in the lesioned spinal cord. *J Neurotrauma* 23:181–192.

Labombarda F, Pianos A, Liere P, Eychenne B, Gonzalez S, Cambourg A, De Nicola AF, Schumacher M, Guennoun R. (2006b) Injury elicited increase in spinal cord neurosteroid content analyzed by gas chromatography mass spectrometry. *Endocrinology* 147:1847–1859.

Lacapere JJ, Papadopoulos V. (2003) Peripheral-type benzodiazepine receptor: Structure and function of a cholesterol-binding protein in steroid and bile acid biosynthesis. *Steroids* 68:569–585.

Lacor P, Gandolfo P, Tonon MC, Brault E, Dalibert I, Schumacher M, Benavides J, Ferzaz B. (1999) Regulation of the expression of peripheral benzodiazepine receptors and their endogenous ligands during rat sciatic nerve degeneration and regeneration: A role for PBR in neurosteroidogenesis. *Brain Res* 815:70–80.

Lafarga M, Palacios G, Perez R. (1975) Morphological aspects of the functional synchronization of supraoptic nucleus neurons. *Experientia* 31:348–349.

Lai M, Horsburgh K, Bae SE, Carter RN, Stenvers DJ, Fowler JH, Yau JL, Gomez-Sanchez CE, Holmes MC, Kenyon CJ, Seckl JR, Macleod MR. (2007) Forebrain mineralocorticoid receptor overexpression enhances memory, reduces anxiety and attenuates neuronal loss in cerebral ischaemia. *Eur J Neurosci* 25:1832–1842.

Lai ZN, Emtner M, Roos P, Nyberg F. (1991) Characterization of putative growth hormone receptors in human choroid plexus. *Brain Res* 546:222–226.

Lam TT, Leranth C. (2003a) Role of the medial septum diagonal band of Broca cholinergic neurons in oestrogen-induced spine synapse formation on hippocampal CA1 pyramidal cells of female rats. *Eur J Neurosci* 17:1997–2005.

Lam TT, Leranth C. (2003b) Gonadal hormones act extrinsic to the hippocampus to influence the density of hippocampal astroglial processes. *Neuroscience* 116:491–498.

Lambert JJ, Belelli D, Peden DR, Vardy AW, Peters JA. (2003) Neurosteroid modulation of GABA$_A$ receptors. *Prog Neurobiol* 71:67–80.

Lamberts SWJ, van den Beld AW, van der Lely AJ. (1997) The endocrinology of aging. *Science* 278:419–424.

Landfield PW. (1988) Hippocampal neurobiological mechanisms of age-related memory dysfunction. *Neurobiol Aging* 9:571–579.

Lang S. (2002) The role of peripheral benzodiazepine receptors (PBRs) in CNS pathophysiology. *Curr Med Chem* 9:1411–1415.

Langle SL, Poulain DA, Theodosis DT. (2003) Induction of rapid, activity-dependent neuronal-glial remodeling in the adult rat hypothalamus in vitro. *Eur J Neurosci* 18:206–214.

Langub MC, Watson RE. (1992) Estrogen receptor-immunoreactive glia, endothelia, and ependyma in guinea pig preoptic area and median eminence: Electron microscopy. *Endocrinology* 130:364–372.

Langub MC, Maley BE, Watson RE. (1994) Estrous cycle-associated axosomatic synaptic plasticity upon estrogen receptive neurons in the rat preoptic area. *Brain Res* 641:303–310.

Lapchak PA, Chapman DF, Nunez SY, Zivin JA. (2000) Dehydroepiandrosterone sulfate is neuroprotective in a reversible spinal cord ischemia model: Possible involvement of GABA(A) receptors. *Stroke* 31:1953–1956.

Lariva-Sahd J. (1991) Ultrastructural evidence of a sexual dimorphism in the neuropil of the medial preoptic nucleus of the rat: A quantitative study. *Neuroendocrinology* 54:416–419.

Larkin JE, Yellon SM, Zucker I. (2003) Melatonin production accompanies arousal from daily torpor in Siberian hamsters. *Physiol Biochem Zool* 76:577–585.

Larsen CM, Kokay IC, Grattan DR. (2008) Male pheromones initiate prolactin-induced neurogenesis and advance maternal behavior in female mice. *Horm Behav* 53:509–517.

Larson J, Jessen RE, Uz T, Arslan AD, Kurtuncu M, Imbesi M, Manev H. (2006) Impaired hippocampal long-term potentiation in melatonin MT2 receptor-deficient mice. *Neurosci Lett* 393:23–26.

Lauder JM. (1978) Effects of early hypo- and hyperthyroidism on development of rat cerebellar cortex. IV. The parallel fibers. *Brain Res* 142:25–39.

Laurin D, Verreault R, Lindsay J, MacPherson K, Rockwood K. (2001) Physical activity and risk of cognitive impairment and dementia in elderly persons. *Arch Neurol* 58:498–504.

Laurino L, Wang XX, de la Houssaye BA, Sosa L, Dupraz S, Caceres A, Pfenninger KH, Quiroga S. (2005) PI3K activation by IGF-1 is essential for the regulation of membrane expansion at the nerve growth cone. *J Cell Sci* 118:3653–3662.

Lautenschlager NT, Almeida OP. (2006) Physical activity and cognition in old age. *Curr Opin Psychiatry* 19:190–193.

Lavado-Autric R, Ausó E, García-Velasco JV, Arufe MC, Escobar del Rey F, Berbel P, Morreale de Escobar G. (2003) Early maternal hypothyroxinemia alters histogenesis and cerebral cortex cytoarchitecture of the progeny. *J Clin Invest* 111:1073–1082.

Lavaque E, Mayen A, Azcoitia I, Tena-Sempere M, Garcia-Segura LM. (2006a) Sex differences, developmental changes, response to injury and cAMP regulation of the mRNA levels of steroidogenic acute regulatory protein, cytochrome p450scc, and aromatase in the olivocerebellar system. *J Neurobiol* 66:308–318.

Lavaque E, Sierra A, Azcoitia I, Garcia-Segura LM. (2006b) Steroidogenic acute regulatory protein in the brain. *Neuroscience* 138:741–747.

Lavenex P, Steele MA, Jacobs LF. (2000) Sex differences, but no seasonal variations in the hippocampus of food-caching squirrels: A stereological study. *J Comp Neurol* 425:152–166.

Lavialle M, Serviere J. (1993) Circadian fluctuations in GFAP distribution in the Syrian hamster suprachiasmatic nucleus. *NeuroReport* 4:1243–1246.

Lavialle M, Begue A, Papillon C, Vilaplana J. (2001) Modifications of retinal afferent activity induce changes in astroglial plasticity in the hamster circadian clock. *Glia* 34:88–100.

Laviola G, Rea M, Morley-Fletcher S, Di Carlo S, Bacosi A, De Simone R, Bertini M, Pacifici R. (2004) Beneficial effects of enriched environment on adolescent rats from stressed pregnancies. *Eur J Neurosci* 20:1655–1664.

LeBlanc AC, Poduslo JF. (1990) Regulation of apolipoprotein E gene expression after injury of the rat sciatic nerve. *J Neurosci Res* 25:162–171.

Lechuga-Sancho AM, Arroba AI, Frago LM, Garcia-Caceres C, de Celix AD, Argente J, Chowen JA. (2006a) Reduction in the number of astrocytes and their projections is associated with increased synaptic protein density in the hypothalamus of poorly controlled diabetic rats. *Endocrinology* 147:5314–5324.

Lechuga-Sancho AM, Arroba AI, Frago LM, Paneda C, Garcia-Caceres C, Delgado Rubin de Celix A, Argente J, Chowen JA. (2006b) Activation of the intrinsic cell death pathway, increased apoptosis and modulation of astrocytes in the cerebellum of diabetic rats. *Neurobiol Dis* 23:290–299.

Ledoux VA, Woolley CS. (2005) Evidence that disinhibition is associated with a decrease in number of vesicles available for release at inhibitory synapses. *J Neurosci* 25:971–976.

Lee DW, Smith GT, Tramontin AD, Soma KK, Brenowitz EA, Clayton NS. (2001) Hippocampal volume does not change seasonally in a non food-storing songbird. *NeuroReport* 12:1925–1928.

Lee DW, Fernando G, Peterson RS, Allen TA, Schlinger BA. (2007) Estrogen mediation of injury-induced cell birth in neuroproliferative regions of the adult zebra finch brain. *Dev Neurobiol* 67:1107–1117.

Lee EJ, Lee MY, Chen HY, Hsu YS, Wu TS, Chen ST, Chang GL. (2005) Melatonin attenuates gray and white matter damage in a mouse model of transient focal cerebral ischemia. *J Pineal Res* 38:42–52.

Lee J, Seroogy KB, Mattson MP. (2002) Dietary restriction enhances neurotrophin expression and neurogenesis in the hippocampus of adult mice. *J Neurochem* 80:539–547.

Lee SJ, McEwen BS. (2001) Neurotrophic and neuroprotective actions of estrogens and their therapeutic implications. *Annu Rev Pharmacol Toxicol* 41:569–591.

Lee ST, Chu K, Sinn DI, Jung KH, Kim EH, Kim SJ, Kim JM, Ko SY, Kim M, Roh JK. (2006) Erythropoietin reduces perihematomal inflammation and cell death with eNOS and STAT3 activations in experimental intracerebral hemorrhage. *J Neurochem* 96:1728–1739.

Lee W, Watanabe M, Glass JD. (1995) Photoperiod affects the expression of neural cell adhesion molecule and polysialic acid in the hypothalamus of the Siberian hamster. *Brain Res* 690:64–72.

Leedom L, Lewis C, Garcia-Segura LM, Naftolin F. (1994) Regulation of arcuate nucleus synaptology by estrogen. *Ann N Y Acad Sci* 743:61–71.

Leedy MG, Beattie MS, Bresnahan JC. (1987) Testosterone induced plasticity of synaptic inputs to adult mammalian motoneurons. *Brain Res* 424:386–390.

Le Goascogne C, Robel P, Gouezou M, Sananes N, Baulieu EE, Waterman M. (1987) Neurosteroids: Cytochrome P-450scc in rat brain. *Science* 237:1212–1215.

Legrand J. (1979) Morphogenetic actions of thyroid hormones. *Trends Neurosci* 2:234–236.

Lehman MN, Durham DM, Jansen HT, Adrian B, Goodman RL. (1996) Dopaminergic A14/A15 neurons are activated during estradiol negative feedback in anestrous, but not breeding season, ewes. *Endocrinology* 137:4443–4450.

Lehman MN, Goodman RL, Karsch FJ, Jackson GL, Berriman SJ, Jansen HT. (1997) The GnRH system of seasonal breeders: Anatomy and plasticity. *Brain Res Bull* 44:445–457.

Lei DL, Long JM, Hengemihle J, O'Neill J, Manaye KF, Ingram DK, Mouton PR. (2003) Effects of estrogen and raloxifene on neuroglia number and morphology in the hippocampus of aged female mice. *Neuroscience* 121:659–666.

Lema SC, Hodges MJ, Marchetti MP, Nevitt GA. (2005) Proliferation zones in the salmon telencephalon and evidence for environmental influence on proliferation rate. *Comp Biochem Physiol A Mol Integr Physiol* 141:327–335.

Lemaire V, Koehl M, Le Moal M, Abrous DN. (2000) Prenatal stress produces learning deficits associated with an inhibition of neurogenesis in the hippocampus. *Proc Natl Acad Sci USA* 97:11032–11037.

Lemaire V, Lamarque S, Le Moal M, Piazza PV, Abrous DN. (2006a) Postnatal stimulation of the pups counteracts prenatal stress-induced deficits in hippocampal neurogenesis. *Biol Psychiatr* 59:786–792.

Lemaire V, Billard JM, Dutar P, George O, Piazza PV, Epelbaum J, Le Moal M, Mayo W. (2006b) Motherhood-induced memory improvement persists across lifespan in rats but is abolished by a gestational stress. *Eur J Neurosci* 23:3368–3374.

Lemkine GF, Raj A, Alfama G, Turque N, Hassani Z, Alegria-Prévot O, Samarut J, Levi G, Demeneix BA. (2005) Adult neural stem cell cycling in vivo requires thyroid hormone and its alpha receptor. *FASEB J* 19:863–865.

Leonard BE, Song C. (1996) Stress and the immune system in the etiology of anxiety and depression. *Pharmacol Biochem Behav* 54:299–303.

Leonelli E, Yague JG, Ballabio M, Azcoitia I, Magnaghi V, Schumacher M, Garcia-Segura LM, Melcangi RC. (2005) Ro5-4864, a synthetic ligand of peripheral benzodiazepine receptor, reduces aging-associated myelin degeneration in the sciatic nerve of male rats. *Mech Ageing Dev* 126:1159–1163.

Leonelli E, Ballabio M, Consoli A, Roglio I, Magnaghi V, Melcangi RC. (2006) Neuroactive steroids: A therapeutic approach to maintain peripheral nerve integrity during neurodegenerative events. *J Mol Neurosci* 28:65–76.

Leonelli E, Bianchi R, Cavaletti G, Caruso D, Crippa D, Garcia-Segura LM, Lauria G, Magnaghi V, Roglio I, Melcangi RC. (2007) Progesterone and its derivatives are neuroprotective agents in experimental diabetic neuropathy: A multimodal analysis. *Neuroscience* 144:1293–1304.

Lephart ED. (1996) A review of brain aromatase cytochrome P450. *Brain Res Rev* 22:1–26.

Leranth C, Shanabrough M, Horvath TL. (2000) Hormonal regulation of hippocampal spine synapse density involves subcortical mediation. *Neuroscience* 101:349–356.

Leranth C, Shanabrough M. (2001) Supramammillary area mediates subcortical estrogenic action on hippocampal synaptic plasticity. *Exp Neurol* 167:445–450.

Leranth C, Shanabrough M, Redmond DE Jr. (2002) Gonadal hormones are responsible for maintaining the integrity of spine synapses in the CA1 hippocampal subfield of female nonhuman primates. *J Comp Neurol* 447:34–42.

Leranth C, Petnehazy O, MacLusky NJ. (2003) Gonadal hormones affect spine synaptic density in the CA1 hippocampal subfield of male rats. *J Neurosci* 23:1588–1592.

Leranth C, Hajszan T, MacLusky NJ. (2004) Androgens increase spine synapse density in the CA1 hippocampal subfield of ovariectomized female rats. *J Neurosci* 24:495–499.

Lesort M, Jope RS, Johnson GVW. (1999) Insulin transiently increases tau phosphorylation: Involvement of glycogen synthase kinase-3β and Fyn tyrosine kinase. *J Neurochem* 72:576–584.

Letechipia-Vallejo G, Lopez-Loeza E, Espinoza-Gonzalez V, Gonzalez-Burgos I, Olvera-Cortes ME, Morali G, Cervantes M. (2007) Long-term morphological and functional evaluation of the neuroprotective effects of post-ischemic treatment with melatonin in rats. *J Pineal Res* 42:138–146.

Leuner B, Mirescu C, Noiman L, Gould E. (2007) Maternal experience inhibits the production of immature neurons in the hippocampus during the postpartum period through elevations in adrenal steroids. *Hippocampus* 17:434–442.

Leung A, Chue P. (2000) Sex differences in schizophrenia, a review of the literature. *Acta Psychiatr Scand Suppl* 401:3–38.

Leverenz JB, Wilkinson CW, Wamble M, Corbin S, Grabber JE, Raskind MA, Peskind ER. (1999) Effect of chronic high-dose exogenous cortisol on hippocampal neuronal number in aged nonhuman primates. *J Neurosci* 19:2356–2361.

Levi G, Broders F, Dunon D, Edelman GM, Thiery JP. (1990) Thyroxine-dependent modulations of the expression of the neural cell adhesion molecule N-CAM during Xenopus laevis metamorphosis. *Development* 108:681–692.

Levine S. (1967) Maternal and environmental influences on the adrenocortical response to stress in weanling rats. *Science* 156:258–260.

Levine S, Wiener SG, Coe CL. (1993) Temporal and social factors influencing behavioral and hormonal responses to separation in mother and infant squirrel monkeys. *Psychoneuroendocrinology* 18:297–306.

Levitt NS, Lindsay RS, Holmes MC, Seckl JR. (1996) Dexamethasone in the last week of pregnancy attenuates hippocampal glucocorticoid receptor gene expression and elevates blood pressure in the adult offspring in the rat. *Neuroendocrinology* 64:412–418.

Levy F, Keller M, Poindron P. (2004) Olfactory regulation of maternal behavior in mammals. *Horm Behav* 46:284–302.

Lewis C, McEwen BS, Frankfurt M. (1995) Estrogen-induction of dendritic spines in ventromedial hypothalamus and hippocampus: Effects of neonatal aromatase blockade and adult GDX. *Dev Brain Res* 87:91–95.

Li H, Klein G, Sun P, Buchan AM. (2001) Dehydroepiandrosterone (DHEA) reduces neuronal injury in a rat model of global cerebral ischemia. *Brain Res* 888:263–266.

Li Q, Puro GD. (2002) Diabetes-induced dysfunction of the glutamate transporter in retinal Müller cells. *Invest Ophthalmol Vis Sci* 43:3109–3116.

Li R, Shen Y, Yang LB, Lue LF, Finch C, Rogers J. (2000) Estrogen enhances uptake of amyloid beta-protein by microglia derived from the human cortex. *J Neurochem* 75:1447–1454.

Li S, Crenshaw BE, Rawson EJ, Simmons DM, Swanson LW, Rosenfeld MG. (1990) Dwarf locus mutants lacking three pituitary cell types result from mutations in the POU-domain gene pit-1. *Nature* 347:528–533.

Li W, Maeda Y, Yuan RR, Elkabes S, Cook S, Dowling P. (2004) Beneficial effect of erythropoietin on experimental allergic encephalomyelitis. *Ann Neurol* 56:767–777.

Li XC, Jarvis ED, Alvarez-Borda B, Lim DA, Nottebohm F. (2000) A relationship between behavior, neurotrophin expression, and new neuron survival. *Proc Natl Acad Sci USA* 97:8584–8589.

Li XL, Aou S, Oomura Y, Hori N, Fukunaga K, Hori T. (2002) Impairment of long-term potentiation and spatial memory in leptin receptor-deficient rodents. *Neuroscience* 113:607–615.

Li ZG, Zhang W, Grunberger G, Sima AA. (2002) Hippocampal neuronal apoptosis in type 1 diabetes. *Brain Res* 946:221–231.

Liang Z, Valla J, Sefidvash-Hockley S, Rogers J, Li R. (2002) Effects of estrogen treatment on glutamate uptake in cultured human astrocytes derived from cortex of Alzheimer's disease patients. *J Neurochem* 80:807–814.

Liao GY, Leonard JP. (1999) Insulin modulation of cloned mouse NMDA receptor currents in Xenopus oocytes. *J Neurochem* 73:1510–1519.

Lichtenwalner RJ, Forbes ME, Bennett SA, Lynch CD, Sonntag WE, Riddle DR. (2001) Intracerebroventricular infusion of insulin-like growth factor-I ameliorates the age-related decline in hippocampal neurogenesis. *Neuroscience* 107:603–613.

Lieth E, Barber AJ, Xu B, Dice C, Ratz MJ, Tanase D, Strother JM. (1998) Glial reactivity and impaired glutamate metabolism in short-term experimental diabetic retinopathy. Penn State Retina Research Group. *Diabetes* 47:815–820.

Lim MM, Young LJ. (2006) Neuropeptidergic regulation of affiliative behavior and social bonding in animals. *Horm Behav* 50:506–517.

Lim MM, Liu Y, Ryabinin AE, Bai Y, Wang Z, Young LJ. (2007) CRF receptors in the nucleus accumbens modulate partner preference in prairie voles. *Horm Behav* 51:508–515.

Lima FR, Gervais A, Colin C, Izembart M, Neto VM, Mallat M. (2000) Regulation of microglial development: A novel role for thyroid hormone. *J Neurosci* 21:2028–2038.

Lindqvist A, Mohapel P, Bouter B, Frielingsdorf H, Pizzo D, Brundin P, Erlanson-Albertsson C. (2006) High-fat diet impairs hippocampal neurogenesis in male rats. *Eur J Neurol* 13:1385–1388.

Liston C, Miller MM, Goldwater DS, Radley JJ, Rocher AB, Hof PR, Morrison JH, McEwen BS. (2006) Stress-induced alterations in prefrontal cortical dendritic morphology predict selective impairments in perceptual attentional set-shifting. *J Neurosci* 26:7870–7874.

Littleton-Kearney MT, Klaus JA, Hurn PD. (2005) Effects of combined oral conjugated estrogens and medroxyprogesterone acetate on brain infarction size after experimental stroke in rat. *J Cereb Blood Flow Metab* 25:421–426.

Liu D, Diorio J, Tannenbaum B, Caldji C, Francis D, Freedman A, Sharma S, Pearson D, Plotsky PM, Meaney MJ. (1997) Maternal care, hippocampal glucocorticoid receptors, and hypothalamic–pituitary–adrenal response to stress. *Science* 277:1659–1662.

Liu J, Yu B, Neugebauer V, Grigoriadis DE, Rivier J, Vale WW, Shinnick-Gallagher P, Gallagher JP. (2004) Corticotropin-releasing factor and Urocortin I modulate excitatory glutamatergic synaptic transmission. *J Neurosci* 24:4020–4029.

Liu L, Brown JC, Webster WW, Morrisett RA, Monaghan DT. (1995) Insulin potentiates N-methyl-D-aspartate receptor activity in Xenopus oocytes and rat hippocampus. *Neurosci Lett* 192:5–8.

Lledo PM, Lazarini F. (2007) Neuronal replacement in microcircuits of the adult olfactory system. *C R Biol* 330:510–520.

Llorens-Martín MV, Rueda N, Martínez-Cué C, Torres-Alemán I, Flórez J, Trejo JL. (2007) Both increases in immature dentate neuron number and decreases of immobility time in the forced swim test occurred in parallel after environmental enrichment of mice. *Neuroscience* 147:631–638.

Llorente R, Arranz L, Marco EM, Moreno E, Puerto M, Guaza C, De la Fuente M, Viveros MP. (2007) Early maternal deprivation and neonatal single administration with a cannabinoid agonist induce long-term sex-dependent psychoimmunoendocrine effects in adolescent rats. *Psychoneuroendocrinology* 32:636–650.

Lloyd D, Aon MA, Cortassa S. (2001) Why homeodynamics, not homeostasis? *Scientific World Journal* 1:133–145.

Lo DC. (1995) Neurotrophic factors and synaptic plasticity. *Neuron* 15:979–981.

Lobie PE, Garcia Aragon J, Lincoln DT, Barnard R, Wilcox JN, Waters MJ. (1993) Localization and ontogeny of growth hormone receptor gene expression in the central nervous system. *Dev Brain Res* 74:225–233.

Lockhart EM, Warner DS, Pearlstein RD, Penning DH, Mehrabani S, Boustany RM. (2002) Allopregnanolone attenuates N-methyl-D-aspartate-induced excitotoxicity and apoptosis in the human NT2 cell line in culture. *Neurosci Lett* 328:33–36.

London SE, Monks DA, Wade J, Schlinger BA. (2006) Widespread capacity for steroid synthesis in the avian brain and song system. *Endocrinology* 147:5975–5987.

London SE, Schlinger BA. (2007) Steroidogenic enzymes along the ventricular proliferative zone in the developing songbird brain. *J Comp Neurol* 502:507–521.

Lopez J, Martinez A. (2002) Cell and molecular biology of the multifunctional peptide, adrenomedullin. *Int Rev Cytol* 221:1–92.

Lopez-Fernandez J, Sanchez-Franco F, Velasco B, Tolon RM, Pazos F, Cacicedo L. (1996) Growth hormone induces somatostatin and insulin-like growth factor I gene expression in the cerebral hemispheres of aging rats. *Endocrinology* 137:4384–4391.

Lord C, Buss C, Lupien SJ, Pruessner JC. (2008) Hippocampal volumes are larger in postmenopausal women using estrogen therapy compared to past users, never users and men: A possible window of opportunity effect. *Neurobiol Aging* 29:95–101.

Lordi B, Protais P, Mellier D, Caston J. (1997) Acute stress in pregnant rats: Effects on growth rate, learning and memory capabilities of the offspring. *Physiol Behav* 63:1092–1097.

Lorente de Nó R. (1933) Vestibulo-ocular reflex arc. *Arch Neurol Psychiatry* 30:245–291.

Lorenz B, Garcia-Segura LM, DonCarlos LL. (2005) Cellular phenotype of androgen receptor-immunoreactive nuclei in the developing and adult rat brain. *J Comp Neurol* 492:456–468.

Lorenzo A, Diaz H, Carrer H, Cáceres, A. (1992) Amygdala neurons in vitro: Neurite growth and effects of estradiol. *J Neurosci Res* 33:418–435.

Lorenzo M, Peino R, Castro AI, Lage M, Popovic V, Dieguez C, Casanueva FF. (2005) Hypopituitarism and growth hormone deficiency in adult subjects after traumatic brain injury: Who and when to test. *Pituitary* 8:233–237.

Louissaint A, Rao S, Leventhal C, Goldman SA. (2002) Coordinated interaction of neurogenesis and angiogenesis in the adult songbird brain. *Neuron* 34:945–960.

Louvart H, Maccari S, Darnaudéry M. (2005) Prenatal stress affects behavioral reactivity to an intense stress in adult female rats. *Brain Res* 1031:67–73.

Love G, Torrey N, McNamara I, Morgan M, Banks M, Hester NW, Glasper ER, Devries AC, Kinsley CH, Lambert KG. (2005) Maternal experience produces long-lasting behavioral modifications in the rat. *Behav Neurosci* 119:1084–1096.

Lovic V, Gonzalez A, Fleming AS. (2001) Maternally separated rats show deficits in maternal care in adulthood. *Dev Psychobiol* 39:19–33.

Lu A, Ran RQ, Clark J, Reilly M, Nee A, Sharp FR. (2002) 17-beta-estradiol induces heat shock proteins in brain arteries and potentiates ischemic heat shock protein induction in glia and neurons. *J Cereb Blood Flow Metab* 22:183–195.

Lu D, Mahmood A, Qu C, Goussev A, Schallert T, Chopp M. (2005) Erythropoietin enhances neurogenesis and restores spatial memory in rats after traumatic brain injury. *J Neurotrauma* 22:1011–1017.

Lu EJ, Brown WJ. (1977) The developing caudate nucleus in the euthyroid and hypothyroid rat. *J Comp Neurol* 171:261–284.

Lu J, Park CS, Lee SK, Shin DW, Kang JH. (2006) Leptin inhibits 1-methyl-4-phenylpyridinium-induced cell death in SH-SY5Y cells. *Neurosci Lett* 407:240–243.

Lucio RA, Garcia JV, Cerezo JR, Pacheco P, Innocenti GM, Berbel P. (1997) The development of auditory callosal connections in normal and hypothyroid rats. *Cereb Cortex* 7:303–306.

Luckman SM, Bicknell RJ. (1990) Morphological plasticity that occurs in the neurohypophysis following activation of the magnocellular neurosecretory system can be mimicked in vitro by beta-adrenergic stimulation. *Neuroscience* 39:701–709.

Lund TD, Salyer DL, Fleming DE, Lephart ED. (2000) Pre- or postnatal testosterone and flutamide effects on sexually dimorphic nuclei of the rat hypothalamus. *Dev Brain Res* 120:261–266.

Luo J, Daniels SB, Lennington JB, Notti RQ, Conover JC. (2006) The aging neurogenic subventricular zone. *Aging Cell* 5:139–152.

Lupien SJ, Maheu F, Tu M, Fiocco A, Schramek TE. (2007) The effects of stress and stress hormones on human cognition: Implications for the field of brain and cognition. *Brain Cogn* 65:209–237.

Luquín S, Naftolin F, Garcia-Segura LM. (1993) Natural fluctuation and gonadal hormone regulation of astrocyte immunoreactivity in dentate gyrus. *J Neurobiol* 24:913–924.

Lustig RH. (1996) In vitro models for the effects of sex hormones on neurons. *Ann NY Acad Sci* 784:370–380.

Lustig RH, Sudol M, Pfaff DW, Federoff HJ. (1991) Estrogenic regulation and sex dimorphism of growth-associated protein 43 kDa (GAP-43) messenger RNA in the rat. *Mol Brain Res* 11:125–132.

Lynch CD, Lyons D, Khan A, Bennett SA, Sonntag WE. (2001) Insulin-like growth factor-1 selectively increases glucose utilization in brains of aged animals. *Endocrinology* 142:506–509.

Lynch G, Rex CS, Gall CM. (2006) Synaptic plasticity in early aging. *Ageing Res Rev* 5:255–280.

Lyons MK, Anderson RE, Meyer FB. (1991) Corticotropin releasing factor antagonist reduces ischemic hippocampal neuronal injury. *Brain Res* 545:339–342.

Ma YJ, Junier M-P, Costa ME, Ojeda SR. (1992) Transforming growth factor alpha (TGFα) gene expression in the hypothalamus is developmentally regulated and linked to sexual maturation. *Neuron* 9:657–670.

Ma YJ, Berg-von der Emde K, Rage F, Wetsel WC, Ojeda SR. (1997) Hypothalamic astrocytes respond to transforming growth factor-alpha with the secretion of neuroactive substances that stimulate the release of luteinizing hormone-releasing hormone. *Endocrinology* 138:19–25.

Ma YJ, Hill DF, Creswick KE, Costa ME, Cornea A, Lioubin MN, Plowman GD, Ojeda SR. (1999) Neuregulins signaling via a glial erbB-2-erbB-4 receptor complex contribute to the neuroendocrine control of mammalian sexual development. *J Neurosci* 19:9913–9927.

Ma ZQ, Santagati S, Patrone C, Pollio G, Vegeto E, Maggi A. (1994) Insulin-like growth factors activate estrogen receptor to control the growth and differentiation of the human neuroblastoma cell line SK-ER3. *Mol Endocrinol* 8:910–918.

Maccari S, Piazza PV, Kabbaj M, Barbazanges A, Simon H, Le Moal M. (1995) Adoption reverses the longterm impairment in glucocorticoid feedback induced by prenatal stress. *J Neurosci* 15:110–116.

Maccari S, Darnaudéry M, Morley-Fletcher S, Zuena AR, Cinque C, Van Reeth O. (2003) Prenatal stress and long-term consequences: Implications of glucocorticoid hormones. *Neurosci Biobehav Rev* 27:119–127.

MacDougall-Shackleton SA, Ball GF. (1999) Comparative studies of sex differences in the song-control system of songbirds. *Trends Neurosci* 22:432–436.

MacKenzie SM, Lai M, Clark CJ, Fraser R, Gómez-Sánchez CE, Seckl JR, Connell JM, Davies E. (2002) 11beta-hydroxylase and aldosterone synthase expression in fetal rat hippocampal neurons. *J Mol Endocrinol* 29:319–325.MacLusky NJ, Naftolin F. (1981) Sexual differentiation of the central nervous system. *Science* 211:1294–1302.

MacLusky NJ, Hajszan T, Leranth C. (2004) Effects of dehydroepiandrosterone and flutamide on hippocampal CA1 spine synapse density in male and female rats: Implications for the role of androgens in maintenance of hippocampal structure. *Endocrinology* 145:4154–4161.

MacLusky NJ, Luine VN, Hajszan T, Leranth C. (2005) The 17alpha and 17beta isomers of estradiol both induce rapid spine synapse formation in the CA1 hippocampal subfield of ovariectomized female rats. *Endocrinology* 146:287–293.

MacLusky NJ, Hajszan T, Johansen JA, Jordan CL, Leranth C. (2006a) Androgen effects on hippocampal CA1 spine synapse numbers are retained in Tfm male rats with defective androgen receptors. *Endocrinology* 147:2392–2398.

MacLusky NJ, Hajszan T, Prange-Kiel J, Leranth C. (2006b) Androgen modulation of hippocampal synaptic plasticity. *Neuroscience* 138:957–965.

MacMaster FP, Mirza Y, Szeszko PR, Kmiecik LE, Easter PC, Taormina SP, Lynch M, Rose M, Moore GJ, Rosenberg DR. (2008) Amygdala and hippocampal volumes in familial early onset major depressive disorder. *Biol Psychiatry* 63:385–390.

MacQueen GM, Ramakrishnan K, Ratnasingan R, Chen B, Young LT. (2003) Desipramine treatment reduces the long-term behavioural and neurochemical sequelae of early-life maternal separation. *Int J Neuropsychopharmacol* 6:391–396.

Madeira MD, Sousa N, Paula-Barbosa MM. (1991) Sexual dimorphism in the mossy fiber synapses of the rat hippocampus. *Exp Brain Res* 87:537–545.

Madeira MD, Sousa N, Lima-Andrade MT, Calheiros F, Cadete-Leite A, Paula-Barbosa MM. (1992) Selective vulnerability of the hippocampal pyramidal neurons to hypothyroidism in male and female rats. *J Comp Neurol* 322:501–518.

Madeira MD, Paula-Barbosa MM. (1993) Reorganization of mossy fiber synapses in male and female hypothyroid rats: A stereological study. *J Comp Neurol* 337:334–352.

Madeira MD, Silva-Ferreira L, Paula-Barbosa MM. (2001) Influence of sex and estrous cycle on the sexual dimorphisms of the hypothalamic ventromedial nucleus: Stereological evaluation and Golgi study. *J Comp Neurol* 432:329–345.

Magariños AM, McEwen BS. (1995) Stress-induced atrophy of apical dendrites of hippocampal CA3c neurons: Involvement of glucocorticoid secretion and excitatory amino acid receptors. *Neuroscience* 69:89–98.

Magariños AM, Verdugo JM, McEwen BS. (1997) Chronic stress alters synaptic terminal structure in hippocampus. *Proc Natl Acad Sci USA* 94:14002–14008.

Magariños AM, McEwen BS. (2000) Experimental diabetes in rats causes hippocampal dendritic and synaptic reorganization and increased glucocorticoid reactivity to stress. *Proc Natl Acad Sci USA* 97:11056–11061.

Magariños AM, McEwen BS, Saboureau M, Pevet P. (2006) Rapid and reversible changes in intrahippocampal connectivity during the course of hibernation in European hamsters. *Proc Natl Acad Sci USA* 103:18775–18780.

Magistretti PJ. (2006) Neuron-glia metabolic coupling and plasticity. *J Exp Biol* 209:2304–2311.

Magnaghi V, Cavarretta I, Zucchi I, Susani L, Rupprecht R, Hermann B, Martini L, Melcangi RC. (1999) Po gene expression is modulated by androgens in the sciatic nerve of adult male rats. *Mol Brain Res* 70:36–44.

Magnaghi V, Cavarretta I, Galbiati M, Martini L, Melcangi RC. (2001) Neuroactive steroids and peripheral myelin proteins. *Brain Res Rev* 37:360–371.

Magnaghi V, Ballabio M, Gonzalez LC, Leonelli E, Motta M, Melcangi RC. (2004) The synthesis of glycoprotein P0 and peripheral myelin protein 22 in sciatic nerve of male rats is modulated by testosterone metabolites. *Mol Brain Res* 126:67–73.

Magnaghi V, Ballabio M, Roglio I, Melcangi RC. (2007) Progesterone derivatives increase expression of Krox-20 and Sox-10 in rat Schwann cells. *J Mol Neurosci* 31:149–157.

Magnus TH, Henderson NE. (1988) Thyroid hormone resistance in hibernating ground squirrels, Spermophilus richardsoni. I. Increased binding of triiodo-L-thyronine and L-thyroxine by serum proteins. *Gen Comp Endocrinol* 69:352–360.

Mahesh VB, Dhandapani KM, Brann DW. (2006) Role of astrocytes in reproduction and neuroprotection. *Mol Cell Endocrinol* 246:1–9.

Mahncke HW, Bronstone A, Merzenich MM. (2006) Brain plasticity and functional losses in the aged: Scientific bases for a novel intervention. *Prog Brain Res* 157:81–109.

Mainen ZF, Sejnowski TJ. (1996) Influence of dendritic structure on firing pattern in model neocortical neurons. *Nature* 382:363–366.

Maiter D, Underwood LE, Martin JB, Koenig JI. (1991) Neonatal treatment with monosodium glutamate: Effects of prolonged growth hormone (GH)-releasing hormone deficiency on pulsatile GH secretion and growth in female rats. *Endocrinology* 128:1100–1106.

Majewska MD. (1992) Neurosteroids: Endogenous bimodal modulators of the GABAA receptor. Mechanism of action and physiological significance. *Prog Neurobiol* 38:379–395.

Mak GK, Enwere EK, Gregg C, Pakarainen T, Poutanen M, Huhtaniemi I, Weiss S. (2007) Male pheromone-stimulated neurogenesis in the adult female brain: Possible role in mating behavior. *Nat Neurosci* 10:1003–1011.

Maki PM. (2005) A systematic review of clinical trials of hormone therapy on cognitive function: Effects of age at initiation and progestin use. *Ann NY Acad Sci* 1052:182–197.

Maki PM. (2006a) Hormone therapy and cognitive function: Is there a critical period for benefit? *Neuroscience* 138:1027–1030.

Maki PM. (2006b) Potential importance of early initiation of hormone therapy for cognitive benefit. *Menopause* 13:6–7.

Maki PM, Rich JB, Rosenbaum RS. (2002) Implicit memory varies across the menstrual cycle: Estrogen effects in young women. *Neuropsychologia* 40:518–529.

Mala H, Alsina CG, Madsen KS, Sibbesen EC, Stick H, Mogensen J. (2005) Erythropoietin improves place learning in an 8-arm radial maze in fimbria-fornix transected rats. *Neural Plast* 12:329–340.

Malenka R, Bear M. (2004). LTP and LTD: An embarrassment of riches. *Neuron* 44:5–21.

Malhotra S, Savitz SI, Ocava L, Rosenbaum DM. (2006) Ischemic preconditioning is mediated by erythropoietin through PI-3 kinase signaling in an animal model of transient ischemic attack. *J Neurosci Res* 83:19–27.

Malinow R, Malenka RC. (2002) AMPA receptor trafficking and synaptic plasticity. *Annu Rev Neurosci* 25:103–126.

Maller JJ, Daskalakis ZJ, Fitzgerald PB. (2007) Hippocampal volumetrics in depression: The importance of the posterior tail. *Hippocampus* 17:1023–1027.

Man HY, Lin JW, Ju WH, Ahmadian G, Liu L, Becker LE, Sheng M, Wang YT. (2000) Regulation of AMPA receptor-mediated synaptic transmission by clathrin-dependent receptor internalization. *Neuron* 25:649–662.

Mani S. (2001) Ligand-independent activation of progestin receptors in sexual receptivity. *Horm Behav* 40:183–190.

Manly JJ, Merchant CA, Jacobs DM, Small SA, Bell K, Ferin M, Mayeux R. (2000) Endogenous estrogen levels and Alzheimer's disease among postmenopausal women. *Neurology* 54:833–837.

Mannella P, Brinton RD. (2006) Estrogen receptor protein interaction with phosphatidylinositol 3-kinase leads to activation of phosphorylated Akt and extracellular signal-regulated kinase 1/2 in the same population of cortical neurons: A unified mechanism of estrogen action. *J Neurosci* 26:9439–9447.

Manzon RG, Youson JH. (1997) The effects of exogenous thyroxine (T4) or triiodothyronine (T3), in the presence and absence of potassium perchlorate, on the incidence of metamorphosis and on serum T4 and T3 concentrations in larval sea lampreys (Petromyzon marinus L.). *Gen Comp Endocrinol* 106:211–220.

Manzon RG, Holmes JA, Youson JH. (2001) Variable effects of goitrogens in inducing precocious metamorphosis in sea lampreys (Petromyzon Marinus). *J Exp Zool* 289:290–303.

Marco EM, Adriani W, Canese R, Podo F, Viveros MP, Laviola G. (2007) Enhancement of endocannabinoid signaling during adolescence: Modulation of impulsivity and long-term consequences on metabolic brain parameters in early maternally deprived rats. *Pharmacol Biochem Behav* 86:334–345.

Maren S. (2005) Synaptic mechanisms of associative memory in the amygdala. *Neuron* 47:783–786.

Maren S, Quirk GJ. (2004) Neuronal signaling of fear memory. *Nat Rev Neurosci* 5:844–852.

Maren S, De Oca B, Fanselow MS. (1994) Sex differences in hippocampal long-term potentiation (LTP) and Pavlovian fear conditioning in rats: Positive correlation between LTP and contextual learning. *Brain Res* 661:25–34.

Marin R, Guerra B, Hernandez-Jimenez JG, Kang XL, Fraser JD, Lopez FJ, Alonso R. (2003) Estradiol prevents amyloid-beta peptide-induced cell death in a cholinergic cell line via modulation of a classical estrogen receptor. *Neuroscience* 121:917–926.

Marin R, Guerra B, Alonso R, Ramirez CM, Diaz M. (2005) Estrogen activates classical and alternative mechanisms to orchestrate neuroprotection. *Curr Neurovasc Res* 2:287–301.

Marin R, Ramírez C, Morales A, González M, Alonso R, Díaz M. (2008) Modulation of Abeta-induced neurotoxicity by estrogen receptor alpha and other associated proteins in lipid rafts. *Steroids* 73:992–996.

Marin-Husstege M, Muggironi M, Raban D, Skoff RP, Casaccia-Bonnefil P. (2004) Oligodendrocyte progenitor proliferation and maturation is differentially regulated by male and female sex steroid hormones. *Dev Neurosci* 26:245–254.

Mariotti S, Franceschi C, Cossarizza A, Pinchera A. (1995) The aging thyroid. *Endocr Rev* 16:686–715.

Markham JA, Juraska JM. (2002) Aging and sex influence the anatomy of the rat anterior cingulate cortex. *Neurobiol Aging* 23:579–588.

Markham JA, Morris JR, Juraska JM. (2007) Neuron number decreases in the rat ventral, but not dorsal, medial prefrontal cortex between adolescence and adulthood. *Neuroscience* 144:961–968.

Markowska AL, Mooney M, Sonntag WE. (1998) Insulin-like growth factor-1 ameliorates age-related behavioral deficits. *Neuroscience* 87:559–569.

Markram K, Gerardy-Schahn R, Sandi C. (2007) Selective learning and memory impairments in mice deficient for polysialylated NCAM in adulthood. *Neuroscience* 144:788–796.

Marselli L, Trincavelli L, Santangelo C, Lupi R, Del Guerra S, Boggi U, Falleni A, Gremigni V, Mosca F, Martini C, Dotta F, Di Mario U, Del Prato S, Marchetti P. (2004) The role of peripheral benzodiazepine receptors on the function and survival of isolated human pancreatic islets. *Eur J Endocrinol* 151:207–214.

Marsh JT, Brown WS, Wolcott D, Carr CR, Harper R, Schweitzer SV, Nissenson AR. (1991) rHuEPO treatment improves brain and cognitive function of anemic dialysis patients. *Kidney Int* 39:155–163.

Marsh-Armstrong N, Huang H, Remo BF, Liu TT, Brown DD. (1999) Asymmetric growth and development of the Xenopus laevis retina during metamorphosis is controlled by type III deiodinase. *Neuron* 24:871–878.

Marsh-Armstrong N, Cai L, Brown DD. (2004) Thyroid hormone controls the development of connections between the spinal cord and limbs during Xenopus laevis metamorphosis. *Proc Natl Acad Sci USA* 101:165–170.

Marti HH, Wenger RH, Rivas LA, Straumann U, Digicaylioglu M, Henn V, Yonekawa Y, Bauer C, Gassmann M. (1996) Erythropoietin gene expression in human, monkey and murine brain. *Eur J Neurosci* 8:666–676.

Martin MB, Franke TF, Stoica GE, Chambon P, Katzenellenbogen BS, Stoica BA, McLemore MS, Olivo SE, Stoica A. (2000) A role for Akt in mediating the estrogenic functions of epidermal growth factor and insulin-like growth factor I. *Endocrinology* 141:4503–4511.

Martinez-Cerdeno V, Noctor SC, Kriegstein AR. (2006) Estradiol stimulates progenitor cell division in the ventricular and subventricular zones of the embryonic neocortex. *Eur J Neurosci* 24:3475–3488.

Martinez-Cue C, Rueda N, Garcia E, Davisson MT, Schmidt C, Florez J. (2005) Behavioral, cognitive and biochemical responses to different environmental conditions in male Ts65Dn mice, a model of Down syndrome. *Behav Brain Res* 163:174–185.

Martinez-Galan JR, Pedraza P, Santacana M, Escobar del Rey F, Morreale de Escobar G, Ruiz-Marcos A. (1997a) Myelin basic protein immunoreactivity in the internal capsule of neonates from rats on a low iodine intake or on methylmercaptoimidazole (MMI). *Dev Brain Res* 101:249–256.

Martinez-Galan JR, Pedraza P, Santacana M, Escobar del Ray F, Morreale de Escobar G, Ruiz-Marcos A. (1997b) Early effects of iodine deficiency on radial glial cells of the hippocampus of the rat fetus. A model of neurological cretinism. *J Clin Invest* 99:2701–2709.

Martinez-Galan JR, Escobar del Rey F, Morreale de Escobar G, Santacana M, Ruiz-Marcos A. (2004) Hypothyroidism alters the development of radial glial cells in the term fetal and postnatal neocortex of the rat. *Dev Brain Res* 153:109–114.

Maruff P, Falleti M. (2005) Cognitive function in growth hormone deficiency and growth hormone replacement. *Horm Res 64* (Suppl 3):100–108.

Maruska KP, Mizobe MH, Tricas TC. (2007) Sex and seasonal co-variation of arginine vasotocin (AVT) and gonadotropin-releasing hormone (GnRH) neurons in the brain of the halfspotted goby. *Comp Biochem Physiol A Mol Integr Physiol* 147:129–144.

Marzban F, Tweedle CD, Hatton GI. (1992) Reevaluation of the plasticity in the rat supraoptic nucleus after chronic dehydration using immunogold for oxytocin and vasopressin at the ultrastructural level. *Brain Res Bull* 28:757–766.

Masliah E, Crews L, Hansen L. (2006) Synaptic remodeling during aging and in Alzheimer's disease. *J Alzheimer's Dis* 9(3 Suppl):91–99.

Matsumoto A. (1991) Synaptogenic action of sex steroids in developing and adult neuroendocrine brain. *Psychoneuroendocrinology* 16:25–40.

Matsumoto A. (1997) Hormonally induced neuronal plasticity in the adult motoneurons. *Brain Res Bull* 44:539–547.

Matsumoto A. (2001) Androgen stimulates neuronal plasticity in the perineal motoneurons of aged male rats. *J Comp Neurol* 430:389–395.

Matsumoto A. (2005) Testosterone prevents synaptic loss in the perineal motoneuron pool in the spinal cord in male rats exposed to chronic stress. *Stress* 8:133–140.

Matsumoto A, Arai Y. (1976) Developmental changes in synaptic formation in the hypothalamic arcuate nucleus of female rats. *Cell Tissue Res* 169:143–156.

Matsumoto A, Arai Y. (1977) Precocious puberty and synaptogenesis in the hypothalamic arcuate nucleus in pregnant mare serum gonadotropin (PMSG) treated immature female rats. *Brain Res* 129:375–378.

Matsumoto A, Arai Y. (1979) Synaptogenic effect of estrogen on the hypothalamic arcuate nucleus of the adult female rat. *Cell Tissue Res* 198:427–433.

Matsumoto A, Arai Y. (1980) Sexual dimorphism in 'wiring pattern' in the hypothalamic arcuate nucleus and its modification by neonatal hormone environment. *Brain Res* 190:238–242.

Matsumoto A, Arai Y. (1981) Neuronal plasticity in the deafferented hypothalamic arcuate nucleus of adult female rats and its enhancement by treatment with estrogen. *J Comp Neurol* 197:197–205.

Matsumoto A, Arai Y, Osanai M. (1985) Estrogen stimulates neuronal plasticity in the deafferented hypothalamic arcuate nucleus in aged female rats. *Neurosci Res* 2:412–418.

Matsumoto A, Arai Y. (1986) Male-female differences in synaptic organization of the ventromedial nucleus of the hypothalamus in the rat. *Neuroendocrinology* 42:232–236.

Matsumoto A, Micevych PE, Arnold AP. (1988) Androgen regulates synaptic input to motoneurons of the adult rat spinal cord. *J Neurosci* 8:4168–4176.

Matsumoto A, Prins GS. (2002) Androgenic regulation of expression of androgen receptor protein in the perineal motoneurons of aged male rats. *J Comp Neurol* 443:383–387.

Matsumoto K, Pinna G, Puia G, Guidotti A, Costa E. (2005) Social isolation stress-induced aggression in mice: A model to study the pharmacology of neurosteroidogenesis. *Stress* 8:85–93.

Mattson MP, Magnus T. (2006) Ageing and neuronal vulnerability. *Nat Rev Neurosci* 7:278–294.

Matys T, Pawlak R, Matys E, Pavlides C, McEwen BS, Strickland S. (2004) Tissue plasminogen activator promotes the effects of corticotropin-releasing factor on the amygdala and anxiety-like behavior. *Proc Natl Acad Sci USA* 101:16345–16350.

Maul B, von Bohlen Und Halbach O, Becker A, Sterner-Kock A, Voigt JP, Siems WE, Grecksch G, Walther T. (2008) Impaired spatial memory and altered dendritic spine morphology in angiotensin II type 2 receptor-deficient mice. *J Mol Med* 86:563–571.

Maurel D, Sage D, Mekaouche M, Bosler O. (2000) Glucocorticoids up-regulate the expression of glial fibrillary acidic protein in the rat suprachiasmatic nucleus. *Glia* 29:212–221.

Maurice T, Urani A, Phan VL, Romieu P. (2001) The interaction between neuroactive steroids and the signal receptor function: Behavioral consequences and therapeutic opportunities. *Brain Res Rev* 37:116–132.

Mayo W, Le Moal M, Abrous DN. (2001) Pregnenolone sulfate and aging of cognitive functions: Behavioral, neurochemical, and morphological investigations. *Horm Behav* 40:215–217.

Mayo W, Lemaire V, Malaterre J, Rodriguez JJ, Cayre M, Stewart MG, Kharouby M, Rougon G, Le Moal M, Piazza PV, Abrous DN. (2005) Pregnenolone sulfate enhances neurogenesis and PSA-NCAM in young and aged hippocampus. *Neurobiol Aging* 26:103–114.

Mazzucco CA, Lieblich SE, Bingham BI, Williamson MA, Viau V, Galea LA. (2006) Both estrogen receptor alpha and estrogen receptor beta agonists enhance cell proliferation in the dentate gyrus of adult female rats. *Neuroscience* 141:1793–1800.

McCauley J, Kern DE, Kolodner K, Dill L, Schroeder AF, DeChant HK, Ryden J, Derogatis LR, Bass EB. (1997) Clinical characteristics of women with a history of childhood abuse: Unhealed wounds. *JAMA* 277:1362–1368.

McCormick CM, Robarts D, Gleason E, Kelsey JE. (2004) Stress during adolescence enhances locomotor sensitization to nicotine in adulthood in female, but not male, rats. *Horm Behav* 46:458–466.

McCullough LD, Hurn PD. (2003) Estrogen and ischemic neuroprotection: An integrated view. *Trends Endocrinol Metab* 14:228–235.

McCullough LD, Blizzard K, Simpson ER, Oz OK, Hurn PD. (2003) Aromatase cytochrome P450 and extragonadal estrogen play a role in ischemic neuroprotection. *J Neurosci* 23:8701–8705.

McEwen BS. (1999) Stress and hippocampal plasticity. *Annu Rev Neurosci* 22:105–122.

McEwen BS. (2002) Sex, stress and the hippocampus: Allostasis, allostatic load and the aging process. *Neurobiol Aging* 23:921–939.

McEwen BS. (2005) Glucocorticoids, depression, and mood disorders: Structural remodeling in the brain. *Metabolism* 54 (Suppl 1):20–23.

McEwen BS. (2007) Physiology and neurobiology of stress and adaptation: Central role of the brain. *Physiol Rev* 87:873–904.

McEwen BS. (2008) Central effects of stress hormones in health and disease: Understanding the protective and damaging effects of stress and stress mediators. *Eur J Pharmacol* 583:174–185.

McEwen BS, Woolley CS. (1994) Estradiol and progesterone regulate neuronal structure and synaptic connectivity in adult as well as developing brain. *Exp Gerontol* 29:431–436.

McEwen BS, Biron CA, Brunson KW, Bulloch K, Chambers WH, Dhabhar FS, Goldfarb RH, Kitson RP, Miller AH, Spencer RL, Weiss JM. (1997) The role of adrenocorticoids as modulators of immune function in health and disease: Neural, endocrine and immune interactions. *Brain Res Rev* 23:79–133.

McEwen BS, Wingfield JC. (2003) The concept of allostasis in biology and biomedicine. *Horm Behav* 43:2–15.

McGaugh JL, Roozendaal B. (2002) Role of adrenal stress hormones in forming lasting memories in the brain. *Cur Opin Neurobiol* 12:205–210.

McIlwain DL, Hoke VB, Kopchick JJ, Fuller CR, Lund PK. (2004) Differential inhibition of postnatal brain, spinal cord and body growth by a growth hormone antagonist. *BMC Neurosci* 5:6.

McKittrick CR, Magariños AM, Blanchard DC, Blanchard RJ, McEwen BS, Sakai RR. (2000) Chronic social stress reduces dendritic arbors in CA3 of hippocampus and decreases binding to serotonin transporter sites. *Synapse* 36:85–94.

McMillan PJ, Singer CA, Dorsa DM. (1996) The effects of ovariectomy and estrogen replacement on trkA and choline acetyltransferase mRNA expression in the basal forebrain of the adult female Sprague-Dawley rat. *J Neurosci* 16:1860–1865.

McNay EC. (2007) Insulin and ghrelin: Peripheral hormones modulating memory and hippocampal function. *Curr Opin Pharmacol* 7:628–632.

Meaney MJ, Sapolsky RM, McEwen BS. (1985) The development of the glucocorticoid receptor system in the rat limbic brain. I. Ontogeny and autoregulation. *Brain Res* 350:159–164.

Medosch CM, Diamond MC. (1982) Rat occipital cortical synapses after ovariectomy. *Exp Neurol* 75:120–133.

Meffre D, Delespierre B, Gouezou M, Leclerc P, Vinson GP, Schumacher M, Stein DG, Guennoun R. (2005) The membrane-associated progesterone-binding protein 25-Dx is expressed in brain regions involved in water homeostasis and is up-regulated after traumatic brain injury. *J Neurochem* 93:1314–1326.

Mehta SH, Dhandapani KM, De Sevilla LM, Webb RC, Mahesh VB, Brann DW. (2003) Tamoxifen, a selective estrogen receptor modulator, reduces ischemic damage caused by middle cerebral artery occlusion in the ovariectomized female rat. *Neuroendocrinology* 77:44–50.

Meijer A. (1985) Child psychiatric sequelae of maternal war stress. *Acta Psychiatr Scand* 72:505–511.

Meisel RL, Luttrell WR. (1990) Estradiol increases the dendritic length of ventromedial hypothalamic neurons in female Syrian hamsters. *Brain Res Bull* 25:165–168.

Meitzen J, Moore IT, Lent K, Brenowitz EA, Perkel DJ. (2007) Steroid hormones act transsynaptically within the forebrain to regulate neuronal phenotype and song stereotypy. *J Neurosci* 27:12045–12057.

Meitzen J, Thompson CK. (2008) Seasonal-like growth and regression of the avian song control system: Neural and behavioral plasticity in adult male Gambel's white-crowned sparrows. *Gen Comp Endocrinol* 157:259–265.

Melcangi RC, Magnaghi V, Cavarretta I, Riva MA, Martini L. (1997) Corticosteroid effects on gene expression of myelin basic protein in oligodendrocytes and of glial fibrillary acidic protein in type 1 astrocytes. *J Neuroendocrinol* 9:729–733.

Melcangi RC, Magnaghi V, Martini L. (1999a) Steroid metabolism and effects in central and peripheral glial cells. *J Neurobiol* 40:471–483.

Melcangi RC, Magnaghi V, Cavarretta I, Zucchi I, Bovolin P, D'Urso D, Martini L. (1999b) Progesterone derivatives are able to influence peripheral myelin protein 22 and P0 gene expression: Possible mechanisms of action. *J Neurosci Res* 56:349–357.

Melcangi RC, Magnaghi V, Galbiati M, Ghelarducci B, Sebastiani L, Martini L. (2000a) The action of steroid hormones on peripheral myelin proteins: A possible new tool for the rebuilding of myelin? *J Neurocytol* 29:327–339.

Melcangi RC, Magnaghi V, Martini L. (2000b) Aging in peripheral nerves: Regulation of myelin protein genes by steroid hormones. *Prog Neurobiol* 60:291–308.

Melcangi RC, Magnaghi V, Galbiati M, Martini L. (2001) Formation and effects of neuroactive steroids in the central and peripheral nervous system. *Int Rev Neurobiol* 46:145–176.

Melcangi RC, Azcoitia I, Ballabio M, Cavarretta I, Gonzalez LC, Leonelli E, Magnaghi V, Veiga S, Garcia-Segura LM. (2003) Neuroactive steroids influence peripheral myelination: A promising opportunity for preventing or treating age-dependent dysfunctions of peripheral nerves. *Prog Neurobiol* 71:57–66.

Melcangi RC, Cavarretta IT, Ballabio M, Leonelli E, Schenone A, Azcoitia I, Garcia-Segura LM, Magnaghi V. (2005) Peripheral nerves: A target for the action of neuroactive steroids. *Brain Res Rev* 48:328–338.

Melcangi RC, Garcia-Segura LM, Mensah-Nyagan AG. (2008) Neuroactive steroids: State of the art and new perspectives. *Cell Mol Life Sci* 65:777–797.

Mellon SH, Griffin LD, Compagnone NA. (2001) Biosynthesis and action of neurosteroids. *Brain Res Rev* 37:3–12.

Mendez P, Azcoitia I, Garcia-Segura LM. (2003) Estrogen receptor alpha forms estrogen-dependent multimolecular complexes with insulin-like growth factor receptor and phosphatidylinositol 3-kinase in the adult rat brain. Mol *Brain Res* 112:170–176.

Mendez P, Azcoitia I, Garcia-Segura LM. (2005) Interdependence of oestrogen and insulin-like growth factor-I in the brain: Potential for analyzing neuroprotective mechanisms. *J Endocrinol* 185:11–17.

Mendez P, Garcia-Segura LM. (2006) Phosphatidylinositol 3-kinase and glycogen synthase kinase 3 regulate estrogen receptor-mediated transcription in neuronal cells. *Endocrinology* 147:3027–3039.

Mendez P, Wandosell F, Garcia-Segura LM. (2006) Cross-talk between estrogen receptors and insulin-like growth factor-I receptor in the brain: Cellular and molecular mechanisms. *Front Neuroendocrinol* 27:391–403.

Merchenthaler I, Dellovade TL, Shughrue PJ. (2003) Neuroprotection by estrogen in animal models of global and focal ischemia. *Ann NY Acad Sci* 1007:89–100.

Mercier G, Turque N, Schumacher M. (2001) Early activation of transcription factor expression in Schwann cells by progesterone. *Mol Brain Res* 97:137–148.

Merrill DA, Roberts JA, Tuszynski MH. (2000) Conservation of neuron number and size in entorhinal cortex layers II, III, and V/VI of aged primates. *J Comp Neurol* 422:396–401.

Merrill DA, Chiba AA, Tuszynski MH. (2001) Conservation of neuronal number and size in the entorhinal cortex of behaviorally characterized aged rats. *J Comp Neurol* 438:445–456.

Merzenich MM, Kaas, JH, Wall J, Nelson RJ, Sur M, Felleman D. (1983a) Topographic reorganization of somatosensory cortical areas 3b and 1 in adult monkeys following restricted deafferentation. *Neuroscience* 8:33–55.

Merzenich MM, Kaas JH, Wall JT, Sur M, Nelson RJ, Felleman DJ. (1983b) Progression of change following median nerve section in the cortical representation of the hand in areas 3b and 1 in adult owl and squirrel monkeys. *Neuroscience* 10:639–665.

Mesenge C, Margaill I, Verrecchia C, Allix M, Boulu RG, Plotkine M. (1998) Protective effect of melatonin in a model of traumatic brain injury in mice. *J Pineal Res* 25:41–46.

Mesches MH, Fleshner M, Heman KL, Rose GM, Diamond DM. (1999) Exposing rats to a predator blocks primed burst potentiation in the hippocampus in vitro. *J Neurosci* 19:RC18.

Meyer D L, von Seydlitz-Kurzbach U, Fiebig E. (1981) Bilaterally asymmetrical uptake of [14C]2-deoxyglucose by the octavo-lateralis complexes in flatfish. *Cell Tissue Res* 214:659–662.

Meyer G, Ferres-Torres R, Mas M. (1978) The effects of puberty and castration on hippocampal dendritic spines of mice. A Golgi study. *Brain Res* 155:108–112.

Miao Y, Xia Q, Hou Z, Zheng Y, Pan H, Zhu S. (2007) Ghrelin protects cortical neuron against focal ischemia/reperfusion in rats. *Biochem Biophys Res Commun* 359:795–800.

Micevych P, Sinchak K. (2008) Synthesis and function of hypothalamic neuroprogesterone in reproduction. *Endocrinology* 149:2739–2742.

Michaloudi HC, el Majdoubi M, Poulain DA, Papadopoulos GC, Theodosis DT. (1997) The noradrenergic innervation of identified hypothalamic magnocellular somata and its contribution to lactation-induced synaptic plasticity. *J Neuroendocrinol* 9:17–23.

Mickley KR, Dluzen DE. (2004) Dose-response effects of estrogen and tamoxifen upon methamphetamine-induced behavioral responses and neurotoxicity of the nigrostriatal dopaminergic system in female mice. *Neuroendocrinology* 79:305–316.

Miklos IH, Kovacs KJ. (2002) GABAergic innervation of corticotropin-releasing hormone (CRH)-secreting parvocellular neurons and its plasticity as demonstrated by quantitative immunoelectron microscopy. *Neuroscience* 113:581–592.

Miller BH, Gore AC. (2001) Alterations in hypothalamic insulin-like growth factor-I and its association with gonadotrophin releasing hormone neurones during reproductive development and ageing. *J Neuroendocrinol* 13:728–736.

Miller DB, Ali SF, O'Callaghan JP, Laws SC. (1998) The impact of gender and estrogen on striatal dopaminergic neurotoxicity. *Ann NY Acad Sci* 844:153–165.

Miller KJ, Parsons TD, Whybrow PC, van Herle K, Rasgon N, van Herle A, Martinez D, Silverman DH, Bauer M. (2006) Memory improvement with treatment of hypothyroidism. *Int J Neurosci* 116:895–906.

Miller RA. (1996) The aging immune system: Primer and prospectus. *Science* 273:70–74.

Milner TA, Ayoola K, Drake CT, Herrick SP, Tabori NE, McEwen BS, Warrier S, Alves SE. (2005) Ultrastructural localization of estrogen receptor beta immunoreactivity in the rat hippocampal formation. *J Comp Neurol* 491:81–95.

Miranda RC, Sohrabji F, Toran-Allerand D. (1993) Neuronal colocalization of mRNAs for neurotrophins and their receptors in the developing central nervous system suggests a potential for autocrine interactions. *Proc Natl Acad Sci USA* 90:6439–6443.

Miranda RC, Sohrabji F, Toran-Allerand D. (1994) Interactions of estrogen with the neurotrophins and their receptors during neural development. *Horm Behav* 28:367–375.

Miranda RC, Sohrabji F, Singh M, Toran-Allerand D. (1996) Nerve growth factor (NGF) regulation of estrogen receptors in explant cultures of the developing forebrain. *J Neurobiol* 31:77–87.

Mirescu C, Peters JD, Gould E. (2004) Early life experience alters response of adult neurogenesis to stress. *Nat Neurosci* 7:841–846.

Mirescu C, Gould E. (2006) Stress and adult neurogenesis. *Hippocampus* 16: 233–238.

Mishra MK, Wilson FE, Scanlan TS, Chiellini G. (2004) Thyroid hormone-dependent seasonality in American tree sparrows (Spizella arborea): Effects of GC-1, a thyroid receptor beta-selective agonist, and of iopanoic acid, a deiodinase inhibitor. *J Comp Physiol* (B) 174:471–479.

Mitome M, Hasegawa T, Shirakawa T. (2005) Mastication influences the survival of newly generated cells in mouse dentate gyrus. *NeuroReport* 16:249–252.

Mitra R, Sapolsky RM. (2008) Acute corticosterone treatment is sufficient to induce anxiety and amygdaloid dendritic hypertrophy. *Proc Natl Acad Sci USA* 105:5573–5578.

Miwa S, Tagawa M, Inui Y, Hirano T. (1988) Thyroxine surge in metamorphosing flounder larvae. *Gen Comp Endocrinol* 70:158–163.

Miyakawa M, Arai Y. (1987) Synaptic plasticity to estrogen in the lateral septum of the adult male and female rats. *Brain Res* 436:184–188.

Miyashita K, Itoh H, Arai H, Suganami T, Sawada N, Fukunaga Y, Sone M, Yamahara K, Yurugi-Kobayashi T, Park K, Oyamada N, Sawada N, Taura D, Tsujimoto H, Chao TH, Tamura N, Mukoyama M, Nakao K. (2006) The neuroprotective and vasculo–neuro–regenerative roles of adrenomedullin in ischemic brain and its therapeutic potential. *Endocrinology* 147:1642–1653.

Miyata S, Nakashima T, Kiyohara T. (1994a) Structural dynamics of neural plasticity in the supraoptic nucleus of the rat hypothalamus during dehydration and rehydration. *Brain Res Bull* 34:169–175.

Miyata S, Itoh T, Matsushima O, Nakashima T, Kiyohara T. (1994b) Not only osmotic stress but also repeated restraint stress causes structural plasticity in the supraoptic nucleus of the rat hypothalamus. *Brain Res Bull* 33:669–675.

Miyata S, Matsushima O, Hatton GI. (1997) Taurine in rat posterior pituitary: Localization in astrocytes and selective release by hypoosmotic stimulation. *J Comp Neurol* 381:513–523.

Miyata M, Okada D, Hashimoto K, Kano M, Ito M. (1999) Corticotropin-releasing factor plays a permissive role in cerebellar long-term depression. *Neuron* 22:763–775.

Miyata S, Hatton GI. (2002) Activity-related, dynamic neuron-glial interactions in the hypothalamo-neurohypophysial system. *Microsc Res Tech* 56:143–157.

Mizutani M, Gerhardinger C, Lorenzi M. (1998) Müller cell changes in human diabetic retinopathy. *Diabetes* 47:445–449.

Moderscheim TA, Gorba T, Pathipati P, Kokay IC, Grattan DR, Williams CE, Scheepens A. (2007) Prolactin is involved in glial responses following a focal injury to the juvenile rat brain. *Neuroscience* 145:963–973.

Moffat SD, Zonderman AB, Metter EJ, Kawas C, Blackman MR, Harman SM, Resnick SM. (2004) Free testosterone and risk for Alzheimer's disease in older men. *Neurology* 62:188–193.

Mogensen J, Miskowiak K, Sorensen TA, Lind CT, Olsen NV, Springborg JB, Mala H. (2004) Erythropoietin improves place learning in fimbria-fornix-transected rats and modifies the search pattern of normal rats. *Pharmacol Biochem Behav* 77:381–390.

Mong JA, Kurzweil RL, Davis AM, Rocca MS, McCarthy MM. (1996) Evidence for sexual differentiation of glia in rat brain. *Horm Behav* 30:553–562.

Mong JA, McCarthy MM. (1999) Steroid-induced developmental plasticity in hypothalamic astrocytes: Implications for synaptic patterning. *J Neurobiol* 40:602–619.

Mong JA, Glaser E, McCarthy MM. (1999) Gonadal steroids promote glial differentiation and alter neuronal morphology in the developing hypothalamus in a regionally specific manner. *J Neurosci* 19:1464–1472.

Mong JA, Roberts RC, Kelly JJ, McCarthy MM. (2001) Gonadal steroids reduce the density of axospinous synapses in the developing rat arcuate nucleus: An electron microscopy analysis. *J Comp Neurol* 432:259–267.

Mong JA, Nunez JL, McCarthy MM. (2002) GABA mediates steroid-induced astrocyte differentiation in the neonatal rat hypothalamus. *J Neuroendocrinol* 14:45–55.

Mong JA, Blutstein T. (2006) Estradiol modulation of astrocytic form and function: Implications for hormonal control of synaptic communication. *Neuroscience* 138:967–975.

Monlezun S, Ouali S, Poulain DA, Theodosis DT. (2005) Polysialic acid is required for active phases of morphological plasticity of neurosecretory axons and their glia. *Mol Cell Neurosci* 29:516–524.

Montagnese C, Poulain DA, Vincent JD, Theodosis DT. (1987) Structural plasticity in the rat supraoptic nucleus during gestation, post-partum lactation and suckling-induced pseudogestation and lactation. *J Endocrinol* 115: 97–105.

Montero-Pedrazuela A, Venero C, Lavado-Autric R, Fernandez-Lamo I, Garcia-Verdugo JM, Bernal J, Guadaño-Ferraz A. (2006) Modulation of adult hippocampal neurogenesis by thyroid hormones: Implications in depressive-like behavior. *Mol Psychiatry* 11:361–371.

Montouris G, Morris GL. (2005) Reproductive and sexual dysfunction in men with epilepsy. *Epilepsy Behav* 7 (Suppl 2):7–14.

Mook-Jung I, Joo I, Sohn S, Kwon HJ, Huh K, Jung MW. (1997) Estrogen blocks neurotoxic effects of β-amyloid (1-42) and induces neurite extension on B103 cells. *Neurosci Lett* 235:101–104.

Moore IT, Bentley GE, Wotus C, Wingfield JC. (2006) Photoperiod-independent changes in immunoreactive brain gonadotropin-releasing hormone (GnRH) in a free-living, tropical bird. *Brain Behav Evol* 68:37–44.

Moosmann B, Behl C. (1999) The antioxidant neuroprotective effects of estrogens and phenolic compounds are independent from their estrogenic properties. *Proc Natl Acad Sci USA* 96:8867–8872.

Mor G, Nilsen J, Horvath T, Bechmann I, Brown S, Garcia-Segura LM, Naftolin
    F. (1999) Estrogen and microglia: A regulatory system that affects the brain.
    J Neurobiol 40:484–496.
Mora F, Segovia G, Del Arco A. (2007) Aging, plasticity and environmental
    enrichment: Structural changes and neurotransmitter dynamics in several areas
    of the brain. *Brain Res Rev* 55:78–88.
Moradpour F, Naghdi N, Fathollahi Y. (2006) Anastrozole improved testosterone-
    induced impairment acquisition of spatial learning and memory in the
    hippocampal CA1 region in adult male rats. *Behav Brain Res* 175:223–232.
Morales AJ, Nolan JJ, Nelson JC, Yen SS. (1994) Effects of replacement dose of
    dehydroepiandrosterone in men and women of advancing age. *J Clin Endocrinol
    Metab* 78:1360–1367.
Morali G, Letechipia-Vallejo G, Lopez-Loeza E, Montes P, Hernandez-Morales L,
    Cervantes M. (2005) Post-ischemic administration of progesterone in rats exerts
    neuroprotective effects on the hippocampus. *Neurosci Lett* 382:286–290.
Morishita E, Masuda S, Nagao M, Yasuda Y, Sasaki R. (1997) Erythropoietin receptor
    is expressed in rat hippocampal and cerebral cortical neurons, and erythropoietin
    prevents in vitro glutamate-induced neuronal death. *Neuroscience* 76:105–116.
Morissette M, Jourdain S, Al Sweidi S, Menniti FS, Ramirez AD, Di Paolo T. (2007)
    Role of estrogen receptors in neuroprotection by estradiol against MPTP toxicity.
    Neuropharmacology 52:1509–1520.
Morissette M, Le Saux M, D'Astous M, Jourdain S, Al Sweidi S, Morin N, Estrada-
    Camarena E, Mendez P, Garcia-Segura LM, Di Paolo T. (2008) Contribution of
    estrogen receptors alpha and beta to the effects of estradiol in the brain. *J Steroid
    Biochem Mol Biol* 108:327–338.
Morley-Fletcher S, Rea M, Maccari S, Laviola G. (2003a) Environmental enrichment
    during adolescence reverses the effects of prenatal stress on play behaviour and
    HPA axis reactivity in rats. *Eur J Neurosci* 18:3367–3374.
Morley-Fletcher S, Darnaudéry M, Koehl M, Casolini P, Van Reeth O, Maccari S.
    (2003b) Prenatal stress in rats predicts immobility behavior in the forced swim
    test. Effects of a chronic treatment with tianeptine. *Brain Res* 989:246–251.
Morreale de Escobar G, Obregon MJ, Calvo R, Escobar del Rey F. (1993) Effects of
    iodine deficiency on thyroid hormone metabolism and the brain in fetal rats: The
    role of the maternal transfer of thyroxin. *Am J Clin Nutr* 57(2 Suppl):280S-285S.
Morreale de Escobar G, Obregon MJ, Escobar del Rey F. (2004a) Role of thyroid
    hormone during early brain development. *Eur J Endocrinol* 151 (Suppl
    3):U25–U37.
Morreale de Escobar G, Obregon MJ, Escobar del Rey F. (2004b) Maternal thyroid
    hormones early in pregnancy and fetal brain development. *Best Pract Res Clin
    Endocrinol Metab* 18:225–248.
Morris JA, Jordan CL, Breedlove SM. (2004) Sexual differentiation of the vertebrate
    nervous system. *Nat Neurosci* 7:1034–1039.
Morris MJ, Tortelli CF, Filippis A, Proietto J. (1998) Reduced BAT function as a
    mechanism for obesity in the hypophagic, neuropeptide Y-deficient monosodium
    glutamate-treated rat. *Regul Pept* 75–76:441–447.
Morse JK, Scheff SW, DeKosky ST. (1986) Gonadal steroids influence axon sprouting
    in the hippocampal dentate gyrus: A sexually dimorphic response. *Exp Neurol*
    94:649–658.

Morse JK, DeKosky ST, Scheff SW. (1992) Neurotrophic effects of steroids on lesion-induced growth in the hippocampus. II. Hormone Replacement. *Exp Neurol* 118:47–52.

Moss RL, Gu Q. (1999) Estrogen: Mechanisms for a rapid action in CA1 hippocampal neurons. *Steroids* 64:14–21.

Mueller NK, Di S, Paden CM, Herman JP. (2005) Activity-dependent modulation of neurotransmitter innervation to vasopressin neurons of the supraoptic nucleus. *Endocrinology* 146:348–354.

Mukai H, Takata N, Ishii HT, Tanabe N, Hojo Y, Furukawa A, Kimoto T, Kawato S. (2006) Hippocampal synthesis of estrogens and androgens which are paracrine modulators of synaptic plasticity: Synaptocrinology. *Neuroscience* 138:757–764.

Mukai H, Tsurugizawa T, Murakami G, Kominami S, Ishii H, Ogiue-Ikeda M, Takata N, Tanabe N, Furukawa A, Hojo Y, Ooishi Y, Morrison JH, Janssen WG, Rose JA, Chambon P, Kato S, Izumi S, Yamazaki T, Kimoto T, Kawato S. (2007) Rapid modulation of long-term depression and spinogenesis via synaptic estrogen receptors in hippocampal principal neurons. *J Neurochem* 100:950–967.

Mukuda T, Sugiyama H. (2007) An angiotensin II receptor antagonist suppresses running-enhanced hippocampal neurogenesis in rat. *Neurosci Res* 58:140–144.

Muller D, Nikonenko I, Jourdain P, Alberi S. (2002) LTP, memory and structural plasticity. *Curr Mol Med* 2:605–611.

Muller D, Nikonenko I. (2003) Dynamic presynaptic varicosities: A role in activity-dependent synaptogenesis. *Trends Neurosci* 26:573–575.

Muller M, Aleman A, Grobbee DE, de Haan EH, van der Schouw YT. (2005) Endogenous sex hormone levels and cognitive function in aging men is there an optimal level? *Neurology* 64:866–871.

Mulnard RA, Cotman CW, Kawas C, van Dyck CH, Sano M, Doody R, Koss E, Pfeiffer E, Jin S, Gamst A, Grundman M, Thomas R, Thal LJ. (2000) Estrogen replacement therapy for treatment of mild to moderate Alzheimer's disease: A randomized controlled trial. Alzheimer's Disease Cooperative Study. *JAMA* 283:1007–1015.

Mungenast AE, Ojeda SR. (2005) Expression of three gene families encoding cell-cell communication molecules in the prepubertal nonhuman primate hypothalamus. *J Neuroendocrinol* 17:208–219.

Muñoz A, Rodriguez-Peña A, Perez-Castillo A, Ferreiro B, Sutcliffe JG, Bernal J. (1991) Effects of neonatal hypothyroidism on rat brain gene expression. *Mol Endocrinol* 5:273–280.

Muñoz-Cueto JA, Garcia-Segura LM, Ruiz-Marcos A. (1990) Developmental sex differences and effect of ovariectomy on the number of cortical pyramidal cell dendritic spines. *Brain Res* 515:64–68.

Muñoz-Cueto JA, Garcia-Segura LM, Ruiz-Marcos A. (1991) Regional sex differences in spine density along the apical shafts of visual cortex pyramids during postnatal development. *Brain Res* 541:41–47.

Murakami K, Nakagawa T, Shozu M, Uchide K, Koike K, Inoue M. (1999) Changes with aging of steroidal levels in the cerebrospinal fluid of women. *Maturitas* 33:71–80.

Murakami K, Fellous A, Baulieu EE, Robel P. (2000) Pregnenolone binds to microtubule-associated protein 2 and stimulates microtubule assembly. *Proc Natl Acad Sci USA* 97:3579–3584.

Murmu MS, Salomon S, Biala Y, Weinstock M, Braun K, Bock J. (2006) Changes of spine density and dendritic complexity in the prefrontal cortex in offspring of mothers exposed to stress during pregnancy. *Eur J Neurosci* 24:1477–1487.

Murphy DD, Segal M. (1996) Regulation of dendritic spine density in cultured rat hippocampal neurons by steroid hormones. *J Neurosci* 16:4059–4068.

Murphy DD, Segal M. (1997) Morphological plasticity of dendritic spines in central neurons is mediated by activation of cAMP response element binding protein. *Proc Natl Acad Sci USA* 94:1482–1487.

Murphy DD, Cole NB, Segal M. (1998a) Brain-derived neurotrophic factor mediates estradiol-induced dendritic spine formation in hippocampal neurons. *Proc Natl Acad Sci USA* 95:11412–11417.

Murphy DD, Cole NB, Greenberger V, Segal M. (1998b) Estradiol increases dendritic spine density by reducing GABA neurotransmission in hippocampal neurons. *J Neurosci* 18:2550–2559.

Murphy DD, Segal M. (2000) Progesterone prevents estradiol-induced dendritic spine formation in cultured hippocampal neurons. *Neuroendocrinology* 72:133–143.

Murphy SJ, Littleton-Kearney MT, Hurn PD. (2002) Progesterone administration during reperfusion, but not preischemia alone, reduces injury in ovariectomized rats. *J Cereb Blood Flow Metab* 22:1181–1188.

Muzumdar RH, Ma X, Yang X, Atzmon G, Barzilai N. (2006) Central resistance to the inhibitory effects of leptin on stimulated insulin secretion with aging. *Neurobiol Aging* 27:1308–1314

Mydlarski MB, Liberman A, Schipper HM. (1995) Estrogen induction of glial heat shock proteins: Implications for hypothalamic aging. *Neurobiol Aging* 16:977–981.

Nacher J, Pham K, Gil-Fernandez V, McEwen BS. (2004) Chronic restraint stress and chronic corticosterone treatment modulate differentially the expression of molecules related to structural plasticity in the adult rat piriform cortex. *Neuroscience* 126:503–509.

Naessen T, Lindmark B, Larsen HC. (1997) Better postural balance in elderly women receiving estrogens. *Am J Obstet Gynecol* 177:412–416.

Naftolin F. (1994) Brain aromatization of androgens. *J Reprod Med* 39:257–261.

Naftolin F, Ryan KJ, Petro Z. (1971a) Aromatization of androstenedione by the diencephalon. *J Clin Endocrinol Metab* 33:368–370.

Naftolin F, Ryan KJ, Petro Z. (1971b) Aromatization of androstenedione by limbic system tissue from human foetuses. *J Endocrinol* 51:795–796.

Naftolin F, Ryan KJ, Petro Z. (1972a) Aromatization of androstenedione by the anterior hypothalamus of adult male and female rats. *Endocrinology* 90:295–298.

Naftolin F, Brown-Grant K, Corkers CS. (1972b) Plasma and pituitary luteinizing hormone and peripheral plasma oestradiol concentrations in the normal oestrus cycle of the rat and after experimental manipulation of the cycle. *J Endocr* 53:17–30.

Naftolin F, Ryan KJ, Davies IJ, Petro Z, Kuhn M. (1975) The formation and metabolism of estrogens in brain tissues. *Adv Biosci* 15:105–121.

Naftolin F, Brawer JR. (1978) The effect of estrogens on hypothalamic structure and function. *Am J Obstet Gynecol* 132:758–765.

Naftolin F, Leranth C, Perez J, Garcia-Segura LM. (1993) Estrogen induces synaptic plasticity in adult primate neurons. *Neuroendocrinology* 57:935–939.

Naftolin F, Bruhlmann-Papazyan M, Baetens D, Garcia-Segura LM. (1985) Neurons with whorl bodies have increased numbers of synapses. *Brain Res* 329:289–293.

Naftolin F, Leranth C, Horvath TL, Garcia-Segura LM. (1996a) Potential neuronal mechanisms of estrogen actions in synaptogenesis and synaptic plasticity. *Cell Mol Neurobiol* 16:213–223.

Naftolin F, Horvath TL, Jakab RL, Leranth C, Harada N, Balthazart J. (1996b) Aromatase immunoreactivity in axon terminals of the vertebrate brain. An immunocytochemical study on quail, rat, monkey and human tissues. *Neuroendocrinology* 63:149–155.

Naftolin F, Garcia-Segura LM, Horvath TL, Zsarnovszky A, Demir N, Fadiel A, Leranth C, Vondracek-Klepper S, Lewis C, Chang A, Párducz A. (2007) Estrogen-induced hypothalamic synaptic plasticity and pituitary sensitization in the control of the estrogen-induced gonadotrophin surge. *Reprod Sci* 14:101–116.

Nair A, Bonneau RH. (2006) Stress-induced elevation of glucocorticoids increases microglia proliferation through NMDA receptor activation. *J Neuroimmunol* 171:72–85.

Nakazato M, Murakami N, Date Y, Kojima M, Matsuo H, Kangawa K, Matrukura S. (2001) A role for ghrelin in the central regulation of feeding. *Nature* 409:194–198.

Nathan BP, Barsukova AG, Shen F, McAsey M, Struble RG. (2004) Estrogen facilitates neurite extension via apolipoprotein E in cultured adult mouse cortical neurons. *Endocrinology* 145:3065–3073.

Navarro VM, Castellano JM, Fernandez-Fernandez R, Barreiro ML, Roa J, Sanchez-Criado JE, Aguilar E, Dieguez C, Pinilla L, Tena-Sempere M. (2004) Developmental and hormonally regulated messenger ribonucleic acid expression of KiSS-1 and its putative receptor, GPR54, in rat hypothalamus and potent luteinizing hormone-releasing activity of KiSS-1 peptide. *Endocrinology* 145:4565–4574.

Navarro VM, Castellano JM, Garcia-Galiano D, Tena-Sempere M. (2007) Neuroendocrine factors in the initiation of puberty: The emergent role of kisspeptin. *Rev Endocr Metab Disord* 8:11–20.

Neeper SA, Gomez-Pinilla F, Choi J, Cotman CW. (1996) Physical activity increases mRNA for brain-derived neurotrophic factor and nerve growth factor in rat brain. *Brain Res* 726:49–56.

Neuman RS, Harley CW. (1983) Long-lasting potentiation of the dentate gyrus population spike by norepinephrine. *Brain Res* 273:162–165.

Nevretdinova Z, Solovenchuk L, Lapinski A. (1992) Some aspects of lipid metabolism and thyroid function in arctic ground squirrel, Citellus parryi during hibernation. *Arctic Med Res* 51:196–204.

Ni Y, Malarkey EB, Parpura V. (2007) Vesicular release of glutamate mediates bidirectional signaling between astrocytes and neurons. *J Neurochem* 103:1273–1284.

Nichols NR, Agolley D, Zieba M, Bye N. (2005) Glucocorticoid regulation of glial responses during hippocampal neurodegeneration and regeneration. *Brain Res Rev* 48:287–301.

Nicholson DA, Yoshida R, Berry RW, Gallagher M, Geinisman Y. (2004) Reduction in size of perforated postsynaptic densities in hippocampal axospinous synapses and age-related spatial learning impairments. *J Neurosci* 24:7648–7653.

Nicholson JL, Altman J. (1972) The effects of early hypo- and hyperthyroidism on the development of the rat cerebellar cortex. I. Cell proliferation and differentiation. *Brain Res* 44:13–23.

Nicol SC, Andersen NA, Tomasi TE. (2000) Seasonal variations in thyroid hormone levels in free-living echidnas (Tachyglossus aculeatus). *Gen Comp Endocrinol* 117:1–7.

Niederland T, Makovi H, Gal V, Andreka B, Abraham CS, Kovacs J. (2007) Abnormalities of pituitary function after traumatic brain injury in children. *J Neurotrauma* 24:119–127.

Nieto-Bona MP, Garcia-Segura LM, Torres-Alemán I. (1993) Orthograde transport and release of insulin-like growth factor I from the inferior olive to the cerebellum. *J Neurosci Res* 36:520–527.

Nieto-Bona MP, Garcia-Segura LM, Torres-Alemán I. (1997) Transynaptic modulation by insulin-like growth factor I of dendritic spines in Purkinje cells. *Int J Dev Neurosci* 15:749–754.

Nilsen J, Brinton RD. (2002a) Impact of progestins on estrogen-induced neuroprotection: Synergy by progesterone and 19-norprogesterone and antagonism by medroxyprogesterone acetate. *Endocrinology* 143:205–212.

Nilsen J, Brinton RD. (2002b). Impact of progestins on estradiol potentiation of the glutamate calcium response. *NeuroReport* 13:825–830.

Nilsen J, Brinton RD. (2003a) Mechanism of estrogen-mediated neuroprotection: Regulation of mitochondrial calcium and Bcl-2 expression. *Proc Natl Acad Sci USA* 100:2842–2847.

Nilsen J, Brinton RD. (2003b) Divergent impact of progesterone and medroxyprogesterone acetate (Provera) on nuclear mitogen-activated protein kinase signaling. *Proc Natl Acad Sci USA* 100:10506–10511.

Nilsen J, Morales A, Brinton RD. (2006) Medroxyprogesterone acetate exacerbates glutamate excitotoxicity. *Gynecol Endocrinol* 22:355–361.

Nishikawa Y, Shibata S, Watanabe S. (1995) Circadian changes in long-term potentiation of rat suprachiasmatic field potentials elicited by optic nerve stimulation in vitro. *Brain Res* 695:158–162.

Nishino H, Nakajima K, Kumazaki M, Fukuda A, Muramatsu K, Deshpande SB, Inubushi T, Morikawa S, Borlongan CV, Sanberg PR. (1998) Estrogen protects against while testosterone exacerbates vulnerability of the lateral striatal artery to chemical hypoxia by 3-nitropropionic acid. *Neurosci Res* 30:303–312.

Nishio H, Kasuga S, Ushijima M, Harada Y. (2001) Prenatal stress and postnatal development of neonatal rats. Sex-dependent effects on emotional behavior and learning ability of neonatal rats. *Int J Dev Neurosci* 19:37–45.

Nishizuka M, Arai Y. (1981a) Sexual dimorphism in synaptic organization in the amygdala and its dependence on neonatal hormone environment. *Brain Res* 212:31–38.

Nishizuka M, Arai Y. (1981b) Organizational action of estrogen on synaptic pattern in the amygdala: Implication for sexual differentiation of the brain. *Brain Res* 213:422–426.

Nishizuka M, Sumida H, Kano Y, Arai Y. (1993) Formation of neurons in the sexually dimorphic anteroventral periventricular nucleus of the preoptic area of the rat: Effects of prenatal treatment with testosterone propionate. *J Neuroendocrinol* 5:569–573.

Nissenson AR. (1992) Epoetin and cognitive function. *Am J Kidney Dis* 20 (Suppl 1):21–24.

Nithianantharajah J, Hannan AJ. (2006) Enriched environments, experience-dependent plasticity and disorders of the nervous system. *Nat Rev Neurosci* 7:697–709.

Nixdorf-Bergweiler BE. (2001) Lateral magnocellular nucleus of the anterior neostriatum (LMAN) in the zebra finch: Neuronal connectivity and the emergence of sex differences in cell morphology. *Microsc Res Tech* 54:335–353.

Nixdorf-Bergweiler BE, Wallhausser-Franke E, DeVoogd TJ. (1995) Regressive development in neuronal structure during song learning in birds. *J Neurobiol* 27:204–215.

Noguchi T. (1991) Retarded cerebral growth of hormone-deficient mice. *Comp Biochem Physiol* 98:239–248.

Noguchi T. (1996) Effects of growth hormone on cerebral development: Morphological studies. *Horm Res* 45:5–17.

Nordeen EJ, Nordeen KW. (1989) Estrogen stimulates the incorporation of new neurons into avian song nuclei during adolescence. *Dev Brain Res* 49:27–32.

Nordeen EJ, Nordeen KW, Sengelaub DR, Arnold AP. (1985) Androgens prevent normally occurring cell death in a sexually dimorphic spinal nucleus. *Science* 229:671–673.

Nordell VL, Lewis DK, Bake S, Sohrabji F. (2005) The neurotrophin receptor p75NTR mediates early anti-inflammatory effects of estrogen in the forebrain of young adult rats. *BMC Neurosci* 6:58.

Norris DO, Gern WA. (1976) Thyroxine-induced activation of hypothalamo-hypophysial axis in neotenic salamander larvae. *Science* 194:525–527.

Nottebohm F. (1980) Testosterone triggers growth of brain vocal control nuclei in adult female canaries. *Brain Res* 189:429–436.

Nottebohm F. (1981) A brain for all seasons: Cyclical anatomical changes in song control nuclei of the canary brain. *Science* 214:1368–1370.

Nottebohm F. (2002) Neuronal replacement in adult brain. *Brain Res Bull* 57:737–749.

Nottebohm F, Arnold AP. (1976) Sexual dimorphism in vocal control areas of the songbird brain. *Science* 194:211–213.

Nottebohm F, Nottebohm ME, Crane LA, Wingfield JC. (1987) Seasonal changes in gonadal hormone levels of adult male canaries and their relation to song. *Behav Neural Biol* 47:197–211.

Nunez JL, Lauschke DM, Juraska JM. (2001) Cell death in the development of the posterior cortex in male and female rats. *J Comp Neurol* 436:32–41.

Nunez JL, Sodhi J, Juraska JM. (2002) Ovarian hormones after postnatal day 20 reduce neuron number in the rat primary visual cortex. *J Neurobiol* 52:312–321.

Oates M, Woodside B, Walker CD. (2000) Chronic leptin administration in developing rats reduces stress responsiveness partly through changes in maternal behavior. *Horm Behav* 37:366–376.

O'Barr SA, Oh JS, Ma C, Brent GA, Schultz JJ. (2006) Thyroid hormone regulates endogenous amyloid-beta precursor protein gene expression and processing in both in vitro and in vivo models. *Thyroid* 16:1207–1213.

Oberlander JG, Schlinger BA, Clayton NS, Saldanha CJ. (2004) Neural aromatization accelerates the acquisition of spatial memory via an influence on the songbird hippocampus. *Horm Behav* 45:250–258.

O'Connor TG, Heron J, Golding J, Glover V, ALSPAC Study Team. (2003) Maternal antenatal anxiety and behavioural/emotional problems in children: A test of a programming hypothesis. *J Child Psychol Psychiatry* 44:1025–1036.

Oestreicher AB, De Graan PN, Gispen WH, Verhaagen J, Schrama LH. (1997) B-50, the growth associated protein-43: Modulation of cell morphology and communication in the nervous system. *Prog Neurobiol* 53:627–686.

Ogata T, Nakamura Y, Tsuji K, Shibata T, Kataoka K. (1993) Steroid hormones protect spinal cord neurons from glutamate toxicity. *Neuroscience* 55:445–449.

Ogiue-Ikeda M, Tanabe N, Mukai H, Hojo Y, Murakami G, Tsurugizawa T, Takata N, Kimoto T, Kawato S. (2008) Rapid modulation of synaptic plasticity by estrogens as well as endocrine disrupters in hippocampal neurons. *Brain Res Rev* 57:363–375.

Ojeda SR, Dissen GA, Junier MP. (1992) Neurotrophic factors and female sexual development. *Front Neuroendocrinol* 13:120–162.

Ojeda SR, Ma YJ. (1998) Epidermal growth factor tyrosine kinase receptors and the neuroendocrine control of mammalian puberty. *Mol Cell Endocrinol* 140:101–106.

Ojeda SR, Ma YJ. (1999) Glial–neuronal interactions in the neuroendocrine control of mammalian puberty: Facilitatory effects of gonadal steroids. *J Neurobiol* 40:528–540.

Ojeda SR, Hill J, Hill DF, Costa ME, Tapia V, Cornea A, Ma YJ. (1999) The Oct-2 POU-domain gene in the neuroendocrine brain: A transcriptional regulator of mammalian puberty. *Endocrinology* 140:3774–3789.

Ojeda SR, Ma YJ, Lee BJ, Prevot V. (2000) Glia-to-neuron signaling and the neuroendocrine control of female puberty. *Recent Prog Horm Res* 55:197–223.

Ojeda SR, Lomniczi A, Mastronardi C, Heger S, Roth C, Parent AS, Matagne V, Mungenast AE. (2006) Minireview: The neuroendocrine regulation of puberty: Is the time ripe for a systems biology approach? *Endocrinology* 147:1166–1174.

O'Kusky JR, Ye P, D'Ercole AJ. (2003) Increased expression of insulin-like growth factor I augments the progressive phase of synaptogenesis without preventing synapse elimination in the hypoglossal nucleus. *J Comp Neurol* 464:382–391.

Oliet SH, Piet R. (2004) Anatomical remodeling of the supraoptic nucleus: Changes in synaptic and extrasynaptic transmission. *J Neuroendocrinol* 16:303–307.

Oliet SH, Panatier A, Piet R. (2006) Functional neuronal-glial anatomical remodeling in the hypothalamus. *Novartis Found Symp* 276:238–248.

Oliet SH, Baimoukhametova DV, Piet R, Bains JS. (2007) Retrograde regulation of GABA transmission by the tonic release of oxytocin and endocannabinoids governs postsynaptic firing. *J Neurosci* 27:1325–1333.

Olmos G, Aguilera P, Tranque P, Naftolin F, Garcia-Segura LM. (1987) Estrogen-induced synaptic remodeling in adult rat brain is accompanied by the reorganization of neuronal membranes. *Brain Res* 425:57–64.

Olmos G, Naftolin F, Perez J, Tranque PA, Garcia-Segura LM. (1989) Synaptic remodeling in the rat arcuate nucleus during the estrous cycle. *Neuroscience* 32:663–667.

Oomura Y, Hori N, Shiraishi T, Fukunaga K, Takeda H, Tsuji M, Matsumiya T, Ishibashi M, Aou S, Li XL, Kohno D, Uramura K, Sougawa H, Yada T, Wayner MJ, Sasaki K. (2006) Leptin facilitates learning and memory performance and enhances hippocampal CA1 long-term potentiation and CaMK II phosphorylation in rats. *Peptides* 27:2738–2749.

Oppenheimer JH, Schwartz HL. (1997) Molecular basis of thyroid hormone-dependent brain development. *Endocr Rev* 18:462–475.

Ord WM. (1888) Report of a committee of the Clinical Society of London nominated December 14, 1883, to investigate the subject of myxoedema. *Trans Clin Soc Lond* 21 (Suppl):1–215.

Ormerod BK, Galea LA. (2001) Reproductive status influences cell proliferation and cell survival in the dentate gyrus of adult female meadow voles: A possible regulatory role for estradiol. *Neuroscience* 102:369–379.

Ormerod BK, Lee TT-Y, Galea LAM. (2003) Estradiol initially enhances but subsequently suppresses (via adrenal steroids) granula cell proliferation in the dentate gyrus of adult female rats. *J Neurobiol* 55:247–260.

Ormerod BK, Lee TT, Galea LA. (2004) Estradiol enhances neurogenesis in the dentate gyri of adult male meadow voles by increasing the survival of young granule neurons. *Neuroscience* 128:645–654.

Osterweil D, Syndulko K, Cohen SN, Pettler-Jennings PD, Hershman JM, Cummings JL, Tourtellotte WW, Solomon DH. (1992) Cognitive function in non-demented older adults with hypothyroidism. *J Am Geriatr Soc* 40:325–335.

Otaegi G, Yusta-Boyo MJ, Vergano-Vera E, Mendez-Gomez HR, Carrera AC, Abad JL, Gonzalez M, de la Rosa EJ, Vicario-Abejon C, de Pablo F. (2006) Modulation of the PI 3-kinase-Akt signaling pathway by IGF-I and PTEN regulates the differentiation of neural stem/precursor cells. *J Cell Sci* 119:2739–2748.

Ozcan M, Yilmaz B, Carpenter DO. (2006) Effects of melatonin on synaptic transmission and long-term potentiation in two areas of mouse hippocampus. *Brain Res* 1111:90–94.

Ozdinler PH, Macklis JD. (2006) IGF-I specifically enhances axon outgrowth of corticospinal motor neurons. *Nat Neurosci* 9:1371–1381.

Paganini-Hill A. (1995) Estrogen replacement therapy and stroke. *Prog Cardiovasc Dis* 38:223–242.

Paganini-Hill A. (2001) Hormone replacement therapy and stroke: Risk, protection or no effect? *Maturitas* 38:243–261.

Paganini-Hill A, Henderson VW. (1996) Estrogen replacement therapy and risk of Alzheimer's disease. *Arch Intern Med* 156:2213–2217.

Pakkenberg B, Gundersen HJ. (1997) Neocortical neuron number in humans: Effect of sex and age. *J Comp Neurol* 384:312–320.

Pan Y, Zhang H, Acharya AB, Patrick PH, Oliver D, Morley JE. (2005) Effect of testosterone on functional recovery in a castrate male rat stroke model. *Brain Res* 1043:195–204.

Panatier A, Theodosis DT, Mothet JP, Touquet B, Pollegioni L, Poulain DA, Oliet SH (2006a). Glia-derived D-serine controls NMDA receptor activity and synaptic memory. *Cell* 125:775–784.

Panatier A, Gentles SJ, Bourque CW, Oliet SH. (2006b) Activity-dependent synaptic plasticity in the supraoptic nucleus of the rat hypothalamus. *J Physiol* 573:711–721.

Paneda C, Arroba AI, Frago LM, Holm AM, Romer J, Argente J, Chowen JA. (2003) Growth hormone-releasing peptide-6 inhibits cerebellar cell death in aged rats. *NeuroReport* 14:1633–1635.

Papadopoulos V, Guarneri P, Kreuger KE, Guidotti A, Costa E (1992) Pregnenolone biosynthesis in C6-2B glioma cell mitochondria: Regulation by a mitochondrial diazepam binding inhibitor receptor. *Proc Natl Acad Sci USA* 89:5113–5117.

Papadopoulos V, Boujrad N, Ikonomovic MD, Ferrara P, Vidic B. (1994) Topography of the Leydig cell mitochondrial peripheral-type benzodiazepine receptor. *Mol Cell Endocrinol* 104:R5–R9.

Papadopoulos V, Amri H, Boujrad N, Cascio C, Culty M, Garnier M, Hardwick M, Li H, Vidic B, Brown AS, Reversa JL, Bernassau JM, Drieu K. (1997) Peripheral benzodiazepine receptor in cholesterol transport and steroidogenesis. *Steroids* 62:21–28.

Papadopoulos V, Baraldi M, Guilarte TR, Knudsen TB, Lacapere JJ, Lindemann P, Norenberg MD, Nutt D, Weizman A, Zhang MR, Gavish M. (2006) Translocator protein (18kDa): New nomenclature for the peripheral-type benzodiazepine receptor based on its structure and molecular function. *Trends Pharmacol Sci* 27:402–409.

Papasozomenos SC. (1997) The heat shock-induced hyperphosphorylation of tau is estrogen-independent and prevented by androgens: Implications for Alzheimer's disease. *Proc Natl Acad Sci USA* 94:6612–6617.

Papasozomenos SCh, Shanavas A. (2002) Testosterone prevents the heat shock-induced overactivation of glycogen synthase kinase-3 beta but not of cyclin-dependent kinase 5 and c-Jun NH2-terminal kinase and concomitantly abolishes hyperphosphorylation of tau: Implications for Alzheimer's disease. *Proc Natl Acad Sci USA* 99:1140–1145.

Párducz A. Garcia-Segura LM. (1993) Sexual differences in the synaptic connectivity in the rat dentate gyrus. *Neurosci Lett* 161:53–56.

Párducz A, Perez J, Garcia-Segura LM. (1993) Estradiol induces plasticity of GABAergic synapses in the hypothalamus. *Neuroscience* 53:395–401.

Párducz A, Hoyk Z, Kis Z, Garcia-Segura LM. (2002) Hormonal enhancement of neuronal firing is linked to structural remodeling of excitatory and inhibitory synapses. *Eur J Neurosci* 16:665–670.

Párducz A, Zsarnovszky A, Naftolin F, Horvath TL. (2003) Estradiol affects axo-somatic contacts of neuroendocrine cells in the arcuate nucleus of adult rats. *Neuroscience* 117:791–794.

Parent AS, Rasier G, Matagne V, Lomniczi A, Lebrethon MC, Gérard A, Ojeda S, Bourguignon JP. (2008) Oxytocin facilitates female sexual maturation through a glia-to-neuron signaling pathway. *Endocrinology* 149:1358–1365.

Park JJ, Tobet SA, Baum MJ. (1998) Cell death in the sexually dimorphic dorsal preoptic area anterior hypothalamus of perinatal male and female ferrets. *J Neurobiol* 34:242–252.

Park MK, Hoang TA, Belluzzi JD, Leslie FM. (2003) Gender specific effect of neonatal handling on stress reactivity of adolescent rats. *J Neuroendocrinol* 15:289–295.

Parkash J, Kaur G. (2005) Neuronal–glial plasticity in gonadotropin-releasing hormone release in adult female rats: Role of the polysialylated form of the neural cell adhesion molecule. *J Endocrinol* 186:397–409.

Parkash J, Kaur G. (2007) Potential of PSA-NCAM in neuron-glial plasticity in the adult hypothalamus: Role of noradrenergic and GABAergic neurotransmitters. *Brain Res Bull* 74:317–328.

Paternostro M, Meisami E. (1989) Selective effects of thyroid hormonal deprivation on growth and development of olfactory receptor sheet during the early postnatal period: A morphometric and cell count study in the rat. *Int J Dev Neurosci* 7:243–255.

Patrone C, Ma ZQ, Pollio G, Agrati P, Parker MG, Maggi A. (1996) Cross-coupling between insulin and estrogen receptor in human neuroblastoma cells. *Mol Endocrinol* 10:499–507.

Patrone C, Gianazza E, Santagati S, Agrati P, Maggi A. (1998) Divergent pathways regulate ligand-independent activation of ERα in SK-N-BE neuroblastoma and COS-1 renal carcinoma cells. *Mol Endocrinol* 12:835–841.

Patrone C, Andersson S, Korhonen L, Lindholm D. (1999) Estrogen receptor-dependent regulation of sensory neuron survival in developing dorsal root ganglion. *Proc Natl Acad Sci USA* 96:10905–10910.

Patte-Mensah C, Kibaly C, Mensah-Nyagan AG. (2005) Substance P inhibits progesterone conversion to neuroactive metabolites in spinal sensory circuit: A potential component of nociception. *Proc Natl Acad Sci USA* 102:9044–9049.

Paus T. (2005) Mapping brain maturation and cognitive development during adolescence. *Trends Cogn Sci* 9:60–68.

Paus T, Collins DL, Evans AC, Leonard G, Pike B, Zijdenbos A. (2001) Maturation of white matter in the human brain: A review of magnetic resonance studies. *Brain Res Bull* 54:255–266.

Pavlides C, Kimura A, Magarinos AM, McEwen BS. (1995) Hippocampal homosynaptic long-term depression/depotentiation induced by adrenal steroids. *Neuroscience* 68:379–385.

Pavlides C, Ogawa S, Kimura A, McEwen BS. (1996) Role of adrenal steroid mineralocorticoid and glucocorticoid receptors in long-term potentiation in the CA1 field of hippocampal slices. *Brain Res* 738:229–235.

Pavlides C, Nivon LG, McEwen BS. (2002) Effects of chronic stress on hippocampal long-term potentiation. *Hippocampus* 12:245–257.

Pawlak R, Magarinos AM, Melchor J, McEwen B, Strickland S. (2003) Tissue plasminogen activator in the amygdala is critical for stress-induced anxiety-like behavior. *Nat Neurosci* 6:168–174.

Pawlak R, Rao BS, Melchor JP, Chattarji S, McEwen B, Strickland S. (2005) Tissue plasminogen activator and plasminogen mediate stress-induced decline of neuronal and cognitive functions in the mouse hippocampus. *Proc Natl Acad Sci USA* 102:18201–18206.

Pawluski JL, Galea LA. (2006) Hippocampal morphology is differentially affected by reproductive experience in the mother. *J Neurobiol* 66:71–81.

Pawluski JL, Walker SK, Galea LA. (2006a) Reproductive experience differentially affects spatial reference and working memory performance in the mother. *Horm Behav* 49:143–149.

Pawluski JL, Vanderbyl BL, Ragan K, Galea LA. (2006b) First reproductive experience persistently affects spatial reference and working memory in the mother and these effects are not due to pregnancy or 'mothering' alone. *Behav Brain Res* 175:157–165.

Pelligrino DA, Santizo R, Baughman VL, Wang Q. (1998) Cerebral vasodilating capacity during forebrain ischemia: Effects of chronic estrogen depletion and repletion and the role of neuronal nitric oxide synthase. *NeuroReport* 9:3285–3291.

Perakis A, Stylianopoulou F. (1986) Effects of a prenatal androgen peak on rat brain sexual differentiation. *J Endocrinol* 108:281–285.

Perea G, Araque A. (2007) Astrocytes potentiate transmitter release at single hippocampal synapses. *Science* 317:1083–1086.

Perera AD, Lageuaur CF, Plant TM. (1993) Postnatal expression of polysialic acid-neural cell adhesion molecule in the hypothalamus of the male Rhesus monkey (Macaca mulatta). *Endocrinology* 133:2729–2735.

Perera AD, Plant TM. (1997) Ultrastructural studies of neuronal correlates of the pubertal reaugmentation of hypothalamic gonadotropin-releasing hormone (GnRH) release in the rhesus monkey (Macaca mulatta). *J Comp Neurol* 385:71–82.

Pereyra ME, Sharbaugh SM, Hahn TP. (2005) Interspecific variation in photo-induced GnRH plasticity among nomadic cardueline finches. *Brain Behav Evol* 66:35–49.

Perez J, Naftolin F, Garcia-Segura LM. (1990b) Sexual differentiation of synaptic connectivity and neuronal plasma membrane in the arcuate nucleus of the rat hypothalamus. *Brain Res* 527:116–122.

Perez J, Hernandez P, Garcia-Segura LM. (1991) Estradiol increases the number of nuclear pores in the arcuate neurons of the rat hypothalamus. *J Comp Neurol* 303:225–232.

Perez J, Luquín S, Naftolin F, Garcia-Segura LM. (1993a) The role of estradiol and progesterone in phased synaptic remodeling of the rat arcuate nucleus. *Brain Res* 608:38–44.

Perez J, Naftolin F, Garcia-Segura LM. (1993b) Cyclohexamide mimics effects of oestradiol that are linked to synaptic plasticity of hypothalamic neurons. *J Neurocytol* 22:233–243.

Perez J, Cohen MA, Kelley DB. (1996) Androgen receptor mRNAexpression in Xenopus laevis CNS: Sexual dimorphism and regulation in laryngeal motor nucleus. *J Neurobiol* 30:556–568.

Perez J, Kelley DB. (1996) Trophic effects of androgen: Receptor expression and the survival of laryngeal motor neurons after axotomy. *J Neurosci* 16:6625–6633.

Perez-Martin M, Azcoitia I, Trejo JL, Sierra A, Garcia-Segura LM. (2003) An antagonist of estrogen receptors blocks the induction of adult neurogenesis by insulin-like growth factor-I in the dentate gyrus of adult female rat. *Eur J Neurosci* 18:923–930.

Perez-Martin M, Salazar V, Castillo C, Ariznavarreta C, Azcoitia I, Garcia-Segura LM, Tresguerres JA. (2005) Estradiol and soy extract increase the production of new cells in the dentate gyrus of old rats. *Exp Gerontol* 40:450–453.

Perez-Otano I, Ehlers MD. (2005) Homeostatic plasticity and NMDA receptor trafficking. *Trends Neurosci* 28:229–238.

Perlmutter LS, Tweedle CD, Hatton GI. (1984) Neuronal/glial plasticity in the supraoptic dendritic zone: Dendritic bundling and double synapse formation at parturition. *Neuroscience* 13:769–779.

Perlmutter LS, Tweedle CD, Hatton GI. (1985) Neuronal/glial plasticity in the supraoptic dendritic zone in response to acute and chronic dehydration. *Brain Res* 361:225–232.

Perls T. (2004) Centenarians who avoid dementia. *Trends Neurosci* 27:633–636.

Perry T, Greig NH. (2003) The glucagon-like peptides: A double-edged therapeutic sword? *Trends Pharmacol Sci* 24:377–383.

Perry T, Lahiri DK, Sambamurti K, Chen D, Mattson MP, Egan JM, Greig NH. (2003) Glucagon-like peptide-1 decreases endogenous amyloid-beta peptide (Abeta) levels and protects hippocampal neurons from death induced by Abeta and iron. *J Neurosci Res* 72:603–612.

Peterfi Z, Churchill L, Hajdu I, Obal Jr F, Krueger JM, Párducz A. (2004) Fos-immunoreactivity in the hypothalamus: Dependency on the diurnal rhythm, sleep, gender, and estrogen. *Neuroscience* 124:695–707.

Peters A, Leahu D, Moss MB, McNally KJ. (1994) The effects of aging on area 46 of the frontal cortex of the rhesus monkey. *Cereb Cortex* 4:621–635.

Peterson RS, Saldanha CJ, Schlinger BA. (2001) Rapid upregulation of aromatase mRNA and protein following neural injury in the zebra finch (Taeniopygia guttata). *J Neuroendocrinol* 13:317–323.

Peterson RS, Lee DW, Fernando G, Schlinger BA. (2004) Radial glia express aromatase in the injured zebra finch brain. *J Comp Neurol* 475:261–269.

Peterson RS, Yarram L, Schlinger BA, Saldanha CJ. (2005) Aromatase is pre-synaptic and sexually dimorphic in the adult zebra finch brain. *Proc Biol Sci* 272:2089–2096.

Peterson RS, Fernando G, Day L, Allen TA, Chapleau JD, Menjivar J, Schlinger BA, Lee DW. (2007) Aromatase expression and cell proliferation following injury of the adult zebra finch hippocampus. *Dev Neurobiol* 67:1867–1878.

Petralia SM, Jahagirdar V, Frye CA. (2005) Inhibiting biosynthesis and/or metabolism of progestins in the ventral tegmental area attenuates lordosis of rats in behavioural oestrus. *J Neuroendocrinol* 17:545–552.

Pfaff DW. (1999) *Drive: Neurobiological and molecular mechanisms of sexual motivation.* Cambridge, MA: MIT Press, 316 pp.

Pfaff DW, Keiner M. (1973) Atlas of estradiol-concentrating cells in the central nervous system of the female rat. *J Comp Neurol* 151:121–158.

Pfaus JG. (2000) Understanding sex in the brain. *Cell* 101:153–155.

Pfefferbaum A, Mathalon DH, Sullivan EV, Rawles JM, Zipursky RB, Lim KO. (1994) A quantitative magnetic resonance imaging study of changes in brain morphology from infancy to late adulthood. *Arch Neurol* 51:874–887.

Pham K, Nacher J, Hof PR, McEwen BS. (2003) Repeated restraint stress suppresses neurogenesis and induces biphasic PSA-NCAM expression in the adult rat dentate gyrus. *Eur J Neurosci* 17:879–886.

Phoenix CH, Goy RW, Garall AA, Young WC. (1959) Organizing action of prenatally administered testosterone propionate on the tissues mediating mating behaviour in the female guinea pig. *Endocrinology* 65:369–382.

Picazo O, Azcoitia I, Garcia-Segura LM. (2003) Neuroprotective and neurotoxic effects of estrogens. *Brain Res* 990:20–27.

Pike CJ. (1999) Estrogen modulates neuronal Bcl-XL expression and beta-amyloid-induced apoptosis: Relevance to Alzheimer's disease. *J Neurochem* 72:1552–1563.

Pike CJ. (2001) Testosterone attenuates beta-amyloid toxicity in cultured hippocampal neurons. *Brain Res* 919:160–165.

Pike CJ, Rosario ER, Nguyen TV. (2006) Androgens, aging, and Alzheimer's disease. *Endocrine* 29:233–241.

Pinos H, Collado P, Rodriguez-Zafra M, Rodriguez C, Segovia S, Guillamon A. (2001) The development of sex differences in the locus coeruleus of the rat. *Brain Res Bull* 56:73–78.

Pinto S, Roseberry AG, Liu H, Diano S, Shanabrough M, Cai X, Friedman JM, Horvath TL. (2004) Rapid rewiring of arcuate nucleus feeding circuits by leptin. *Science* 304:110–115.

Place NJ, Kenagy GJ. (2000) Seasonal changes in plasma testosterone and glucocorticoids in free-living male yellow-pine chipmunks and the response to capture and handling. *J Comp Physiol B* 170:245–251.

Plassart-Schiess E, Baulieu EE. (2001) Neurosteroids: Recent findings. *Brain Res Rev* 37:133–140.

Platania P, Seminara G, Aronica E, Troost D, Catania MV, Sortino MA. (2005) 17beta-estradiol rescues spinal motoneurons from AMPA-induced toxicity: A role for glial cells. *Neurobiol Dis* 20:461–470.

Plitzko D, Rumpel S, Gottmann K. (2001) Insulin promotes functional induction of silent synapses in differentiating rat neocortical neurons. *Eur J Neurosci* 14:1412–1415.

Plotsky PM, Meaney MJ. (1993) Early, postnatal experience alters hypothalamic corticotropin-releasing factor (CRF) mRNA, median eminence CRF content and stress-induced release in adult rats. *Mol Brain Res* 18:195–200.

Poirier J. (1994) Apolipoprotein E in animal models of CNS injury and in Alzheimer's disease. *Trends Neurosci* 17:525–530.

Pollock GS, Vernon E, Forbes ME, Yan Q, Ma YT, Hsieh T, Robichon R, Frost DO, Johnson JE. (2001) Effects of early visual experience and diurnal rhythms on BDNF mRNA and protein levels in the visual system, hippocampus, and cerebellum. *J Neurosci* 21:3923–3931.

Poltyrev T, Keshet GI, Kay G, Weinstock M. (1996) Role of experimental conditions in determining differences in exploratory behavior of prenatally stressed rats. *Dev Psychobiol* 29:453–462.

Pompolo S, Pereira A, Kaneko T, Clarke IJ. (2003) Seasonal changes in the inputs to gonadotropin-releasing hormone neurones in the ewe brain: An assessment by conventional fluorescence and confocal microscopy. *J Neuroendocrinol* 15:538–545.

Popken GJ, Hodge RD, Ye P, Zhang J, Ng W, O'Kusky JR, D'Ercole AJ. (2004) In vivo effects of insulin-like growth factor-I (IGF-I) on prenatal and early postnatal development of the central nervous system. *Eur J Neurosci* 19:2056–2068.

Popko B, Goodrum JF, Bouldin TW, Zhang SH, Maeda N. (1993) Nerve regeneration occurs in the absence of apolipoprotein E in mice. *J Neurochem* 60:1155–1158.

Popov VI, Bocharova LS. (1992) Hibernation-induced structural changes in synaptic contacts between mossy fibres and hippocampal pyramidal neurons. *Neuroscience* 48: 53–62.

Popov VI, Bocharova LS, Bragin AG. (1992) Repeated changes of dendritic morphology in the hippocampus of ground squirrels in the course of hibernation. *Neuroscience* 48:45–51.

Popovic V. (2005) GH Deficiency as the most common pituitary defect after TBI: Clinical implications. *Pituitary* 8:239–243.

Popovic V, Aimaretti G, Casanueva FF, Ghigo E. (2005) Hypopituitarism following traumatic brain injury. *GH & IGF Res* 15:177–184.

Porterfield SP, Hendrich CE. (1993) The role of thyroid hormones in prenatal and neonatal neurological development-current perspectives. *Endocr Rev* 14:94–106.

Post RM, Weiss SR, Li H, Smith MA, Zhang LX, Xing G, Osuch EA, McCann UD. (1998) Neural plasticity and emotional memory. *Dev Psychopathol* 10:829–855.

Potter E, Sutton S, Donaldson C, Chen R, Perrin M, Sawchenko PE, Vale W. (1994) Distribution of corticotropin-releasing factor receptor mRNA expression in the rat brain and pituitary. *Proc Natl Acad Sci USA* 91:8777–8781.

Prange-Kiel J, Rune GM, Leranth C. (2004) Median raphe mediates estrogenic effects to the hippocampus in female rats. *Eur J Neurosci* 19:309–317.

Prange-Kiel J, Fester L, Zhou L, Lauke H, Carretero J, Rune GM. (2006) Inhibition of hippocampal estrogen synthesis causes region-specific downregulation of synaptic protein expression in hippocampal neurons. *Hippocampus* 16:464–471.

Prange-Kiel J, Rune GM. (2006) Direct and indirect effects of estrogen on rat hippocampus. *Neuroscience* 138:765–772.

Prange-Kiel J, Jarry H, Schoen M, Kohlmann P, Lohse C, Zhou L, Rune GM. (2008) Gonadotropin-releasing hormone regulates spine density via its regulatory role in hippocampal estrogen synthesis. *J Cell Biol* 180:417–426.

Prass K, Scharff A, Ruscher K, Lowl D, Muselmann C, Victorov I, Kapinya K, Dirnagl U, Meisel A. (2003) Hypoxia-induced stroke tolerance in the mouse is mediated by erythropoietin. *Stroke* 34:1981–1986.

Prevot V. (2002) Glial-neuronal-endothelial interactions are involved in the control of GnRH secretion. *J Neuroendocrinol* 14:247–255.

Prevot V, Croix D, Bouret S, Dutoit S, Tramu G, Stefano GB, Beauvillain JC. (1999) Definitive evidence for the existence of morphological plasticity in the external zone of the median eminence during the rat estrous cycle: Implication of neuro–glio–endothelial interactions in gonadotropin-releasing hormone release. *Neuroscience* 94:809–819.

Prevot V, Cornea A, Mungenast A, Smiley G, Ojeda SR. (2003) Activation of erbB-1 signaling in tanycytes of the median eminence stimulates transforming growth factor beta1 release via prostaglandin E2 production and induces cell plasticity. *J Neurosci* 23:10622–10632.

Prevot V, Dehouck B, Poulain P, Beauvillain JC, Buée-Scherrer V, Bouret S. (2007) Neuronal–glial–endothelial interactions and cell plasticity in the postnatal hypothalamus: Implications for the neuroendocrine control of reproduction. *Psychoneuroendocrinology* 32 (Suppl 1):S46–S51.

Prokai L, Simpkins JW. (2007) Structure-nongenomic neuroprotection relationship of estrogens and estrogen-derived compounds. *Pharmacol Ther* 114:1–12.

Proulx K, Clavel S, Nault G, Richard D, Walker CD. (2001) High neonatal leptin exposure enhances brain GR expression and feedback efficacy on the adrenocortical axis of developing rats. *Endocrinology* 142:4607–4616.

Pruessner JC, Champagne F, Meaney MJ, Dagher A. (2004) Dopamine release in response to a psychological stress in humans and its relationship to early life maternal care: A positron emission tomography study using [11C]raclopride. *J Neurosci* 24:2825–2831.

Puia G, Santi MR, Vicini S, Pritchett DB, Purdy RH, Paul SM, Seeburg PH, Costa E. (1990) Neurosteroids act on recombinant human GABAA receptors. *Neuron* 4:759–765.

Purves D, Hadley RD. (1985) Changes in the dendritic branching of adult mammalian neurones revealed by repeated imaging in situ. *Nature* 315:404–406.

Pyter LM, Reader BF, Nelson RJ. (2005) Short photoperiods impair spatial learning and alter hippocampal dendritic morphology in adult male white-footed mice (Peromyscus leucopus). *J Neurosci* 25:4521–4526.

Qin Y, Xu G, Wang W. (2006) Dendritic abnormalities in retinal ganglion cells of three-month diabetic rats. *Curr Eye Res* 31:967–974.

Quesada A, Micevych PE. (2004) Estrogen interacts with the IGF-1 system to protect nigrostriatal dopamine and maintain motoric behavior after 6-hydroxdopamine lesions. *J Neurosci Res* 75:107–116.

Quintanilla RA, Munoz FJ, Metcalfe MJ, Hitschfeld M, Olivares G, Godoy JA, Inestrosa NC. (2005) Trolox and 17beta-estradiol protect against amyloid beta-peptide neurotoxicity by a mechanism that involves modulation of the Wnt signaling pathway. *J Biol Chem* 280:11615–1625.

Rabbani O, Panickar KS, Rajakumar G, King MA, Bodor N, Meyer EM, Simpkins JW. (1997) 17 beta-estradiol attenuates fimbrial lesion-induced decline of ChAT-immunoreactive neurons in the rat medial septum. *Exp Neurol* 146:179–186.

Raber J, Bongers G, LeFevour A, Buttini M, Mucke L. (2002) Androgens protect against apolipoprotein E4-induced cognitive deficits. *J Neurosci* 22:5204–5209.

Racagni G, Apud JA, Cocchi D, Locatelli V, Iuliano E, Casanueva F, Muller EE. (1984) Regulation of prolactin secretion during suckling: Involvement of the hypothalamo-pituitary GABAergic system. *J Endocrinol Invest* 7:481–487.

Racchi M, Govoni S, Solerte SB, Galli CL, Corsini E. (2001) Dehydroepiandrosterone and the relationship with aging and memory: A possible link with protein kinase C functional machinery. *Brain Res Rev* 37:287–293.

Radley JJ, Morrison JH. (2005). Repeated stress and structural plasticity in the brain. *Ageing Res Rev* 4:271–287.

Radley JJ, Sisti HM, Hao J, Rocher AB, McCall T, Hof PR, McEwen BS, Morrison JH. (2004) Chronic behavioral stress induces apical dendritic reorganization in pyramidal neurons of the medial prefrontal cortex. *Neuroscience* 125:1–6.

Radley JJ, Rocher AB, Janssen WG, Hof PR, McEwen BS, Morrison JH. (2005) Reversibility of apical dendritic retraction in the rat medial prefrontal cortex following repeated stress. *Exp Neurol* 196:199–203.

Radley JJ, Rocher AB, Rodriguez A, Ehlenberger DB, Dammann M, McEwen BS, Morrison JH, Wearne SL, Hof PR. (2008) Repeated stress alters dendritic spine morphology in the rat medial prefrontal cortex. *J Comp Neurol* 507:1141–1150.

Rage F, Lee BJ, Ma YJ, Ojeda SR. (1997) Estradiol enhances prostaglandin E2 receptor gene expression in luteinizing hormone-releasing hormone (LHRH) neurons and facilitates the LHRH response to PGE2 by activating a glia-to-neuron signaling pathway. *J Neurosci* 17:9145–9156.

Raggenbass M. (2008) Overview of cellular electrophysiological actions of vasopressin. *Eur J Pharmacol* 583:243–254.

Raghavan AV, Horowitz JM, Fuller CA. (1999) Diurnal modulation of long-term potentiation in the hamster hippocampal slice. *Brain Res* 833:311–314.

Rainnie DG, Bergeron R, Sajdyk TJ, Patil M, Gehlert DR, Shekhar A. (2004). Corticotrophin releasing factor-induced synaptic plasticity in the amygdala translates stress into emotional disorders. *J Neurosci* 24:3471–3479.

Raisman G, Field PM. (1973) Sexual dimorphism in the neuropil of the preoptic area of the rat and its dependence on neonatal androgen. *Brain Res* 54:1–29.

Rajkowska G, Miguel-Hidalgo JJ. (2007) Gliogenesis and glial pathology in depression. *CNS Neurol Disord Drug Targets* 6:219–233.

Ralph MR, Foster RG, Davis FC, Menaker M. (1990) Transplanted suprachiasmatic nucleus determines circadian period. *Science* 247:975–978.

Rami A, Patel AJ, Rabie A. (1986) Thyroid hormone and development of the rat hippocampus: Morphological altercations in granule and pyramidal cells. *Neuroscience* 19:1217–1226.

Rami A, Rabie A. (1990) Delayed synaptogenesis in the dentate gyrus of the thyroid-deficient developing rat. *Dev Neurosci* 12:398–405.

Ramirez VD, Zheng J. (1996) Membrane sex-steroid receptors in the brain. *Front Neuroendocrinol* 17:402–439.

Ramón y Cajal S. (1888) Estructura de los centros nerviosos de las aves. *Rev Trim Histol Norm Pat* 1:1–10.

Ramón y Cajal S. (1891) Significación fisiológica de las expansiones protoplásmicas y nerviosas de la sustancia gris. *Revista de Ciencias Médicas de Barcelona* 22: 671–679, 715–723.

Ramón y Cajal S. (1894) The Croonian lecture: La fine structure desc centres nerveux. *Proc Roy Soc London* 55:444–467.

Ramón y Cajal S. (1896a) Le bleu de methylene dans les centres nerveaux. *Rev Trim Microgr* 1:21–82.

Ramón y Cajal S. (1896b) Les épines collaterales des cellules du cerveau colorées au bleu de méthylene. *Rev Trim Microgr* 1:5–19.

Ramón y Cajal S. (1899) Estudios sobre la cortexa cerebral humana: Corteza visual. *Rev Trim Microgr* 4:1–63.

Ramón y Cajal S. (1913) Contribución al conocimiento de la neuroglia del cerebro humano. *Trab Lab Invest Biol* 11:255–315.

Rampon C, Tang YP, Goodhouse J, Shimizu E, Kyin M, Tsien JZ. (2000) Enrichment induces structural changes and recovery from nonspatial memory deficits in CA1 NMDAR1-knockout mice. *Nat Neurosci* 3:238–244.

Ramsey MM, Weiner JL, Moore TP, Carter CS, Sonntag WE. (2004) Growth hormone treatment attenuates age-related changes in hippocampal short-term plasticity and spatial learning. *Neuroscience* 129:119–127.

Ramsey MM, Adams MM, Ariwodola OJ, Sonntag WE, Weiner JL. (2005) Functional characterization of des-IGF-1 action at excitatory synapses in the CA1 region of rat hippocampus. *J Neurophysiol* 94:247–254.

Rand MN, Breedlove SM. (1995) Androgen alters the dendritic arbors of SNB motoneurons by acting upon their target muscles. *J Neurosci* 15:4408–4416.

Randell KM, Honkanen RJ, Komulainen MH, Tuppurainen MT, Kroger H, Saarikoski S. (2001) Hormone replacement therapy and risk of falling in early postmenopausal women—a population-based study. *Clin Endocrinol* (Oxf) 54:769–774.

Rankin SL, Partlow GD, McCurdy RD, Giles ED, Fisher KR. (2003) Postnatal neurogenesis in the vasopressin and oxytocin-containing nucleus of the pig hypothalamus. *Brain Res* 971:189–196.

Ransome MI, Goldshmit Y, Bartlett PF, Waters MJ, Turnley AM. (2004) Comparative analysis of CNS populations in knockout mice with altered growth hormone responsiveness. *Eur J Neurosci* 19:2069–2079.

Rapp PR, Gallagher M. (1996) Preserved neuron number in the hippocampus of aged rats with spatial learning deficits. *Proc Natl Acad Sci USA* 93:9926–9930.

Rasia-Filho AA, Fabian C, Rigoti KM, Achaval M. (2004) Influence of sex, estrous cycle and motherhood on dendritic spine density in the rat medial amygdala revealed by the Golgi method. *Neuroscience* 126:839–847.

Rasika S, Nottebohm F, Alvarez-Buylla A. (1994) Testosterone increases the recruitment and/or survival of new high vocal center neurons in adult female canaries. *Proc Natl Acad Sci USA* 89:8591–8595.

Rasika S, Alvarez-Buylla A, Nottebohm F. (1999) BDNF mediates the effects of testosterone on the survival of new neurons in an adult brain. *Neuron* 22:53–62.

Rasmussen T, Schliemann T, Sorensen JC, Zimmer J, West MJ. (1996) Memory impaired aged rats: No loss of principal hippocampal and subicular neurons. *Neurobiol Aging* 17:143–147.

Rauch SL, Shin LM. (1997) Functional neuroimaging studies in posttraumatic stress disorder. *Ann NY Acad Sci* 821:83–98.

Rauch SL, Savage CR, Alpert NM, Fischman AJ, Jenike MA. (1997) The functional neuroanatomy of anxiety: A study of three disorders using positron emission tomography and symptom provocation. *Biol Psychiatry* 42:446–452.

Rayner DV, Dalgliesh GD, Duncan JS, Hardie LJ, Hoggard N, Trayhurn P. (1997) Postnatal development of the ob gene system: Elevated leptin levels in suckling fa/ fa rats. *Am J Physiol* 273:R446–R450.

Reagan LP. (2007) Insulin signaling effects on memory and mood. *Curr Opin Pharmacol* 7:633–637.

Regan RF, Guo Y. (1997) Estrogens attenuate neuronal injury due to hemoglobin, chemical hypoxia, and excitatory amino acids in murine cortical cultures. *Brain Res* 764:133–140.

Regard E, Taurog A, Nakashima T. (1978) Plasma thyroxine and triiodothyronine levels in spontaneously metamorphosing Rana catesbeiana tadpoles and in adult anuran amphibia. *Endocrinology* 102:674–684.

Reibel S, Andre V, Chassagnon S, Andre G, Marescaux C, Nehlig A, Depaulis A. (2000) Neuroprotective effects of chronic estradiol benzoate treatment on hippocampal cell loss induced by status epilepticus in the female rat. *Neurosci Lett* 281:79–82.

Reid SN, Juraska JM. (1992) Sex differences in neuron number in the binocular area of the rat visual cortex. *J Comp Neurol* 321:448–455.

Reiner A, Perkel DJ, Bruce LL, Butler AB, Csillag A, Kuenzel W, Medina L, Paxinos G, Shimizu T, Striedter G, Wild M, Ball GF, Durand S, Güntürkün O, Lee DW, Mello CV, Powers A, White SA, Hough G, Kubikova L, Smulders TV, Wada K, Dugas-Ford J, Husband S, Yamamoto K, Yu J, Siang C, Jarvis ED; Avian Brain Nomenclature Forum. (2004) Revised nomenclature for avian telencephalon and some related brainstem nuclei. *J Comp Neurol* 473:377–414.

Reisert I, Pilgrim C. (1991) Sexual differentiation of monoaminergic neurons— genetic or epigenetic. *Trends Neurosci* 14:467–473.

Resnick SM, Maki PM. (2001) Effects of hormone replacement therapy on cognitive and brain aging. *Ann NY Acad Sci* 949:203–214.

Revankar CM, Cimino DF, Sklar LA, Arterburn JB, Prossnitz ER. (2005) A transmembrane intracellular estrogen receptor mediates rapid cell signaling. *Science* 307:1625–1630.

Reymond MJ. (1990) Age-related loss of the responsiveness of the tuberoinfundibular dopaminergic neurons to prolactin in the female rat. *Neuroendocrinology* 52:490–496.

Reyna-Neyra A, Camacho-Arroyo I, Ferrera P, Arias C. (2002) Estradiol and progesterone modify microtubule associated protein 2 content in the rat hippocampus. *Brain Res Bull* 58:607–612.

Rhodes ME, Frye CA. (2004) Progestins in the hippocampus of female rats have antiseizure effects in a pentylenetetrazole seizure model. *Epilepsia* 45:1531–1538.

Rhodes ME, McCormick CM, Frye CA. (2004) 3alpha,5alpha-THP mediates progestins' effects to protect against adrenalectomy-induced cell death in the dentate gyrus of female and male rats. *Pharmacol Biochem Behav* 78:505–512.

Rissman EF. (1996) Behavioral regulation of gonadotropin-releasing hormone. *Biol Reprod* 54:413–419.

Rivas M, Naranjo JR. (2007) Thyroid hormones, learning and memory. *Genes Brain Behav* 6 (Suppl 1):40–44.

Robertson CL, Puskar A, Hoffman GE, Murphy AZ, Saraswati M, Fiskum G. (2006) Physiologic progesterone reduces mitochondrial dysfunction and hippocampal cell loss after traumatic brain injury in female rats. *Exp Neurol* 197:235–243.

Robertson DM, van Amelsvoort T, Daly E, Simmons A, Whitehead M, Morris RG, Murphy KC, Murphy DG. (2001) Effects of estrogen replacement therapy on human brain aging: An in vivo 1H MRS study. *Neurology* 57:2114–2117.

Robertson JC, Watson JT, Kelley DB. (1994) Androgen directs sexual differentiation of laryngeal innervation in developing Xenopus laevis. *J Neurobiol* 25:1625–1636.

Robertson JC, Kelley DB. (1996) Thyroid hormone controls the onset of androgen sensitivity in the developing larynx of Xenopus laevis. *Dev Biol* 176:108–123.

Robinson J. (2006) Prenatal programming of the female reproductive neuroendocrine system by androgens *Reproduction* 132:539–547.

Rodriguez EM, Blazquez JL, Pastor FE, Pelaez B, Pena P, Peruzzo B, Amat P. (2005) Hypothalamic tanycytes: A key component of brain-endocrine interaction. *Int Rev Cytol* 247:89–164.

Rodriguez JJ, Montaron MF, Petry KG, Aurousseau C, Marinelli M, Premier S, Rougon G, Le Moal M, Abrous DN. (1998) Complex regulation of the expression of the polysialylated form of the neuronal cell adhesion molecule by glucocorticoids in the rat hippocampus. *Eur J Neurosci* 10:2994–3006.

Rodriguez-Peña A. (1999) Oligodendrocyte development and thyroid hormone. *J Neurobiol* 40:497–512.

Rodriquez de Fonseca F, Navarro M, Alvarez E, Roncero I, Chowen JA, Maestre O, Gomez R, Munoz RM, Eng J, Blazquez E. (2000) Peripheral versus central effects of glucagon-like peptide-1 receptor agonists on satiety and body weight loss in Zucker obese rats. *Metabolism* 49:709–717.

Rogan MT, Stäubli UV, Ledoux JE. (1997) Fear conditioning induces associative long-term potentiation in the amygdala. *Nature* 390:604–607.

Rogerio F, de Souza Queiroz L, Teixeira SA, Oliveira AL, de Nucci G, Langone F. (2002) Neuroprotective action of melatonin on neonatal rat motoneurons after sciatic nerve transection. *Brain Res* 926:33–41.

Roglio I, Bianchi R, Giatti S, Cavaletti G, Caruso D, Scurati S, Crippa D, Garcia-Segura LM, Camozzi F, Lauria G, Melcangi RC. (2007) Testosterone derivatives are neuroprotective agents in experimental diabetic neuropathy. *Cell Mol Life Sci* 64:1158–1168.

Romeo RD, Sisk CL. (2001) Pubertal and seasonal plasticity in the amygdale. *Brain Res* 889:71–77.

Romeo RD, Lee SJ, Chhua N, McPherson CR, McEwen BS. (2004) Testosterone cannot activate an adult-like stress response in prepubertal male rats. *Neuroendocrinology* 79:125–132.

Romeo RD, Bellani R, Karatsoreos IN, Chhua N, Vernov M, Conrad CD, McEwen BS. (2006) Stress history and pubertal development interact to shape hypothalamic–pituitary–adrenal axis plasticity. *Endocrinology* 147:1664–1674.

Romeo RD, McEwen BS. (2006) Stress and the adolescent brain. *Ann N Y Acad Sci* 1094:202–214.

Roof RL, Duvdevani R, Stein DG. (1993a) Gender influences outcome of brain injury: Progesterone plays a protective role. *Brain Res* 607:333–336.

Roof RL, Duvdevani R, Braswell L, Stein DG. (1994) Progesterone facilitates cognitive recovery and reduces secondary neuronal loss caused by cortical contusion injury in male rats. *Exp Neurol* 129:64–69.

Roof RL, Duvdevani R, Heyburn JW, Stein DG. (1996) Progesterone rapidly decreases brain edema: Treatment delayed up to 24 hours is still effective. *Exp Neurol* 138:246–251.

Roof RL, Hoffman SW, Stein DG. (1997) Progesterone protects against lipid peroxidation following traumatic brain injury in rats. *Mol Chem Neuropathol* 31:1–11.

Roozendaal B, Okuda S, de Quervain DJ, McGaugh JL. (2006) Glucocorticoids interact with emotion-induced noradrenergic activation in influencing different memory functions. *Neuroscience* 138:901–910.

Roselli CE, Horton LE, Resko JA. (1985) Distribution and regulation of aromatase activity in the rat hypothalamus and limbic system. *Endocrinology* 117:2471–2477.

Rosenzweig ES, Barnes CA. (2003) Impact of aging on hippocampal function: Plasticity, network dynamics, and cognition. *Prog Neurobiol* 69:143–179.

Rosenzweig MR, Krech D. Bennett EL, Diamond MC. (1962) Effects of environmental complexity and training on brain chemistry and anatomy: A replication and extension. *J Comp Physiol Psychol* 55:429–437.

Rosenzweig MR, Bennett EL. (1996) Psychobiology of plasticity: Effects of training and experience on brain and behavior. *Behav Brain Res* 78:57–65.

Rossberg MI, Murphy SJ, Traystman RJ, Hurn PD. (2000) LY353381.HCl, a selective estrogen receptor modulator, and experimental stroke. *Stroke* 31:3041–3046.

Rosselet C, Zennou-Azogui Y, Xerri C. (2006) Nursing-induced somatosensory cortex plasticity: Temporally decoupled changes in neuronal receptive field properties are accompanied by modifications in activity-dependent protein expression. *J Neurosci* 26:10667–10676.

Rossi GL, Bestetti GE, Reymond MJ. (1992) Tuberoinfundibular dopaminergic neurons and lactotropes in young and old female rats. *Neurobiol Aging* 13:275–281.

Roth CL, McCormack AL, Lomniczi A, Mungenast AE, Ojeda SR. (2006) Quantitative proteomics identifies a change in glial glutamate metabolism at the time of female puberty. *Mol Cell Endocrinol* 254–255:51–59.

Rotwein P, Burgess SK, Milbrandt JD, Krause JE. (1988) Differential expression of insulin-like growth factor genes in rat central nervous system. *Proc Natl Acad Sci USA* 85:265–269.

Roubenoff R, Harris TB, Abad LW, Wilson PW, Dallal GE, Dinarello CA. (1998) Monocyte cytokine production in an elderly population: Effect of age and inflammation. *J Gerontol A Biol Sci Med Sci* 53:M20–M26.

Rudick CN, Woolley CS. (2000) Estradiol induces a phasic Fos response in the hippocampal CA1 and CA3 regions of adult female rats. *Hippocampus* 10:274–228.

Rudick CN, Woolley CS. (2001) Estrogen regulates functional inhibition of hippocampal CA1 pyramidal cells in the adult female rat. *J Neurosci* 21:6532–6543.

Rudick CN, Gibbs RB, Woolley CS. (2003) A role for the basal forebrain cholinergic system in estrogen-induced disinhibition of hippocampal pyramidal cells. *J Neurosci* 23:4479–4490.

Rudick CN, Woolley CS. (2003) Selective estrogen receptor modulators regulate phasic activation of hippocampal CA1 pyramidal cells by estrogen. *Endocrinology* 144:179–187.

Ruediger J, Van der Zee EA, Strijkstra AM, Aschoff A, Daan S, Hut RA. (2007) Dynamics in the ultrastructure of asymmetric axospinous synapses in the frontal cortex of hibernating European ground squirrels (Spermophilus citellus). *Synapse* 61:343–352.

Ruiz-Marcos A, Valverde F (1969) The temporal evolution of the distribution of dendritic spines in the visual cortex of normal and dark raised mice. *Exp Brain Res* 8:284–294.

Ruiz-Marcos A, Sanchez-Toscano F, Escobar del Rey F, Morreale de Escobar G. (1979) Severe hypothyroidism and the maturation of the rat cerebral cortex. *Brain Res* 162:315–329.

Ruiz Marcos A, Sanchez-Toscano F, Morreale de Escobar G. (1982a) Reversible morphological alterations of cortical neurons in juvenile and adult hypothyroidism on the rat. *Brain Res* 185:91–102.

Ruiz-Marcos A, Sanchez-Toscano F, Obregon MJ, Escobar del Rey F, Morreale de Escobar G. (1982b) Thyroxine treatment and recovery of hypothyroidism-induced pyramidal cell damage. *Brain Res* 239:559–574.

Ruiz-Marcos A, Ipina SL. (1986) Hypothyroidism affects preferentially the dendritic densities on the more superficial region of pyramidal neurons of the rat cerebral cortex. *Brain Res* 393:259–262.

Ruiz-Marcos A, Cartagena Abella P, Garcia Garcia A, Escobar del Rey F, Morreale de Escobar G. (1988) Rapid effects of adult-onset hypothyroidism on dendritic spines of pyramidal cells of the rat cerebral cortex. *Exp Brain Res* 73:583–588.

Ruiz-Marcos A, Sanchez-Toscano F, Muñoz-Cueto JA. (1992) Aging reverts to juvenile conditions the synaptic connectivity of cerebral cortical pyramidal shafts. *Dev Brain Res* 69:41–49.

Ruiz-Marcos A, Cartagena-Abella P, Martinez-Galan JR, Calvo R, Morreale de Escobar G, Escobar del Rey F. (1994) Thyroxine treatment and the recovery of pyramidal cells of the cerebral cortex from changes induced by juvenile-onset hypothyroidism. *J Neurobiol* 25:808–818.

Rune GM, Frotscher M. (2005) Neurosteroid synthesis in the hippocampus: Role in synaptic plasticity. *Neuroscience* 136:833–842.

Ruppenthal GC, Arling GL, Harlow HF, Sackett GP, Suomi SJ. (1976) A 10-year perspective of motherless–mother monkey behavior. *J Abnorm Psychol* 85:341–349.

Rupprecht R, Reul JM, Trapp T, van SB, Wetzel C, Damm K, Zieglgansberger W, Holsboer F. (1993) Progesterone receptor-mediated effects of neuroactive steroids. *Neuron* 11:523–530.

Rusa R, Alkayed NJ, Crain BJ, Traystman RJ, Kimes AS, London ED, Klaus J.A, Hurn PD. (1999) 17β-estradiol reduces stroke injury in estrogen-deficient female animals. *Stroke* 30:1665–1670.

Rush ME, Blake CA. (1982) Serum testosterone concentrations during the 4-day estrous cycle in normal and adrenalectomized rats. *Proc Soc Exp Biol Med* 169:216–221.

Russell JA, Douglas AJ, Ingram CD. (2001) Brain preparations for maternity-adaptive changes in behavioral and neuroendocrine systems during pregnancy and lactation. An overview. *Prog Brain Res* 133:1–38.

Russo VC, Metaxas S, Kobayashi K, Harris M, Werther GA. (2004) Antiapoptotic effects of leptin in human neuroblastoma cells. *Endocrinology* 145:4103–4112.

Russo VC, Gluckman PD, Feldman EL, Werther GA. (2005) The insulin-like growth factor system and its pleiotropic functions in brain. *Endocr Rev* 26:916–943.

Ryan KJ, Naftolin F, Reddy V, Flores F, Petro Z. (1972) Estrogen formation in the brain. *Am J Obstet Gynecol* 114:454–460.

Rygula R, Abumaria N, Flugge G, Fuchs E, Ruther E, Havemann-Reinecke U. (2005) Anhedonia and motivational deficits in rats: Impact of chronic social stress. *Behav Brain Res* 162:127–134.

Sá SI, Madeira MD. (2005) Estrogen modulates the sexually dimorphic synaptic connectivity of the ventromedial nucleus. *J Comp Neurol* 484:68–79.

Saarela S, Reiter RJ. (1994) Function of melatonin in thermoregulatory processes. *Life Sci* 54:295–311.

Saavedra JM. (2005) Brain angiotensin II: New developments, unanswered questions and therapeutic opportunities. *Cell Mol Neurobiol* 25:485–512.

Saavedra JM, Ando H, Armando I, Baiardi G, Bregonzio C, Juorio A, Macova M. (2005) Anti-stress and anti-anxiety effects of centrally acting angiotensin II AT1 receptor antagonists. *Regul Pept* 128:227–238.

Saavedra JM, Benicky J. (2007) Brain and peripheral angiotensin II play a major role in stress. *Stress* 10:185–193.

Saccheti B, Scelfo B, Tempia F, Strata P. (2004) Long-term synaptic changes induced in the cerebellar cortex by fear conditioning. *Neuron* 42:973–982.

Sadamoto Y, Igase K, Sakanaka M, Sato K, Otsuka H, Sakaki S, Masuda S, Sasaki R. (1998) Erythropoietin prevents place navigation disability and cortical infarction in rats with permanent occlusion of the middle cerebral artery. *Biochem Biophys Res Commun* 253:26–32.

Sadow TF, Rubin RT. (1992) Effects of hypothalamic peptides on the aging brain. *Psychoneuroendocrinology* 17:293–314.

Sagales T, Gimeno V, Planella MJ, Raguer N, Bartolome J. (1993) Effects of rHuEPO on Q-EEG and event-related potentials in chronic renal failure. *Kidney Int* 44:1109–1115.

Sahay A, Hen R. (2007) Adult hippocampal neurogenesis in depression. *Nat Neurosci* 10:1110–1115.

Sakamoto H, Mezaki Y, Shikimi H, Ukena K, Tsutsui K. (2003) Dendritic growth and spine formation in response to estrogen in the developing Purkinje cell. *Endocrinology* 144:4466–4477.

Sakanaka M, Wen TC, Matsuda S, Masuda S, Morishita E, Nagao M, Sasaki R. (1998) In vivo evidence that erythropoietin protects neurons from ischemic damage. *Proc Natl Acad Sci USA* 95:4635–4640.

Sakuma Y, Pfaff DW. (1979) Mesencephalic mechanisms for integration of female reproductive behavior in the rat. *Am J Physiol* 237:R285–R290.

Sakurai T, Amemiya A, Ishii M, Matsuzaki I, Chemelli RM, Tanaka H, Williams SC, Richarson JA, Kozlowski GP, Wilson S, Arch JR, Buckingham RE, Haynes AC, Carr SA, Annan RS, McNulty DE, Liu WS, Terrett JA, Elshourbagy NA, Bergsma DJ, Yanagisawa M. (1998) Orexins and orexin receptors: A family of hypothalamic neuropeptides and G protein-coupled receptors that regulate feeding behavior. *Cell* 92:573–585.

Sakurai T, Gil OD, Whittard JD, Gazdoiu M, Joseph T, Wu J, Waksman A, Benson DL, Salton SR, Felsenfeld DP. (2008) Interactions between the L1 cell adhesion molecule and ezrin support traction-force generation and can be regulated by tyrosine phosphorylation. *J Neurosci Res* 86:2602–2614.

Salat DH, Tuch DS, Greve DN, van der Kouwe AJ, Hevelone ND, Zaleta AK, Rosen BR, Fischl B, Corkin S, Rosas HD, Dale AM. (2005) Age-related alterations in white matter microstructure measured by diffusion tensor imaging. *Neurobiol Aging* 26:1215–1227.

Saldanha CJ, Tuerk MJ, Kim YH, Fernandes AO, Arnold AP, Schlinger BA. (2000) Distribution and regulation of telencephalic aromatase expression in the zebra finch revealed with a specific antibody. *J Comp Neurol* 423:619–630.

Saldanha CJ, Silverman AJ, Silver R. (2001) Direct innervation of GnRH neurons by encephalic photoreceptors in birds. *J Biol Rhythms* 16:39–49.

Saldanha CJ, Rohmann KN, Coomaralingam L, Wynne RD. (2005) Estrogen provision by reactive glia decreases apoptosis in the zebra finch (Taeniopygia guttata). *J Neurobiol* 64:192–201.

Salm AK, Smithson KG, Hatton GI. (1985) Lactation-associated redistribution of the glial fibrillary acidic protein within the supraoptic nucleus. An immunocytochemical study. *Cell Tissue Res* 242:9–15.

Sanchez MM, Hearn EF, Do D, Rilling JK, Herndon JG. (1998) Differential rearing affects corpus callosum size and cognitive function of rhesus monkeys. *Brain Res* 812:38–49.

Sanchez MM, Young LJ, Plotsky PM, Insel TR. (2000) Distribution of corticosteroid receptors in the rhesus brain: Relative absence of glucocorticoid receptors in the hippocampal formation. *J Neurosci* 20:4657–4668.

Sanchez MM, Ladd CO, Plotsky PM. (2001) Early adverse experience as a developmental risk factor for later psychopathology: Evidence from rodent and primate models. *Dev Psychopathol* 13:419–449.

Sanchez-Toscano F, Escobar del Rey F, Morreale de Escobar G, Ruiz-Marcos A. (1977) Measurement of the effects of hypothyroidism on the number and distribution of spines along the apical shaft of pyramidal neurons of the rat cerebral cortex. *Brain Res* 126:547–550.

Sandi C. (2004) Stress, cognitive impairment and cell adhesion molecules. *Nat Rev Neurosci* 5:917–930.

Sandi C, Merino JJ, Cordero MI, Touyarot K, Venero C. (2001) Effects of chronic stress on contextual fear conditioning and the hippocampal expression of the neural cell adhesion molecule, its polysialylation, and L1. *Neuroscience* 102:329–339.

Sandi C, Davies HA, Cordero MI, Rodriguez JJ, Popov VI, Stewart MG. (2003) Rapid reversal of stress induced loss of synapses in CA3 of rat hippocampus following water maze training. *Eur J Neurosci* 17:2447–2456.

Sandi C, Woodson JC, Haynes VF, Park CR, Touyarot K, Lopez-Fernandez MA, Venero C, Diamond DM. (2005) Acute stress-induced impairment of spatial memory is associated with decreased expression of neural cell adhesion molecule in the hippocampus and prefrontal cortex. *Biol Psychiatry* 57:856–864.

Santarelli L, Saxe M, Gross C, Surget A, Battaglia F, Dulawa S, Weisstaub N, Lee J, Duman R, Arancio O, Belzung C, Hen R. (2003) Requirement of hippocampal neurogenesis for the behavioral effects of antidepressants. *Science* 301:805–809.

Sanz A, Carrero P, Carrero P, Pernía O, Garcia-Segura LM. (2008) Pubertal maturation modifies the regulation of insulin-like growth factor-I receptor signaling by estradiol in the rat prefrontal cortex. *Dev Neurobiol* 68:1018–1028.

Sapolsky RM. (1992) *Stress, the Aging Brain and the Mechanisms of Neuron Death.* MIT Press, Cambridge, MA, pp. 1–429.

Sapolsky RM, Krey LC, McEwen BS. (1985) Prolonged glucocorticoid exposure reduces hippocampal neuron number: Implications for aging. *J Neurosci* 5:1222–1227.

Sapolsky RM, Krey LC, McEwen BS. (1986) The neuroendocrinology of stress and aging: The glucocorticoid cascade hypothesis. *Endocr Rev* 7:284–301.

Saravia FE, Revsin Y, Lux-Lantos V, Beauquis J, Homo-Delarche F, De Nicola AF. (2004) Oestradiol restores cell proliferation in dentate gyrus and subventricular zone of streptozotocin-diabetic mice. *J Neuroendocrinol* 16:704–710.

Saravia FE, Beauquis J, Revsin Y, Homo-Delarche F, de Kloet ER, De Nicola AF. (2006) Hippocampal neuropathology of diabetes mellitus is relieved by estrogen treatment. *Cell Mol Neurobiol* 26:941–955.

Saravia FE, Beauquis J, Pietranera L, De Nicola AF. (2007) Neuroprotective effects of estradiol in hippocampal neurons and glia of middle age mice. *Psychoneuroendocrinology* 32:480–492.

Sarkey S, Azcoitia I, Garcia-Segura LM, Garcia-Ovejero D, DonCarlos LL. (2008) Classical androgen receptors in non-classical sites in the brain. *Horm Behav* 53:753–764.

Sasahara K, Shikimi H, Haraguchi S, Sakamoto H, Honda S, Harada N, Tsutsui K. (2007) Mode of action and functional significance of estrogen-inducing dendritic growth, spinogenesis, and synaptogenesis in the developing Purkinje cell. *J Neurosci* 27:7408–7417.

Sasaki F, Kawai T, Ohta M. (1994) Immunohistochemical evidence of neurons with GHRH or LHRH in the arcuate nucleus of male mice and their possible role in the postnatal development of adenohypophysial cells. *Anat Rec* 240:255–260.

Sasano H, Takashashi K, Satoh F, Nagura H, Harada N. (1998) Aromatase in the human central nervous system. *Clin Endocrinol* (Oxf) 48:325–329.

Sathiavageeswaran M, Burman P, Lawrence D, Harris AG, Falleti MG, Maruff P, Wass J. (2007) Effects of GH on cognitive function in elderly patients with adult-onset GH deficiency: A placebo-controlled 12-month study. *Eur J Endocrinol* 156:439–447.

Sato M, Nakahara K, Goto S, Kaiya H, Miyazato M, Date Y, Nakazato M, Kangawa K, Murakami N. (2006) Effects of ghrelin and des-acyl ghrelin on neurogenesis of the rat fetal spinal cord. *Biochem Biophys Res Commun* 350:598–603.

Saunders-Pullman R. (2003) Estrogens and Parkinson disease: Neuroprotective, symptomatic, neither, or both? *Endocrine* 21:81–87.

Saunders-Pullman R, Gordon-Elliott J, Parides M, Fahn S, Saunders HR, Bressman S. (1999) The effect of estrogen replacement on early Parkinson's disease. *Neurology* 52:1417–1421.

Savino W, Arzt E, Dardenne M. (1999) Immunoneuroendocrine connectivity: The paradigm of the thymus–hypothalamus–pituitary axis. *Neuroimmunomodulation* 6:126–136.

Sawada, H, Ibi M, Kihara T, Urushitani M, Akaike A, Shimohama S. (1998) Estradiol protects mesencephalic dopaminergic neurons from oxidative stress-induced neuronal death. *J Neurosci Res* 54:707–719.

Sawada M, Alkayed NJ, Goto S, Crain BJ, Traystman RJ, Shaivitz A, Nelson RJ, Hurn PD. (2000) Estrogen receptor antagonist ICI 182,780 exacerbates ischemic injury in female mouse. *J Cereb Blood Flow Metab* 20:112–118.

Sayeed I, Guo Q, Hoffman SW, Stein DG. (2006) Allopregnanolone, a progesterone metabolite, is more effective than progesterone in reducing cortical infarct volume after transient middle cerebral artery occlusion. *Ann Emerg Med* 47:381–389.

Sayeed I, Wali B, Stein DG. (2007) Progesterone inhibits ischemic brain injury in a rat model of permanent middle cerebral artery occlusion. *Restor Neurol Neurosci* 25:151–159.

Scarpace PJ, Matheny M, Tümer N. (2001) Hypothalamic leptin resistance is associated with impaired leptin signal transduction in aged obese rats. *Neuroscience* 104:1111–1117.

Schaap J, Albus H, Eilers PH, Detari L, Meijer JH. (2001) Phase differences in electrical discharge rhythms between neuronal populations of the left and right suprachiasmatic nuclei. *Neuroscience* 108:359–363.

Schaap J, Albus H, VanderLeest HT, Eilers PH, Detari L, Meijer JH. (2003) Heterogeneity of rhythmic suprachiasmatic nucleus neurons: Implications for circadian waveform and photoperiodic encoding. *Proc Natl Acad Sci USA* 100:15994–15999.

Schaefer AT, Larkum ME, Sakmann B, Roth A. (2003) Coincidence detection in pyramidal neurons is tuned by their dendritic branching pattern. *J Neurophysiol* 89:3143–3154.

Schafe GE, Nader K, Blair HT, Ledoux JE. (2001) Memory consolidation of Pavlovian fear conditioning: A cellular and molecular perspective. *Trends Neurosci* 24:540–546.

Schaible R, Gowen JW. (1961) A new dwarf mouse. *Genetics* 46:896.

Scharfman HE, MacLusky NJ. (2005) Similarities between actions of estrogen and BDNF in the hippocampus: Coincidence or clue? *Trends Neurosci* 28:79–85.

Scheepens A, Sirimanne ES, Breier BH, Clark RG, Gluckman PD, Williams CE. (2001) Growth hormone as a neuronal rescue factor during recovery from CNS injury. *Neuroscience* 104:677–687.

Scheepens A, Moderscheim TA, Gluckman PD. (2005) The role of growth hormone in neural development. *Horm Res* 64 (Suppl 3):66–72.

Scheibel ME, Lindsay RD, Tomiyasu U, Scheibel AB. (1976) Progressive dendritic changes in the aging human limbic system. *Exp Neurol* 53:420–430.

Scheibel AB. (1979) The hippocampus: Organizational patterns in health and senescence. *Mech Ageing Dev* 9:89–102.

Schlinger BA. (1998) Sexual differentiation of avian brain and behavior: Current views on gonadal hormone-dependent and independent mechanisms. *Annu Rev Physiol* 60:407–429.

Schlinger BA, Callard GV. (1989) Localization of aromatase in synaptosomal and microsomal subfractions of quail (Coturnix coturnix japonica) brain. *Neuroendocrinology* 49:434–441.

Schlinger BA, Arnold AP. (1992) Plasma sex steroids and tissue aromatization in hatchling zebra finches: Implications for the sexual differentiation of singing behavior. *Endocrinology* 130:289–299.

Schmidt KE, Kelley KM. (2001) Down-regulation in the insulin-like growth factor (IGF) axis during hibernation in the golden-mantled ground squirrel, Spermophilus lateralis: IGF-I and the IGF-binding proteins (IGFBPs). *J Exp Zool* 289:66–73.

Schmitz C, Rhodes ME, Bludau M, Kaplan S, Ong P, Ueffing I, Vehoff J, Korr H, Frye CA. (2002) Depression: Reduced number of granule cells in the hippocampus of female but not male, rats due to prenatal restraint stress. *Mol Psychiatr* 7:810–813.

Schnedl WJ, Ferber S, Johnson JH, Newgard CB. (1994) STZ transport and cytotoxicity. Specific enhancement in GLUT2-expressing cells. *Diabetes* 43:1326–1333.

Schneider ML. (1992) Prenatal stress exposure alters postnatal behavioral expression under conditions of novelty challenge in rhesus monkey infants. *Dev Psychobiol* 25:529–540.

Schneider ML, Roughton EC, Koehler AJ, Lubach GR. (1999) Growth and development following prenatal stress exposure in primates: An examination of ontogenetic vulnerability. *Child Dev* 70:263–274.

Schonknecht P, Pantel J, Klinga K, Jensen M, Hartmann T, Salbach B, Schroder J. (2001) Reduced cerebrospinal fluid estradiol levels are associated with increased beta-amyloid levels in female patients with Alzheimer's disease. *Neurosci Lett* 307:122–124.

Schoonover CM, Seibel MM, Jolson DM, Stack MJ, Rahman RJ, Jones SA, Mariash CN, Anderson GW. (2004) Thyroid hormone regulates oligodendrocyte accumulation in developing rat brain white matter tracts. *Endocrinology* 145:5013–5020.

Schreiber AM, Specker JL. (1998) Metamorphosis in the summer flounder (Paralichthys dentatus): Stage-specific developmental response to altered thyroid status. *Gen Comp Endocrinol* 111:156–166.

Schreiber AM, Das B, Huang H, Marsh-Armstrong N, Brown DD. (2001) Diverse developmental programs of Xenopus laevis metamorphosis are inhibited by a dominant negative thyroid hormone receptor. *Proc Natl Acad Sci USA* 98:10739–10744.

Schulkin J. (2003) *Rethinking homeostasis. Allostatic regulation in physiology and pathophysiology.* MIT press, Cambridge, MA.

Schumacher M, Balthazart J. (1987) Neuroanatomical distribution of testosterone-metabolizing enzymes in the Japanese quail. *Brain Res* 422:137–148.

Schumacher M, Guennoun R, Mercier G, Désarnaud F, Lacor P, Bénavides J, Ferzaz B, Robert F, Baulieu EE. (2001) Progesterone synthesis and myelin formation in peripheral nerves. *Brain Res Rev* 37:343–359.

Schumacher M, Guennoun R, Robert F, Carelli C, Gago N, Ghoumari A, Gonzalez Deniselle MC, Gonzalez SL, Ibanez C, Labombarda F, Coirini H, Baulieu EE, De Nicola AF. (2004) Local synthesis and dual actions of progesterone in the nervous system: Neuroprotection and myelination. *Growth Horm IGF Res* 14 (Suppl) A:S18–S33.

Schumacher M, Guennoun R, Stein DG, De Nicola AF. (2007) Progesterone: Therapeutic opportunities for neuroprotection and myelin repair. *Pharmacol Ther* 116:77–106.

Schutter DJ, van Honk J. (2005) The cerebellum on the rise in human emotion. *Cerebellum* 4:290–294.

Seckl JR. (2004) Prenatal glucocorticoids and long-term programming. *Eur J Endocrinol* 151:49–62.

Secoli SR, Teixeira N. (1998) Chronic prenatal stress affects development and behavioral depression in rats. *Stress* 2:273–280.

Seeman TE, Robbins RJ. (1994) Aging and hypothalamic-pituitary-adrenal response to challenge in humans. *Endocr Rev* 15:233–260.

Segal M. (2005) Dendritic spines and long-term plasticity. *Nat Rev Neurosci* 6:277–284.

Segal M, Murphy D. (2001) Estradiol induces formation of dendritic spines in hippocampal neurons: Functional correlates. *Horm Behav* 40:156–159.

Segarra AC, McEwen BS. (1991) Estrogen increases spine density in ventromedial hypothalamic neurons of peripubertal rats. *Neuroendocrinology* 54:365–372.

Segovia S, Guillamon A. (1993) Sexual dimorphism in the vomeronasal pathway and sex differences in reproductive behaviors. *Brain Res Rev* 18:51–74.

Segovia S, Guillamon A, del Cerro MC, Ortega E, Perez-Laso C, Rodriguez-Zafra M, Beyer C. (1999) The development of brain sex differences: A multisignaling process. *Behav Brain Res* 105:69–80.

Seki T, Arai Y. (1995) Age-related production of new granule cells in the adult dentate gyrus. *NeuroReport* 6:2479–2482.

Selye H. (1936) A syndrome produced by diverse nocuous agents. *Nature* 138:32.

Seminara SB, Messager S, Chatzidaki EE, Thresher RR, Acierno JS, Shagoury JK, Bo-Abbas Y, Kuohung W, Schwinof KM, Hendrick AG, Zahn D, Dixon J, Kaiser UB, Slaugenhaupt SA, Gusella JF, O'Rahilly S, Carlton MB, Crowley WF, Aparicio SA, Colledge WH. (2003) The GPR54 gene as a regulator of puberty. *N Engl J Med* 349:1614–1627.

Sengelaub DR, Arnold AP. (1989) Hormonal control of neuron number in sexually dimorphic spinal nuclei of the rat: I. Testosterone-regulated cell death in the dorsolateral nucleus. *J Comp Neurol* 280:622–629.

Sengelaub DR, Jordan CL, Kurz EM, Arnold AP. (1989a) Hormonal control of neuron number in sexually dimorphic spinal nuclei of the rat: I1. Development of the spinal nucleus of the bulbocavernosus in androgen-insensitive (Tfm) rats. *J Comp Neurol* 280:630–636.

Sengelaub DR, Nordeen EJ, Nordeen KW, Arnold AP. (1989b) Hormonal control of neuron number in sexually dimorphic spinal nuclei of the rat: III. Differential effects of the androgen dihydrotestosterone. *J Comp Neurol* 280:637–644.

Seoane LM, Al-Massadi O, Lage M, Dieguez C, Casanueva FF. (2004) Ghrelin: From a GH-secretagogue to the regulation of food intake, sleep and anxiety. *Pediatr Endocrinol Rev 1* (Suppl) 3:432–437.

Seress L, Basco E, Hajos F, Fulop Z. (1978) The effect of thyroid hormone on the formation of rat cerebellar Bergmann-glia. *Acta Morphol Acad Sci Hung* 26:95–100.

Shah S, Bell RJ, Savage G, Goldstat R, Papalia MA, Kulkarni J, Donath S, Davis SR. (2006) Testosterone aromatization and cognition in women: A randomized, placebo-controlled trial. *Menopause* 13:600–608.

Shahab M, Mastronardi C, Seminara SB, Crowley WF, Ojeda SR, Plant TM. (2005) Increased hypothalamic GPR54 signaling: A potential mechanism for initiation of puberty in primates. *Proc Natl Acad Sci USA* 102:2129–2134.

Shamlian NT, Cole MG. (2006) Androgen treatment of depressive symptoms in older men: A systematic review of feasibility and effectiveness. *Can J Psychiatry* 51:295–299.

Shanley LJ, Irving AJ, Harvey J. (2001) Leptin enhances NMDA receptor function and modulates hippocampal synaptic plasticity. *J Neurosci* 21:RC186.

Sharma R, McMillan CR, Tenn CC, Niles LP. (2006) Physiological neuroprotection by melatonin in a 6-hydroxydopamine model of Parkinson's disease. *Brain Res* 1068:230–236.

Shaw P, Greenstein D, Lerch J, Clasen L, Lenroot R, Gogtay N, Evans A, Rapoport J, Giedd J. (2006) Intellectual ability and cortical development in children and adolescents. *Nature* 440:676–679.

Shaywitz BA, Shaywitz SE. (2000) Estrogen and Alzheimer's disease: Plausible theory, negative clinical trial. *JAMA* 283:1055–1056.

Shear DA, Galani R, Hoffman SW, Stein DG. (2002) Progesterone protects against necrotic damage and behavioral abnormalities caused by traumatic brain injury. *Exp Neurol* 178:59–67.

Shekhar A, Truitt W, Rainnie D, Sajdyk T. (2005) Role of stress, corticotrophin releasing factor (CRF) and amygdala plasticity in chronic anxiety. *Stress* 8:209–219.

Shen H, Watanabe M, Tomasiewicz H, Rutishauser U, Magnuson T, Glass JD. (1997) Role of neural cell adhesion molecule and polysialic acid in mouse circadian clock function. *J Neurosci* 17:5221–5229.

Sheng H, Laskowitz DT, Mackensen GB, Kudo M, Pearlstein RD, Warner DS. (1999) Apolipoprotein E deficiency worsens outcome from global cerebral ischemia in the mouse. *Stroke* 30:1118–1124.

Sherman BM, West JH, Korenman SG. (1976) The menopausal transition: Analysis of LH, FSH, estradiol, and progesterone concentrations during menstrual cycles of older women. *J Clin Endocrinol Metab* 42:629–636.

Sherman BM, Wysham C, Pfohl B. (1985) Age-related changes in the circadian rhythm of plasma cortisol in man. *J Clin Endocrinol Metab* 61:439–443.

Sherwin BB, Henry JF. (2008) Brain aging modulates the neuroprotective effects of estrogen on selective aspects of cognition in women: A critical review. *Front Neuroendocrinol* 29:88–113.

Shi J, Panickar KS, Yang SH, Rabbani O, Day AL, Simpkins JW. (1998) Estrogen attenuates over-expression of beta-amyloid precursor protein messager RNA in an animal model of focal ischemia. *Brain Res* 810:87–92.

Shi L, Linville MC, Tucker EW, Sonntag WE, Brunso-Bechtold JK. (2005) Differential effects of aging and insulin-like growth factor-1 on synapses in CA1 of rat hippocampus. *Cereb Cortex* 15:571–577.

Shi YB. (1999) *Amphibian metamorphosis: From morphology to molecular biology.* Wiley & Sons, New York.

Shin CY, Choi JW, Jang ES, Ryu JH, Kim WK, Kim HC, Ko KH. (2001) Glucocorticoids exacerbate peroxynitrite mediated potentiation of glucose deprivation-induced death of rat primary astrocytes. *Brain Res* 923:163–171.

Shin DH, Lee E, Kim JW, Kwon BS, Jung MK, Jee YH, Kim J, Bae SR, Chang YP. (2004) Protective effect of growth hormone on neuronal apoptosis after hypoxia-ischemia in the neonatal rat brain. *Neurosci Lett* 354:64–68.

Shin LM, McNally RJ, Kosslyn SM, Thompson WL, Rauch SL, Alpert NM, Metzger LJ, Lasko NB, Orr SP, Pitman RK. (1999) Regional cerebral blood flow during script driven imagery in childhood sexual abuse-related PTSD: A PET investigation. *Am J Psychiat* 156:575–584.

Shin LM, Rauch SL, Pitman RK. (2006) Amygdala, medial prefrontal cortex, and hippocampal function in PTSD. *Ann N Y Acad Sci* 1071:67–79.

Shingo T, Sorokan ST, Shimazaki T, Weiss S. (2001) Erythropoietin regulates the in vitro and in vivo production of neuronal progenitors by mammalian forebrain neural stem cells. *J Neurosci* 21:9733–9743.

Shingo T, Gregg C, Enwere E, Fujikawa H, Hassam R, Geary C, Cross JC, Weiss S. (2003) Pregnancy-stimulated neurogenesis in the adult female forebrain mediated by prolactin. *Science* 299:117–120.

Shinoda K, Nagano M, Osawa Y. (1994) Neuronal aromatase expression in preoptic, strial, and amygdaloid regions during late prenatal and early postnatal development in the rat. *J Comp Neurol* 343:113–129.

Shintani M, Tamura Y, Monden M, Shiomi H. (2005) Thyrotropin-releasing hormone induced thermogenesis in Syrian hamsters: Site of action and receptor subtype. *Brain Res* 1039:22–29.

Shintani N, Nohira T, Hikosaka A, Kawahara A. (2002) Tissue-specific regulation of type III iodothyronine 5-deiodinase gene expression mediates the effects of prolactin and growth hormone in Xenopus metamorphosis. *Dev Growth Differ* 44:327–335.

Shivatcheva TM, Ankov VK, Hadjioloff AI. (1988) Circannual fluctuations of the serum cortisol in the European ground squirrel, Citellus citellus L. *Comp Biochem Physiol* 90A:515–518.

Shors TJ, Seib TB, Levine S, Thompson RF. (1989) Inescapable versus escapable shock modulates long-term potentiation in the rat hippocampus. *Science* 244:224–226.

Shughrue PJ, Dorsa DM. (1993) Estrogen modulates the growth-associated protein GAP-43 (Neuromodulin) mRNA in the rat preoptic area and basal hypothalamus. *Neuroendocrinology* 57:439–447.

Shughrue PJ, Lane MV, Merchenthaler I. (1997) Comparative distribution of estrogen receptor-alpha and -beta mRNA in the rat central nervous system. *J Comp Neurol* 388:507–525.

Shumaker SA, Legault C, Rapp SR, Thal L, Wallace RB, Ockene JK, Hendrix SL, Jones BN, III, Assaf AR, Jackson RD, Kotchen JM, Wassertheil-Smoller S, Wactawski-Wende J. (2003) Estrogen plus progestin and the incidence of dementia and mild cognitive impairment in postmenopausal women: The Women's Health Initiative Memory Study: A randomized controlled trial. *JAMA* 289:2651–2662.

Sierra A. (2004) Neurosteroids: The StAR protein in the brain. *J Neuroendocrinol* 16:787–793.

Sierra A, Azcoitia I, Garcia-Segura LM. (2003a) Endogenous estrogen formation is neuroprotective in a model of cerebellar ataxia. *Endocrine* 21:43–52.

Sierra A, Lavaque E, Perez-Martin M, Azcoitia I, Hales DB, Garcia-Segura LM. (2003b) Steroidogenic acute regulatory protein in the rat brain: Cellular distribution, developmental regulation and overexpression after injury. *Eur J Neurosci* 18:1458–1467.

Sigurdsson T, Doyere V, Cain CK, Ledoux JE. (2006) Long-term potentiation in the amygdala: A cellular mechanism of fear learning and memory. *Neuropharmacology* 52:215–227.

Silverman RC, Gibson MJ, Silverman AJ. (1991) Relationship of glia to GnRH axonal outgrowth from third ventricular grafts in hpg hosts. *Exp Neurol* 114: 259–274.

Simerly RB. (2002) Wired for reproduction: Organization and development of sexually dimorphic circuits in the mammalian forebrain. *Annu Rev Neurosci* 25:507–536.

Simerly RB, Chang C, Muramatsu M, Swanson LW. (1990) Distribution of androgen and estrogen receptor mRNA-containing cells in the rat brain: An in situ hybridization study. *J Comp Neurol* 294:76–95.

Simerly RB, Zee MC, Pendleton JW, Lubahn DB, Korach KS. (1997) Estrogen receptor dependent sexual differentiation of dopaminergic neurons in the preoptic region of the mouse. *Proc Natl Acad Sci USA* 94:14077–14082.

Simpkins JW, Green PS, Gridley KE, Singh M, de Fiebre NC, Rajakumar G.
    (1997a) Role of estrogen replacement therapy in memory enhancement and
    the prevention of neuronal loss associated with Alzheimer's disease. *Am J Med*
    103:19S–25S.

Simpkins JW, Rajakumar G, Zhang YQ, Simpkins CE, Greenwald D, Yu CJ, Bodor N,
    Day AL. (1997b) Estrogens may reduce mortality and ischemic damage caused by
    middle cerebral artery occlusion in the female rat. *J Neurosurg* 87:724–730.

Simpkins JW, Yang SH, Liu R, Perez E, Cai ZY, Covey DF, Green PS. (2004)
    Estrogen-like compounds for ischemic neuroprotection. *Stroke* 35(11 Suppl
    1):2648–2651.

Simpkins JW, Wang J, Wang X, Perez E, Prokai L, Dykens JA. (2005) Mitochondria
    play a central role in estrogen-induced neuroprotection. *Curr Drug Targets CNS
    Neurol Disord* 4:69–83.

Simpson ER, Davis SR. (2001) Minireview: Aromatase and the regulation of estrogen
    biosynthesis-some new perspectives. *Endocrinology* 142:4589–4594.

Singer CA, Pang PA, Dobie DJ, Dorsa DM. (1996a) Estrogen increases GAP-43
    (neuromodulin) mRNA in the preoptic area of aged rats. *Neurobiol Aging*
    17:661–663.

Singer CA, Rogers KL, Strickland TM, Dorsa DM. (1996b) Estrogen protects primary
    cortical neurons from glutamate toxicity. *Neurosci Lett* 212:13–16.

Singer CA, Rogers KL, Dorsa DM. (1998) Modulation of Bcl-2 expression: A potential
    component of estrogen protection in NT2 neurons. *NeuroReport* 9:2565–2568.

Singer CA, Figueroa-Masot XA, Batchelor RH, Dorsa DM. (1999) The mitogen-
    activated protein kinase pathway mediates estrogen neuroprotection after
    glutamate toxicity in primary cortical neurons. *J Neurosci* 19:2455–2463.

Singh M. (2001) Ovarian hormones elicit phosphorylation of Akt and extracellular-
    signal regulated kinase in explants of the cerebral cortex. *Endocrine* 14:407–415.

Singh M. (2005) Mechanisms of progesterone-induced neuroprotection. *Ann NY
    Acad Sci* 1052:145–151.

Sinopoli KJ, Floresco SB, Galea LA. (2006) Systemic and local administration of
    estradiol into the prefrontal cortex or hippocampus differentially alters working
    memory. *Neurobiol Learn Mem* 86:293–304.

Siren AL, Fratelli M, Brines M, Goemans C, Casagrande S, Lewczuk P, Keenan
    S, Gleiter C, Pasquali C, Capobianco A, Mennini T, Heumann R, Cerami A,
    Ehrenreich H, Ghezzi P. (2001) Erythropoietin prevents neuronal apoptosis after
    cerebral ischemia and metabolic stress. *Proc Natl Acad Sci USA* 98:4044–4049.

Siren AL, Radyushkin K, Boretius S, Kammer D, Riechers CC, Natt O, Sargin D,
    Watanabe T, Sperling S, Michaelis T, Price J, Meyer B, Frahm J, Ehrenreich H.
    (2006) Global brain atrophy after unilateral parietal lesion and its prevention by
    erythropoietin. *Brain* 129:480–489.

Sisk CL, Zehr JL. (2005) Pubertal hormones organize the adolescent brain and
    behavior. *Front Neuroendocrinol* 26:163–174.

Skaper SD, Ancona B, Facci L, Franceschini D, Giusti P. (1998) Melatonin prevents
    the delayed death of hippocampal neurons induced by enhanced excitatory
    neurotransmission and the nitridergic pathway. *FASEB J* 12:725–731.

Skeberdis VA, Lan J, Zheng X, Zukin RS, Bennett MV. (2001) Insulin promotes rapid
    delivery of N-methyl-D-aspartate receptors to the cell surface by exocytosis. *Proc
    Natl Acad Sci USA* 98:3561–3566.

Skinner DC, Herbison AE. (1997) Effects of photoperiod on estrogen receptor, tyrosine hydroxylase, neuropeptide Y, and β-endorphin immunoreactivity in the ewe hypothalamus. *Endocrinology* 138:2585–2595.

Smith BL, Wills G, Naylor D. (1981) The effects of prenatal stress on rat offsprings' learning ability. *J Physiol* 107:45–51.

Smith CC, McMahon LL. (2005) Estrogen-induced increase in the magnitude of long-term potentiation occurs only when the ratio of NMDA transmission to AMPA transmission is increased. *J Neurosci* 25:7780–7791.

Smith CC, McMahon LL. (2006) Estradiol-induced increase in the magnitude of long-term potentiation is prevented by blocking NR2B-containing receptors. *J Neurosci* 26:8517–8522.

Smith DE, Rapp PR, McKay HM, Roberts JA, Tuszynski MH. (2004) Memory impairment in aged primates is associated with focal death of cortical neurons and atrophy of subcortical neurons. *J Neurosci* 24:4373–4381.

Smith GT. (1996) Seasonal plasticity in the song nuclei of wild rufous-sided towhees. *Brain Res* 734:79–85.

Smith GT, Brenowitz EA, Wingfield JC, Baptista LF. (1995) Seasonal changes in song nuclei and song behavior in Gambel's whitecrowned sparrows. *J Neurobiol* 28:114–125.

Smith GT, Brenowitz EA, Wingfield JC. (1997) Roles of photoperiod and testosterone in seasonal plasticity of the avian song control system. *J Neurobiol* 32:426–442.

Smith JT. (2008) Kisspeptin signaling in the brain: Steroid regulation in the rodent and ewe. *Brain Res Rev* 57:288–298.

Smith RG, Betancourt L, Sun Y. (2005) Molecular endocrinology and physiology of the aging nervous system. *Endocr Rev* 26:203–250.

Smith RG, Sun Y, Jiang H, Albarran-Zeckler R, Timchenko N. (2007) Ghrelin receptor (GHS-R1A) agonists show potential as interventive agents during aging. *Ann N Y Acad Sci* 1119:147–164.

Smith SS. (1998) Estrous hormones enhance coupled, rhythmic olivary discharge in correlation with facilitated limb stepping. *Neuroscience* 82:83–95.

Smulders TV, Sasson AD, DeVoogd TJ. (1995) Seasonal variation in hippocampal volume in a food-storing bird, the black capped chickadee. *J Neurobiol* 27:15–25.

Snell GD. (1929) Dwarf, a new mendelian recessive character of the house mouse. *Proc Natl Acad Sci USA* 15:733–734.

Sohrabji F, Greene LA, Miranda RC, Toran-Allerand CD. (1994a) Reciprocal regulation of estrogen and NGF receptors by their ligands in PC12 cells. *J Neurobiol* 25:974–988.

Sohrabji F, Miranda RC, Toran-Allerand CD. (1994b) Estrogen differentially regulates estrogen and nerve growth factor receptor mRNAs in adult sensory neurons. *J Neurosci* 14:459–471.

Sohrabji F, Lewis DK. (2006) Estrogen-BDNF interactions: Implications for neurodegenerative diseases. *Front Neuroendocrinol* 27:404–414.

Soma KK. (2006) Testosterone and aggression: Berthold, birds and beyond. *J Neuroendocrinol* 18:543–551.

Son GH, Geum D, Chung S, Kim EJ, Jo JH, Kim CM, Lee KH, Kim H, Choi S, Kim HT, Lee CJ, Kim K. (2006) Maternal stress produces learning deficits associated with impairment of NMDA receptor-mediated synaptic plasticity. *J Neurosci* 26:3309–3318.

Sonntag WE, Lynch CD, Cooney PT, Hutchins PM. (1997) Decreases in cerebral microvasculature with age are associated with the decline in growth hormone and insulin-like growth factor 1. *Endocrinology* 138:3515–3520.

Sonntag WE, Lynch CD, Bennett SA, Khan AS, Thornton PL, Cooney PT, Ingram RL, McShane T, Brunso-Bechtold JK. (1999) Alterations in insulin-like growth factor-1 gene and protein expression and type 1 insulin-like growth factor receptors in the brains of ageing rats. *Neuroscience* 88:269–279.

Sonntag WE, Bennett SA, Khan AS, Thornton PL, Xu X, Ingram RL, Brunso-Bechtold JK. (2000a) Age and insulin-like growth factor-1 modulate N-methyl-D-aspartate receptor subtype expression in rats. *Brain Res Bull* 51:331–338.

Sonntag WE, Lynch C, Thornton P, Khan A, Bennett S, Ingram R. (2000b) The effects of growth hormone and IGF-1 deficiency on cerebrovascular and brain ageing. *J Anat* 197: 575–585.

Sortino MA, Chisari M, Merlo S, Vancheri C, Caruso M, Nicoletti F, Canonico PL, Copani A. (2004) Glia mediates the neuroprotective action of estradiol on beta-amyloid-induced neuronal death. *Endocrinology* 145:5080–5086.

Soto-Moyano R, Burgos H, Flores F, Valladares L, Sierralta W, Fernandez V, Perez H, Hernandez P, Hernandez A. (2006) Melatonin administration impairs visuo-spatial performance and inhibits neocortical long-term potentiation in rats. *Pharmacol Biochem Behav* 85:408–414.

Sotres-Bayon F, Cain CK, LeDoux JE. (2006) Brain mechanisms of fear extinction: Historical perspectives on the contribution of prefrontal cortex. *Biol Psychiatry* 60:329–336.

Sousa N, Lukoyanov NV, Madeira MD, Almeida OF, Paula-Barbosa MM. (2000) Reorganization of the morphology of hippocampal neurites and synapses after stress-induced damage correlates with behavioral improvement. *Neuroscience* 97:253–266.

Sousa N, Almeida OF. (2002) Corticosteroids: Sculptors of the hippocampal formation. *Rev Neurosci* 13:59–84.

Sousa N, Cerqueira JJ, Almeida OF. (2008) Corticosteroid receptors and neuroplasticity. *Brain Res Rev* 57:561–570.

Sowell ER, Thompson PM, Holmes CJ, Jernigan TL, Toga AW. (1999) In vivo evidence for post-adolescent brain maturation in frontal and striatal regions. *Nat Neurosci* 2:859–861.

Spear LP. (2000) The adolescent brain and age-related behavioral manifestations. *Neurosci Biobehav Rev* 24:417–463.

Speert DB, Konkle AT, Zup SL, Schwarz JM, Shiroor C, Taylor ME, McCarthy MM. (2007) Focal adhesion kinase and paxillin: Novel regulators of brain sexual differentiation? *Endocrinology* 148:3391–3401.

Sporn AL, Greenstein DK, Gogtay N, Jeffries NO, Lenane M, Gochman P, Clasen LS, Blumenthal J, Giedd JN, Rapoport JL. (2003) Progressive brain volume loss during adolescence in childhood-onset schizophrenia. *Am J Psychiatry* 160:2181–2189.

Srinivasan V, Pandi-Perumal SR, Maestroni GJ, Esquifino AI, Hardeland R, Cardinali DP. (2005) Role of melatonin in neurodegenerative diseases. *Neurotox Res* 7:293–318.

Stanton TL, Daley JC, Salzman SK. (1987) Prolongation of hibernation bout duration by continuous intracerebroventricular infusion of melatonin in hibernating ground squirrels. *Brain Res* 413:350–355.

Stanton TL, Caine SB, Winokur A. (1992) Seasonal and state-dependent changes in brain TRH receptors in hibernating ground squirrels. *Brain Res Bull* 28:877–886.

Steckelbroeck S, Heidrich DD, Stoffel-Wagner B, Hans VH, Schramm J, Bidlingmaier F, Klingmüller D. (1999) Characterization of aromatase cytochrome P450 activity in the human temporal lobe. *J Clin Endocrinol Metab* 84:2795–2801.

Stefanovic I, Adrian B, Jansen HT, Lehman MN, Goodman RL. (2000) The ability of estradiol to induce Fos expression in a subset of estrogen receptor-alpha-containing neurons in the preoptic area of the ewe depends on reproductive status. *Endocrinology* 141:190–196.

Stein DG. (2005) The case for progesterone. *Ann NY Acad Sci* 1052:152–169.

Stein DG. (2007) Sex differences in brain damage and recovery of function: Experimental and clinical findings. *Prog Brain Res* 161:339–351.

Stein MB, Keller SE, Schleifer SJ. (1988) Immune system. Relationship to anxiety disorders. *Psychiatr Clin North Am* 11:349–360.

Stein MB, Koverola C, Hanna C, Torchia MG, McClarty B. (1997) Hippocampal volume in women victimized by childhood sexual abuse. *Psychol Med* 27:951–959.

Steinberg L. (2005) Cognitive and affective development in adolescence. *Trends Cogn Sci* 9:69–74.

Sterling P. (2004) Principles of allostasis: Optimal design, predictive regulation, pathophysiology and rational therapeutics. In: J Schulkin (Ed.) *Allostasis, homeostasis and the cost of adaptation.* Cambridge University Press, Cambridge, pp. 1–36.

Sterling P, Eyer J. (1988) Allostasis, a new paradigm to explain arousal pathology. In: S. Fisher and J. Reason (Eds.) *Handbook of life stress, cognition and health.* John Wiley & Sons, New York, pp. 629–649.

Stern JE, Armstrong WE. (1998) Reorganization of the dendritic trees of oxytocin and vasopressin neurons of the rat supraoptic nucleus during lactation. *J Neurosci* 18:841–853.

Stern PC, Carstensen LL. (2000) *The aging mind.* Washington, DC, National Academy Press.

Stevens JR. (2002) Schizophrenia: Reproductive hormones and the brain. *Am J Psychiatry* 159:713–719.

Stewart J, Kolb B. (1994) Dendritic branching in cortical pyramidal cells in response to ovariectomy in adult female rats: Suppression by neonatal exposure to testosterone. *Brain Res* 654:149–154.

Stewart J, Rajabi H. (1994) Estradiol derived from testosterone in prenatal life affects the development of catecholamine systems in the frontal cortex in the male rat. *Brain Res* 646:157–160.

Stewart MG, Davies HA, Sandi C, Kraev IV, Rogachevsky VV, Peddie CJ, Rodriguez JJ, Cordero MI, Donohue HS, Gabbott PL, Popov VI. (2005) Stress suppresses and learning induces plasticity in CA3 of rat hippocampus: A three-dimensional ultrastructural study of thorny excrescences and their postsynaptic densities. *Neuroscience* 131:43–54.

Stocco DM. (2001) StAR protein and the regulation of steroid hormone biosynthesis. *Annu Rev Physiol* 63:193–213.

Stoffel-Wagner B. (2001) Neurosteroid metabolism in the human brain. *Eur J Endocrinol* 145:669–679.

Stoffel-Wagner B. (2003) Neurosteroid biosynthesis in the human brain and its clinical implications. *Ann N Y Acad Sci* 1007:64–78.

Stoffel-Wagner B, Watzka M, Steckelbroeck S, Wickert L, Schramm J, Romalo G, Klingmuller D, Schweikert HU. (1998) Expression of 5alpha-reductase in the human temporal lobe of children and adults. *J Clin Endocrinol Metab* 83:3636–3642.

Stoffel-Wagner B, Watzka M, Schramm J, Bidlingmaier F, Klingmuller D. (1999) Expression of CYP19 (aromatase) mRNA in different areas of the human brain. *J Steroid Biochem Mol Biol* 70:237–241.

Stone DJ, Rozovsky I, Morgan TE, Anderson CP, Hajian H, Finch CE. (1997) Astrocytes and microglia respond to estrogen with increased apoE mRNA in vivo and in vitro. *Exp Neurol* 143:313–318.

Stone DJ, Rozovsky I, Morgan TE, Anderson CP, Finch CE. (1998) Increased synaptic sprouting in response to estrogen via an apolipoprotein E-dependent mechanism: Implications for Alzheimer's disease. *J Neurosci* 18:3180–3185.

Storer PD, Jones KJ. (2003) Glial fibrillary acidic protein expression in the hamster red nucleus: Effects of axotomy and testosterone treatment. *Exp Neurol* 184:939–946.

Storm EE, Tecott LH. (2005) Social circuits: Peptidergic regulation of mammalian social behavior. *Neuron* 47:483–486.

Stranahan AM, Arumugam TV, Cutler RG, Lee K, Egan JM, Mattson MP. (2008) Diabetes impairs hippocampal function through glucocorticoid-mediated effects on new and mature neurons. *Nat Neurosci* 11:309–317.

Strijbos PJ, Relton JK, Rothwell NJ. (1994) Corticotrophin-releasing factor antagonist inhibits neuronal damage induced by focal cerebral ischaemia or activation of NMDA receptors in the rat brain. *Brain Res* 656:405–408.

Struble RG, Rosario ER, Kircher ML, Ludwig SM, McAdamis PJ, Watabe K, McAsey ME, Cady C, Nathan BP. (2003) Regionally specific modulation of brain apolipoprotein E in the mouse during the estrous cycle and by exogenous 17beta estradiol. *Exp Neurol* 183:638–644.

Struble RG, Nathan BP, Cady C, Cheng X, McAsey M. (2007) Estradiol regulation of astroglia and apolipoprotein E: An important role in neuronal regeneration. *Exp Gerontol* 42:54–63.

Strumwasser F. (1959) Regulatory mechanisms, brain activity and behavior during deep hibernation in the squirrel, Citellus beecheyi. *Am J Physiol* 196:23–30.

Sudo S, Wen TC, Desaki J, Matsuda S, Tanaka J, Arai T, Maeda N, Sakanaka M. (1997) β-Estradiol protects hippocampal CA1 neurons against transient forebrain ischemia in gerbil. *Neurosci Res* 29:345–354.

Sui L, Wang F, Li BM. (2006) Adult-onset hypothyroidism impairs paired-pulse facilitation and long-term potentiation of the rat dorsal hippocampo-medial prefrontal cortex pathway in vivo. *Brain Res* 1096:53–60.

Sullivan SD, Moenter SM. (2004) Prenatal androgens alter GABAergic drive to gonadotropin-releasing hormone neurones: Implications for a common fertility disorder. *Proc Natl Acad Sci USA* 101:7129–7134.

Sumida H, Nishizuka M, Kano Y, Arai Y. (1993) Sex differences in the anteroventral periventricular nucleus of the preoptic area and in the related effects of androgen in prenatal rats. *Neurosci Lett* 151:41–44.

Sun FY, Lin X, Mao LZ, Ge WH, Zhang LM, Huang YL, Gu J. (2002) Neuroprotection by melatonin against ischemic neuronal injury associated with modulation of DNA damage and repair in the rat following a transient cerebral ischemia. *J Pineal Res* 33:48–56.

Sun LY, Al-Regaiey K, Masternak MM, Wang J, Bartke A. (2005a) Local expression of GH and IGF-1 in the hippocampus of GH-deficient long-lived mice. *Neurobiol Aging* 26:929–937.

Sun LY, Evans MS, Hsieh J, Panici J, Bartke A. (2005b) Increased neurogenesis in dentate gyrus of long-lived Ames dwarf mice. *Endocrinology* 146:1138–1144.

Sun LY, Bartke A. (2007) Adult neurogenesis in the hippocampus of long-lived mice during aging. *J Gerontol A Biol Sci Med Sci* 62:117–125.

Surget A, Belzung C. (2008) Involvement of vasopressin in affective disorders. *Eur J Pharmacol* 583:340–349.

Sutcliffe JG, de Lecea L. (2002) The hypocretins: Setting the arousal threshold. *Nat Rev Neurosci* 3:339–349.

Suzuki C, Ozaki I, Tanosaki M, Suda T, Baba M, Matsunaga M. (2000) Peripheral and central conduction abnormalities in diabetes mellitus. *Neurology* 54:1932–1937.

Suzuki S, Brown CM, Dela Cruz CD, Yang E, Bridwell DA, Wise PM. (2007a) Timing of estrogen therapy after ovariectomy dictates the efficacy of its neuroprotective and antiinflammatory actions. *Proc Natl Acad Sci USA* 104:6013–6018.

Suzuki S, Gerhold LM, Bottner M, Rau SW, Dela Cruz C, Yang E, Zhu H, Yu J, Cashion AB, Kindy MS, Merchenthaler I, Gage FH, Wise PM. (2007b) Estradiol enhances neurogenesis following ischemic stroke through estrogen receptors alpha and beta. *J Comp Neurol* 500:1064–1075.

Swaab DF, Bao AM, Lucassen PJ. (2005) The stress system in the human brain in depression and neurodegeneration. *Ageing Res Rev* 4:141–194.

Swinny JD, Kalicharan D, Blaauw EH, Ijkema-Paassen J, Shi F, Gramsbergen A, van der Want JJ. (2003) Corticotropin-releasing factor receptor types 1 and 2 are differentially expressed in pre- and post-synaptic elements in the post-natal developing rat cerebellum. *Eur J Neurosci* 18:549–562.

Swinny JD, Valentino RJ. (2006) Corticotropin-releasing factor promotes growth of brain norepinephrine neuronal processes through Rho GTPase regulators of the actin cytoskeleton in rat. *Eur J Neurosci* 24:2481–2490.

Szuran TF, Pliska V, Pokorny J, Welzl H. (2000) Prenatal stress in rats: Effects on plasma corticosterone, hippocampal glucocorticoid receptors, and maze performance. *Physiol Behav* 71:353–362.

Takamatsu N, Ohba KI, Kondo J, Kondo N, Shiba T. (1993) Hibernation-associated gene regulation of plasma proteins with a collagen-like domain in mammalian hibernators. *Mol Cell Biol* 13:1516–1521.

Takamatsu N, Kojima M, Taniyama M, Ohba KI, Uematsu T, Segawa C, Tsutou S, Watanabe M, Kondo J, Kondo N, Shiba T. (1997) Expression of multiple α1-antitrypsin-like genes in hibernating species of the squirrel family. *Gene* 204:127–132.

Talge NM, Neal C, Glover V. (2007) Antenatal maternal stress and long-term effects on child neurodevelopment: How and why? *J Child Psychol Psychiatry* 48:245–261.

Tamura Y, Shintani M, Nakamura A, Monden M, Shiomi H. (2005) Phase-specific central regulatory systems of hibernation in Syrian hamsters. *Brain Res* 1045:88–96.

Tanapat P, Hastings NB, Reeves AJ, Gould E. (1999) Estrogen stimulates a transient increase in the number of new neurons in the dentate gyrus of the adult female rat. *J Neurosci* 19:5792–5801.

Tanapat P, Hastings NB, Rydel TA, Galea LA, Gould E. (2001) Exposure to fox odor inhibits cell proliferation in the hippocampus of adult rats via an adrenal hormone-dependent mechanism. *J Comp Neurol* 437:496–504.

Tanapat P, Hastings NB, Gould E. (2005) Ovarian steroids influence cell proliferation in the dentate gyrus of the adult female rat in a dose and time-dependent manner. *J Comp Neurol* 481:252–265.

Tanriverdi F, Senyurek H, Unluhizarci K, Selcuklu A, Casanueva FF, Kelestimur F. (2006) High risk of hypopituitarism after traumatic brain injury: A prospective investigation of anterior pituitary function in the acute phase and 12 months after trauma. *J Clin Endocrinol Metabol* 91:2105–2111.

Tanriverdi F, Unluhizarci K, Coksevim B, Selcuklu A, Casanueva FF, Kelestimur, F.(2007) Kickboxing sport as a new cause of traumatic brain injury-mediated hypopituitarism. *Clin Endocrinol* 66:360–366.

Tanzer L, Jones KJ. (1997) Gonadal steroid regulation of hamster facial nerve regeneration: Effects of dihydrotestosterone and estradiol. *Exp Neurol* 146:258–264.

Tanzer L, Jones KJ. (2004) Neurotherapeutic action of testosterone on hamster facial nerve regeneration: Temporal window of effects. *Horm Behav* 45:339–344.

Tapia-Gonzalez S, Carrero P, Pernia O, Garcia-Segura LM, Diz-Chaves Y. (2008) Selective oestrogen receptor (ER) modulators reduce microglia reactivity in vivo after peripheral inflammation: Potential role of microglial ERs. *J Endocrinol* 198:219–230.

Tata DA, Marciano VA, Anderson BJ. (2006) Synapse loss from chronically elevated glucocorticoids: Relationship to neuropil volume and cell number in hippocampal area CA3. *J Comp Neurol* 498:363–374.

Tatar M, Kopelman A, Epstein D, Tu MP, Yin CM, Garofalo RS. (2001) A mutant Drosophila insulin receptor homolog that extends life-span and impairs neuroendocrine function. *Science* 292:107–110.

Tatar M, Bartke A, Antebi A. (2003) The endocrine regulation of aging by insulin-like signals. *Science* 299:1346–1351.

Taziaux M, Keller M, Bakker J, Balthazart J. (2007) Sexual behavior activity tracks rapid changes in brain estrogen concentrations. *J Neurosci* 27:6563–6572.

Tchekalarova J, Albrecht D. (2007) Angiotensin II suppresses long-term depression in the lateral amygdala of mice via L-type calcium channels. *Neurosci Lett* 415:68–72.

Teicher MH, Andersen SL, Hostetter JC. (1995) Evidence for dopamine receptor pruning between adolescence and adulthood in striatum but not nucleus accumbens. *Dev Brain Res* 89:167–172.

Teixeira C, Reed JC, Pratt MAC. (1995) Estrogen promotes hemotherapeutic drug resistance by a mechanism involving bcl-2 proto-oncogene expression in human breast cancer cells. *Cancer Res* 55:3902–3907.

Tekumalla PK, Tontonoz M, Hesla MA, Kirn JR. (2002) Effects of excess thyroid hormone on cell death, cell proliferation, and new neuron incorporation in the adult zebra finch telencephalon. *J Neurobiol* 51:323–341.

Telegdy G, Adamik A. (2002) The action of orexin A on passive avoidance learning. Involvement of transmitters. *Regul Pept* 104:105–110.

Tena-Sempere M. (2006) The roles of kisspeptins and G protein-coupled receptor-54 in pubertal development. *Curr Opin Pediatr* 18:442–447.

Tena-Sempere M. (2008) Ghrelin and reproduction: Ghrelin as novel regulator of the gonadotropic axis. *Vitam Horm* 77:285–300.

Terentini GP, Botticelli A, Sannicola Botticelli C. (1974) Effect of monosodium glutamate on the endocrine glands and on the reproductive function of the rat. *Fertil Steril* 6:478–483.

Teter B, Harris-White ME, Frautschy SA, Cole GM. (1999) Role of apolipoprotein E and estrogen in mossy fiber sprouting in hippocampal slice cultures. *Neuroscience* 91:1009–1016.

Tetzlaff JE, Huppenbauer CB, Tanzer L, Alexander TD, Jones KJ. (2006) Motoneuron injury and repair: New perspectives on gonadal steroids as neurotherapeutics. *J Mol Neurosci* 28:53–64.

Teyler TJ, Vardaris RM, Lewis D, Rawitch AB. (1980) Gonadal steroids: Effects on excitability of hippocampal pyramidal cells. *Science* 209:1017–1018.

Theodosis DT. (1985) Oxytocin-immunoreactive terminals synapse on oxytocin neurones in the supraoptic nucleus. *Nature* 313:682–684.

Theodosis DT. (2002) Oxytocin-secreting neurons: A physiological model of morphological neuronal and glial plasticity in the adult hypothalamus. *Front Neuroendocrinol* 23:101–135.

Theodosis DT, Poulain DA, Vincent JD. (1981) Possible morphological bases for synchronization of neuronal firing in the rat supraoptic nucleus during lactation. *Neuroscience* 6:919–929.

Theodosis DT, Poulain DA. (1984a) Evidence for structural plasticity in the supraoptic nucleus of the rat hypothalamus in relation to gestation and lactation. *Neuroscience* 11:183–193.

Theodosis DT, Poulain DA. (1984b) Evidence that oxytocin-secreting neurones are involved in the ultrastructural reorganization of the rat supraoptic nucleus apparent at lactation. *Cell Tissue Res* 235:217–219.

Theodosis DT, Chapman DB, Montagnese C, Poulain DA, Morris JF. (1986a) Structural plasticity in the hypothalamic supraoptic nucleus at lactation affects oxytocin-, but not vasopressin-secreting neurones. *Neuroscience* 17:661–678.

Theodosis DT, Montagnese C, Rodriguez F, Vincent JD, Poulain DA. (1986b) Oxytocin induces morphological plasticity in the adult hypothalamo-neurohypophysial system. *Nature* 322:738–740.

Theodosis DT, Paut L, Tappaz ML. (1986c) Immunocytochemical analysis of the GABAergic innervation of oxytocin- and vasopressin-secreting neurons in the rat supraoptic nucleus. *Neuroscience* 19:207–222.

Theodosis DT, Poulain DA. (1987) Oxytocin-secreting neurones: A physiological model for structural plasticity in the adult mammalian brain. *Trends Neurosci* 10:426–430.

Theodosis DT, Rougon G, Poulain A. (1991) Retention of embryonic features by an adult neuronal system capable of plasticity: Polysialylated neural cell adhesion molecule in the hypothalamus-neurohypophysial system. *Proc Natl Acad Sci USA* 88:5494–5498.

Theodosis DT, Poulain DA. (1993) Activity-dependent neuronal-glial and synaptic plasticity in the adult mammalian hypothalamus. *Neuroscience* 57:501–535.

Theodosis DT, Bonfanti L, Olive S, Rougon G, Poulain DA. (1994) Adhesion molecules and structural plasticity of the adult hypothalamo-neurohypophysial system. *Psychoneuroendocrinology* 19:455–62.

Theodosis DT, el Majdoubi M, Gies U, Poulain DA. (1995) Physiologically-linked structural plasticity of inhibitory and excitatory synaptic inputs to oxytocin neurons. *Adv Exp Med Biol* 395:155–171.

Theodosis DT, MacVicar B. (1996) Neurone–glia interactions in the hypothalamus and pituitary. *Trends Neurosci* 19:363–367.

Theodosis DT, Bonhomme R, Vitiello S, Rougon G, Poulain DA. (1999) Cell surface expression of polysialic acid on NCAM is a prerequisite for activity-dependent morphological neuronal and glial plasticity. *J Neurosci* 19:10228–10236.

Theodosis DT, Trailin A, Poulain DA. (2006a) Remodeling of astrocytes, a prerequisite for synapse turnover in the adult brain? Insights from the oxytocin system of the hypothalamus. *Am J Physiol Regul Integr Comp Physiol* 290:R1175–R1182.

Theodosis DT, Koksma JJ, Trailin A, Langle SL, Piet R, Lodder JC, Timmerman J, Mansvelder H, Poulain DA, Oliet SH, Brussaard AB. (2006b) Oxytocin and estrogen promote rapid formation of functional GABA synapses in the adult supraoptic nucleus. *Mol Cell Neurosci* 31:785–794.

Theodosis DT, Poulain DA, Oliet SH. (2008) Activity-dependent structural and functional plasticity of astrocyte-neuron interactions. *Physiol Rev* 88:983–1008.

Thomas AJ, Nockels RP, Pan HQ, Shaffrey CI, Chopp M. (1999) Progesterone is neuroprotective after acute experimental spinal cord trauma in rats. *Spine* 24:2134–2138.

Thompson CK, Bentley GE, Brenowitz EA. (2007) Rapid seasonal-like regression of the adult avian song control system. *Proc Natl Acad Sci USA* 104:15520–15525.

Thompson PM, Giedd JN, Woods RP, MacDonald D, Evans AC, Toga AW. (2000) Growth patterns in the developing brain detected by using continuum mechanical tensor maps. *Nature* 404:190–193.

Thompson RR, Adkins-Regan E. (1994) Photoperiod affects the morphology of a sexually dimorphic nucleus within the preoptic area of male Japanese quail. *Brain Res* 667:201–208.

Thompson WR. (1957) Influence of prenatal maternal anxiety on emotionality in young rats. *Science* 125:698–699.

Thornton PL, Ingram RL, Sonntag WE. (2000) Chronic [d-Ala2]-growth hormone-releasing hormone administration attenuates age-related deficits in spatial memory. *J Gerontol A Biol Sci Med Sci* 55:B106–B112.

Tobet SA, Zahniser DJ, Baum MJ. (1986) Differentiation in male ferrets of a sexually dimorphic nucleus of the preoptic/anterior hypothalamic area requires prenatal estrogen. *Neuroendocrinology* 44:299–308.

Toescu EC, Verkhratsky A, Landfield PW. (2004) Ca²⁺ regulation and gene expression in normal brain aging. *Trends Neurosci* 27:614–620.

Tomas-Camardiel M, Sanchez-Hidalgo MC, Sanchez del Pino MJ, Navarro A, Machado A, Cano J. (2002) Comparative study of the neuroprotective effect of dehydroepiandrosterone and 17beta-estradiol against 1-methyl-4-phenylpyridium toxicity on rat striatum. *Neuroscience* 109:569–584.

Tomas-Camardiel M, Venero JL, Herrera AJ, De Pablos RM, Pintor-Toro JA, Machado A, Cano J. (2005) Blood-brain barrier disruption highly induces aquaporin-4 mRNA and protein in perivascular and parenchymal astrocytes: Protective effect by estradiol treatment in ovariectomized animals. *J Neurosci Res* 80:235–246.

Tomasi TE, Hellgren EC, Tucker TJ. (1998) Thyroid hormone concentrations in black bears (Ursus americanus): Hibernation and pregnancy effects. *Gen Comp Endocrinol* 109:192–199.

Tomizawa K, Iga N, Lu YF, Moriwaki A, Matsushita M, Li ST, Miyamoto O, Itano T, Matsui H. (2003) Oxytocin improves long-lasting spatial memory during motherhood through MAP kinase cascade. *Nat Neurosci* 6:384–390.

Toni N, Buchs PA, Nikonenko I, Bron CR, Muller D. (1999) LTP promotes formation of multiple spine synapses between a single axon terminal and a dendrite. *Nature* 402:421–425.

Topalli I, Etgen AM. (2004) Insulin-like growth factor-I receptor and estrogen receptor crosstalk mediates hormone-induced neurite outgrowth in PC12 cells. *Brain Res* 1030: 116–124.

Toran-Allerand CD. (1976) Sex steroids and the development of the newborn mouse hypothalamus and preoptic area in vitro: Implications for sexual differentiation. *Brain Res* 106:407–412.

Toran-Allerand CD. (1980) Sex steroids and the development of the newborn mouse hypothalamus and preoptic area in vitro. II. Morphological correlates and hormonal specificity. *Brain Res* 189:413–427.

Toran-Allerand CD. (1996) Mechanisms of estrogen action during neural development: Mediation by interactions with the neurotrophins and their receptors? *J Steroid Biochem Mol Biol* 56:169–78.

Toran-Allerand CD. (2004) Minireview: A plethora of estrogen receptors in the brain: Where will it end? *Endocrinology* 145:1069–1074.

Toran-Allerand CD, Hashimoto K, Greenough WT, Saltarelli N. (1983) Sex steroids and the development of the newborn mouse hypothalamus in vitro: III. Effects of estrogen on dendritic differentiation. *Dev Brain Res* 7:97–101.

Toran-Allerand CD, Ellis L, Pfenninger KH. (1988) Estrogen and insulin synergism in neurite growth enhancement in vitro: Mediation of steroid effects by interactions with growth factors? *Brain Res* 469:87–100.

Toran-Allerand CD, Miranda RC, Bentham WD, Sohrabji F, Brown TJ, Hochberg RB, MacLusky NJ. (1992) Estrogen receptors colocalize with low-affinity nerve growth factor receptors in cholinergic neurons of the basal forebrain. *Proc Natl Acad Sci USA* 89:4668–7462.

Toran-Allerand CD, Singh M, Setalo G. (1999) Novel mechanisms of estrogen action in the brain: New players in an old story. *Front Neuroendocrinol* 20:97–121.

Toran-Allerand CD, Tinnikov AA, Singh RJ, Nethrapalli IS. (2005) 17alpha-estradiol: A brain-active estrogen? *Endocrinology* 146:3843–3850.

Torres-Alemán I. (1999) Insulin-like growth factors as mediators of functional plasticity in the adult brain. *Horm Metab Res* 31:114–119.

Torres-Alemán I, Pons S, Garcia-Segura LM. (1991) Climbing fiber deafferentation reduces insulin-like growth factor I (IGF-I) content in cerebellum. *Brain Res* 564:348–351.

Torres-Alemán I, Rejas MT, Pons S, Garcia-Segura LM. (1992) Estradiol promotes cell shape changes and glial fibrillary acidic protein redistribution in hypothalamic astrocytes in vitro: A neuronal-mediated effect. *Glia* 6:180–187.

Toufexis DJ, Myers KM, Davis M. (2006) The effect of gonadal hormones and gender on anxiety and emotional learning. *Horm Behav* 50:539–549.

Toung TJ, Traystman RJ, Hurn PD. (1998) Estrogen-mediated neuroprotection after experimental stroke in male rats. *Stroke* 29:1666–1670.

Towart LA, Alves SE, Znamensky V, Hayashi S, McEwen BS, Milner TA. (2003) Subcellular relationships between cholinergic terminals and estrogen receptor-alpha in the dorsal hippocampus. *J Comp Neurol* 463:390–401.

Trachtenberg JT, Chen BE, Knott GW, Feng G, Sanes JR, Welker E, Svoboda K. (2002) Long-term in vivo imaging of experience-dependent synaptic plasticity in adult cortex. *Nature* 420:19–26.

Trainor BC, Kyomen HH, Marler CA. (2006) Estrogenic encounters: How interactions between aromatase and the environment modulate aggression. *Front Neuroendocrinol* 27:170–179.

Tramontin AD, Brenowitz EA. (2000) Seasonal plasticity in the adult brain. *Trends Neurosci* 23:251–258.

Tranque PA, Suarez I, Olmos G, Fernandez B, Garcia-Segura LM. (1987) Estradiol-induced redistribution of glial fibrillary acidic protein immunoreactivity in the rat brain. *Brain Res* 406:348–351.

Trejo JL, Carro E, Torres-Alemán I. (2001) Circulating insulin-like growth factor I mediates exercise-induced increases in the number of new neurons in the adult hippocampus. *J Neurosci* 21:1628–1634.

Trejo JL, Carro E, Garcia-Galloway E, Torres-Alemán I. (2004) Role of insulin-like growth factor I signaling in neurodegenerative diseases. *J Mol Med* 82:156–162.

Trejo JL, Piriz J, Llorens-Martin MV, Fernandez AM, Bolos M, Leroith D, Nunez A, Torres-Alemán I. (2007) Central actions of liver-derived insulin-like growth factor I underlying its pro-cognitive effects. *Mol Psychiatry* 12:1118–1128.

Trejo JL, Llorens-Martín MV, Torres-Alemán I. (2008) The effects of exercise on spatial learning and anxiety-like behavior are mediated by an IGF-I-dependent mechanism related to hippocampal neurogenesis. *Mol Cell Neurosci* 37:402–411.

Trentani A, Kuipers SD, Ter Horst GJ, Den Boer JA. (2002) Selective chronic stress-induced in vivo ERK1/2 hyperphosphorylation in medial prefrontocortical dendrites: Implications for stress-related cortical pathology? *Eur J Neurosci* 15:1681–1691.

Trentin AG. (2006) Thyroid hormone and astrocyte morphogenesis. *J Endocrinol* 189:189–197.

Trudeau F, Gagnon S, Massicotte G. (2004) Glucose, insulin and the brain: Modulation of cognition and synaptic plasticity in health and disease. *Eur J Pharmacol* 490:177–186.

Tsai PT, Ohab JJ, Kertesz N, Groszer M, Matter C, Gao J, Liu X, Wu H, Carmichael ST. (2006) A critical role of erythropoietin receptor in neurogenesis and post-stroke recovery. *J Neurosci* 26:1269–1274.

Tsang KL, Ho SL, Lo SK. (2000) Estrogen improves motor disability in parkinsonian postmenopausal women with motor fluctuations. *Neurology* 54:2292–2298.

Tseng KY, O'Donnell P. (2005) Post-pubertal emergence of prefrontal cortical up states induced by D1-NMDA co-activation. *Cereb Cortex* 15:49–57.

Tsutsui K. (2006) Biosynthesis, mode of action and functional significance of neurosteroids in the developing Purkinje cell. *J Steroid Biochem Mol Biol* 102:187–194.

Tsutsui K, Sakamoto H, Shikimi H, Ukena K. (2004) Organizing actions of neurosteroids in the Purkinje neuron. *Neurosci Res* 49:273–279.

Tweedle CD, Hatton GI. (1976) Ultrastructural comparisons of neurons of supraoptic and circularis nuclei in normal and dehydrated rats. *Brain Res Bull* 1:103–121.

Tweedle CD, Hatton GI. (1977) Ultrastructural changes in rat hypothalamic neurosecretory cells and their associated glia during minimal dehydration and rehydration. *Cell Tissue Res* 181:59–72.

Tweedle CD, Hatton GI. (1980) Evidence for dynamic interactions between pituicytes and neurosecretory axons in the rat. *Neuroscience* 5:661–671.

Tweedle CD, Hatton GI. (1982) Magnocellular neuropeptidergic terminals in neurohypophysis: Rapid glial release of enclosed axons during parturition. *Brain Res Bull* 8:205–209.

Tweedle CD, Hatton GI. (1984) Synapse formation and disappearance in adult rat supraoptic nucleus during different hydration states. *Brain Res* 309:373–376.

Tweedle CD, Hatton GI. (1987) Morphological adaptability at neurosecretory axonal endings on the neurovascular contact zone of the rat neurohypophysis. *Neuroscience* 20:241–246.

Ugrumov MV, Ivanova IP, Mitskevich MS, Liposits ZS, Setalo G, Flerko B. (1985) Axovascular relationships in developing median eminence of perinatal rats with special reference to luteinizing hormone-releasing hormone projections. *Neuroscience* 16:897–908.

Ugrumov MV, Hisano S, Daikoku S. (1989) Topographic relations between tyrosine hydroxylase- and luteinizing hormone-releasing hormone-immunoreactive fibers in the median eminence of adult rats. *Neurosci Lett* 102:159–164.

Urban IJ. (1998) Effects of vasopressin and related peptides on neurons of the rat lateral septum and ventral hippocampus. *Prog Brain Res* 119:285–310.

Uylings HB, de Brabander JM. (2002) Neuronal changes in normal human aging and Alzheimer's disease. *Brain Cogn* 49:268–276.

Valastro B, Cossette J, Lavoie N, Gagnon S, Trudeau F, Massicotte G. (2002) Up-regulation of glutamate receptors is associated with LTP defects in the early stages of diabetes mellitus. *Diabetologia* 45:642–650.

Valcana T, Einstein ER, Csejtey J, Dalal KB, Timiras PS. (1975) Influence of thyroid hormones on myelin proteins in the developing rat brain. *J Neurol Sci* 25:19–27.

Valenciano AI, Corrochano S, de Pablo F, de la Villa P, de la Rosa EJ. (2006) Proinsulin/insulin is synthesized locally and prevents caspase- and cathepsin-mediated cell death in the embryonic mouse retina. *J Neurochem* 99:524–536.

Vallée M, Mayo W, Darnaudéry M, Corpéchot C, Young J, Koehl M, Le Moal M, Baulieu EE, Robel P, Simon H. (1997a) Neurosteroids: Deficient cognitive performance in aged rats depends on low pregnenolone sulfate levels in the hippocampus. *Proc Natl Acad Sci USA* 94:14865–14870.

Vallée M, Mayo W, Dellu F, Le Moal M, Simon H, Maccari S. (1997b) Prenatal stress induces high anxiety and postnatal handling induces low anxiety in adult offspring: Correlation with stress-induced corticosterone secretion. *J Neurosci* 17:2626–2636.

Vallée M, MacCari S, Dellu F, Simon H, Le Moal M, Mayo W. (1999) Long-term effects of prenatal stress and postnatal handling on age-related glucocorticoid secretion and cognitive performance: A longitudinal study in the rat. *Eur J Neurosci* 11:2906–2916.

Vallée M, Mayo W, Le Moal M. (2001) Role of pregnenolone, dehydroepiandrosterone and their sulfate esters on learning and memory in cognitive aging. *Brain Res Rev* 37:301–312.

Valverde F. (1967) Apical dendritic spines of the visual cortex and light deprivation in the mouse. *Exp Brain Res* 3:337–352.

Valverde F. (1968) Structural changes in the area striata of the mouse after enucleation. *Exp Brain Res* 5:274–292.

Van CE, Leproult R, Kupfer DJ. (1996) Effects of gender and age on the levels and circadian rhythmicity of plasma cortisol. *J Clin Endocrinol Metab* 81:2468–2473.

Vanbesien-Mailliot CC, Wolowczuk I, Mairesse J, Viltart O, Delacre M, Khalife J, Chartier-Harlin MC, Maccari S. (2007) Prenatal stress has pro-inflammatory consequences on the immune system in adult rats. *Psychoneuroendocrinology* 32:114–124.

van Dam PS. (2005) Neurocognitive function in adults with growth hormone deficiency. *Horm Res* 64 (Suppl) 3:109–114.

van Dellen A, Blakemore C, Deacon R, York D, Hannan AJ. (2000) Delaying the onset of Huntington's in mice. *Nature* 404:721–722.

van den Hooff P, Urban IJ, de Wied D. (1989) Vasopressin maintains long-term potentiation in rat lateral septum slices. *Brain Res* 505:181–186.

van der Heide LP, Kamal A, Artola A, Gispen WH. (2005) Ramakers GM. Insulin modulates hippocampal activity-dependent synaptic plasticity in a N-methyl-d-aspartate receptor and phosphatidyl-inositol-3-kinase-dependent manner. *J Neurochem* 94:1158–1166.

van der Kroon PH, Speijers GJ. (1979) Brain deviations in adult obese-hyperglycemic mice (ob/ob). *Metabolism* 28:1–3.

Vanecek J, Jansky L, Illnerova H, Hoffmann K. (1984) Pineal melatonin in hibernating and aroused golden hamsters (Mesocricetus auratus). *Comp Biochem Physiol A* 77:759–762.

VanLandingham JW, Cutler SM, Virmani S, Hoffman SW, Covey DF, Krishnan K, Hammes SR, Jamnongjit M, Stein DG. (2006) The enantiomer of progesterone acts as a molecular neuroprotectant after traumatic brain injury. *Neuropharmacology* 51:1078–85.

van Londen L, Goekoop JG, van Kempen GM, Frankhuijzen-Sierevogel AC, Wiegant VM, van der Velde EA, De Wied D. (1997) Plasma levels of arginine vasopressin elevated in patients with major depression. *Neuropsychopharmacology* 17:284–292.

van Niekerk JK, Huppert FA, Herbert J. (2001) Salivary cortisol and DHEA: Association with measures of cognition and well-being in normal older men, and effects of three months of DHEA supplementation. *Psychoneuroendocrinology* 26:591–612.

van Os J, Selten JP. (1998) Prenatal exposure to maternal stress and subsequent schizophrenia. The May 1940 invasion of The Netherlands. *Br J Psychiatr* 172:324–326.

van Praag H. (2008) Neurogenesis and exercise: Past and future directions. *Neuromolecular Med* 10:128–140.

van Praag H, Kempermann G, Gage FH. (1999) Running increases cell proliferation and neurogenesis in the adult mouse dentate gyrus. *Nat Neurosci* 2:266–270.

Vardimon L, Ben-Dror I, Avisar N, Oren A, Shiftan L. (1999) Glucocorticoid control of glial gene expression. *J Neurobiol* 40:513–527.

Varela-Nieto I, Morales-Garcia JA, Vigil P, Diaz-Casares A, Gorospe I, Sanchez-Galiano S, Canon S, Camarero G, Contreras J, Cediel R, Leon Y. (2004) Trophic effects of insulin-like growth factor-I (IGF-I) in the inner ear. *Hear Res* 196:19–25.

Vaynman S, Ying Z, Gomez-Pinilla F. (2003) Interplay between brain-derived neurotrophic factor and signal transduction modulators in the regulation of the effects of exercise on synaptic-plasticity. *Neuroscience* 122:647–657.

Vedder H, Anthes N, Stumm G, Wurz C, Behl C, Krieg JC. (1999) Estrogen hormones reduce lipid peroxidation in cells and tissues of the central nervous system. *J Neurochem* 72:2531–2538.

Veenman L, Levin E, Weisinger G, Leschiner S, Spanier I, Snyder SH, Weizman A, Gavish M. (2004) Peripheral-type benzodiazepine receptor density and in vitro tumorigenicity of glioma cell lines. *Biochem Pharmacol* 68:689–698.

Vega-Naredo I, Poeggeler B, Sierra-Sanchez V, Caballero B, Tomas-Zapico C, Alvarez-Garcia O, Tolivia D, Rodriguez-Colunga MJ, Coto-Montes A. (2005) Melatonin neutralizes neurotoxicity induced by quinolinic acid in brain tissue culture. *J Pineal Res* 39:266–275.

Vegeto E, Pollio G, Pellicciari C, Maggi A. (1999) Estrogen and progesterone induction of survival of monoblastoid cells undergoing TNF-alpha-induced apoptosis. *FASEB J* 13:793–803.

Vegeto E, Bonincontro C, Pollio G, Sala A, Viappiani S, Nardi F, Brusadelli A, Viviani B, Ciana P, Maggi A. (2001) Estrogen prevents the lipopolysaccharide-induced inflammatory response in microglia. *J Neurosci* 21:1809–1818.

Vegeto E, Belcredito S, Etteri S, Ghisletti S, Brusadelli A, Meda C, Krust A, Dupont S, Ciana P, Chambon P, Maggi A. (2003) Estrogen receptor-alpha mediates the brain antiinflammatory activity of estradiol. *Proc Natl Acad Sci USA* 100: 9614–9619.

Vegeto E, Belcredito S, Ghisletti S, Meda C, Etteri S, Maggi A. (2006) The endogenous estrogen status regulates microglia reactivity in animal models of neuroinflammation. *Endocrinology* 147:2263–2272.

Veiga S, Garcia-Segura LM, Azcoitia I. (2003) Neuroprotection by the steroids pregnenolone and dehydroepiandrosterone is mediated by the enzyme aromatase. *J Neurobiol* 56:398–406.

Veiga S, Azcoitia I, Garcia-Segura LM. (2005a) Extragonadal synthesis of estradiol is protective against kainic acid excitotoxic damage to the hippocampus. *NeuroReport* 16:1599–1603.

Veiga S, Azcoitia I, Garcia-Segura LM. (2005b) Ro5–4864, a peripheral benzodiazepine receptor ligand, reduces reactive gliosis and protects hippocampal hilar neurons from kainic acid excitotoxicity. *J Neurosci Res* 80:129–137.

Veiga S, Leonelli E, Beelke M, Garcia-Segura LM, Melcangi RC. (2006) Neuroactive steroids prevent peripheral myelin alterations induced by diabetes. *Neurosci Lett* 402:150–153.

Veiga S, Carrero P, Pernia O, Azcoitia I, Garcia-Segura LM. (2007) Translocator protein (18 kDa) is involved in the regulation of reactive gliosis. *Glia* 55:1426–1436.

Veliskova J, Velisek L, Galanopoulou AS, Sperber EF. (2000) Neuroprotective effects of estrogens on hippocampal cells in adult female rats after status epilepticus. *Epilepsia* 41(Suppl 6):S30–S35.

Venero C, Herrero AI, Touyarot K, Cambon K, Lopez-Fernandez MA, Berezin V, Bock E, Sandi C. (2006) Hippocampal up-regulation of NCAM expression and polysialylation plays a key role on spatial memory. *Eur J Neurosci* 23:1585–1595.

Venters HD, Tang Q, Liu Q, VanHoy RW, Dantzer R, Kelley KW. (1999) A new mechanism of neurodegeneration: A proinflammatory cytokine inhibits receptor signaling by a survival peptide. *Proc Natl Acad Sci USA* 96:9879–9884.

Verdonck O, Lahrech H, Francony G, Carle O, Farion R, Van de Looij Y, Remy C, Segebarth C, Payen JF. (2007) Erythropoietin protects from post-traumatic edema in the rat brain. *J Cereb Blood Flow Metab* 27:1369–1376.

Vicario-Abejon C, Yusta-Boyo MJ, Fernandez-Moreno C, de Pablo F. (2003) Locally born olfactory bulb stem cells proliferate in response to insulin-related factors and require endogenous insulin-like growth factor-I for differentiation into neurons and glia. *J Neurosci* 23:895–906.

Viguie C, Jansen HT, Glass JD, Watanabe M, Billings HJ, Coolen L, Lehman MN, Karsch FJ. (2001) Potential for polysialylated form of neural cell adhesion molecule-mediated neuroplasticity within the gonadotropin-releasing hormone neurosecretory system of the ewe. *Endocrinology* 142:1317–1324.

Villa P, Bigini P, Mennini T, Agnello D, Laragione T, Cagnotto A, Viviani B, Marinovich M, Cerami A, Coleman TR, Brines M, Ghezzi P. (2003) Erythropoietin selectively attenuates cytokine production and inflammation in cerebral ischemia by targeting neuronal apoptosis. *J Exp Med* 198:971–975.

Viscoli CM, Brass LM, Kernan WN, Sarrel PM, Suissa S, Horwitz RI. (2001) A clinical trial of estrogen-replacement therapy after ischemic stroke. *N Engl J Med* 345:1243–1249.

Viveros MP, Marco EM, Llorente R, López-Gallardo M. (2007) Endocannabinoid system and synaptic plasticity: Implications for emotional responses. *Neural Plast* 2007:52908.

Viviani B, Bartesaghi S, Corsini E, Villa P, Ghezzi P, Garau A, Galli CL, Marinovich M. (2005) Erythropoietin protects primary hippocampal neurons increasing the expression of brain-derived neurotrophic factor. *J Neurochem* 93:412–421.

Volkmar FR, Greenough WT. (1972) Rearing complexity affects branching of dendrites in the visual cortex of the rat. *Science* 176:1445–1447.

Vollmann-Honsdorf GK, Flügge G, Fuchs E. (1997) Chronic psychosocial stress does not affect the number of pyramidal neurons in tree shrew hippocampus. *Neurosci Lett* 233:121–124.Volterra A, Meldolesi J. (2005) Astrocytes, from brain glue to communication elements: The revolution continues. *Nat Rev Neurosci* 6:626–640.

von der Ohe CG, Darian-Smith C, Garner CC, Heller HC. (2006) Ubiquitous and temperature-dependent neural plasticity in hibernators. *J Neurosci* 26:10590–10598.

von der Ohe CG, Garner CC, Darian-Smith C, Heller HC. (2007) Synaptic protein dynamics in hibernation. *J Neurosci* 27:84–92.

Vongher JM, Frye CA. (1999) Progesterone in conjunction with estradiol has neuroprotective effects in an animal model of neurodegeneration. *Pharmacol Biochem Behav* 64:777–785.

Voogt JL, Lee Y, Yang S, Arbogast L. (2001) Regulation of prolactin secretion during pregnancy and lactation. *Prog Brain Res* 133:173–185.

Vouimba RM, Munoz C, Diamond DM. (2006) Differential effects of predator stress and the antidepressant tianeptine on physiological plasticity in the hippocampus and basolateral amygdala. *Stress* 9:29–40.

Vowinckel E, Reutens D, Becher B, Verge G, Evans A, Owens T, Antel JP. (1997) PK11195 binding to the peripheral benzodiazepine receptor as a marker of microglia activation in multiple sclerosis and experimental autoimmune encephalomyelitis. *J Neurosci Res* 50:345–353.

Vyas A, Mitra R, Shankaranarayana Rao BS, Chattarji S. (2002) Chronic stress induces contrasting patterns of dendritic remodeling in hippocampal and amygdaloid neurons. *J Neurosci* 22:6810–6818.

Vyas A, Pillai AG, Chattarji S. (2004) Recovery after chronic stress fails to reverse amygdaloid neuronal hypertrophy and enhanced anxiety-like behavior. *Neuroscience* 128:667–673.

Wade J, Arnold AP. (2004) Sexual differentiation of the zebra finch song system. *Ann NY Acad Sci* 1016:540–559.

Wadhwa PD, Sandman CA, Garite TJ. (2001) The neurobiology of stress in human pregnancy: Implications for prematurity and development of the fetal central nervous system. *Prog Brain Res* 133:131–142.

Wakshlak A, Weinstock M. (1990) Neonatal handling reverses behavioral abnormalities induced in rats by prenatal stress. *Physiol Behav* 48:289–292.

Walf AA, Sumida K, Frye CA. (2006) Inhibiting 5alpha-reductase in the amygdala attenuates antianxiety and antidepressive behavior of naturally receptive and hormone-primed ovariectomized rats. *Psychopharmacology* (Berl) 186:302–311.

Walker CD, Deschamps S, Proulx K, Tu M, Salzman C, Woodside B, Lupien S, Gallo-Payet N, Richard D. (2004a) Mother to infant or infant to mother? Reciprocal regulation of responsiveness to stress in rodents and the implications for humans. *J Psychiatry Neurosci* 29:364–382.

Walker CD, Salzmann C, Long H, Otis M, Roberge C, Gallo-Payet N. (2004b) Direct inhibitory effects of leptin on the neonatal adrenal and potential consequences for brain glucocorticoid feedback. *Endocr Res* 30:837–844.

Walker EF, Sabuwalla Z, Huot R. (2004) Pubertal neuromaturation, stress sensitivity, and psychopathology. *Dev Psychopathol* 16:807–824.

Walker JM, Glotzbach SF, Berger RJ, Heller HC. (1977) Sleep and hibernation in ground squirrels (Citellus spp): Electrophysiological observations. *Am J Physiol* 233:R213–R221.

Wallhausser-Franke E, Nixdorf-Bergweiler BE, DeVoogd TJ. (1995) Song isolation is associated with maintaining high spine frequencies on zebra finch 1MAN neurons. *Neurobiol Learn Mem* 64:25–35.

Walling SG, Nutt DJ, Lalies MD, Harley CW. (2004) Orexin-A infusion in the locus ceruleus triggers norepinephrine (NE) release and NE-induced long-term potentiation in the dentate gyrus. *J Neurosci* 24:7421–7426.

Walsh RN. (1980) Effects of environmental complexity and deprivation on brain chemistry and physiology: A review. *Int J Neurosci* 11:77–89.

Walsh RN. (1981) Effects of environmental complexity and deprivation on brain anatomy and histology: A review. *Int J Neurosci* 12:33–51.

Walters JK, Hatton GI. (1974) Supraoptic neuronal activity in rats during five days of water deprivation. *Physiol Behav* 13:661–667.

Walters SN, Morell P. (1981) Effects of altered thyroid states on myelinogenesis. *J Neurochem* 36:1792–1801.

Waltman C, Blackman MR, Chrousos GP, Riemann C, Harman SM. (1991) Spontaneous and glucocorticoid-inhibited adrenocorticotropic hormone and cortisol secretion are similar in healthy young and old men. *J Clin Endocrinol Metab* 73:495–502.

Wan Q, Xiong ZG, Man HY, Ackerley CA, Braunton J, Lu WY, Becker LE, MacDonald JF, Wang YT. (1997) Recruitment of functional GABA(A) receptors to postsynaptic domains by insulin. *Nature* 388:686–690.

Wang HL, Wayner MJ, Chai CY, Lee EH. (1998) Corticotrophin-releasing factor produces a long-lasting enhancement of synaptic efficacy in the hippocampus. *Eur J Neurosci* 10:3428–3437.

Wang JM, Irwin RW, Brinton RD. (2006) Activation of estrogen receptor alpha increases and estrogen receptor beta decreases apolipoprotein E expression in hippocampus in vitro and in vivo. *Proc Natl Acad Sci USA* 103:16983–16988.

Wang LM, Suthana NA, Chaudhury D, Weaver DR, Colwell CS. (2005) Melatonin inhibits hippocampal long-term potentiation. *Eur J Neurosci* 22:2231–2237.

Wang M, Chen JT, Ruan DY, Xu YZ. (2001) Vasopressin reverses aluminum-induced impairment of synaptic plasticity in the rat dentate gyrus in vivo. *Brain Res* 899:193–200.

Wang MJ, Huang HM, Chen HL, Kuo JS, Jeng KC. (2001) Dehydroepiandrosterone inhibits lipopolysaccharide-induced nitric oxide production in BV-2 microglia. *J Neurochem* 77:830–838.

Wang PN, Liao SQ, Liu RS, Liu CY, Chao HT, Lu SR, Yu HY, Wang SJ, Liu HC. (2000) Effects of estrogen on cognition, mood, and cerebral blood flow in AD: A controlled study. *Neurology* 54:2061–2066.

Wang Q, Santizo R, Baughman VL, Pelligrino DA, Iadecola C. (1999) Estrogen provides neuroprotection in transient forebrain ischemia through perfusion-independent mechanisms in rats. *Stroke* 30:630–637.

Wang R, Zhang QG, Han D, Xu J, Lu Q, Zhang GY. (2006) Inhibition of MLK3-MKK4/7-JNK1/2 pathway by Akt1 in exogenous estrogen-induced neuroprotection against transient global cerebral ischemia by a non-genomic mechanism in male rats. *J Neurochem* 99:1543–1554.

Wang XL, Zhang HM, Chen SR, Pan HL. (2007) Altered synaptic input and GABA(B) receptor function in spinal superficial dorsal horn neurons in rats with diabetic neuropathy. *J Physiol* 579:849–861.

Wang Z, Aragona BJ. (2004) Neurochemical regulation of pair bonding in male prairie voles. *Physiol Behav* 83:319–328.

Ward IL, Stehm KE. (1991) Prenatal stress feminizes juvenile play patterns in male rats. *Physiol Behav* 50:601–605.

Warren SG, Humphreys AG, Juraska JM, Greenough WT. (1995) LTP varies across the estrous cycle: Enhanced synaptic plasticity in proestrus rats. *Brain Res* 703:26–30.

Wassertheil-Smoller S, Hendrix SL, Limacher M, Heiss G, Kooperberg C, Baird A, Kotchen T, Curb JD, Black H, Rossouw JE, Aragaki A, Safford M, Stein E, Laowattana S, Mysiw WJ. (2003) Effect of estrogen plus progestin on stroke in postmenopausal women: The Women's Health Initiative: A randomized trial. *JAMA* 289:2673–2684.

Watanabe Y, Gould E, McEwen BS. (1992) Stress induces atrophy of apical dendrites of hippocampal CA3 pyramidal neurons. *Brain Res* 588:341–345.

Watson RE, Hoffmann GE, Wiegand SJ. (1986) Sexually dimorphic opioid distribution in the preoptic area: Manipulation by gonadal steroids. *Brain Res* 398:157–163.

Wayner MJ, Armstrong DL, Polan-Curtain JL, Denny JB. (1993) Ethanol and diazepam inhibition of hippocampal LTP is mediated by angiotensin II and AT1 receptors. *Peptides* 14:441–444.

Wayner MJ, Armstrong DL, Phelix CF. (1996) Nicotine blocks angiotensin II inhibition of LTP in the dentate gyrus. *Peptides* 17:1127–1133.

Wayner MJ, Armstrong DL, Phelix CF, Wright JW, Harding JW. (2001) Angiotensin IV enhances LTP in rat dentate gyrus in vivo. *Peptides* 22:1403–1414.

Wayner MJ, Armstrong DL, Phelix CF, Oomura Y. (2004) Orexin-A (Hypocretin-1) and leptin enhance LTP in the dentate gyrus of rats in vivo. *Peptides* 25:991–996.

Weaver CE, Park-Chung M, Gibbs TT, Farb DH. (1997) 17β-Estradiol protects against NMDA-induced excitotoxicity by direct inhibition of NMDA receptors. *Brain Res* 761:338–341.

Webster JI, Tonelli l, Sternberg EM. (2002) Neuroendocrine regulation of immunity. *Annu Rev Immunol* 20:125–163.

Wehrenberg U, Prange-Kiel J, Rune GM. (2001) Steroidogenic factor-1 expression in marmoset and rat hippocampus: Co-localization with StAR and aromatase. *J Neurochem* 76:1879–1886.

Wei J, Xu H, Davies JL, Hemmings GP. (1992) Increase of plasma IL-6 concentration with age in healthy subjects. *Life Sci* 51:1253–1956.

Weiland NG, Cohen IR, Wise PM. (1989) Age-associated alterations in catecholaminergic concentrations, neuronal activity, and alpha 1 receptor densities in female rats. *Neurobiol Aging* 10:323–329.

Weinstock M. (1997) Does prenatal stress impair coping and regulating of the hypothalamic–pituitary–adrenal axis? *Behav Neurosci* 21:1–10.

Weinstock M. (2001) Alterations induced by gestational stress in brain morphology and behaviour of the offspring. *Prog Neurobiol* 65:427–451.

Weinstock M. (2007) Gender differences in the effects of prenatal stress on brain development and behaviour. *Neurochem Res* 32:1730–1740.

Weinstock M, Matlina E, Maor GI, Rosen H, McEwen BS. (1992) Prenatal stress selectively alters the reactivity of the hypothalamic–pituitary–adrenal system in the female rat. *Brain Res* 595:195–200.

Weinstock M, Poltyrev T, Schorer-Apelbaum D, Men D, McCarty R. (1998) Effect of prenatal stress on plasma corticosterone and catecholamines in response to footshock in rats. *Physiol Behav* 64:439–444.

Weishaupt JH, Bartels C, Polking E, Dietrich J, Rohde G, Poeggeler B, Mertens N, Sperling S, Bohn M, Huther G, Schneider A, Bach A, Siren AL, Hardeland R, Bahr M, Nave KA, Ehrenreich H. (2006) Reduced oxidative damage in ALS by high-dose enteral melatonin treatment. *J Pineal Res* 41:313–323.

Welberg LA, Seckl JR. (2001) Prenatal stress, glucocorticoids, and the programming of the brain. *J Neuroendocrinol* 13:113–128.

Welberg LA, Seckl JR, Holmes MC. (2001) Prenatal glucocorticoid programming of brain corticosteroid receptors and corticotrophin-releasing hormone: Possible implications for behaviour. *Neuroscience* 104:71–79.

Welker E, Rao SB, Dorfl J, Melzer P, van der Loos H. (1992) Plasticity in the barrel cortex of the adult mouse: Effects of chronic stimulation upon deoxyglucose uptake in the behaving animal. *J Neurosci* 12:153–170.

Wellman CL. (2001) Dendritic reorganization in pyramidal neurons in medial prefrontal cortex after chronic corticosterone administration. *J Neurobiol* 49:245–253.

Wen TC, Sadamoto Y, Tanaka J, Zhu PX, Nakata K, Ma YJ, Hata R, Sakanaka M. (2002) Erythropoietin protects neurons against chemical hypoxia and cerebral ischemic injury by up-regulating Bcl-xL expression. *J Neurosci Res* 67:795–803.

Werther GA, Hogg A, McKinley M, Oldfield B, Figdor R, Mendelsohn FAO. (1989) Localization and characterization of insulin-like growth factor-I receptors in rat brain and pituitary gland, using in vitro autoradiography and computerized densitometry, a distinct distribution from insulin receptors. *J Neuroendocrinol* 1:369–377.

Werther GA, Abate M, Hogg A, Cheesman H, Oldfield B, Hards D, Hudson P, Power B, Freed K, Herington AC. (1990) Localization of insulin-like growth factor-I mRNA in rat brain by in situ hybridization-relationship to IGF-I receptors. *Mol Endocrinol* 4:773–778.

West MJ, Coleman PD, Flood DG, Troncoso JC. (1994) Differences in the pattern of hippocampal neuronal loss in normal ageing and Alzheimer's disease. *Lancet* 344:769–772.

Whalley LJ, Dick FD, McNeill G. (2006) A life-course approach to the aetiology of late-onset dementias. *Lancet Neurol* 5:87–96.

Whitfield-Rucker MG, CassoneVM. (1996) Melatonin binding in the house sparrow song control system: Sexual dimorphism and the effect of photoperiod. *Horm Behav* 30:528–537.

Wickelgren I (1998) Tracking insulin to the mind. *Science* 280:517–519.

Wide JK, Hanratty K, Ting J, Galea LA. (2004) High level estradiol impairs and low level estradiol facilitates non-spatial working memory. *Behav Brain Res* 155:45–53.

Wiegratz I, Kuhl H. (2004) Progestogen therapies: Differences in clinical effects? *Trends Endocrinol Metab* 15:277–285.

Wiesel TN, Hubel DH. (1963) Effects of visual deprivation on morphology and physiology of cells in the cat's lateral geniciilate body. *J Neurophysiol* 26:978–993.

Wigley R, Hamilton N, Nishiyama A, Kirchhoff F, Butt AM. (2007) Morphological and physiological interactions of NG2-glia with astrocytes and neurons. *J Anat* 210:661–670.

Wilms H, Claasen J, Rohl C, Sievers J, Deuschl G, Lucius R. (2003) Involvement of benzodiazepine receptors in neuroinflammatory and neurodegenerative diseases: Evidence from activated microglial cells in vitro. *Neurobiol Dis* 14:417–424.

Wilson C, Finch C, Cohen H. (2002) Cytokines and cognition—the case for a head-to-toe inflammatory paradigm. *J Am Geriatr Soc* 50:2041–2056.

Wilson IA, Gallagher M, Eichenbaum H, Tanila H. (2006) Neurocognitive aging: Prior memories hinder new hippocampal encoding. *Trends Neurosci* 29:662–670.

Wilson JD. (2001) Androgens, androgen receptors, and male gender role behavior. *Horm Behav* 40: 358–366.

Wilson ME, Dubal DB, Wise PM. (2000) Estradiol protects against injury-induced cell death in cortical explant cultures: A role for estrogen receptors. *Brain Res* 873:235–242.

Wilson ME, Liu Y, Wise PM. (2002) Estradiol enhances Akt activation in cortical explant cultures following neuronal injury. *Mol Brain Res* 102:48–54.

Wilson RS, Beckett LA, Barnes LL, Schneider JA, Bach J, Evans DA, Bennett DA. (2002) Individual differences in rates of change in cognitive abilities of older persons. *Psychol Aging* 17:179–193.

Winsky-Sommerer R, Yamanaka A, Diano S, Borok E, Roberts AJ, Sakurai T, Kilduff TS, Horvath TL, de Lecea L. (2004) Interaction between the corticotropin-releasing factor system and hypocretins (orexins): A novel circuit mediating stress response. *J Neurosci* 24:11439–11448.

Wise PM. (1987) The role of the hypothalamus in aging of the female reproductive system. *J Steroid Biochem* 27:713–719.

Wise PM. (1999) Neuroendocrine modulation of the 'menopause': Insights into the aging brain. *Am J Physiol* 277:E965–E970.

Wise PM, Smith MJ, Dubal DB, Wilson ME, Krajnak KM, Rosewell KL. (1999) Neuroendocrine influences and repercussions of the menopause. *Endocr Rev* 20:243–248.

Wise PM, Dubal DB, Wilson ME, Rau SW, Liu Y. (2001) Estrogens: Trophic and protective factors in the adult brain. *Front Neuroendocrinol* 22:33–66.

Witkin JW, Ferin M, Popilskis SJ, Silverman AJ. (1991) Effects of gonadal steroids on the ultrastructure of GnRH neurons in the Rhesus monkey: Synaptic input and glial apposition. *Endocrinology* 19:1083–1092.

Witt ED. (2007) Puberty, hormones, and sex differences in alcohol abuse and dependence. *Neurotoxicol Teratol* 29:81–95.

Wong M, Eaton MJ, Moss RL. (1990) Electrophysiological actions of luteinizing hormone-releasing hormone: Intracellular studies in the rat hippocampal slice preparation. *Synapse* 5:65–70.

Wong M, Moss RL. (1992) Long-term and short-term electrophysiological effects of estrogen on the synaptic properties of hippocampal CA1 neurons. *J Neurosci* 12:3217–3225.

Woods AG, Poulsen FR, Gall CM. (1999) Dexamethasone selectively suppresses microglial trophic responses to hippocampal deafferentation. *Neuroscience* 91:1277–1289.

Woods SC, Porte D. (1977) Relationship between plasma and cerebrospinal fluid insulin levels of dogs. *Am J Physiol* 233:E331–E334.

Woolley CS. (1998) Estrogen-mediated structural and functional synaptic plasticity in the female rat hippocampus. *Horm Behav* 34:140–148.

Woolley CS. (2007) Acute effects of estrogen on neuronal physiology. *Annu Rev Pharmacol Toxicol* 47:657–680.

Woolley CS, Gould E, Frankfurt M. McEwen BS. (1990a) Naturally occurring fluctuation in dendritic spine density on adult hippocampal pyramidal neurons. *J Neurosci* 10:4035–4039.

Woolley CS, Gould E, McEwen BS. (1990b) Exposure to excess glucocorticoids alters dendritic morphology of adult hippocampal pyramidal neurons. *Brain Res* 531:225–231.

Woolley CS, McEwen BS. (1992) Estradiol mediates fluctuation in hippocampal synapse density during the estrous cycle in the adult rat. *J Neurosci* 12:2549–2554.

Woolley CS, McEwen BS. (1993) Roles of estradiol and progesterone in regulation of hippocampal dendritic spine density during the estrous cycle in the rat. *J Comp Neurol* 336:293–306.

Woolley CS, McEwen BS. (1994) Estradiol regulates hippocampal dendritic spine density via an N-methyl-D-aspartate receptor-dependent mechanism. *J Neurosci* 14:7680–7687.

Woolley CS, Wenzel HJ, Schwartzkroin PA. (1996) Estradiol increases the frequency of multiple synapse boutons in the hippocampal CA1 region of the adult female rat. *J Comp Neurol* 373:108–117.

Woolley CS, Weiland NG, McEwen BS, Schwartzkroin PA. (1997) Estradiol increases the sensitivity of hippocampal CA1 pyramidal cells to NMDA receptor-mediated synaptic input: Correlation with dendritic spine density. *J Neurosci* 17:1848–1859.

Wosik K, Cayrol R, Dodelet-Devillers A, Berthelet F, Bernard M, Moumdjian R, Bouthillier A, Reudelhuber TL, Prat A. (2007) Angiotensin II controls occludin function and is required for blood brain barrier maintenance: Relevance to multiple sclerosis. *J Neurosci* 27:9032–9042.

Wright JW, Reichert JR, Davis CJ, Harding JW. (2002) Neural plasticity and the brain renin-angiotensin system. *Neurosci Biobehav Rev* 26:529–552.

Wright JW, Harding JW. (2004) The brain angiotensin system and extracellular matrix molecules in neural plasticity, learning, and memory. *Prog Neurobiol* 72:263–293.

Wu FS, Gibbs TT, Farb DH. (1991) Pregnenolone sulphate: A positive allosteric modulator at the N-methyl-D-aspartate receptor. *Mol Pharmacol* 40:333–336.

Wu TW, Wang JM, Chen S, Brinton RD. (2005) 17Beta-estradiol induced Ca^{2+} influx via L-type calcium channels activates the Src/ERK/cyclic-AMP response element binding protein signal pathway and BCL-2 expression in rat hippocampal neurons: A potential initiation mechanism for estrogen-induced neuroprotection. *Neuroscience* 135:59–72.

Wynne RD, Saldanha CJ. (2004) Glial aromatization decreases neural injury in the zebra finch (Taeniopygia guttata): Influence on apoptosis. *J Neuroendocrinol* 16:676–683.

Xerri C, Stern JM, Merzenich MM. (1994) Alterations of the cortical representation of the rat ventrum induced by nursing behavior. *J Neurosci* 14:1710–1721.

Xiong JJ, Karsch FJ, Lehman MN. (1997) Evidence for seasonal plasticity in the gonadotropin-releasing hormone (GnRH) system of the ewe: Changes in synaptic inputs onto GnRH neurons. *Endocrinology* 138:1240–1250.

Xu H, Wang R, Zhang YW, Zhang X. (2006) Estrogen, beta-amyloid metabolism/trafficking, and Alzheimer's disease. *Ann N Y Acad Sci* 1089:324–342.

Xu J, Gingras KM, Bengston L, Di Marco A, Forger NG. (2001) Blockade of endogenous neurotrophic factors prevents the androgenic rescue of rat spinal motoneurons. *J Neurosci* 21:4366–4372.

Xu L, Anwyl R, Rowan MJ. (1997) Behavioural stress facilitates the induction of long-term depression in the hippocampus. *Nature* 387:497–500.

Xu L, Holscher C, Anwyl R, Rowan MJ. (1998) Glucocorticoid receptor and protein/RNA synthesis-dependent mechanisms underlie the control of synaptic plasticity by stress. *Proc Natl Acad Sci USA* 95:3204–3208.

Yaffe K. (2003) Hormone therapy and the brain: Déjà vu all over again? *JAMA* 289:2717–2719.

Yaffe K, Sawaya G, Lieberburg I, Grady D. (1998) Estrogen therapy in postmenopausal women: Effects on cognitive function and dementia. *JAMA* 279:688–695.

Yaffe K, Haan M, Byers A, Tangen C, Kuller L. (2000) Estrogen use, APOE, and cognitive decline: Evidence of gene-environment interaction. *Neurology* 54:1949–1954.

Yague JG, Lavaque E, Carretero J, Azcoitia I, Garcia-Segura LM. (2004) Aromatase, the enzyme responsible for estrogen biosynthesis, is expressed by human and rat glioblastomas. *Neurosci Lett* 368:279–284.

Yague JG, Munoz A, de Monasterio-Schrader P, DeFelipe J, Garcia-Segura LM, Azcoitia I. (2006) Aromatase expression in the human temporal cortex. *Neuroscience* 138:389–401.

Yamada KA, Rensing N, Izumi Y, De Erausquin GA, Gazit V, Dorsey DA, Herrera DG. (2004) Repetitive hypoglycemia in young rats impairs hippocampal long-term potentiation. *Pediatr Res* 55:372–379.

Yamaji R, Okada T, Moriya M, Naito M, Tsuruo T, Miyatake K, Nakano Y. (1996) Brain capillary endothelial cells express two forms of erythropoietin receptor mRNA. *Eur J Biochem* 239:494–500.

Yamamura T, Hirunagi K, Ebihara S, Yoshimura T. (2004) Seasonal morphological changes in the neuro-glial interaction between gonadotropin-releasing hormone nerve terminals and glial endfeet in Japanese quail. *Endocrinology* 145:4264–4267.

Yamamura T, Yasuo S, Hirunagi K, Ebihara S, Yoshimura T. (2006) T(3) implantation mimics photoperiodically reduced encasement of nerve terminals by glial processes in the median eminence of Japanese quail. *Cell Tissue Res* 324:175–179.

Yang CH, Huang CC, Hsu KS. (2004) Behavioral stress modifies hippocampal synaptic plasticity through corticosterone-induced sustained extracellular signal-regulated kinase/mitogen-activated protein kinase activation. *J Neurosci* 24:11029–11034.

Yang CH, Huang CC, Hsu KS. (2006) Novelty exploration elicits a reversal of acute stress-induced modulation of hippocampal synaptic plasticity in the rat. *J Physiol* 577:601–615.

Yang J, Hou C, Ma N, Liu J, Zhang Y, Zhou J, Xu L, Li L. (2007) Enriched environment treatment restores impaired hippocampal synaptic plasticity and cognitive deficits induced by prenatal chronic stress. *Neurobiol Learn Mem* 87:257–263.

Yang LY, Verhovshek T, Sengelaub D. (2004) Brain-derived neurotrophic factor and androgen interact in the maintenance of dendritic morphology in a sexually dimorphic rat spinal nucleus. *Endocrinology* 145:161–168.

Yang PC, Yang CH, Huang CC, Hsu KS. (2008) Phosphatidylinositol 3 kinase activation is required for stress protocol-induced modification of hippocampal synaptic plasticity. *J Biol Chem* 283:2631–2643.

Yang RJ, Mozhui K, Karlsson RM, Cameron HA, Williams RW, Holmes A. (2008) Variation in mouse basolateral amygdala volume is associated with differences in stress reactivity and fear learning. *Neuropsychopharmacology* 33:2595–2604.

Yang SH, Liu R, Perez EJ, Wang X, Simpkins JW. (2005) Estrogens as protectants of the neurovascular unit against ischemic stroke. *Curr Drug Targets CNS Neurol Disord* 4:169–177.

Yang SN, Lu F, Wu JN, Liu DD, Hsieh WY. (1999) Activation of gonadotropin-releasing hormone receptors induces a long-term enhancement of excitatory postsynaptic currents mediated by ionotropic glutamate receptors in the rat hippocampus. *Neurosci Lett* 260:33–36.

Yankova M, Hart SA, Woolley CS. (2001) Estrogen increases synaptic connectivity between single presynaptic inputs and multiple postsynaptic CA1 pyramidal cells: A serial electron-microscopic study. *Proc Natl Acad Sci USA* 98:3525–3530.

Yao M, Nguyen TV, Pike CJ. (2007) Estrogen regulates Bcl-w and Bim expression: Role in protection against beta-amyloid peptide-induced neuronal death. *J Neurosci* 27:1422–1433.

Yao XL, Liu J, Lee E, Ling GS, McCabe JT. (2005) Progesterone differentially regulates pro- and anti-apoptotic gene expression in cerebral cortex following traumatic brain injury in rats. *J Neurotrauma* 22:656–668.

Yap JJ, Takase LF, Kochman LJ, Fornal CA, Miczek KA, Jacobs BL. (2006) Repeated brief social defeat episodes in mice: Effects on cell proliferation in the dentate gyrus. *Behav Brain Res* 172:344–350.

Yaskin VA. (1984) Seasonal changes in brain morphology in small mammals. *Carnegie Mus Nat Hist Spec Publ* 10:183–193.

Yaskin VA. (1994) Variation in brain morphology of the common shrew. *Carnegie Mus Nat Hist Spec Publ* 18:155–161.

Yates FE. (1994) Order and complexity in dynamic systems: Homeodynamics as a generalized mechanism for biology. *Mathematics and Computer Modeling* 14:49–74.

Yates MA, Juraska JM. (2008) Pubertal ovarian hormone exposure reduces the number of myelinated axons in the splenium of the rat corpus callosum. *Exp Neurol* 209:284–287.

Yates MA, Markham JA, Anderson SE, Morris JR, Juraska JM. (2008) Regional variability in age-related loss of neurons from the primary visual cortex and medial prefrontal cortex of male and female rats. *Brain Res* 1218:1–12.

Yatsiv I, Grigoriadis N, Simeonidou C, Stahel PF, Schmidt OI, Alexandrovitch AG, Tsenter J, Shohami E. (2005) Erythropoietin is neuroprotective, improves functional recovery, and reduces neuronal apoptosis and inflammation in a rodent model of experimental closed head injury. *FASEB J* 19:1701–1703.

Ye P, D'Ercole AJ. (2006) Insulin-like growth factor actions during development of neural stem cells and progenitors in the central nervous system. *J Neurosci Res* 83:1–6.

Yeoman RR, Jenkins AJ. (1989) Arcuate area of the female rat maintained in vitro exhibits increased afternoon electrical activity. *Neuroendocrinology* 49:144–149.

Yi CX, van der Vliet J, Dai J, Yin G, Ru L, Buijs RM. (2006) Ventromedial arcuate nucleus communicates peripheral metabolic information to the suprachiasmatic nucleus. *Endocrinology* 147:283–294.

Yildirim M, Mapp OM, Janssen WG, Yin W, Morrison JH, Gore AC. (2008) Postpubertal decrease in hippocampal dendritic spines of female rats. *Exp Neurol* 210:339–348.

Yorek MA, Coppey LJ, Gellett JS, Davidson EP, Bing X, Lund DD, Dillon JS. (2002) Effect of treatment of diabetic rats with dehydroepiandrosterone on vascular and neural function. *Am J Physiol Endocrinol Metab* 283:E1067–E1075.

Youssoufian H, Longmore G, Neumann D, Yoshimura A, Lodish HF. (1993) Structure, function, and activation of the erythropoietin receptor. *Blood* 81:2223–2236.

Yu WH. (1982) Effect of testosterone on the regeneration of the hypoglossal nerve in rats. *Exp Neurol* 77:129–141.

Yu WH. (1989) Survival of motoneurons following axotomy is enhanced by lactation or by progesterone treatment. *Brain Res* 491:379–382.

Yu X, Rajala RV, McGinnis JF, Li F, Anderson RE, Yan X, Li S, Elias RV, Knapp RR, Zhou X, Cao W. (2004) Involvement of insulin/phosphoinositide 3-kinase/Akt signal pathway in 17 beta-estradiol-mediated neuroprotection. *J Biol Chem* 279:13086–13094.

Yu YL, Wagner GC. (1994) Influence of gonadal hormones on sexual differences in sensitivity to methamphetamine-induced neurotoxicity. *J Neural Transm Park Dis Dement Sect* 8:215–221.

Yue X, Lu M, Lancaster T, Cao P, Honda S, Staufenbiel M, Harada N, Zhong Z, Shen
    Y, Li R. (2005) Brain estrogen deficiency accelerates Abeta plaque formation in an
    Alzheimer's disease animal model. *Proc Natl Acad Sci USA* 102:19198–19203.
Yun SH, Park KA, Kwon S, Woolley CS, Sullivan PM, Pasternak JF, Trommer BL.
    (2007) Estradiol enhances long term potentiation in hippocampal slices from
    aged apoE4-TR mice. *Hippocampus* 17:1153–1157.
Yuste R, Bonhoeffer T. (2001) Morphological changes in dendritic spines associated
    with long-term synaptic plasticity. *Ann Rev Neurosci* 24:1071–1089.
Yuzuriha H, Inui A, Asakawa A, Ueno N, Kasuga M, Meguid MM, Miyazaki
    JI, Ninomiya M, Herzog H, Fujimiya M. (2007) Gastrointestinal hormones
    (anorexigenic peptide YY and orexigenic ghrelin) influence neural tube
    development. *FASEB J* 21:2108–2112.
Zaulyanov LL, Green PS, Simpkins JW. (1999) Glutamate receptor requirement for
    neuronal cell death from anoxia-reoxygenation: An in vitro model for assessment
    of the neuroprotective effects of estrogens. *Cell Mol Neurobiol* 19:705–718.
Zecevic N, Rakic P. (1991) Synaptogenesis in monkey somatosensory cortex. *Cereb
    Cortex* 1:510–523.
Zeger M, Popken G, Zhang J, Xuan S, Lu QR, Schwab MH, Nave KA, Rowitch
    D, D'Ercole AJ, Ye P. (2007) Insulin-like growth factor type 1 receptor
    signaling in the cells of oligodendrocyte lineage is required for normal in vivo
    oligodendrocyte development and myelination. *Glia* 55:400–411.
Zehr JL, Todd BJ, Schulz KM, McCarthy MM, Sisk CL. (2006) Dendritic pruning of
    the medial amygdala during pubertal development of the male Syrian hamster.
    J Neurobiol 66:578–590.
Zeutzius I, Probst W, Rahmannn H. (1984) Influence of dark-rearing on the
    ontogenetic development of Sarotherodon mossambicus (Cichlidae, Teleostei): II.
    Effects on allometrical growth relations and differentiation of the optic tectum.
    Exp Biol 43:87–96.
Zhang F, Signore AP, Zhou Z, Wang S, Cao G, Chen J. (2006) Erythropoietin
    protects CA1 neurons against global cerebral ischemia in rat: Potential signaling
    mechanisms. *J Neurosci Res* 83:1241–1251.
Zhang F, Wang S, Signore AP, Chen J. (2007) Neuroprotective effects of leptin
    against ischemic injury induced by oxygen-glucose deprivation and transient
    cerebral ischemia. *Stroke* 38:2329–2336.
Zhang J, Li Y, Cui Y, Chen J, Lu M, Elias SB, Chopp M. (2005) Erythropoietin
    treatment improves neurological functional recovery in EAE mice. *Brain Res*
    1034:34–39.
Zhang L, Rubinow DR, Xaing G, Li BS, Chang YH, Maric D, Barker JL, Ma W. (2001)
    Estrogen protects against beta-amyloid-induced neurotoxicity in rat hippocampal
    neurons by activation of Akt. *NeuroReport* 12:1919–1923.
Zhang L, Li B, Zhao W, Chang YH, Ma W, Dragan M, Barker JL, Hu Q, Rubinow
    DR. (2002) Sex-related differences in MAPKs activation in rat astrocytes: Effects
    of estrogen on cell death. *Mol Brain Res* 103:1–11.
Zhang P, Rodriguez H, Mellon SH. (1995) Transcriptional regulation of P450scc
    gene expression in neural and steroidogenic cells: Implications for regulation of
    neurosteroidogenesis. *Mol Endocrinol* 9:1571–1582.
Zhang W, Lin TR, Hu Y, Fan Y, Zhao L, Stuenkel EL, Mulholland MW. (2004)
    Ghrelin stimulates neurogenesis in the dorsal motor nucleus of the vagus.
    J Physiol 559:729–737.

Zhang W, Hu Y, Lin TR, Fan Y, Mulholland MW. (2005) Stimulation of neurogenesis in rat nucleus of the solitary tract by ghrelin. *Peptides* 26:2280–2288.

Zhang Y, Proenca R, Maffei M, Barone M, Leopold L, Friedman JM. (1994) Positional cloning of the mouse obese gene and its human homologue. *Nature* 372:425–432.

Zhang Y, Milatovic D, Aschner M, Feustel PJ, Kimelberg HK. (2007) Neuroprotection by tamoxifen in focal cerebral ischemia is not mediated by an agonist action at estrogen receptors but is associated with antioxidant activity. *Exp Neurol* 204:819–827.

Zhang YQ, Shi J, Rajakumar G, Day AL, Simpkins JW. (1998) Effects of gender and estradiol treatment on focal brain ischemia. *Brain Res* 784:321–324.

Zhao L, Wu TW, Brinton RD. (2004) Estrogen receptor subtypes alpha and beta contribute to neuroprotection and increased Bcl-2 expression in primary hippocampal neurons. *Brain Res* 1010:22–34.

Zhao L, O'Neill K, Brinton RD. (2005) Selective estrogen receptor modulators (SERMs) for the brain: Current status and remaining challenges for developing NeuroSERMs. *Brain Res Rev* 49:472–493.

Zhao L, O'Neill K, Brinton RD. (2006) Estrogenic agonist activity of ICI 182,780 (Faslodex) in hippocampal neurons: Implications for basic science understanding of estrogen signaling and development of estrogen modulators with a dual therapeutic profile. *J Pharmacol Exp Ther* 319:1124–1132.

Zhao W, Chen H, Xu H, Moore E, Meiri N, Quon MJ, Alkon DJ. (1999) Brain insulin receptors and spatial memory. Correlated changes in gene expression, tyrosine phosphorylation, and signaling molecules in the hippocampus of water maze trained rats. *J Biol Chem* 274:34893–34902.

Zhou J, Ando H, Macova M, Dou J, Saavedra JM. (2005) Angiotensin II AT1 receptor blockade abolishes brain microvascular inflammation and heat shock protein responses in hypertensive rats. *J Cereb Blood Flow Metab* 25:878–886.

Zhou L, Lehan N, Wehrenberg U, Disteldorf E, von Lossow R, Mares U, Jarry H, Rune GM. (2007) Neuroprotection by estradiol: A role of aromatase against spine synapse loss after blockade of GABA(A) receptors. *Exp Neurol* 203:72–81.

Zhou Y, Xu BC, Maheshwari HG, He L, Reed M, Lozykowski M, Okada S, Wagner TE, Cataldo LA, Coschigano K, Baumann G, Kopchick JJ. (1997) A mammalian model for Laron syndrome produced by targeted disruption of the mouse growth hormone receptor/binding protein gene (the Laron mouse). *Proc Natl Acad Sci USA* 94:13215–13220.

Zhu DF, Wang ZX, Zhang DR, Pan ZL, He S, Hu XP, Chen XC, Zhou JN. (2006) fMRI revealed neural substrate for reversible working memory dysfunction in subclinical hypothyroidism. *Brain* 129:2923–2930.

Zhu Y, Rice CD, Pang Y, Pace M, Thomas P. (2003) Cloning, expression, and characterization of a membrane progestin receptor and evidence it is an intermediary in meiotic maturation of fish oocytes. *Proc Natl Acad Sci USA* 100:2231–2236.

Znamensky V, Akama KT, McEwen BS, Milner TA. (2003) Estrogen levels regulate the subcellular distribution of phosphorylated Akt in hippocampal CA1 dendrites. *J Neurosci* 23:2340–2347.

Zsarnovszky A, Horvath TL, Garcia-Segura LM, Horvath B, Naftolin F. (2001) Oestrogen-induced changes in the synaptology of the monkey (Cercopithecus aethiops) arcuate nucleus during gonadotropin feedback. *J Neuroendocrinol* 13:22–28.

Zuloaga DG, Morris JA, Monks DA, Breedlove SM, Jordan CL. (2007) Androgen-sensitivity of somata and dendrites of spinal nucleus of the bulbocavernosus (SNB) motoneurons in male C57BL6J mice. *Hormones Behav* 51:207–212.

Zupanc GKH. (2001) A comparative approach towards the understanding of adult neurogenesis. *Brain Behav Evol* 58:246–249.

Zwain IH, Yen SSC. (1999a) Dehydroepiandrosterone: Biosynthesis and metabolism in the brain. *Endocrinology* 140:880–887.

Zwain IH, Yen SSC. (1999b) Neurosteroidogenesis in astrocytes, oligodendrocytes, and neurons of cerebral cortex of rat brain. *Endocrinology* 140:3843–3852.

Author Index

Subject Index

Note: Page numbers in *italics* refer to figures.

Printed and bound by CPI Group (UK) Ltd, Croydon, CR0 4YY